Table of Contents

FUNDAMENTALS OF PEDIATRIC ORTHOPEDICS

FIFTH EDITION

Lynn T. Staheli, M.D.

Emeritus Professor, Department of Orthopedics
University of Washington School of Medicine
Seattle, Washington

Emeritus Editor, *Journal of Pediatric Orthopaedics*

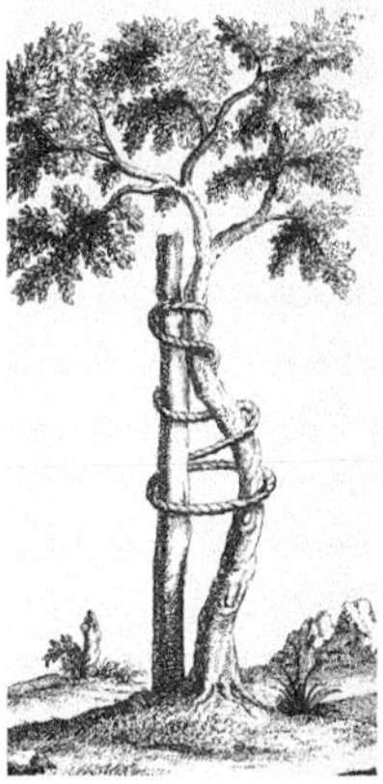

Wolters Kluwer

Philadelphia • Baltimore • New York • London
Buenos Aires • Hong Kong • Sydney • Tokyo

Acquisitions Editor: Jamie M. Elfrank
Product Development Editor: Ashley Fischer
Editorial Assistant: Brian Convery
Marketing Manager: Stephanie Kindlick
Production Project Manager: David Orzechowski
Design Coordinator: Doug Smock
Manufacturing Coordinator: Beth Welsh
Prepress Vendor: SPi Global

Fifth edition

9 8

Printed in The United States of America

Library of Congress Cataloging-in-Publication Data
Staheli, Lynn T., author.
Fundamentals of pediatric orthopedics / Lynn T. Staheli. — Fifth edition.
p. ; cm.
Includes bibliographical references and index.
ISBN 978-1-4511-9393-0 (alk. paper)
I. Title.
[DNLM: 1. Bone Diseases. 2. Child. 3. Infant. 4. Athletic Injuries. 5. Musculoskeletal Abnormalities. 6. Orthopedic Procedures. WS 270]
RD732.3.C48
618.92'7—dc23

2015005261

LWW.com

Consultants

This fifth edition of the ***Fundamentals of Pediatric Orthopedics*** **(FPO)** was prepared with the help of five consultants who practice as Seattle Children's Hospital in the Department of Pediatric Orthopedics and Sports Medicine.

Their academic appointments are with the University of Washington School of Medicine or Nursing, Seattle.

They provided different perspectives in making this fifth edition relevant for the varied Care Providers for children with musculoskeletal problems.

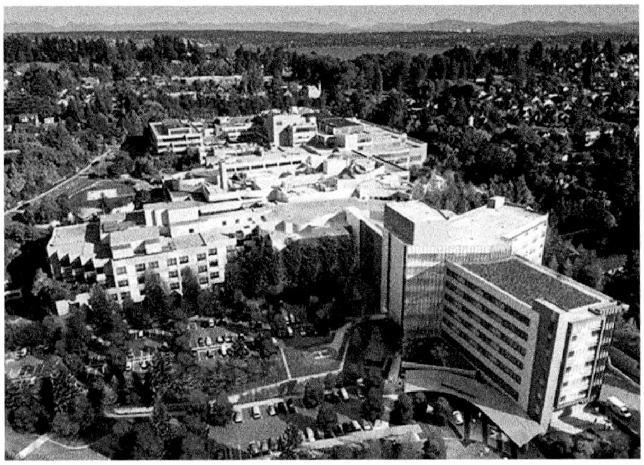

Seattle Children's Hospital and Regional Medical Center, Seattle, Washington.

Monique Burton, MD
Sports Medicine Pediatrician
Director of Sports Medicine

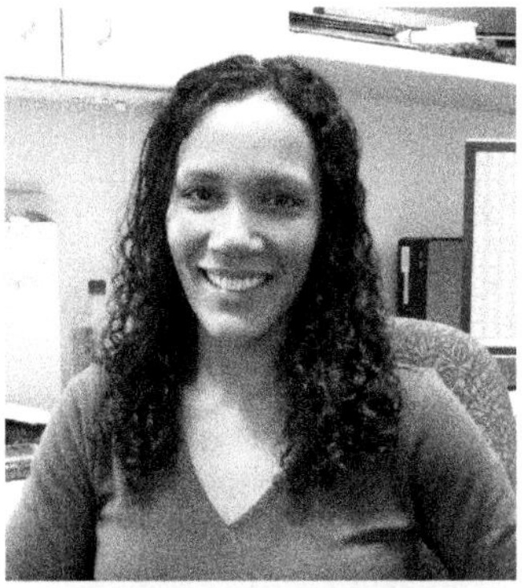

Brenda Eng, MN, CPNP, ARNP
Pediatric Nurse Practitioner

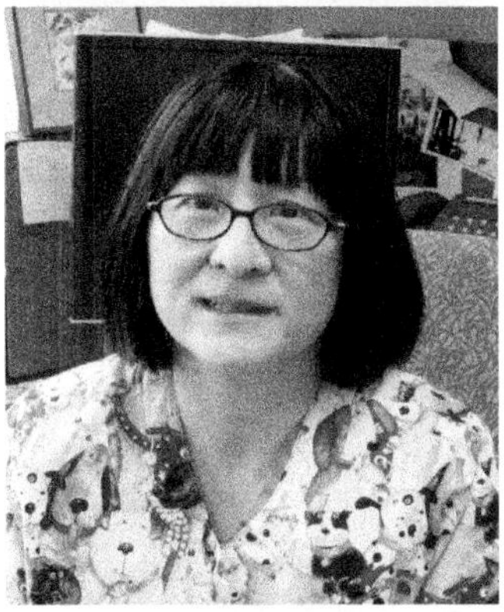

Thomas Jinguji, MD
Pediatrician
Pediatric Orthopedic Musculoskeletal Medicine Practitioner

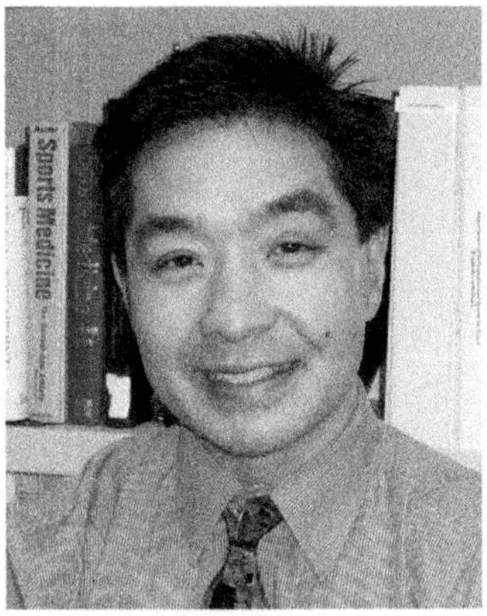

Cheryl Parker, PA
Physician Assistant
Supervisor PA/NP Team

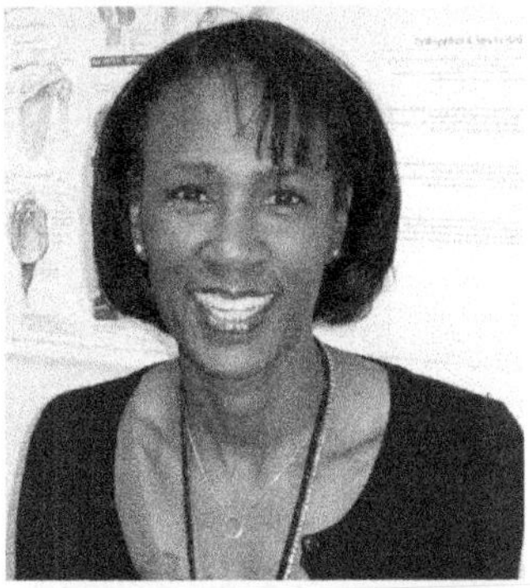

Gregory Schmale, MD
Pediatric Orthopaedic Surgeon
Clinic Chief, Sports Program
Director, Orthopaedic Education

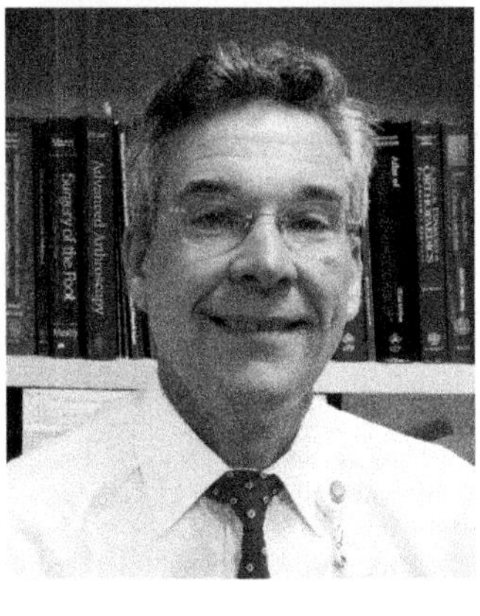

Preface to First Edition

Fundamentals of Pediatric Orthopedics was designed to make learning the basics of pediatric orthopedics a rapid and pleasant experience. Features:

1. This book is designed for the primary care physician. It may be useful for orthopedists as a rapid review of children's problems.
2. An effort was made to control production costs to make the book affordable.
3. The book was produced in color, not only to make it engaging but also to make it most efficient in communicating information.
4. Suggested treatment is scientifically based, current, and child oriented. I suggest management that emphasizes the welfare of the whole child. Special attention is given to natural history.
5. More emphasis is placed on principles than details.
6. Parent education and reference material are included in the last chapter.
7. The book was computer generated. It was conceptualized, designed, and written in my office. This made possible the integration of the text and illustrations to cover each topic efficiently.

Credit is due many hundreds of colleagues whose research and ideas contribute to our knowledge of children's orthopedics. My contribution is based on more than two decades of experience in clinical practice and as head of our university-based teaching program in pediatric orthopedics.

Preface to the Second Edition

Fundamentals of Pediatric Orthopedics has been updated, modified, and supplemented by a chapter on sports medicine. Although the book has been made more comprehensive, it has been condensed to keep the price affordable.

My reviews have been guided by feedback from residents, students, and practicing physicians.

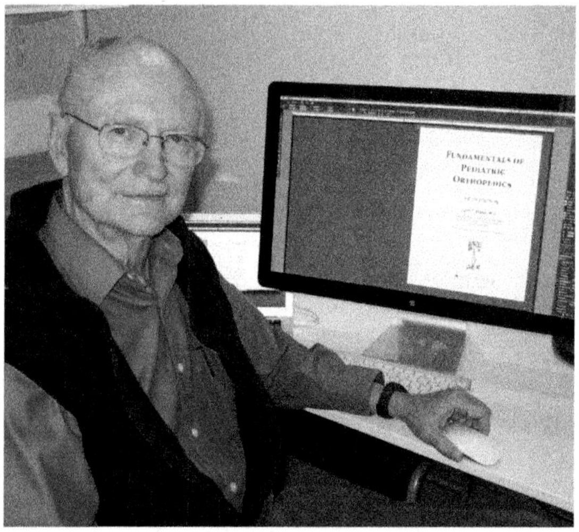

Lynn Staheli, MD
Please e-mail me comments and corrections
staheli@uw.edu

Diva
More help

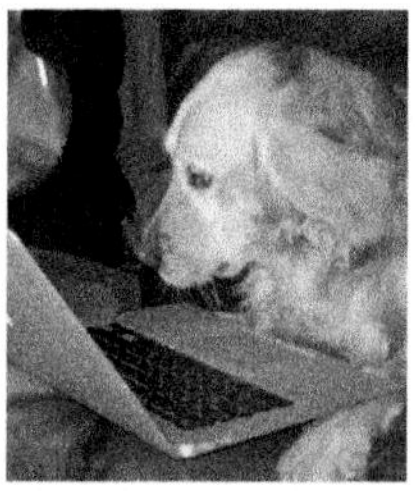

Preface to the Third Edition

This edition is expanded and enhanced with inclusion of content from *Practice of Pediatric Orthopedics,* my companion text produced for orthopedic surgeons.

In addition to expanding content, the designation of illustrations has been simplified. Text reference to illustrations is designed as [A], [B], etc. Illustrations nearly always appear on the same page as the associated text. If it's necessary to identify individual illustrations, list the page number followed by the letter (i.e., illustration B on page 126 is 126B).

Preface to the Fourth Edition

This edition is substantially more comprehensive than previous editions. I expanded this edition as primary care providers manage an increasingly larger number of orthopedic problems.

This book draws from the second edition of the *Practice of Pediatric Orthopedics*, the companion publication designed for practicing orthopedics. The details of surgery are not included, but new text and illustrations are added to detail management of conditions best managed in primary care.

I wish to thank the numerous contributors to this edition. These include the primary care consultants who provided advice and clinical images; the text editor, Sandra Rush; and my design consultant, Jeffery McCord.

I appreciate the advice from orthopedists doctors, Carl Stanitski and Vince Mosca, and support from LWW, especially Ryan Shaw, Sonya Seigafuse, and Brian Convery.

Preface to the Fifth Edition

This edition updates the contents of *Fundamentals of Pediatric Orthopedics*. The material was updated and the chapter on sports medicine expanded. The changes and additions were guided by my colleagues who reviewed the fourth edition and made recommendations to improve this new edition. I valued their varied perspectives as the goal was to make the information as current and relevant. They were ideally qualified as all are actively involved in the care of children with musculoskeletal problems and serve with differing perspectives.

I wish to thank Ms. Jamie Elfrank, Pediatric Acquisitions Editor of Lippincott Williams & Wilkins, for inviting me to create the new edition and providing support during the upgrade.

Dedication

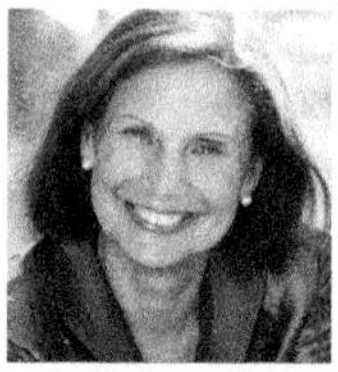

Lana Staheli, wife and best friend

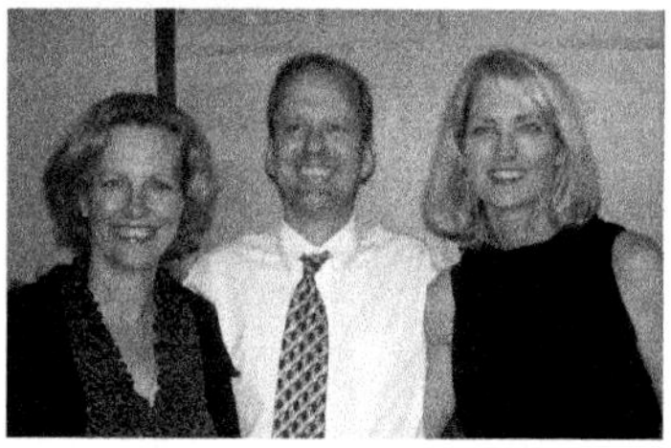

My children: Linda, Todd, and Diane

CHAPTER 1

GROWTH

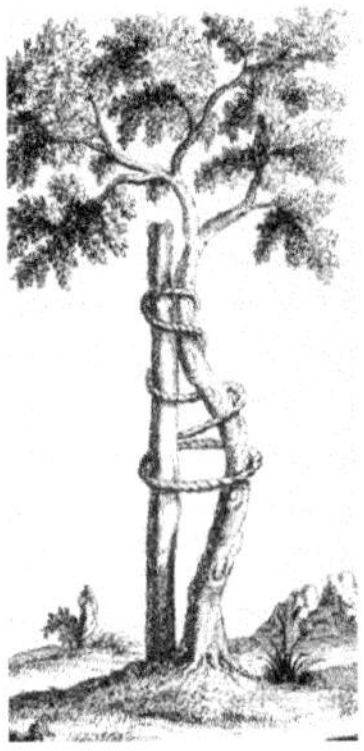

A Andry's Tree

Pediatric orthopedics is a subspecialty of medicine that deals with the prevention and treatment of musculoskeletal disorders in children. In 1741, Nicholas Andry, professor of medicine at the University of Paris, published his treatise describing different methods of preventing and correcting deformities in children [A]. He combined two Greek words, *orthos*, or straight, and *paidios*, child, into one word, "orthopedics," which became the name of the specialty concerned with the preservation and restoration of the musculoskeletal system. Pediatric orthopedics is central to this specialty based on Andry's original focus on childhood problems, due to the large proportion of orthopedic problems that originate during the early period of growth, and finally, because pediatric orthopedics offers a dynamic and inherently interesting subspecialty.

A knowledge of normal and abnormal growth and development is vital to an understanding of pediatric orthopedics [B]. This knowledge increases our comprehension of the musculoskeletal system, improves our understanding of the causes of disease, and makes us better able to manage the varied orthopedic problems of childhood.

Dividing the period of growth into six stages provides a convenient framework to review both normal and abnormal growth and development [C]. During the first stage, reproductive cells or gametes are formed.

Normal Growth

During normal development, cells proliferate, undergo differentiation, move, and even in some cases die in order to produce a normal, mature individual.

Gamete

Gamete is a collective term for ovum and sperm. During gametogenesis, meiotic division halves the chromosome number. Genetic material, which may include defective genes, is shuffled, and mature ova and sperm are formed [D].

Early Embryo

This early embryonic phase encompasses the 2-week period from fertilization to the implantation of the embryo.

First week During the first week following fertilization, the zygote repeatedly divides as it moves through the fallopian tubes to the uterus. The zygote becomes a morula, then a blastocyst. The blastocyst implants itself on the posterior uterine wall.

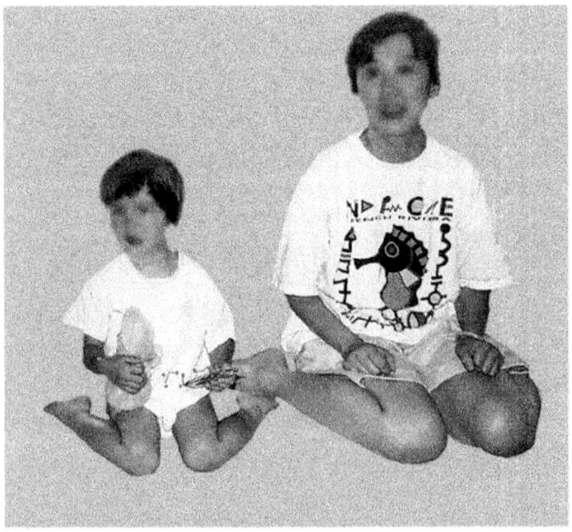

B Femoral torsion Femoral torsion is often familial. Many common musculoskeletal problems have a genetic basis.

Category	Period
Early Embryo	0–2 weeks
Embryo	2–8 weeks
Fetus	8 weeks to birth
Infant	Birth to 2 years
Child	2 years to puberty
Adolescent	Transition to maturity

C Growth phase The period of growth can be divided into six phases.

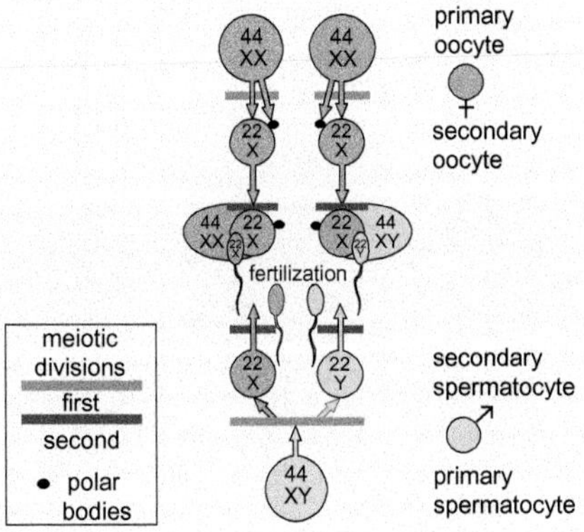

D Gametogenesis The ovum and sperm are formed by two meiotic divisions that halve the chromosome number and shuffle genetic material. Fertilization combines the traits of both parents to create a unique individual.

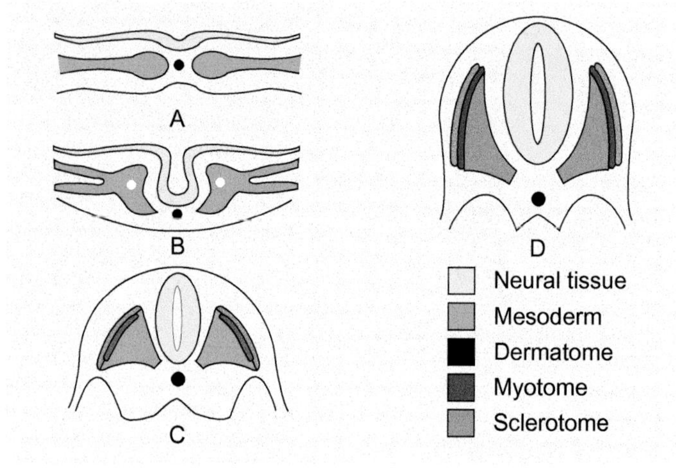

A Trilaminar disc The neural tube closes. The mesoderm differentiates into dermatome, myotome, and sclerotome.

Second week During this week, the amniotic cavity and trilaminar embryonic disc are formed [A]. The early embryo is usually aborted if a lethal or serious genetic defect is present. During these first two weeks, the early embryo is less susceptible to teratogens than during the following embryonic period.

Embryo

The embryonic period is characterized by rapid cell activity and organ formation. Cells differentiate and mature, often through induction, a process by which surrounding cells act on other cells to produce entirely new cells or tissue.

Third week This is the first week of organogenesis. During this week, the trilaminar embryonic disc develops, somites begin to form, and the neural plate closes to form a neural tube.

Fourth week During this week, the limb buds become recognizable [B]. Somites differentiate into three segments. The dermatome becomes skin, the myotome becomes muscle, and the sclerotome becomes cartilage and bone. The apical ectodermal ridge develops in the distal end of each limb bud. The ridge has an inductive influence on limb mesenchyme, which promotes growth and development of the limb. Serious defects in limb development may originate at this time.

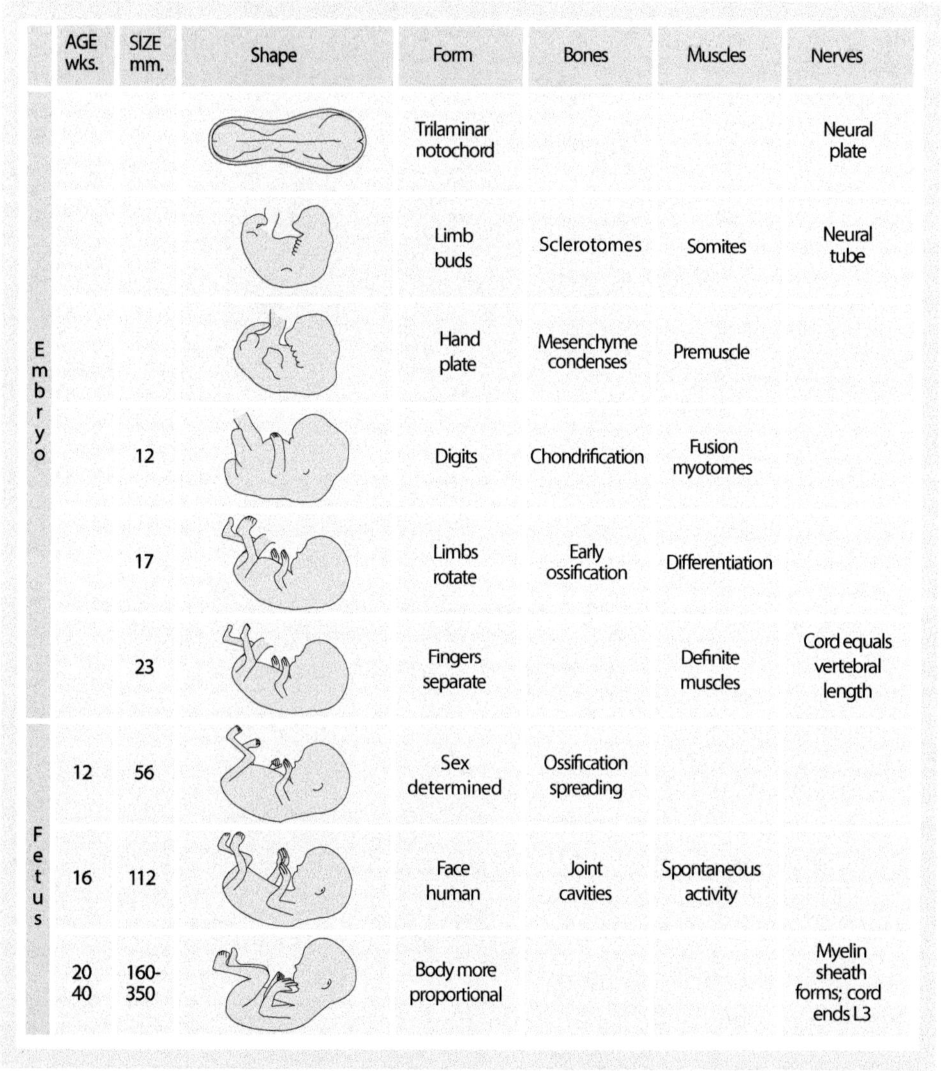

	AGE wks.	SIZE mm.	Shape	Form	Bones	Muscles	Nerves
Embryo				Trilaminar notochord			Neural plate
				Limb buds	Sclerotomes	Somites	Neural tube
				Hand plate	Mesenchyme condenses	Premuscle	
		12		Digits	Chondrification	Fusion myotomes	
		17		Limbs rotate	Early ossification	Differentiation	
		23		Fingers separate		Definite muscles	Cord equals vertebral length
Fetus	12	56		Sex determined	Ossification spreading		
	16	112		Face human	Joint cavities	Spontaneous activity	
	20 40	160- 350		Body more proportional			Myelin sheath forms; cord ends L3

B Prenatal development This chart summarizes musculoskeletal development during embryonic and fetal life.

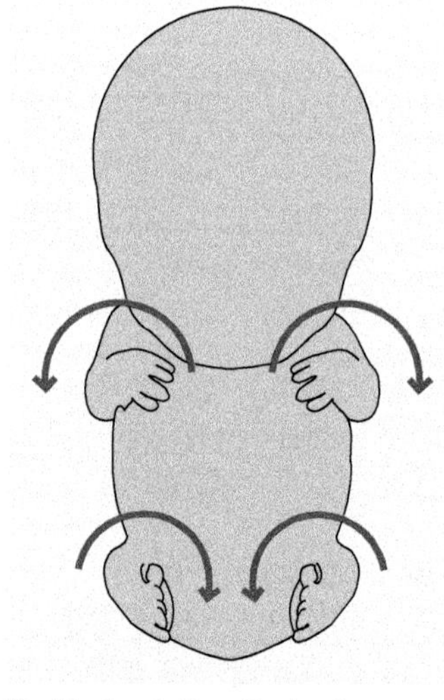

C Limb rotation During the seventh week, the upper limb rotates laterally. The lower limb rotates medially to bring the great toes to the midline.

Fifth week The hand plate forms and mesenchymal condensations occur in the limbs.

Sixth week The rays of the digits become evident and chondrification of mesenchymal condensations occurs.

Seventh week The notches appear between the digit rays. This process, responsible for joint formation, results from cell death. Failure of the separation of rays results in syndactylism. During this week, the upper and lower limbs rotate in opposite directions [C, previous page]. The lower limb rotates medially to bring the great toes to the midline, whereas the upper limb rotates about 90° laterally to position the thumb on the lateral side of the limb.

Eighth week The fingers separate completely, the embryo assumes a human appearance, and the basic organ systems are completed.

Fetus

The fetal period is characterized by rapid growth and changes in body proportions.

Ninth to twelfth weeks The first bone, the clavicle, ossifies by a process of intramembranous deposition of calcium. The skeleton develops in a cranial to caudad sequence, with the upper extremities developing before the lower limbs. This results in the upper limbs becoming proportionate compared to the rest of the body, but the lower limbs remaining short.

Thirteenth to twentieth weeks Growth continues to be rapid. The lower limbs become proportionate, and most bones ossify. The fetal period is characterized by rapid growth and changes in body proportions

Twentieth to fortieth weeks Growth continues and body proportions become more infant-like.

Connective Tissue

During early fetal life, the basic structure of connective tissue is formed largely of two families of macromolecules: collagens and proteoglycans.

Collagen

Collagen is a family of proteins containing a triple helix of peptide chains [A]. Although at least fifteen different types of collagen are known, five types are most common [B].

The biosynthesis of collagen starts in the endoplasmic reticulum, where the basic molecule is assembled. In the extracellular space, procollagen is formed. It is arranged into fibrils and reinforced by cross-linkages to become collagen. Collagen is the major component of connective tissue.

Disorders of collagen are common They may be minor, producing only increased joint laxity [C], or severe, causing considerable disability. The major collagen disorders are classified according to the site of the defect in the pathway of collagen biosynthesis.

Proteoglycans (mucopolysaccharides)

Proteoglycans are macromolecules that form the intracellular matrix of hyaline cartilage and the other connective tissues. Polypeptides or proteins attach to glycosaminoglycan to become proteoglycans [D]. Proteoglycans attach to a hyaluronic acid by a link protein to become an aggregate with a molecular weight in excess of one million. Proteoglycans are highly hydrophilic, and in water they combine with many times their weight of water to create an elastic matrix that is ideal for joint lining. Hyaline cartilage is composed of about equal amounts of proteoglycans and collagen, and it combines with about three times its weight of water, providing a resilient tissue with excellent shock absorbing characteristics. Defects in the formation of these complex molecules produce a variety of diseases.

Mucopolysaccharide (MPS) storage diseases result from a deficiency of specific lysosomal enzymes necessary for the degradation of glycosaminoglycans. These diseases are caused by excessive intracellular accumulation of partially degraded molecules that result in conditions such as avascular necrosis or spinal cord compression.

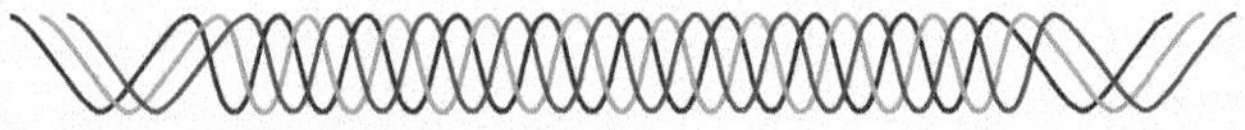

A Collagen helix A triple helix of peptide chains forms the basic collagen structure.

Type	Tissue involved	Disorders
I	Bone, tendon, skin	Osteogenesis imperfecta
II	Cartilage, nucleus pulposus	Spondyloepiphyseal dysplasia
III	Blood vessels	Ehlers-Danlos syndrome
IV	Basement membranes	
V	Minor component of bone	

B Collagen types Of the numerous collagen types, five are most widely distributed.

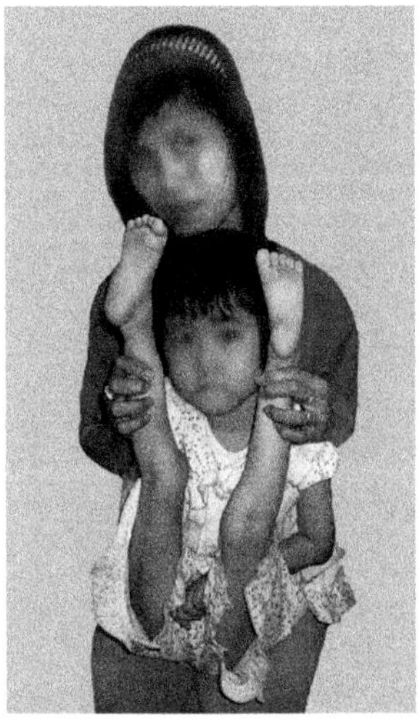

C Clinical manifestations of collagen types Variations of collagen types are common in pediatric orthopedics. This child has developmental hip dysplasia with extreme joint laxity.

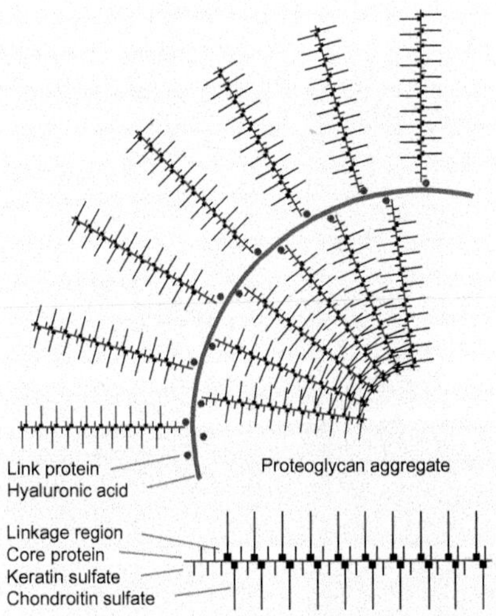

D Proteoglycan aggregate These massive molecules combine with water to form a resilient matrix such as that of hyaline cartilage.

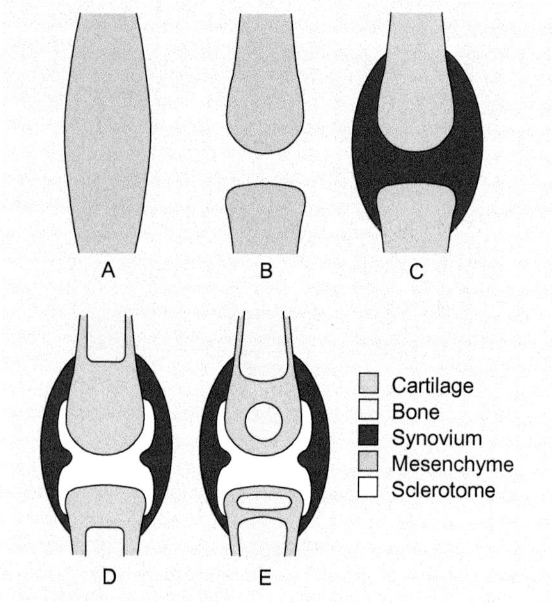

A Synovial joint formation The synovial joints form first as condensations of mesenchyme. Cavitation, chondrification, synovial differentiation, and finally ossification complete the basic structure.

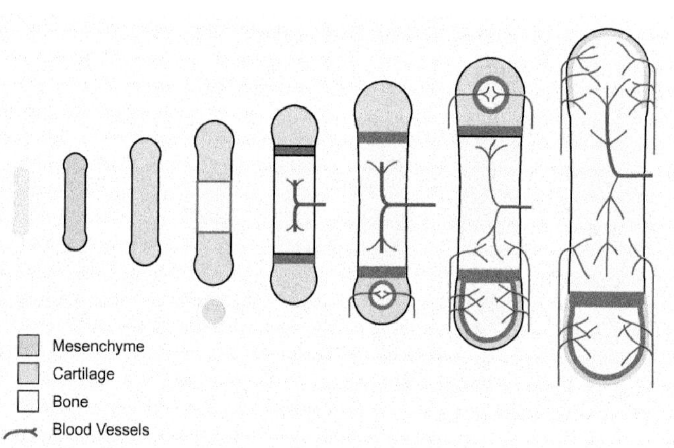

B Endochondral ossification A typical long bone is preformed in mesenchyme. Chondrification precedes ossification.

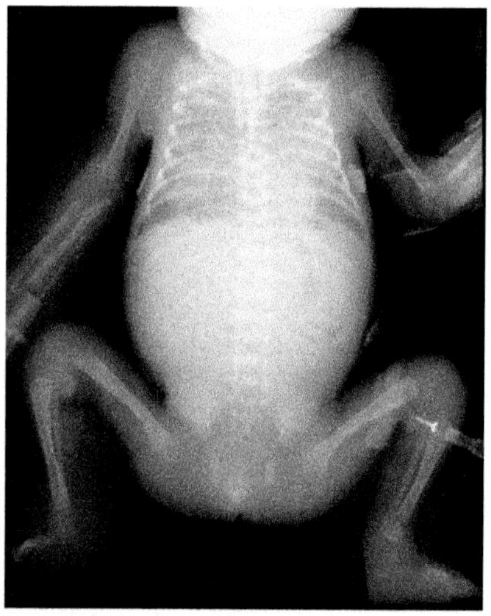

C Radiograph of bones of a newborn infant This radiograph shows primary ossification of the skeleton. Much of the skeleton is cartilage at this age.

Joints

Synovial joints develop first as a cleft in the mesenchyme, which then chondrifies and cavitates [A]. Cavitation is completed by about the fourteenth gestational week, with the inner mesenchyme becoming synovium and the outer mesenchyme becoming the joint capsule. Normal joint development requires motion, and motion requires a functioning neuromuscular system. Thus, defective joints are often seen in infants with neuromuscular disorders such as myelodysplasia or amyoplasia.

Bone

Bones are formed by osteogenesis. The mandible and clavicle are first formed starting in the seventh gestational week by intramembranous ossification.

Intramembranous Ossification

Osteoblasts differentiate from mesenchyme to form bone directly without a cartilaginous stage. Further growth occurs by appositional bone formation.

Endochondral Ossification

During the sixth gestational week, mesenchymal cells differentiate, condense, and transform into chondrocytes to form a model of the future skeleton. In the center of this model, chondrocytes hypertrophy and begin to calcify. During the next week, a periosteal sleeve of bone is formed, and by the eighth week, vascularization is under way [B].

During the fetal period, primary ossification centers develop in long bones within the diaphysis [C]. Ossification first occurs under the perichondrium. Within the cartilage, hypertrophied cells degenerate. Next, vascular ingrowth occurs, and then the core of the cartilage model is ossified to form the primary ossification center. Endochondral ossification proceeds at the cartilage–bone interphase. Later, secondary ossification centers develop at the ends of the bones, and the cartilage interposed between the primary and secondary ossification centers becomes the growth plate.

Except for the clavicle, all bones of the axial and appendicular skeleton are preformed in cartilage and converted to bone by enchondral ossification. This process begins in the scapula, humerus, radius, and ulna. Ossification continues in an orderly fashion, with centers appearing at different ages. Ossification is earlier in girls than boys [D].

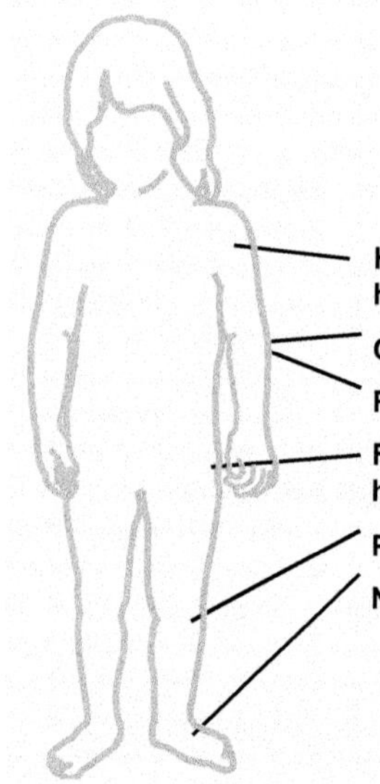

	Girls	Boys
Humeral head	0–2 mo	0–3 mo
Capitellum	1–6 mo	0–8 mo
Radial head	3–5 yrs	4–5 yrs
Femoral head	1–6 mo	2–8 mo
Patella	1.5–3.5 yrs	2.5–6 yrs
Navicular	1.5–3 yrs	1.5–5.5 yrs

D Ossification Appearance of important ossification centers in girls and boys.

Periosteum

The periosteum seems to develop from the perichondrium. The periosteum is osteogenic, allowing appositional bone growth, and provides a thick sleeve adding resilience and strength to the growing skeleton. This osteogenic capability results in rapid fracture healing and bone regeneration.

Bone Types

Growing bone possesses special characteristics, providing the infant and child with greater flexibility and resilience than that of the adult.

Woven bone is formed during the fetal period. This bone has less structure, a relatively higher collagen content, and more flexibility than lamellar bone. Woven bone makes up the metaphysis of growing bones, and the type of bone making up the *callus* following fracture. This flexibility becomes essential during the traverse of the birth canal.

Lamellar bone Once the need for this high degree of flexibility has passed, woven bone is gradually replaced by lamellar bone starting soon after birth. By four years of age, most woven bone has been converted to lamellar bone.

Ossification Centers

Primary ossification centers for long bones usually develop before birth [C, previous page], whereas primary ossification centers for smaller bones, such as the patella and most carpal and tarsal bones, develop during infancy [A].

Secondary ossification centers develop during infancy and early childhood. They fuse with the primary centers during late childhood, adolescence, and early adult life. Because osseous maturation continues throughout childhood and adolescence in a reasonably orderly fashion, the extent of ossification, as radiographically documented, has become the standard for assessing maturation.

Bone Growth

Cortical thickness increases throughout childhood. For example, the diameter of the diaphysis of the femur increases faster than does the diameter of the medullary canal. This produces an increasing diaphyseal thickness with advancing age. This increasing thickness, lamellar structure, and proportion of calcium give mature bone great tensile strength but little flexibility. These changes are important factors in producing the varying patterns of skeletal injury seen during infancy, childhood, and adult life.

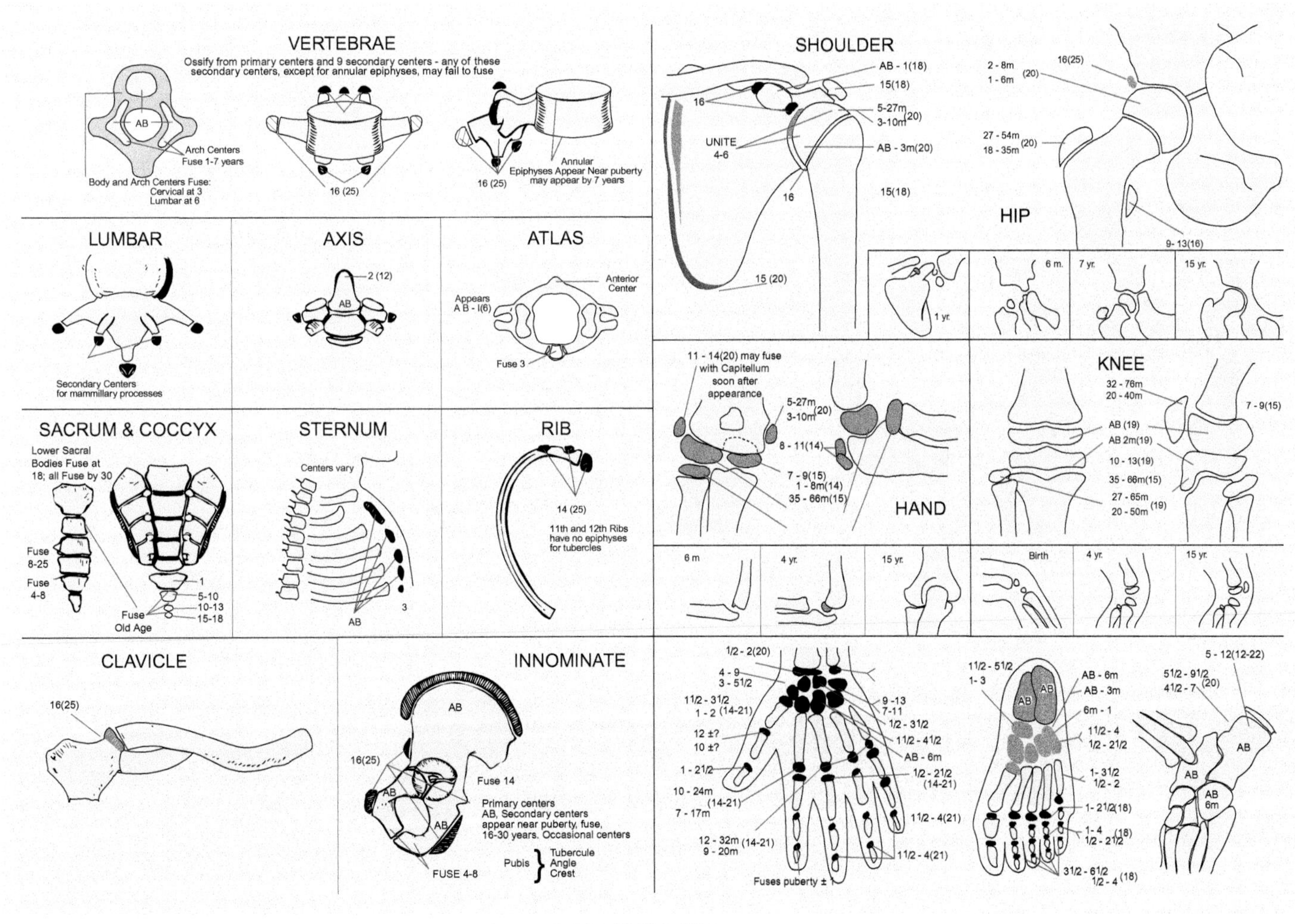

A Ossification centers Redrawn from Girdany BR and Golden R AJR 68:922, 1952.

Growth Plate

The growth plate of long bones develops between the primary and secondary ossification centers [A]. The growth plate is responsible for the longitudinal growth of long bones. Growth plate chondrocytes go through an orderly process of proliferation and differentiation followed by terminal differentiation and the formation of new bone. Growth plates with more limited growth potential develop at other sites. These include the periphery of round bones, such as the tarsal bones or vertebral bodies, and the sites of muscle attachments, such as the margins of the ilium. Such sites are referred to as *apophyses.*

The typical long bone epiphysis is divided into zones that reflect morphological, metabolic, and functional differences.

The Reserve Zone (RZ)

This zone is adjacent to the secondary ossification centers and is a zone of relative inactivity. The RZ does not participate in the longitudinal growth of the bone, but it does provide some matrix production and storage functions. This zone contains proteins and genes important in specifying the chondrocyte phenotype, such as SOX–9.

The Proliferative Zone (PZ)

This is the zone of cartilage cell replication and growth. A high metabolic rate and abundant blood supply, oxygen, glycogen, ATP, and collagen make this rapid growth possible. Signaling pathways, important in regulating cell proliferation, are found in this zone. These include insulin-like growth factors and fibroblastic growth factors; both factors are active in this zone.

The Hypertrophic Zone (HZ)

This zone consists of three sub-zones: maturation, degeneration, and provisional calcification segments. In the HZ, the cartilage cells increase in size and the matrix is prepared for calcification. This is associated with a decline in blood supply, oxygenation, and glycogen stores, and with a disintegration of aggregated mucopolysaccharides and chondrocytes. In the sub-zone of provisional calcification, a unique collagen X that accepts calcium deposition is synthesized.

The Metaphysis

This zone is the site of vascularization, bone formation, and remodeling. The calcified matrix is removed, and fiber bone is formed and replaced by lamellar bone.

The Periphery

This zone includes the growth plate and metaphysis, which are the primary sites for infections, neoplasms, fractures, and metabolic and endocrine disorders. Problems in the growth plate constitute a significant portion of diseases of the musculoskeletal system in childhood.

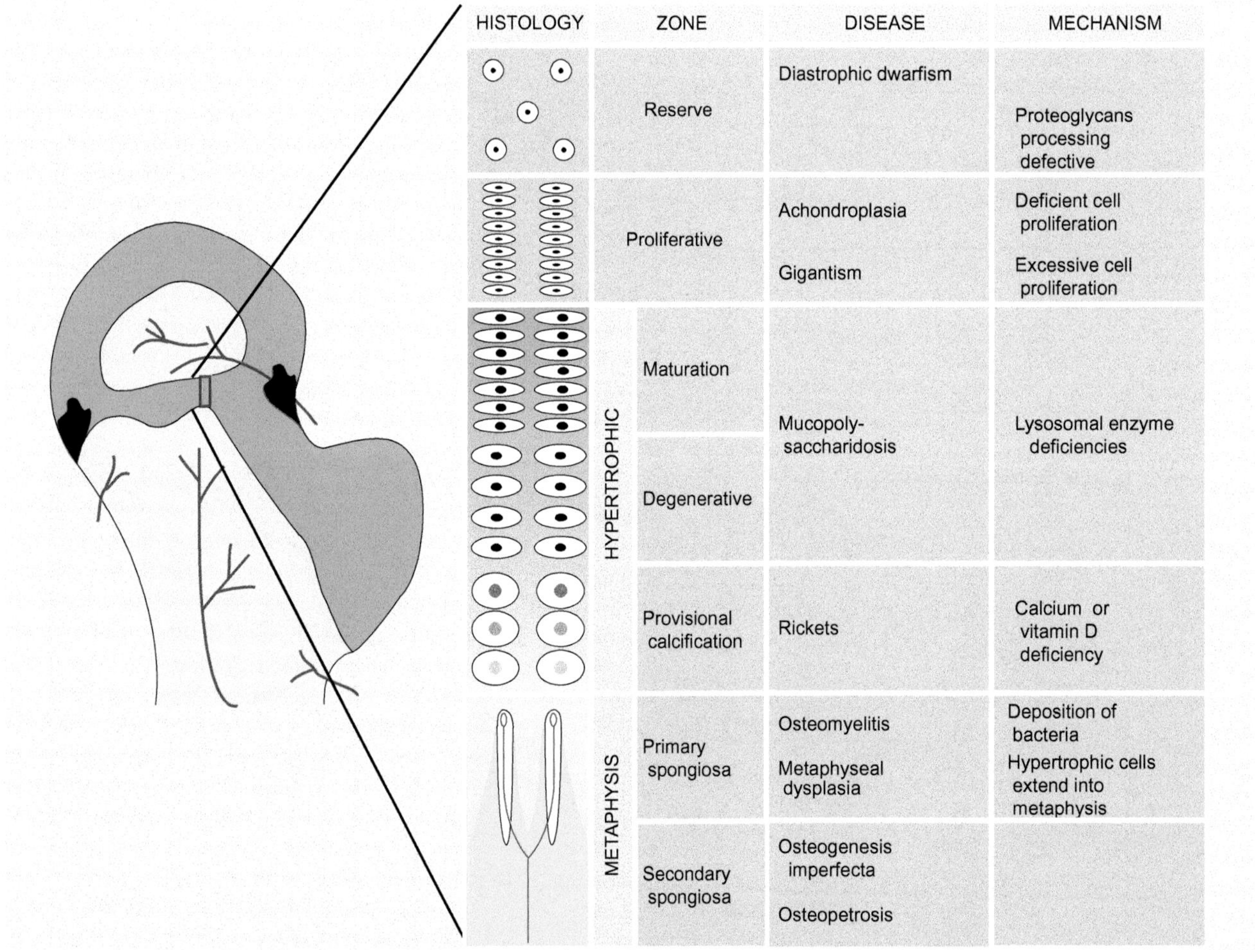

A Growth plate This section from the proximal femoral epiphysis is enlarged to show the histology and disordered growth that occurs at various levels of the growth plate.

Perichondral Ring

The perichondral ring of LaCroix and the ossification groove of the Ranvier ring surround the growth plate [B]. These structures support and expand the width of the growth plate.

The perichondral ring of LaCroix is continuous with the metaphyseal periosteum, increasing the strength of the metaphyseal–physeal interphase.

The ossification groove of Ranvier is an accumulation of chondrocytes, providing the reserve cells necessary for appositional growth of the growth plate.

Growth Plate Types

Growth plates form in a number of patterns, depending upon the shape of the bone [C]. These include:

Epiphyseal plate forms at the end of long bones, providing longitudinal growth.

Ring epiphyses surround round bones such as the tarsals or metatarsals. The bones grow circumferentially.

Apophyses are growth plates applied to the surface of a bone such as the iliac crest.

Traction apophyses are growth plates to which a muscle is attached. Examples include the tibial tubercle and greater trochanter.

Bone Growth

Bone growth rate is precisely regulated with each growth center contributing a prescribed percentage of the final growth. These values are important to know due to their clinical significance [D].

Growth rates from various epiphyses vary. In the upper limb, growth is most rapid at the shoulder and wrist, in contrast to the lower limb where most growth occurs just above and below the knee. To help remember the different growth rates in extremities, a commonly used memory aid is imaging a child in a bathtub. The growth plates that would be above water are the most fast growing [E]. Alterations in the general health of the child are often recorded by growth arrest lines [A]. These are linear calcifications from slowing of growth.

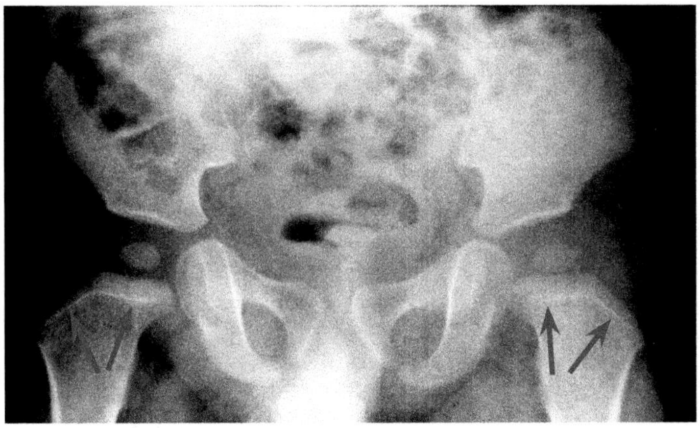

A Growth lines Note the growth arrest lines (red arrows) in this child with developmental hip dysplasia. Presumably, the anesthetic and closed reduction caused the slowing of growth. Bone growth since the event is shown by the width of the new metaphyseal bone.

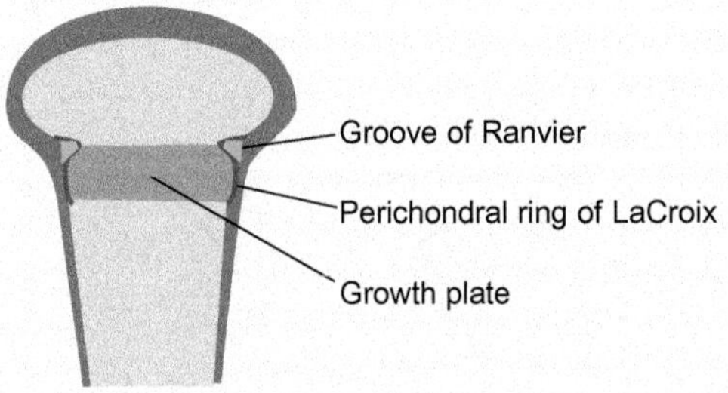

B Perichondral ring This ring consists of elements that provide strength and the capacity of the growth plate to expand in width. The groove of Ranvier (green) and perichondral ring of LaCroix (red) are shown. Based on Gamble, JG 1988.

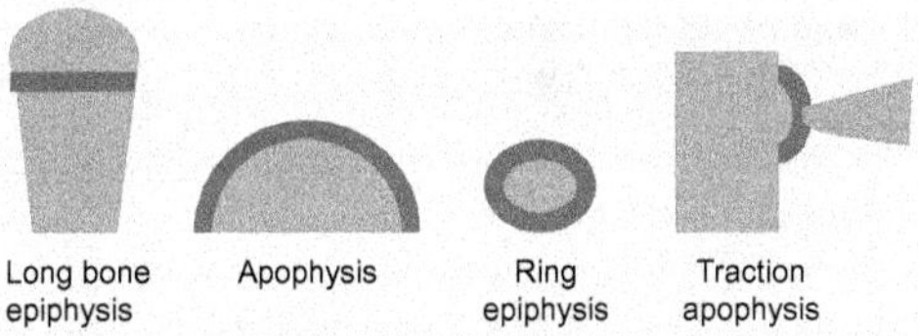

C Types of growth plates The common types include the long bone epiphysis that may be present at one or both ends. The apophysis is applied to the edge of a bone such as the iliac crest. Examples of ring epiphyses include the carpals or tarsal bones.

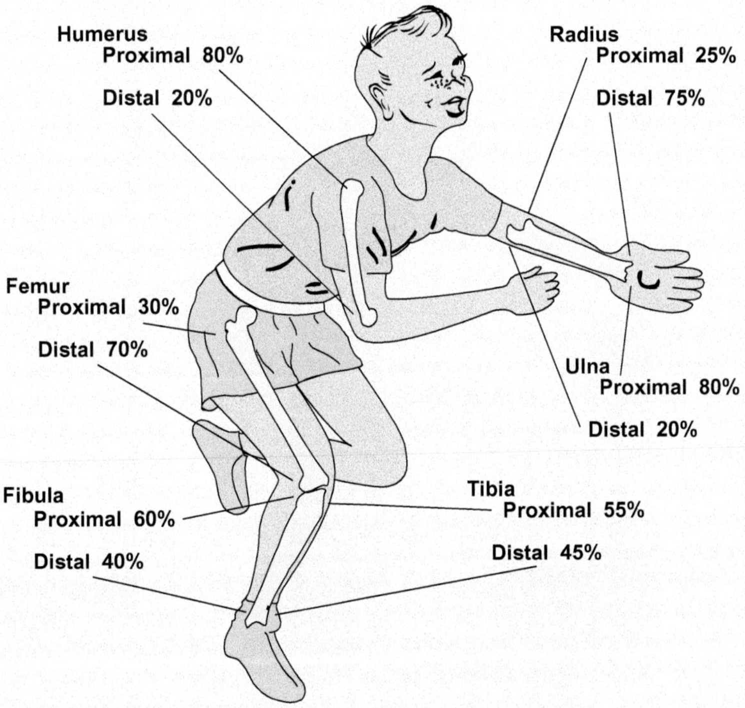

D Epiphyseal contribution of long bone growth From Blount (1955).

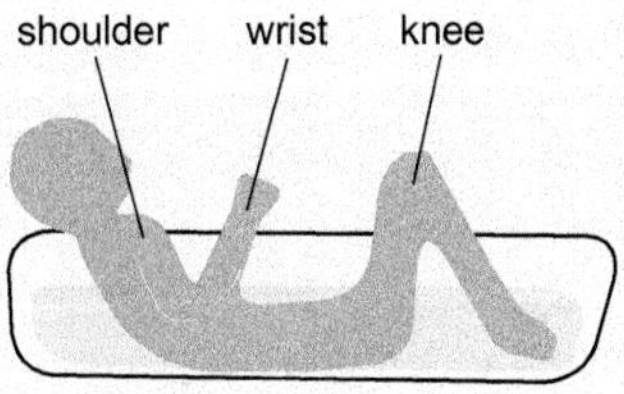

E Growth memory aid Child in a tub. The growth centers around the shoulder, wrist, and knee (the parts out of water in this drawing) are the fastest-growing centers in the limbs.

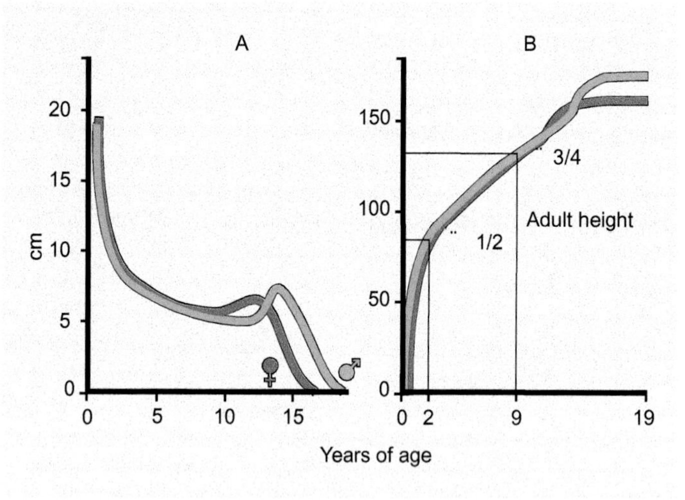

A Growth Rate A Growth rates for girls (red) and boys (blue) by age. The greatest rate of growth occurs during infancy. B Growth rate as a fraction of adult height. About half of an individual's adult height is reached by age 2 years and three-fourths by age 9 years.

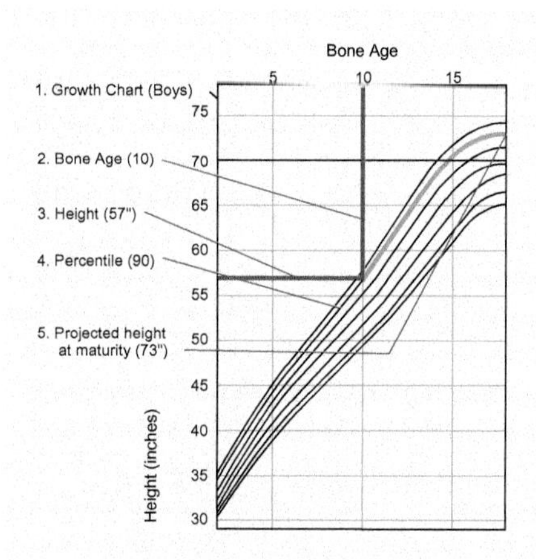

B Prediction of adult height Predict adult height by plotting the child's bone age (vertical red line) against the current height (horizontal red line) to determine the percentile value (green). Follow the percentile (green line) to skeletal maturation to estimate final adult height.

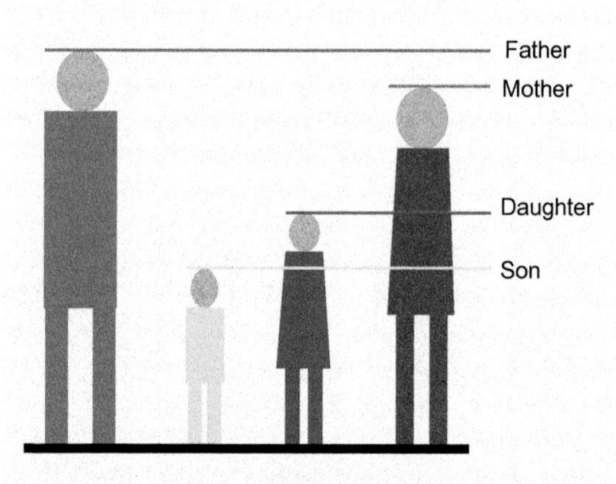

C To estimate adult height Add heights of father and mother. For daughters subtract 5 in. (13 cm) and divide in two. For sons add 5 in. (13 cm) and divide in two.

Growth and Development

Infancy extends from birth to 2 years of age. It encompasses the period of most rapid growth and development after birth.

Growth Rates

The growth rate varies with age and is greatest in early infancy, declines during childhood, and briefly increases again during the adolescent growth spurt. A child is about half his or her adult height at 2 years of age and about three-fourths by 9 years of age [A].

Predicting Adult Height

Estimating adult height is valuable in managing certain deformities, particularly anisomelia (limb length inequality). A variety of methods for predicting adult height are available.

The simplest method is to double the child's height at two years [A].

Another way involves establishing the percentile of height by plotting the child's height on the growth chart by bone age rather than by chronological age. This percentile is projected out to skeletal maturity to provide an estimate of adult height [B].

The most commonly used method [C] is to add the mother's and father's heights in either inches or centimeters. Add 5 in. (13 cm) for boys and subtract 5 in. (13 cm) for girls. Then divide in two. Using this method, most children will reach an adult height within 4 in. (10 cm) of this estimation.

Growth of Different Tissues

The growth rate of tissues varies with age. Subcutaneous fat, which provides nutritional reserve and protection from cold and injury, develops during the first year. The fat obscures the longitudinal arch of the foot, giving the infant a flatfooted appearance [D]. The percentage of muscle increases with age, but the percentage of neural tissue declines with advancing age.

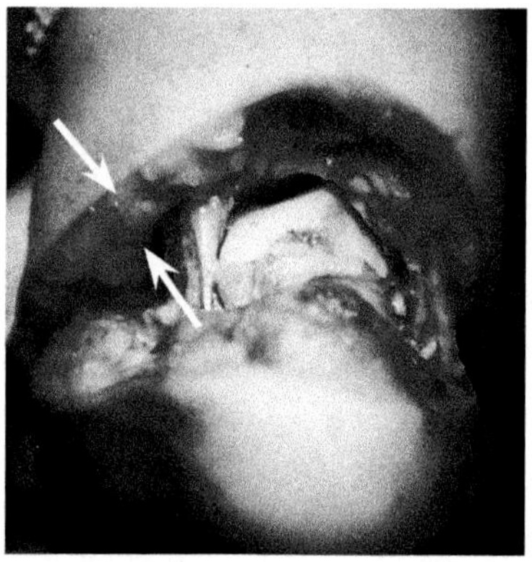

D Subcutaneous fat in infancy Note the thickness in the subcutaneous fat (arrows) in this infant undergoing clubfoot correction.

Body Proportions

Growth of various body parts are different from one another. Upper limb growth occurs earlier than lower limb growth, and the foot grows earlier than the rest of the lower limb. In childhood, the trunk grows most rapidly; in adolescence, the lower limbs grow the fastest. Throughout growth, body proportions gradually assume adult form [A].

Determining Maturation Level

Knowing the amount of growth remaining is important to the timing of physeal fusion and thus in correcting leg length inequality [B] and in managing patients with scoliosis.

Hand–wrist radiographs Use the Greulich–Pyle atlas to estimate the bone age.

Risser sign is based on the extent of ossification of the iliac crest as assessed on the AP radiograph [C]. This sign has been commonly used in assessing maturity when managing scoliosis.

Tanner stages The level of maturation is based on physical examination. Because this assessment requires an assessment of breast and genital development [D] in a sensitive age group, its use is limited.

Other signs, such as the velocity of height gain and the status of the triradiate cartilage (acetabulum), are becoming useful maturational indices.

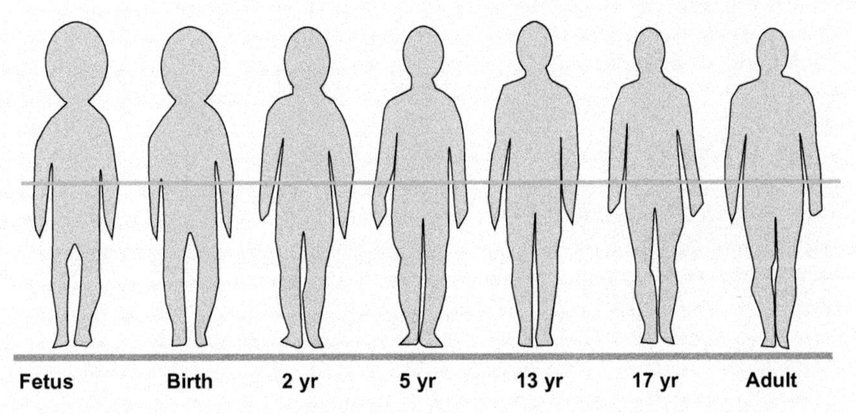

A Changes in body proportions with growth At maturity, the position of the center of gravity (green line) is the level of the sacrum. From Palmer (1944).

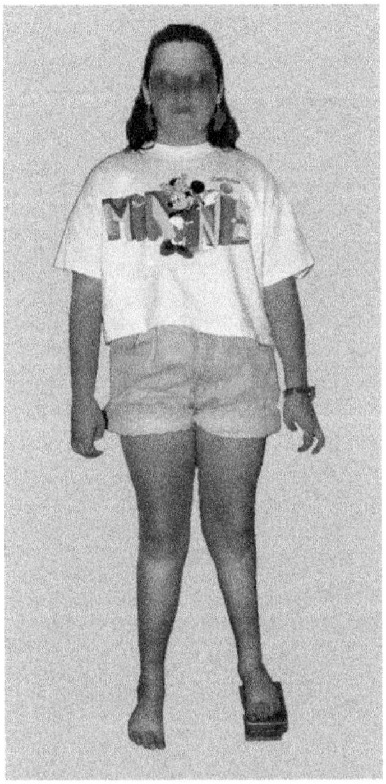

B Leg length inequality Bone age determination is helpful in planning correction by epiphysiodesis.

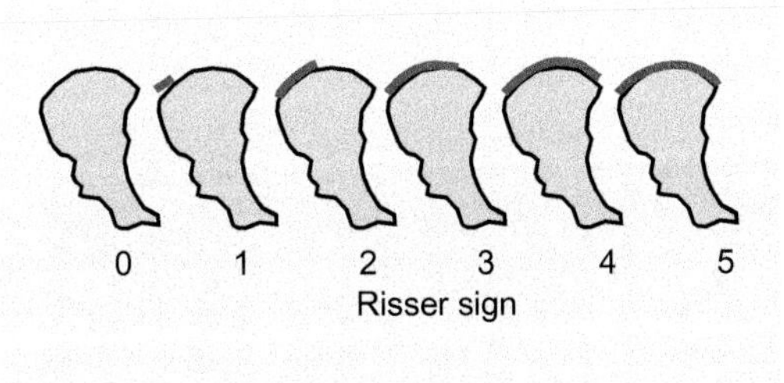

C Risser sign The extent of ossification of the iliac apophysis is commonly used to assess the skeletal maturation of patients with scoliosis. Risser 0 = no iliac apophysis; Risser 5 = fusion of the apophysis with the ilium.

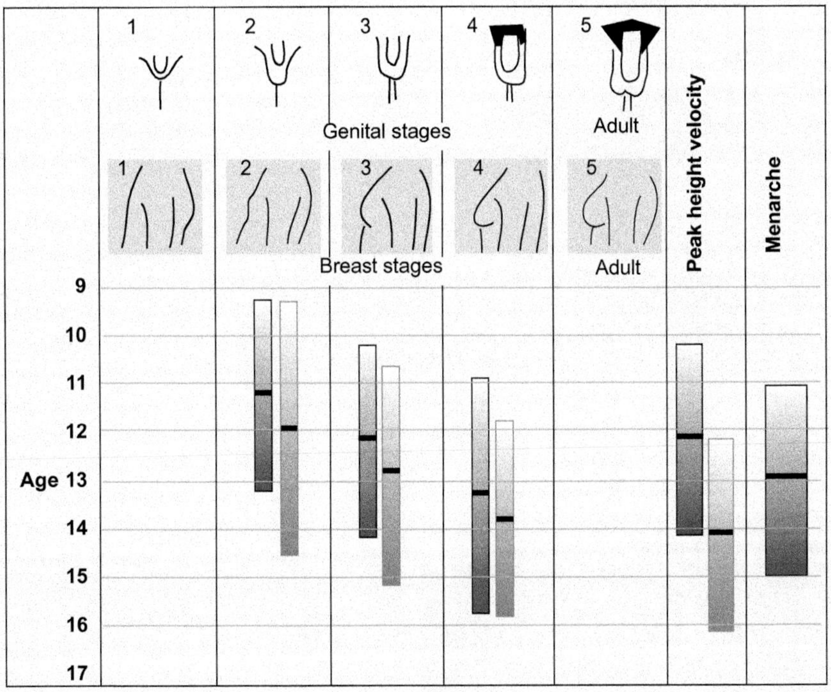

D Tanner maturation index Using physical signs, the level of maturation is assessed for males (blue) and females (red). The columns show the 3–97% levels. Mean values are shown by the black bars.

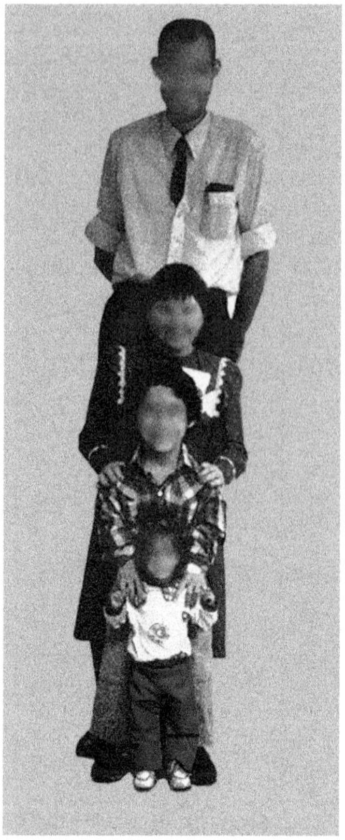

A Growth variations These individuals show the wide variations in growth. Courtesy of Dr Judy Hall.

Extremes in Growth

Wide ranges of normal exist in normal individuals [A]. However, orthopedic problems are more likely to occur in excessively heavy or short children. We define excessive as being either above the 95th percentile in weight or below the 5th percentile in height [B].

Obesity in children is becoming more common. The added weight is a factor in the development of several orthopedic problems. These include slipped capital femoral epiphysis and tibia vara [C].

Short stature below the 5th percentile is common in children with bone dysplasias or metabolic disorders.

Developmental Variations

Developmental variations occur during infancy and childhood [D]. They are commonly mistaken for deformities. They include flatfeet, in-toeing, out-toeing, bowlegs, and knock-knees. These conditions resolve with time and seldom require any treatment. These conditions are covered in more detail in Chapters 4 and 5.

	< 5% Height	> 95% weight
Girls –10 yr	< 50 inches	> 100 pounds
Boys –10 yr	< 50 inches	> 100 pounds
Girls – end of growth	< 60 inches	> 180 pounds
Boys – end of growth	< 65 inches	> 210 pounds

B Extremes of height and weight Orthopedic problems are more common in children who are excessively short (below the 5th percentile) or excessively heavy (above the 95th percentile). These values are given for girls and boys based on North American standards.

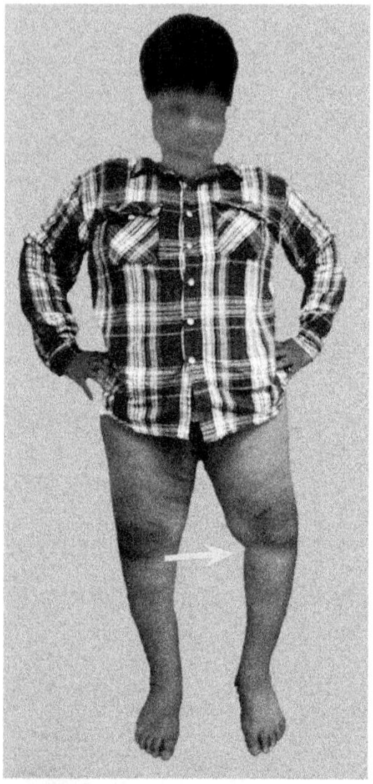

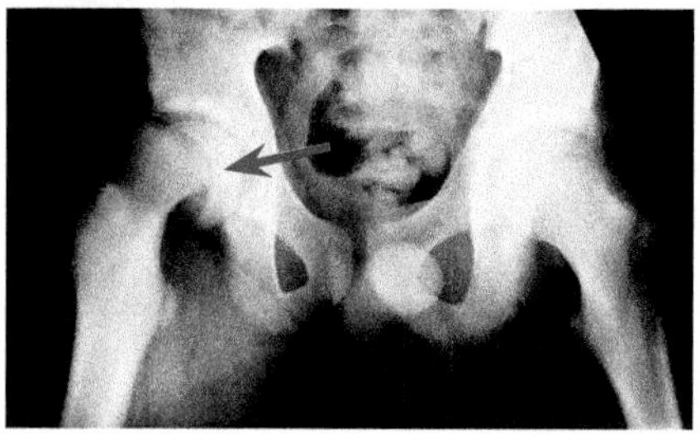

C Obesity and orthopedic problems Two common serious orthopedic problems, slipping of the capital femoral epiphysis (red arrow) and tibia vara (yellow arrow), are commonly associated with obesity.

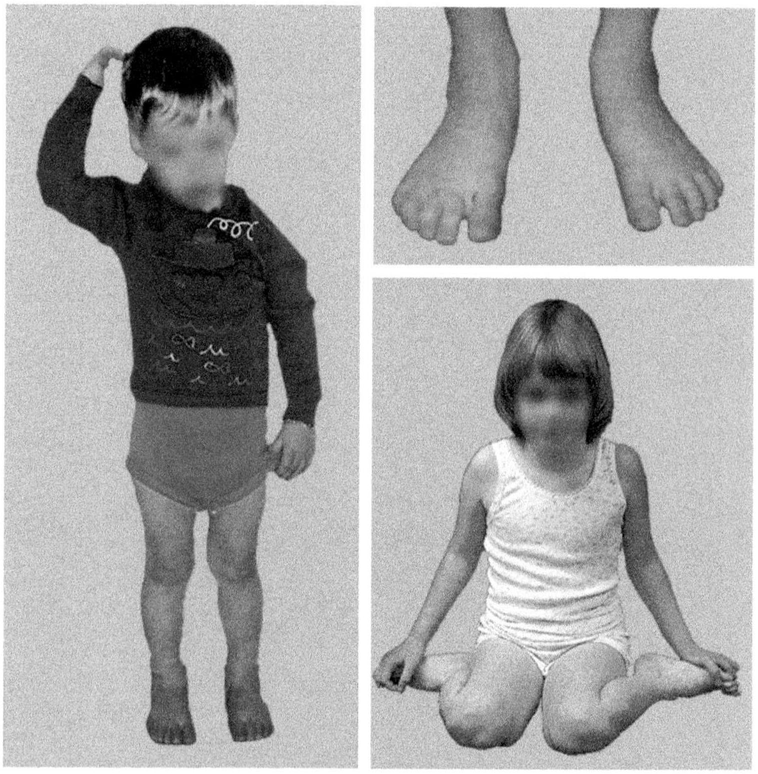

D Developmental variation in normal children Common variations include knock-knees (left), flatfeet (top right), and femoral torsion (lower right).

Gait

Gait during infancy is less stable and efficient than during childhood or adulthood [A]. Early gait is characterized by a wide-base irregular cadence, instability, and poor energy efficiency. The instability of gait in the infant is due to a high center of gravity, low muscle-to-body weight ratio, and immaturity of the nervous system and posture control mechanisms.

Motor Development

The standard for assessing motor development is the age of acquisition of gross motor skills. Such skills are easily measured and useful in assessing development [B]. Infants usually show head control by about 3 months, sit by 6 months, stand with support by 12 months, and walk unsupported by 15 months. The range of normal is broad, and tables showing the normal range and mean values for activities of daily living (ADLS), language, and motor development are widely used. These general guidelines are useful when screening.

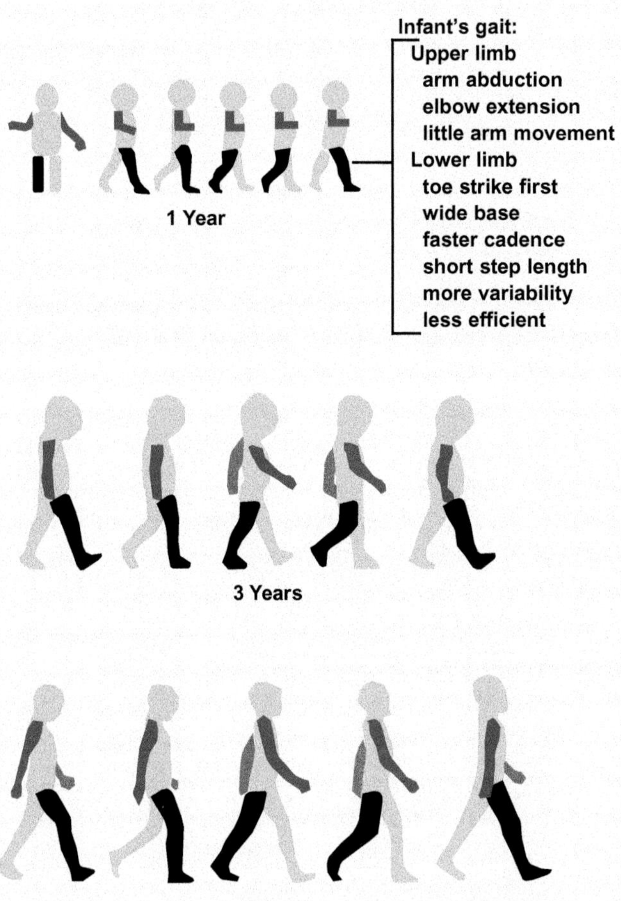

A Development of normal gait Adult gait pattern is achieved by about 7 years of age in the normal child. From Sutherland (1980).

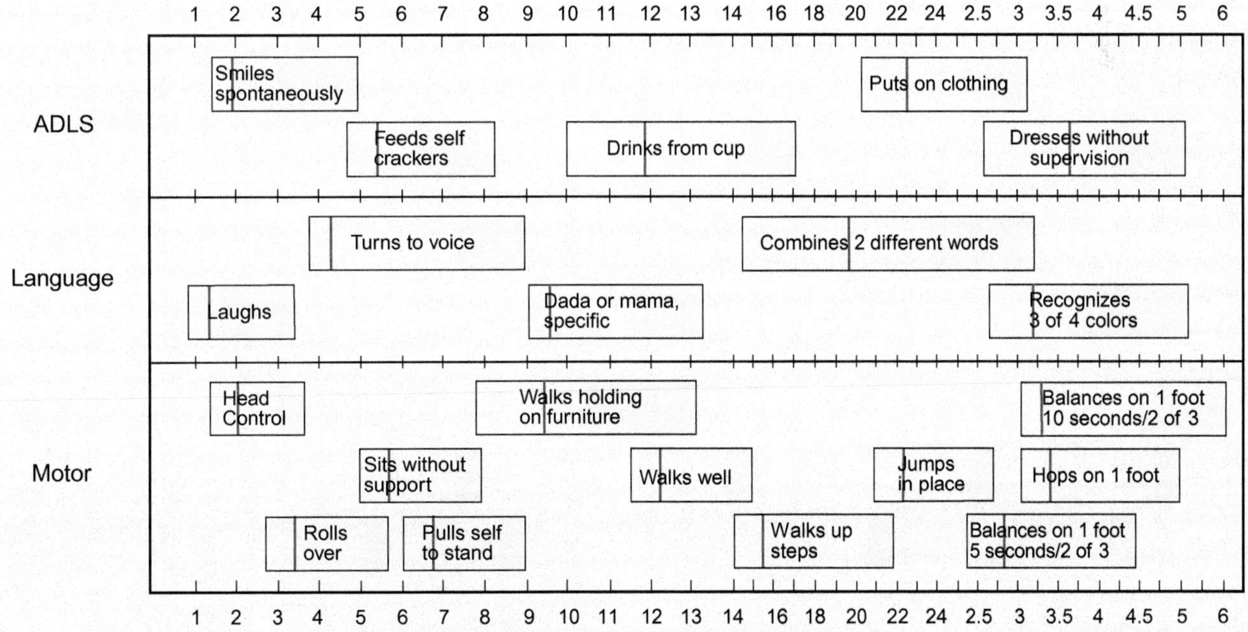

B Denver developmental screening test Shows abilities from 1 to 24 months and then to 6 years of age. Mean values are shown by red lines. Yellow shading shows values beyond 2 stand deviations from the mean. From Frankenberg (1967).

Abnormal Growth

Disorders affecting the musculoskeletal system often run in families [A] and are relatively common [B]. These and other conditions that cause limitation of activity in children have tripled during the past four decades because children with disabilities are more likely to survive today than in the past.

Classification of disorders is enhanced by a better understanding of molecular biology as well as a determination of the time of onset by prenatal ultrasound examinations. Historically, disorders were classified as being either congenital or acquired. This classification overemphasizes the importance of birth as a landmark. Many statistics acquired based on this classification are reported as congenital defects.

Statistics

Congenital defects can be caused by a variety of factors. Some are genetic, and others are environmental in origin. Some are multifactorial. Multifactorial inheritance is the most common cause of congenital defects [C]. Of newborn infants, 3% show major defects and an additional 3% are discovered later during infancy. About 20% of perinatal deaths are attributable to congenital problems. Single minor defects are present in many newborns. Because infants with multiple minor defects have a higher incidence of major malformations, the finding of minor defects should prompt a careful search for more serious problems. Musculoskeletal problems account for about one-third of congenital defects. Hip dysplasia and clubfeet make up half of the primary musculoskeletal defects.

Although inherited disorders may manifest themselves during infancy, the majority of musculoskeletal problems of infancy are due to environmental factors, such as malnutrition, infection, and trauma.

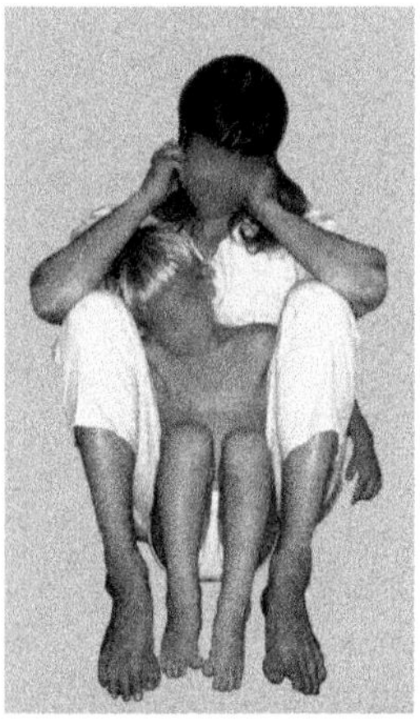

A Familial toe deformities The mother and child have the same toe abnormalities. Toe and finger deformities are often familial.

Disease	Prevalence/1000
Cerebral palsy	25
Trisomy 21	11
Developmental hip dysplasia	10
Clubfoot	10
Sickle cell disease	0.46
Muscular dystrophy	0.06

B Prevalence of orthopedic disorders.

Cause	Percentage
Chromosomal aberrations	6
Environmental factors	7
Monogenic or single gene	8
Multifactorial inheritance	25
Unknown	54

C Causes of congenital defects From Moore (1988).

Classification of Abnormal Morphogenesis

Abnormal morphogenesis has been classified into four categories [D]. These are significant for a number of reasons. The classification helps in understanding the mechanism or origin and also helps in anticipating how difficult correction will be to achieve. Deformities of earliest onset are the most difficult to correct.

Malformations

Malformations are defects that arise in the period of organogenesis and are of teratogenic or genetic origin. Phocomelia and congenital hypoplasia [E] are examples. These deformities are rigid and serious and require operative correction.

Disruptions

Disruptions occur later in gestation when teratogenic, traumatic, or other physical assaults to the fetus interfere with growth. Ring constriction due to amniotic banding [F] is an example.

Deformations

Deformations occur at the end of gestation and are due to intrauterine crowding or position. These deformities are milder and usually resolve spontaneously during early infancy. Breech position is associated with a higher incidence of congenital problems.

Dysplasias

Dysplasias result from altered growth that occurs before and/or after birth.

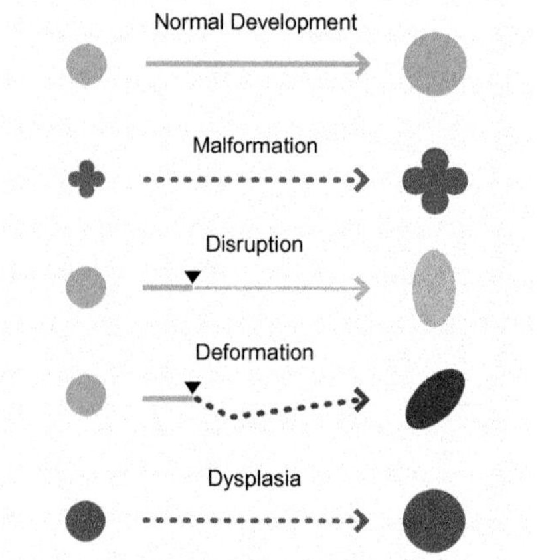

D Classification of abnormal morphogenesis These categories provide a practical basis for understanding congenital defects. From Dunne (1986).

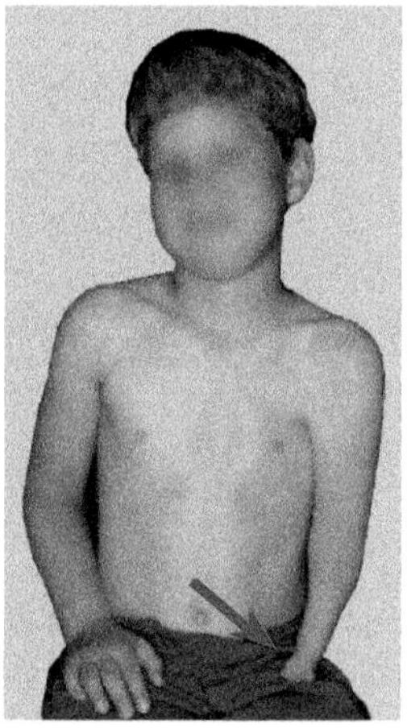

E Limb hypoplasia Major limb defects are malformations arising from interruption of limb development.

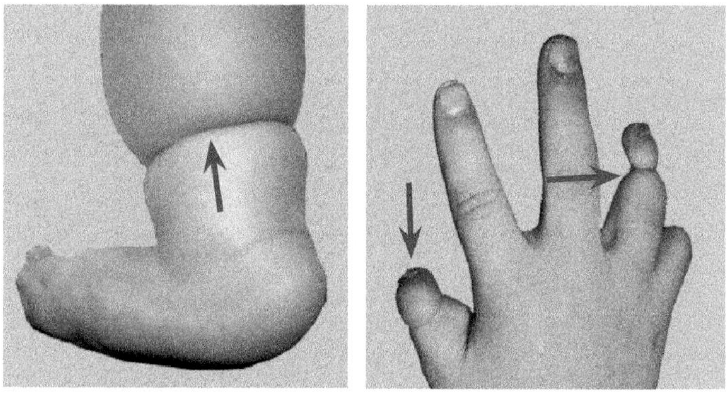

F Congenital constriction bands Intrauterine adhesion caused these deep circumferential bands.

Chromosomal Abnormalities

Chromosomes have been mapped to show the location of defective genes that create disorders often seen in orthopedic clinics [A]. The linkage of genes causing diseases with genes controlling distinguishable characteristics makes possible the identification of individuals at risk for certain diseases. For example, on chromosome 9, the gene carrying nail–patella syndrome is linked to the gene of ABO blood type. Offspring with the same ABO blood type as an affected parent will carry the syndrome.

Many chromosomal abnormalities are due to changes in number, structure, or content of chromosomes. Numerical changes in chromosomes are due to a failure of separation or nondisjunction during cell division. Nondisjunction results in monosomy or trisomy gametes. Monosomy of sex chromosomes produces the XO pattern of Turner syndrome.

Chromosomal Structural Defects

Chromosomal structural defects [B] occur spontaneously or secondarily to the effects of teratogens. Teratogens are agents that induce defects and cause a variety of syndromes. Deletions of portions of chromosomes 4, 5, 18, and 21 produce specific syndromes. For example, deletion of the terminal portion of the short end of chromosome 5 causes the "cri du chat" syndrome. Other common changes include translocations, duplications, and inversions.

Trisomy of Sex Chromosomes

Trisomy of sex chromosomes causes 47XXX females who may have only mild mental retardation, whereas 47XXY causes Klinefelter syndrome and 47XYY causes a disorder characterized by aggressive behavior. Trisomy of autosomes (non-sex chromosomes) is common and frequently affects chromosome 21, which causes Down syndrome [C]. Trisomy of chromosomes 13 and 18 causes significant defects but is less common.

Polygenic Inheritance

Polygenic or multifactorial inheritance involves multiple genes and an environmental "trigger" [F]. Such common conditions as clubfeet [D] and hip dysplasia [E] are transmitted by this mechanism. These disorders make up a large portion of the patients seen in pediatric orthopedic clinics.

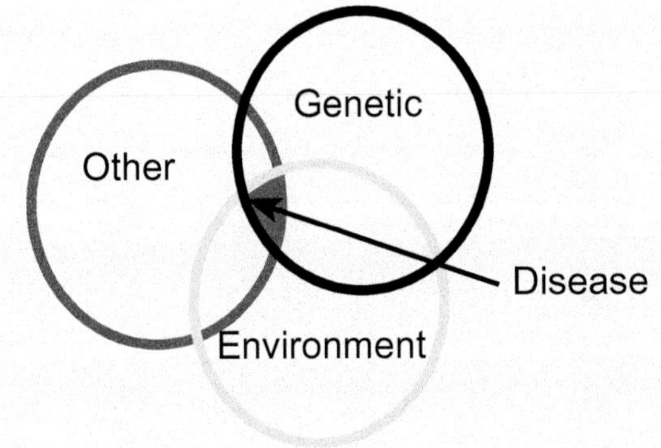

F Multifactorial inheritance Many common orthopedic problems are transmitted by this mode. Genetic, environmental, and possibly other factors combine to cause the problems.

Chromosome	Disorder
1	Rh blood group, Gaucher, CMT diseases
5	MPS VI, cri du chat syndrome
6	Histocompatibility complex
7	MPS VII, Ehlers–Danlos VII, some Marfan
9	ABO typing, nail–patella syndrome
15	Prader–Willi syndrome
X	Duchenne dystrophy, chondrodysplasia

A Chromosome disorder location Localization of musculoskeletal disorders to specific chromosomes.

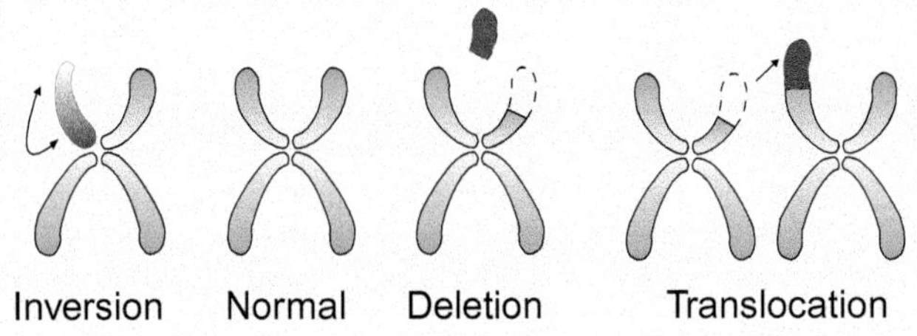

B Chromosomal structural defects Various structural defects include inversions, deletions, and translocations.

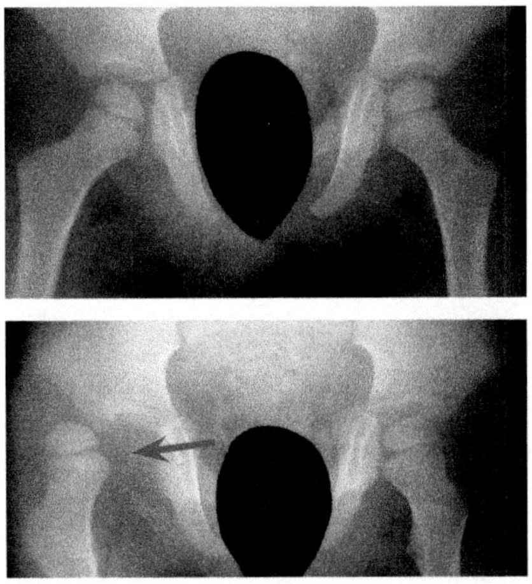

C Down syndrome hip instability Due to the excessive joint laxity, recurrent dislocations (red arrow) may occur in these children.

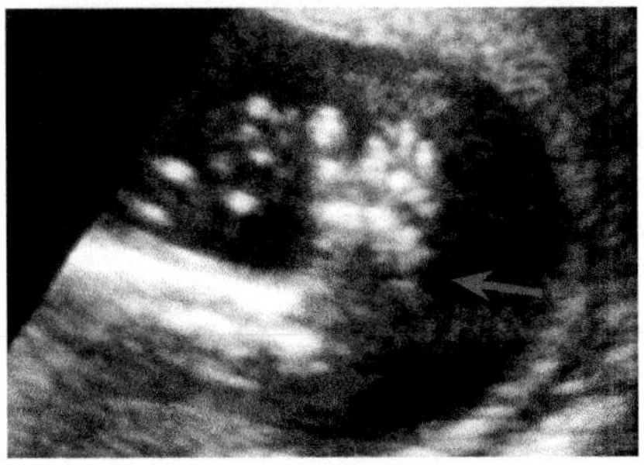

D Clubfoot in utero High-resolution ultrasound shows a clubfoot deformity. Clubfeet are common deformities with a multifactorial etiology.

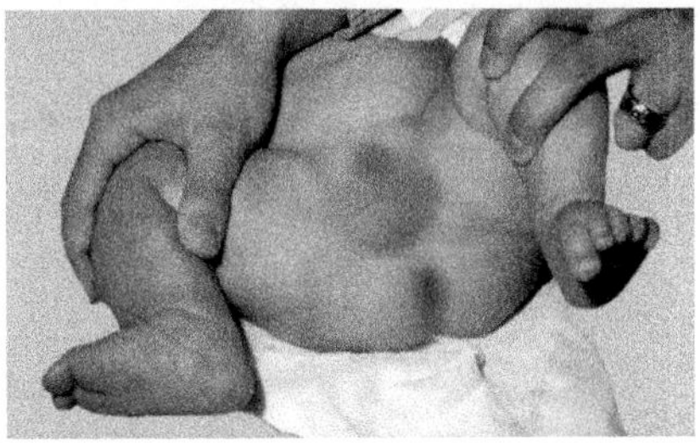

E Hip dysplasia Developmental hip dysplasia is a common condition with a multifactorial etiology.

Mechanism of Inheritance

Fertilization restores the diploid number of chromosomes and composites the traits of both parents. Fertilization may produce an abnormal zygote if the ovum or sperm carries defective genes. These conditions are transmitted by several mechanisms.

Dominant Inheritance

Dominant inheritance results in a disorder caused by a single abnormal gene [A]. Autosomal dominant conditions usually produce structural abnormalities. Variable expressivity and incomplete penetrance suppress or minimize the expression of dominant inheritance.

Recessive Inheritance

Recessive inheritance is expressed only if both gene pairs are affected [B]. Metabolic or enzymatic defects that cause diseases such as the mucopolysaccharidoses are often inherited by autosomal recessive inheritance.

X-linked Inheritance

X-linked inheritance involves only the X chromosome [C]. In the male, the genetic inactivity of the Y chromosome allows even the recessive abnormal gene of the X chromosome to be manifested. A classic example of. X-linked recessive inheritance is pseudohypertrophic muscular dystrophy. The female is the carrier, but only male offspring are affected. In recessive X-linked inheritance, the female is affected only in the rare situation in which both genes of the genetic pair are abnormal.

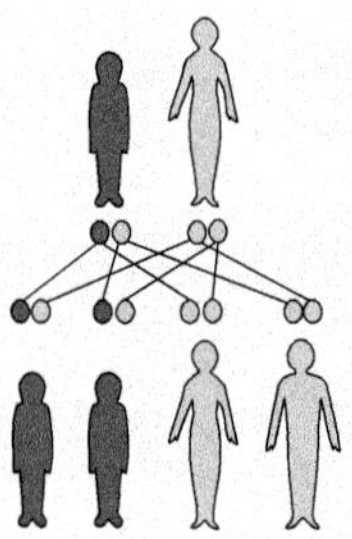

Achondroplasia
Brachydactyly
Cleidocranial dysostosis
Marfan syndrome
Multiple epiphyseal dysplasia
Nail-patella syndrome
Neurofibromatosis
Polydactyly

A Dominant inheritance The dominant gene (red) causes structural defects in both parent and offspring. Musculoskeletal disorders transmitted by dominant inheritance are listed.

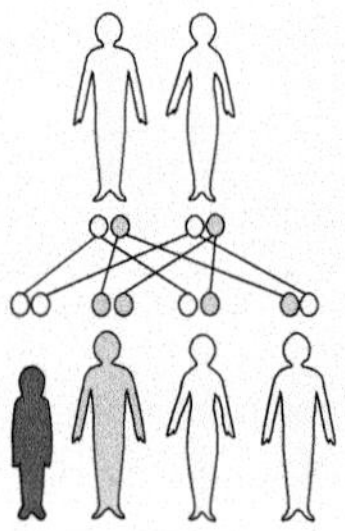

Congenital insensitivity to pain
Diastrophic dwarfism
Gaucher disease
Hurler syndrome
Morquio syndrome
Scheie syndrome
Hypophosphatasia

B Recessive inheritance Carriers of the recessive genes (yellow) are expressed (red) only if both gene pairs are abnormal. Musculoskeletal disorders transmitted by recessive inheritance are listed.

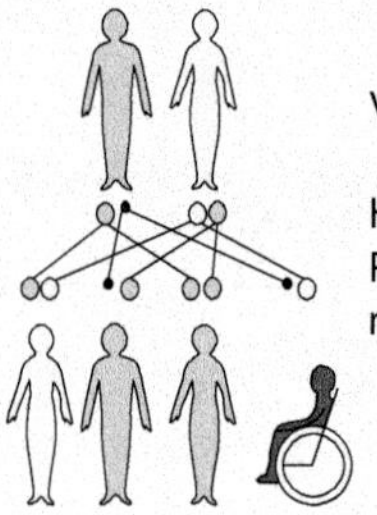

X-linked Dominant
Vitamin D refractory rickets
X-linked Recessive
Hemophilia
Pseudohypertrophic muscular dystrophy

C X-linked inheritance X-linked defects (yellow) are carried by the female and expressed in the female if the gene is dominant. Most defects are recessive and are expressed only in the male (red).

Skeletal Dysplasias

Hundreds of genetic disorders affect skeletal growth. This large number has made classification difficult. Historically, dysplasias were classified by location or radiographic appearance. It is now possible to determine the molecular structure of genes and to classify disorders based on gene types. Gene typing is clinically useful because the features of each disorder from each class of abnormal genes are similar, which makes possible the prediction of how the growth plate is affected by a specific genetic defect. Skeletal dysplasias have been classified into five categories that group disorders with similar features [A, next page]. These five categories list gene defects with similar clinical features:

1. Structural Genes

These gene defects cause proteins necessary for the structural properties of the musculoskeletal system to be abnormal.

2. Tumor-Related or Cell Control Genes

These gene defects cause abnormalities in the control of cell growth, differentiation, or cell death. This usually results in overgrowth of a specific tissue type.

3. Developmental Patterning Genes

Normally, cell proliferation, movement, and disintegration are controlled by a cell signaling system. Failure of this system results in the development of malformations.

4. Nerve or Muscle Function Genes

These genes normally encode proteins that regulate neuron or muscle function or peripheral nerve conduction. These defects often result in paresis with secondary osteopenia.

5. Protein Processing Genes

Defects in these genes result in defective enzymes. Such defects often result in accumulation of substances that normally would have been transformed for use or discarded. This results in an abnormal accumulation of substances in cells that interfere with function.

Chromosomal Defects

These syndromes are included here for comparison. These disorders are not inherited and are the result of any of a large number of defective genes. Examples include Down and Turner syndromes [D].

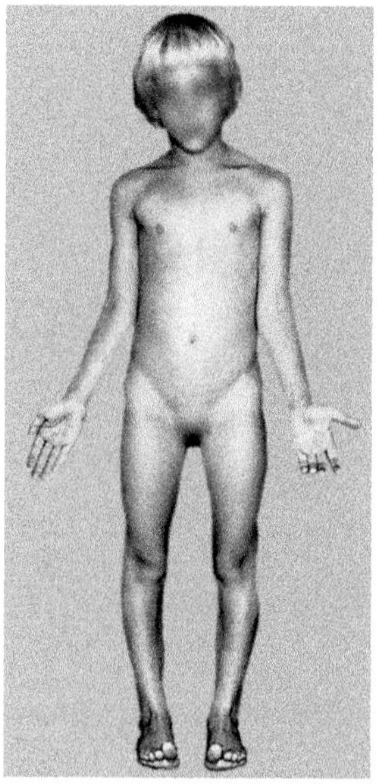

D Turner syndrome This girl shows features of the syndrome, which include an increased carrying angle of the upper limb, slight bowing of the legs, and short stature.

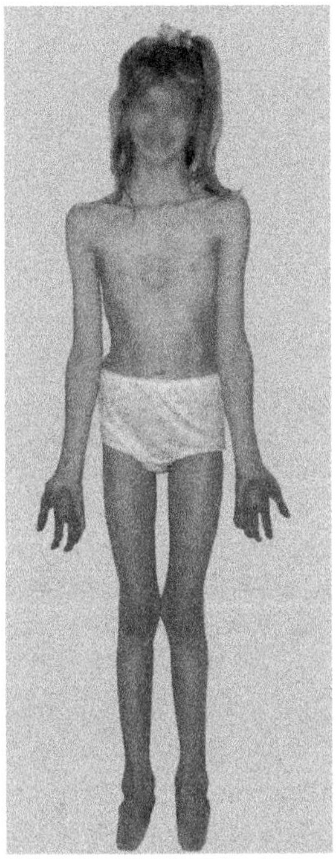
Marfan syndrome

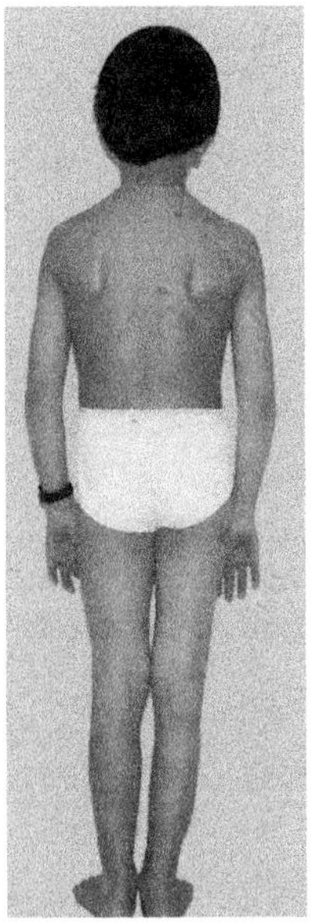
Neurofibromatosis

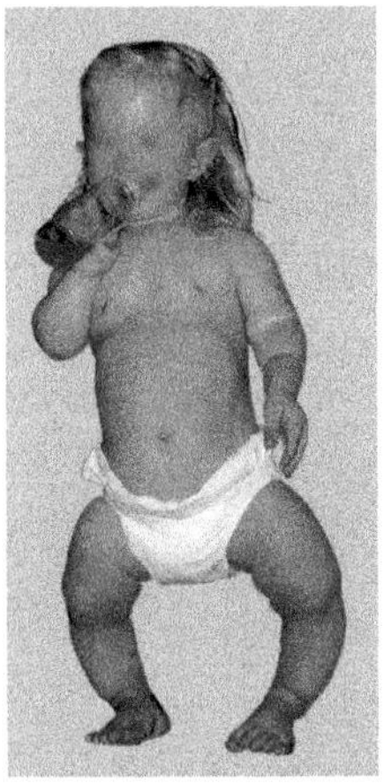
Achondroplasia

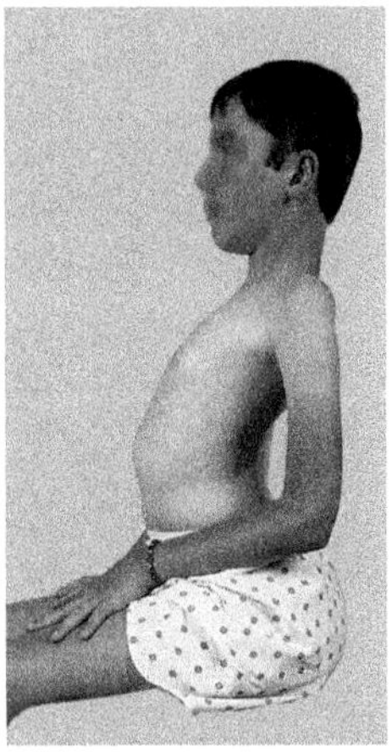
Duchenne syndrome

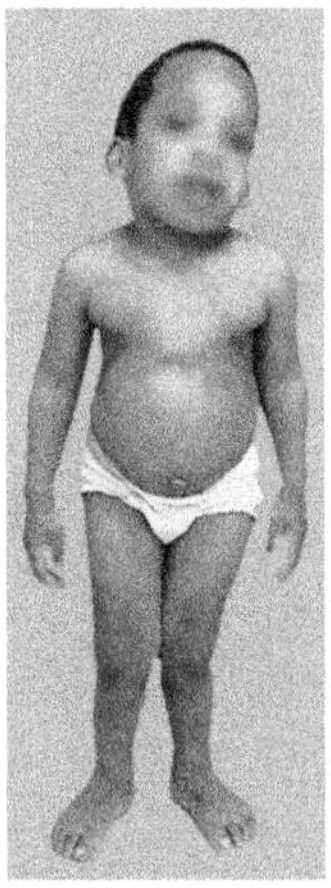
Morquio syndrome

Class	Representative disorder	Clinical features	Inheritance	Natural history
1. Structural Genes	Ehlers-Danlos syndrome Kniest syndrome Marfan syndrome Multiple epiphyseal dysplasia Osteogenesis imperfecta Spondyloepiphyseal dysplasia	Phenotypes develop with time Deformity recurs after surgery Clinical heterogeneity within disorder		Tissue fails or wears out with use Mild cases have normal lifespan Severe cases have shortened lifespan
2. Tumor-Related or Cell Control Genes	Beckwith-Wiedemann syndrome Li-Fraumeni Multiple hereditary exostosis Neurofibromatosis Retinoblastoma-osteosarcoma	Overgrowth of select tissue types Overgrowth worsens with growth Overgrowth may occur after surgery	Autosomal dominant	Risk of malignant degeneration May significantly shorten lifespan
3. Developmental Patterning Gene	Achondroplasia Cleidocranial dysplasia Metaphyseal dysplasia Nail-patella syndrome Spondylocostal dysplasia	Malformation present at birth Other organs involved Subtle joint changes common Corrective alignment osteotomies successful	Dominant, some with other modes of inheritance	Abnormal shape bone and joints Causes early degenerative arthritis
4. Nerve or Muscle Function Genes	Charcot-Marie-Tooth syndrome Duchenne syndrome Rett syndrome Spinal muscular atrophy Spinocerebellar ataxia	Musculoskeletal system usually normal at birth Osteopenia Scoliosis Contractures Weakness	Often linked to X chromosome	Bone and joint abnormalities often develop with time Often shortened lifespan
5. Protein Processing Genes	Diastrophic dysplasia Gaucher syndrome Menkes syndrome Mucopolysaccharidosis (Morquio syndrome) Niemann-Pick syndrome Osteopetrosis	Multiple organ involvement Osteonecrosis common Spinal instability and cord compression in some	Usually autosomal recessive	May shorten lifespan Medical management may improve outlook
Chromosomal defects	Down syndrome Turner syndrome	Mental deficiency common Involves multiple systems High complication rate following surgery	Not inherited	Lifespan nearly normal

A Classification of skeletal dysplasia This etiological and clinically useful classification divides dysplasias into five categories. Chromosomal defects are added for comparison. Based on Alman CO 401:17, 2002.

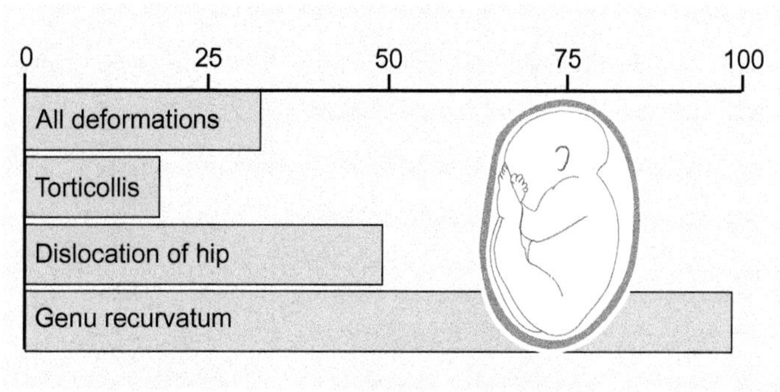

A Breech position Common musculoskeletal defects associated with breech position. From Clarren (1977).

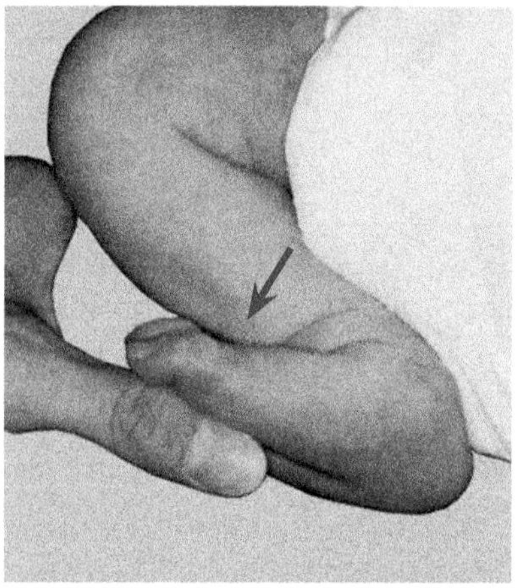

B Molding deformity Intrauterine crowding caused this calcaneovalgus foot deformity.

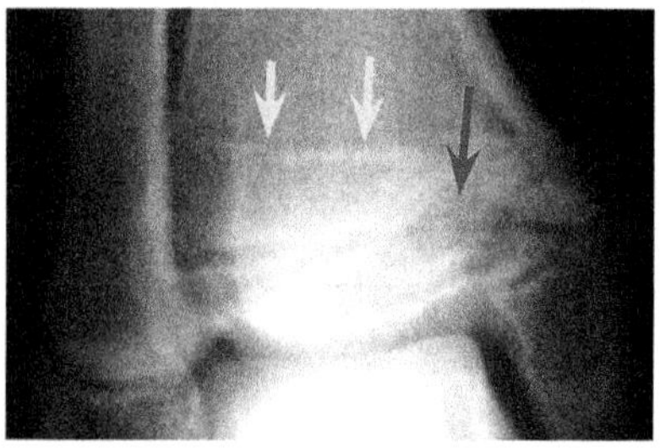

C Growth arrest lines This post-traumatic physeal bridge (red arrow) caused asymmetrical growth of the distal tibia, as shown by the growth arrest line (yellow arrows).

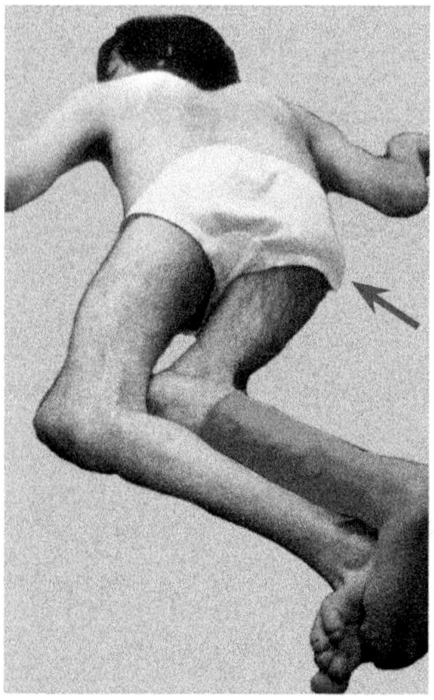

D Hip deformity in cerebral palsy This boy with cerebral palsy (left) developed an adduction deformity (red arrows) and a secondary dislocation (yellow arrow) of the right hip.

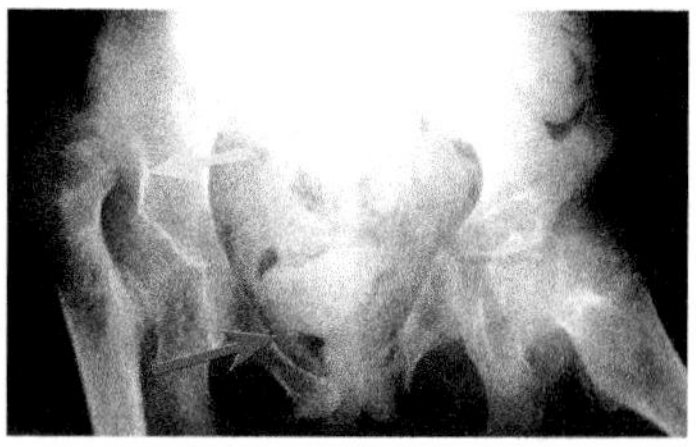

Developmental Deformities

Deformations

Deformations occur at the end of gestation and are due to intrauterine crowding or position. Breech position contributes to this crowding, resulting in a higher incidence of certain deformations [A]. These deformities are milder and usually resolve spontaneously during early infancy. A classic example is the calcaneovalgus foot deformity [B].

Metabolic Disorders

Metabolic disorders such as rickets cause osteopenia and a gradual bowing of long bones.

Inflammatory Disorders

Inflammatory disorders may damage the growth plate or articular cartilage, causing shortening or angular deformity. Less commonly, chronic inflammation that does not affect the growth plate from conditions such as rheumatoid arthritis or chronic osteomyelitis may induce hyperemia and accelerate bone growth, thus causing bone lengthening.

Trauma

Trauma may cause deformity by malunion or growth plate damage [C]. If the growth plates are not damaged, growth contributes to the correction of residual malunion deformity through the process of *remodeling*.

Physical Activity

Physical activity may alter bone growth. For example, long-term non-weight-bearing activity, as was once prescribed in treating Perthes disease, resulted in slight shortening of the involved leg. Similarly, professional tennis players who start their careers as children show relative overgrowth of the dominant upper limb.

Neuromuscular Deformity

Neuromuscular deformity may occur from muscle imbalance such as in the child with spasticity from cerebral palsy. Adductor spasm positions the head of the femur on the lateral acetabular rim, causing deformity and erosion of the cartilage of the labrum, which in turn causes subluxation and eventual dislocation of the hip [D]. The combination of contractures, immobility, gravity, and time create the so-called windswept deformity common in spastic quadriplegia.

Cascading Deformity

Deformity may arise in a series of steps. For example, cerebral palsy causes a sequence of abnormalities:

- Change in muscle tone with imbalance
- Chronic change in joint position leading to contracture formation
- Articular cartilage shape and finally bone shape are altered
- Joints may dislocate
- Pain may follow with accentuation of the muscle imbalance
- Function is affected
- Degenerative arthritis may develop

Osteochondroses

Describes a large group of heterogeneous conditions characterized by variations in enchondral ossification that occurs in epiphyses during growth and involves cartilage and bone [A, next page]. The title osteochondroses is preferred as not all conditions are inflammatory, making the term osteochondritis inappropriate.

Over 50 eponymic conditions have been described; the distinction between a disorder and normal variations of ossification and the local manifestation of systemic disorders adds to the confusion. These conditions are sometimes familial, occur at multiple sites, and show varied clinical manifestations from nothing to others that cause serious deformity and disability. The conditions have certain features in common. They heal spontaneously, have varied onsets, and have varied clinical significance. The conditions may be simple variations of normal ossification, be the consequence of trauma, or result from variations in regional vascularity of bone. Osteochondroses are classified in varied ways. These have been classified anatomically by Siffert (1981).

Articular Osteochondroses

These conditions have the greatest potential for disability because of the potential for residual articular irregularity. These forms concern the orthopedist because of their potential for disability. Two types of articular lesions are differentiated based on the anatomic site of origin:

Primary involvement of articular and epiphyseal cartilage as seen in conditions such as occurs in the metatarsal head (Freiberg disease) or capitellum

Secondary involvement as a consequence of avascular necrosis of subjacent bone as seen in Perthes disease or typical forms of osteochondritis dissecans

Nonarticular Osteochondroses

Pain, swelling, and tenderness characterized these lesions. They are often considered as overuse syndromes. They tend to heal with time and leave little or no residual deformity. They may be classified based on the anatomic features:

At tendon attachments such as Osgood-Schlatter disease and trochanteric osteochondritis.

At ligament attachments such as medial epicondyle at the elbow or the vertebral ring apophysis.

At impact sites such as present over the calcaneum. Variation in ossification of the tubercle of the calcaneum is common. Some describe this as Sever disease.

Physeal Osteochondroses

Primary involvement of the growth plate may cause significant problems that often require treatment.

Long bones may have physes with disordered growth as with tibia vara or Blount disease when involving the proximal medial tibial physis or Madelung deformity when involving the distal radius. Because the shape and length of the bone are altered, both conditions may cause significant disability.

Vertebral involvement, as with Scheuermann disease, leads to increased kyphosis due to wedging of the vertebral bodies.

Clinical Management

No generalizations may be made regarding management as the conditions are so different. A knowledge of the natural history for each lesion is essential. Some conditions such as ischiopubic synchondrosis are important, as they may be confused with a bone tumor and overtreated. Others, such as Osgood-Schlatter disease, require symptomatic management. Tibia vara, osteochondritis dissecans of the knee, Perthes disease, and others may cause considerable deformity and disability.

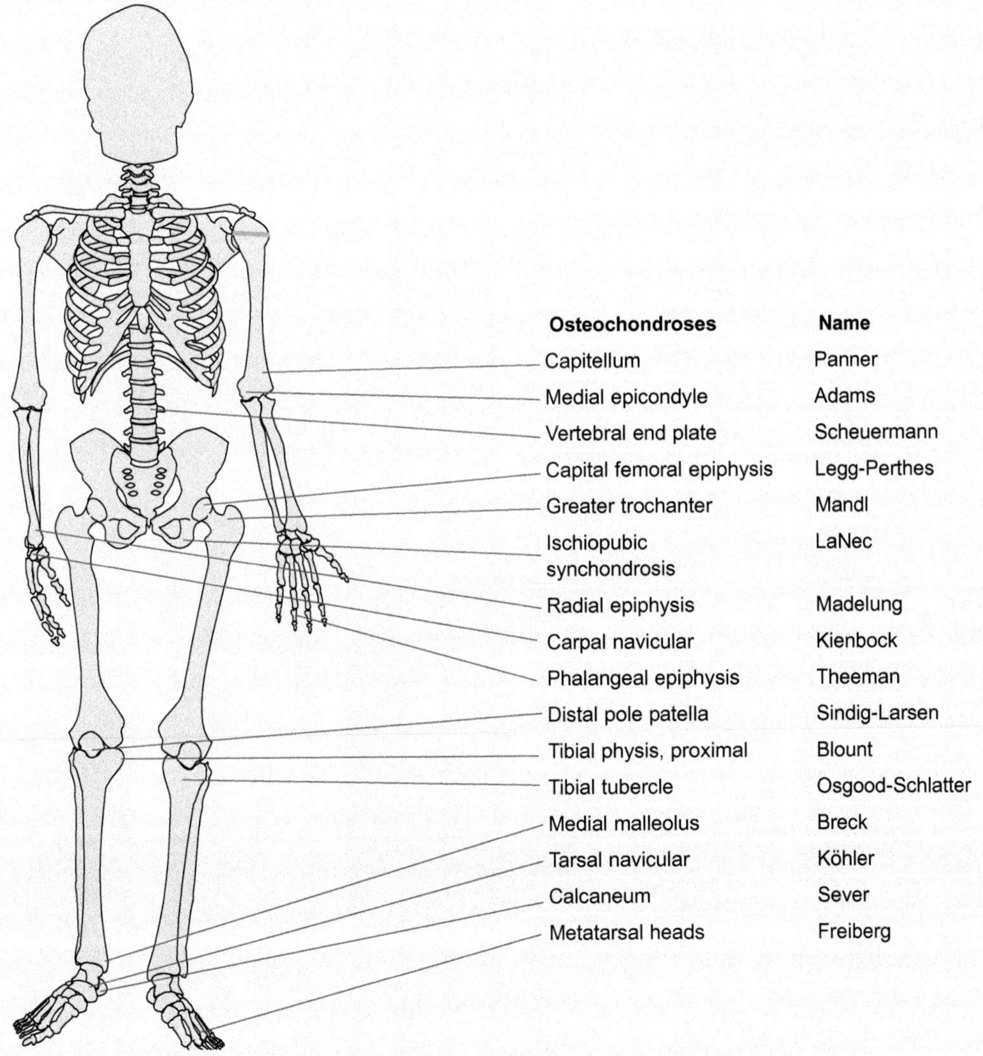

A Osteochondrosis This is a partial list for this condition.

Retards Growth	Accelerates Growth
Osteochondral dystrophies	Pituitary tumors
Neuromuscular disorders	Marfan syndrome
Physeal compression	Sympathectomy
Denervation	AV fistula
Physeal ischemic injury	Periosteal stripping
Metabolic disorders	Diaphyseal fractures
Nutritional deficiencies	Chronic osteomyelitis
	Foreign body reaction

A Factors affecting growth These are common factors that retard or accelerate growth.

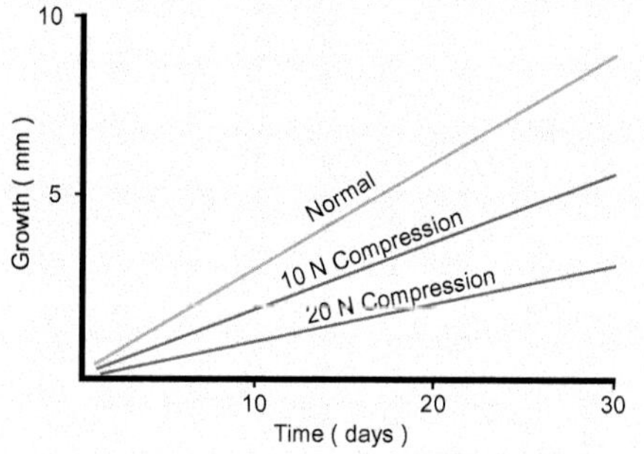

B Physeal compression effect on growth Growth rate is reduced by compression (N = Newtons). From Bonnell (1983).

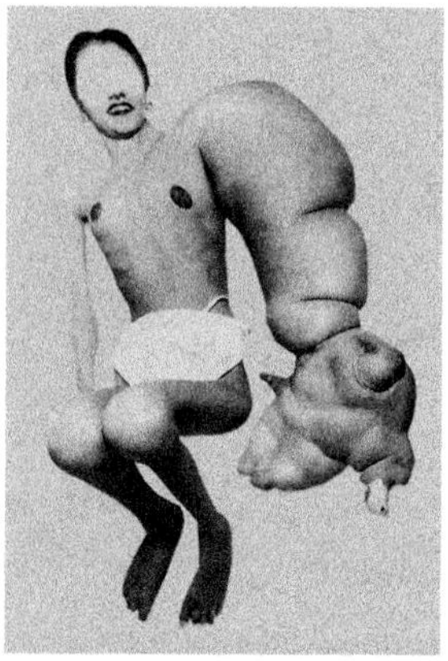

C Idiopathic growth acceleration This girl pictured in the 1940s has massive overgrowth of the left upper extremity, producing a grotesque disability. The girl died during the operation to remove the extremity.

Features of the Immature Skeleton

Many factors control bone growth in the child. These include endocrine, nutritional, and metabolic disorders, which significantly alter growth.

Growth Rate

Numerous factors may retard or accelerate growth [A]. Procedures known to accelerate growth have been used in an attempt to lengthen the short limb due to poliomyelitis. Unfortunately, the gain in length is not predictable and is not enough to be clinically useful.

Compression of the physis retards growth in proportion to the load applied [B]. This has been studied in rats. Forelimb amputations result in upright walking. This bipedal walking causes significant anterior wedging of the lower lumbar vertebrae, presumably due to the greater loads applied to the anterior portion of the vertebral bodies.

Growth control factors are inherent in each growth plate. When juvenile limbs are transplanted onto adult rats, they continue to grow.

Idiopathic disorders Sometimes the cause of the developmental deformity is not determined [C].

Intracapsular Metaphysis

The proximal portion of the metaphysis of several long bones falls within the joint capsule. This anatomic feature has clinical significance in the mechanism of spread of infection, the circulation of the epiphysis, and the healing of fractures.

Proximal femur The hip joint encompasses the entire proximal femoral epiphysis and some of the femoral neck [D]. This feature has significance in several disorders:

Osteomyelitis of proximal femur may penetrate the cortex and spread directly into the joint, causing septic arthritis.

Avascular necrosis of the epiphysis is a greater risk because the vascularity to the epiphysis must traverse the joint, making the vessels at risk for injury or thrombosis. Avascular necrosis of the epiphysis is a common and serious cause of disability in childhood.

Fractures of the femoral neck or physis may be slower to heal and be complicated by avascular necrosis. Drainage of any hematoma of the hip joint may reduce this risk.

Proximal radius This epiphysis is within the elbow joint. This position makes the epiphysis susceptible to avascular necrosis.

Other Features of Immature Bone

Immature bone has several characteristics that have clinical relevance.

The physis as a barrier The physis is usually a barrier to the spread of most tumors and osteomyelitis of the metaphysis [E]. Aggressive tumors may penetrate this barrier.

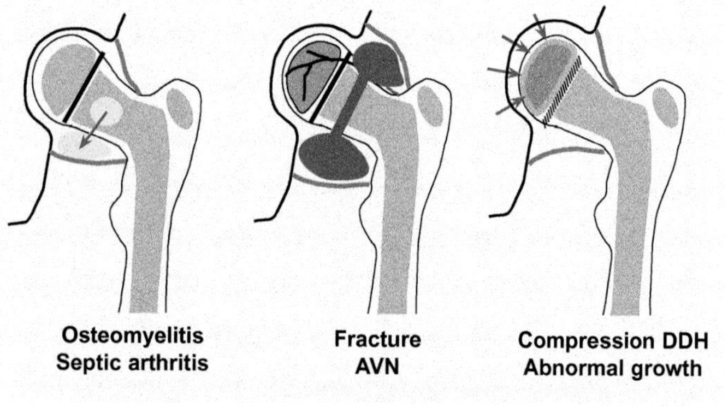

D Intracapsular metaphysis effects The intracapsular location of the metaphysis results in the potential spread of infection from the bone to the joint. Fracture hematoma or joint compression during management of developmental hip dysplasia (DDH) may reduce blood flow to the femoral epiphysis, causing avascular necrosis (AVN) or physeal damage and abnormal growth.

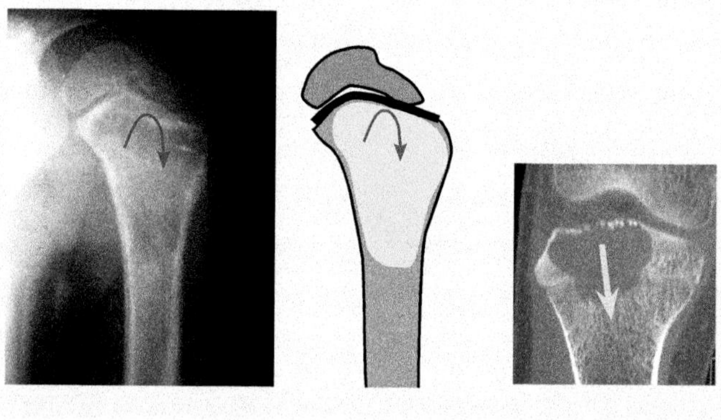

E Growth plate as a barrier The plate is a barrier to the extension of tumors such as this benign cyst (red arrows). This effect is observed for osteomyelitis. Sometimes, aggressive tumors such as this chondroblastoma may traverse the plate (yellow arrow).

Periosteum The periosteum in the immature skeleton is very osteogenic. Fractures heal quickly; bone regenerates following bone loss in trauma or infection. If the periosteum is destroyed, bone regeneration does not occur. This occurs most commonly in severe infection [A].

Circulation Bone blood flow is usually excellent in children, allowing rapid healing of fractures. Diaphyseal and metaphyseal circulation may be compromised by infections or rarely trauma. A cold bone scan segment is a source of concern in osteomyelitis [B].

Flexibility Immature bone is flexible. An example is the bending rather than the fracture of bones of the forearm. Ulnar bending allows the traumatic dislocation of the radial head without an apparent fracture of the ulna. Spinal trauma may result in cord severance with paraplegia without apparent vertebral fractures. Preserve the flexibility of bone by avoiding large, rigid internal fixation if the fixation is to be left in place for long periods.

Iatrogenic Deformities

The cradleboard, by positioning the infant's hip in extension, is a known cause of developmental hip dysplasia [C]. In some cultures, iatrogenic deformities are created in girls to enhance their beauty. Placing rings around the necks [D] of young girls has produced deformity and severe disability. Binding of the feet [E] was once practiced in China.

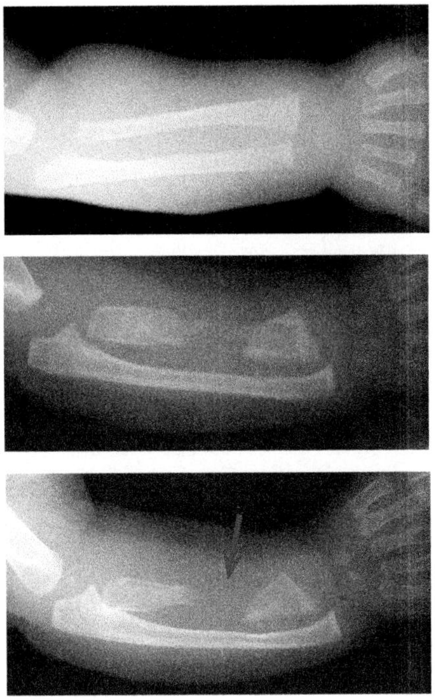

A Loss of periosteum This infant underwent an excision of a desmoid tumor at age 2 months. The excision included the periosteum. Bone formation failed and a bone graft was placed. This also resorbed [middle]. Due to the loss of the periosteum, a persisting nonunion occurred (red arrow).

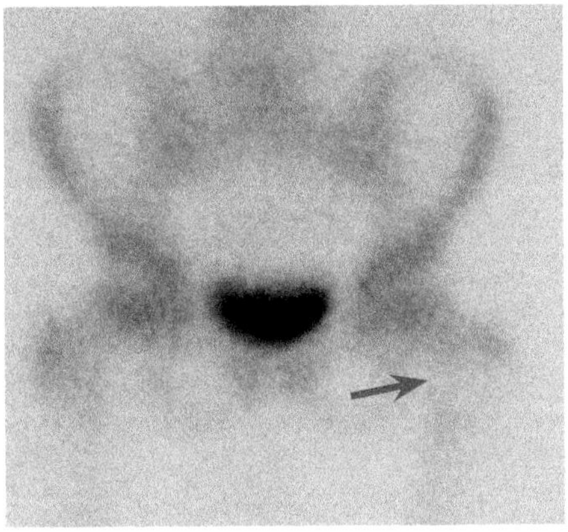

B Cold bone scan segment Note the reduction of uptake in the proximal femoral metaphysis (arrow) in this patient with osteomyelitis. This area was surrounded by a soft tissue abscess.

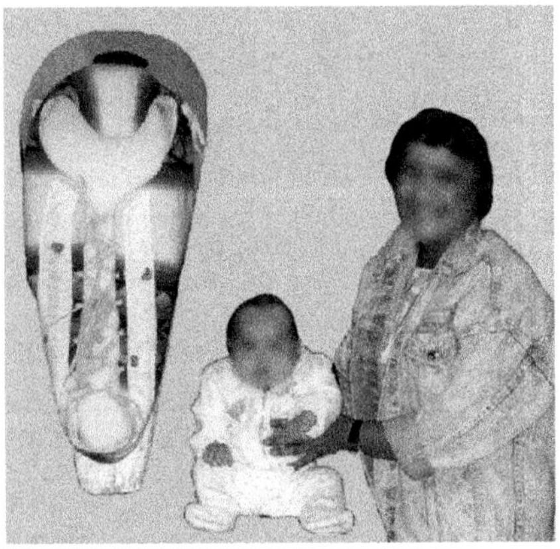

C Cradleboard Cradleboards extend the infant's hips, causing an increased incidence of hip dysplasia.

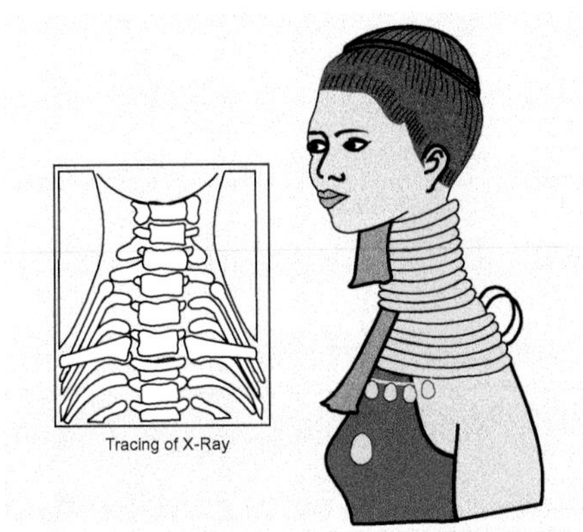

D Thoracic deformity Rings placed around the neck in childhood produce constriction of the upper thorax in the adult woman (Padaung tribe, east Burma / Myanmar). From Roaff (1961).

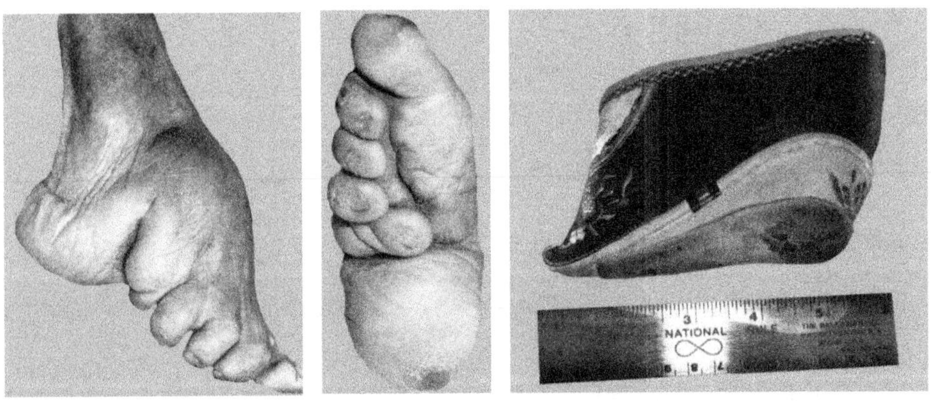

E Bound feet A woman's feet show the effect of foot binding during childhood. The foot becomes triangular in shape (left and middle) and small in size so that it fits the shoe (right). The shoe is less than 6 inches in length.

Aaron RK, Boyan BD, Ciombor DM, Schwartz Z; Simon BJ. Stimulation of growth factor synthesis by electric and electromagnetic fields. Clin Orthop 2004 Feb (419): p30-7.

Alman BA. A classification for genetic disorders of interest to orthopaedists. Clin Orthop 2002 Aug;(401): p17-26.

Anderson M, Green WT, Messner MB. Growth and predictions of growth in the lower extremities. J Bone Joint Surg 1963 45A:1-14.

Andry M. Orthopaedia: or the art of correcting and preventing deformities in children London: A Miller.

Arriola F, Forriol F, Canadell J. Histomorphometric study of growth plate subjected to different mechanical conditions (compression, tension and neutralization): an experimental study in lambs. Mechanical growth plate behavior. J Pediatr Orthop B 2001 Oct;10(4): p334-8.

Baitner AC, Maurer SG, Gruen MB, Di Cesare PE. The genetic basis of the osteochondrodysplasias. J Pediatr Orthop 2000 Sep-Oct;20(5): p594-605

Ballock RT. Molecular and genetic approaches to musculoskeletal diseases. J Pediatr Orthop 2003 Jan-Feb;23(1): p131-7.

Ballock RT; O'Keefe RJ. The biology of the growth plate. J Bone Joint Surg Am 2003 Apr;85-A(4): p715-26.

Blount, W. Fractures in Children, Williams & Wilkins Co, Baltimore, 1955.

Brookes M, Wardle EN. Muscle action and the shape of the femur. J Bone Joint Surg 1962 44B:398-411.

Buckwalter JA, Cooper RR. Bone structure and function. AAOS Instruc Course Lect 1987 34:27-48.

Buxton P; Edwards C; Archer CW; Francis-West P. Growth/differentiation factor-5 (GDF-5) and skeletal development. J Bone Joint Surg Am 2001;83-A Suppl 1(Pt 1): pS23-30.

Bylski-Austrow DI, Wall EJ, Rupert MP, Roy DR, Crawford AH. Growth plate forces in the adolescent human knee: a radiographic and mechanical study of epiphyseal staples. J Pediatr Orthop 2001 Nov-Dec;21(6): p817-23.

Carvell JE. The relationship of the periosteum to angular deformities of long bones: experimental observations of rabbits. Clin Orthop 1983 173:262-74.

Cassidy JD, Yong-Hing K, Kirkaldy-Willis WH. A study of the effects of bipedism and upright posture on the lumbosacral spine and paravertebral muscles of the rat. Spine 1988 13:301-8.

Chen F, Hui JH, Chan WK, Lee EH. Cultured mesenchymal stem cell transfers in the treatment of partial growth arrest. J Pediatr Orthop 2003 Jul-Aug;23(4): p425-9.

Clarren SK, Smith DW. Congenital deformities. Ped Clin North Am 1977 24:665-77.

Crossan JF, Wynne-Davies R. Research for genetic and environmental factors in orthopedic diseases. Clin Orthop 1986 210:97-105.

Damron TA, Horton JA, Naqvi A, Margulies B, Strauss J, Grant W, Farnum CE, Spadaro JA. Decreased proliferation precedes growth factor changes after physeal irradiation. Clin Orthop 2004 May;(422): p233-42.

De Deyne PG. Lengthening of muscle during distraction osteogenesis. Clin Orthop 2002 Oct;(403 Suppl): pS171-7.

Dietz F. The genetics of idiopathic clubfoot. Clin Orthop 2002 Aug;(401): p39-48.

Dietz FR. Effect of denervation on limb growth. J Orthop Res 1989 7:292-303.

Dimeglio A. Growth in pediatric orthopaedics. J Pediatr Orthop 2001 Jul-Aug;21(4): p549-55.

Dunne, KB, Clarren, SK. The origin of prenatal and postnatal deformities. Ped Clin North Am 1986 33:1277-1297.

Edwards TB, Greene CC, Baratta RV, Zieske A, Willis RB. The effect of placing a tensioned graft across open growth plates. A gross and histologic analysis. J Bone Joint Surg Am 2001 May;83-A(5): p725-34.

Egol KA, Karunakar M, Phieffer L, Meyer R; Wattenbarger JM. Early versus late reduction of a physeal fracture in an animal model. J Pediatr Orthop 2002 Mar-Apr;22(2): p208-11.

Ganjavi H, Malkin D. Genetics of childhood cancer. Clin Orthop 2002 Aug;(401): p75-87.

Goldberg MJ, Yassir W, Sadeghi-Nejad A, Stanitski CL. Clinical analysis of short stature. J Pediatr Orthop 2002 Sep-Oct;22(5): p690-6.

Hasler CC, Foster BK. Secondary tethers after physeal bar resection: a common source of failure?. Clin Orthop 2002 Dec;(405): p242-9.

Hensinger RN Standards in pediatric orthopedics: tables, charts, and graphs illustrating growth New York: Raven Press 1986.

Houshian S, Holst AK, Larsen MS, Torfing T. Remodeling of Salter-Harris type II epiphyseal plate injury of the distal radius. J Pediatr Orthop 2004 Sep-Oct;24(5): p472-6.

Iannotti JP. Growth plate physiology and pathology. Orthop Clin North Am 1990 21:1-17.

Izumi Y. The accuracy of Risser staging. Spine 1995 20:1868.

Kealey WD, Lappin KJ, Leslie H, Sheridan B, Cosgrove AP. Endocrine profile and physical stature of children with Perthes disease. J Pediatr Orthop 2004 Mar-Apr;24(2): p161-6.

Kevern L, Warwick D, Wellesley D, Senbaga R, Clarke NM. Prenatal ultrasound: detection and diagnosis of limb abnormalities. J Pediatr Orthop 2003 Mar-Apr;23(2): p251-3.

Khrouf N, Spang R, Podgorna T, Miled SB, Moussaoui M, Chibani M Malformations in 10,000 consecutive births in Tunis Acta Paediatr Scand 1986 75:534-9

Lee CW, Martinek V, Usas A, Musgrave D, Pickvance EA, Robbins P, Moreland MS, Fu FH, Huard J. Muscle-based gene therapy and tissue engineering for treatment of growth plate injuries. J Pediatr Orthop 2002 Sep-Oct;22(5): p565-72.

Little DG, Song KM, Katz D, Herring JA. Relationship of peak height velocity to other maturity indicators in idiopathic scoliosis in girls. J Bone Joint Surg Am 2000 May;82(5): p685-93.

Luvalle P, Ma Q, Beier F. The role of activating transcription factor-2 in skeletal growth control. J Bone Joint Surg Am 2003;85-A Suppl 2:133-6.

Marshall WA, Tanner JM. Variations in pattern of pubertal changes in boys. Arch Dis Child 1970: 45:13-23

Martos-Rodriguez A, Santos-Alvarez I, Campo-Ruiz V, Gonzalez S, Garcia-Ruiz JP, Delgado-Baeza E. Expression of CCAAT/enhancer-binding protein-beta (C/EBPbeta) and CHOP in the murine growth plate. Two possible key modulators of chondrocyte differentiation. J Bone Joint Surg Br 2003 Nov;85(8): p1190-5.

Minamide A, Boden SD, Viggeswarapu M, Hair GA, Oliver C, Titus L. Mechanism of bone formation with gene transfer of the cDNA encoding for the intracellular protein LMP-1. J Bone Joint Surg Am 2003 Jun;85-A(6): p1030-9.

Moore KL. The developing human: clinically oriented embryology, 4th ed Philadelphia: WB Saunders, 1988.

Namba Y, Kawai A, Naito N, Morimoto Y, Hanakawa S, Inoue H. Intraarticular synovial sarcoma confirmed by SYT-SSX fusion transcript. Clin Orthop 2002 Feb;(395): p221-6.

Pritchett JW. Growth and predictions of growth in the upper extremity. J Bone Joint Surg 1988 70A:520-25.

Purkiss SB, Driscoll B, Cole WG, Alman B. Idiopathic scoliosis in families of children with congenital scoliosis. Clin Orthop 2002 Aug;(401): p27-31.

Puzas JE, O'Keefe RJ, Lieberman JR. The orthopaedic genome: what does the future hold and are we ready? J Bone Joint Surg Am 2002 Jan;84-A(1): p133-41.

Siffert, RS, Classification of the osteochondroses Clin Orthop 1981 158:20

Song KM, Little DG. Peak height velocity as a maturity indicator for males with idiopathic scoliosis. J Pediatr Orthop 2000 May-Jun;20(3): p286-8.

Spadaro JA, Baesl MT, Conta AC, Margulies BM, Damron TA. Effects of irradiation on the appositional and longitudinal growth of the tibia and fibula of the rat with and without radioprotectant. J Pediatr Orthop 2003 Jan-Feb;23(1): p35-40.

Stanley G, McLoughlin S, Beals RK. Observations on the cause of bowlegs in achondroplasia. J Pediatr Orthop 2002 Jan-Feb;22(1): p112-6.

Stokes IA, Mente PL, Iatridis JC, Farnum CE, Aronsson DD. Enlargement of growth plate chondrocytes modulated by sustained mechanical loading. J Bone Joint Surg Am 2002 Oct;84-A(10): p1842-8.

Sutherland D, Olshen R, Cooper L, Woo S. The development of mature gait. J Bone Joint Surg Am 1980 62:336.

Tanner JM, Whitehouse RH, Takaishi M. Standards from birth to maturity for height, weight, height velocity and weight velocity: British children. 1965 Part I Arch Dis Child 1966 41:454-71.

Trueta J. Studies of the development and decay of the human frame. Philadelphia: WB Saunders, 1968.

Tuan RS. Biology of developmental and regenerative skeletogenesis. Clin Orthop 2004 Oct;(427 Suppl): pS105-17.

Unger S. A genetic approach to the diagnosis of skeletal dysplasia. Clin Orthop 2002 Aug;(401): p32-8.

Vidil A, Journeau P, Soulie A, Padovani JP, Pouliquen JC. Evolution of scoliosis in six children treated with growth hormone. J Pediatr Orthop B 2001 Jul;10(3): p197-200.

Warman ML. Human genetic insights into skeletal development, growth, and homeostasis. Clin Orthop 2000 Oct;(379 Suppl): pS40-54.

White SC; Gilchrist LA; Wilk BE. Asymmetric limb loading with true or simulated leg-length differences. Clin Orthop 2004 Apr;(421): p287-92.

Wynne-Davies R. Acetabular dysplasia and familial joint laxity JBJSb 1970 52:704.

EVALUATION

CHAPTER 2

Evaluation leading to an accurate diagnosis [A] is the first and most important step in optimal management. Every condition requires a diagnosis, but only some require active treatment. The evaluation of the child is often more difficult than that of the adult. The child is a poor historian, and examination of the child can be difficult. Dealing with the family may be challenging. The history given by the parents is often laced with emotion. Reporting may be complicated by varying gender and generational hierarchy. The physician often finds that managing the child's problem is easier than dealing with the family. Establishing rapport during the first visit is essential.

Establishing Rapport

The goal is to reduce the fear in the child and establish confidence with the parents and family [B].

Dress

Studies have shown that casual dress promotes approachability and more formal dress enhances confidence. Dress in a way that suggests you have good judgment and are appropriate for the situation. More formal dress may be more appropriate in a major referral center than elsewhere. Avoid making a statement by dress. This usually translates into selecting conservative clothing that promotes an image of good taste.

Initial Introduction

On entering the examination room, acknowledge everyone in the room. Consider the cultural background of the family and conform to gender order for introductions. Shake hands with everyone, including the child. Determine the relationship of each person with the patient.

Be professional, yet friendly. Establishing a good rapport with *everyone* in the family may be critical to properly managing the child. Later, when difficult management decisions must be made, having rapport with every member of the family is necessary to avoid pressure on the parents to seek additional opinions. Once started, serial consultations usually end with some unnecessary treatment of the child.

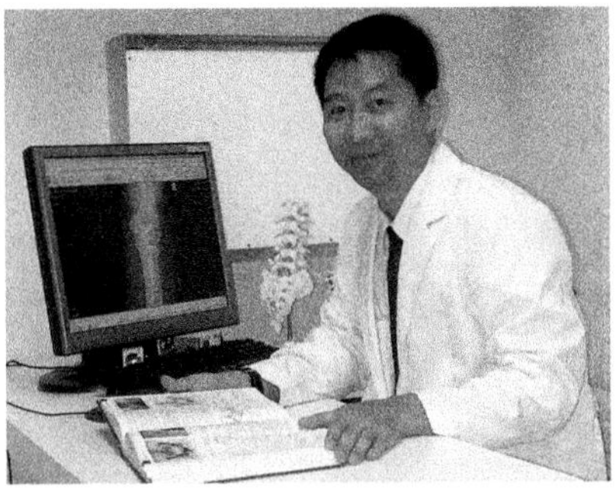

A Diagnosis Evaluation requires integration of clinical, imaging, and laboratory findings.

Tips for the Physician

1. Knock on the door before entering to give anyone undressed a chance to cover up before you go in.
2. Touch the patient either with a handshake or with a pat on the shoulder.
3. Introduce yourself and your colleagues to everyone in the examining room. Attempt to identify the cultural expectations to establish the order of introductions. Shake everyone's hand.
4. Establish the reason for the clinic visit.
5. Sit down in the room, preferably lower than the patient.
6. Show the family the x-ray, especially if it is normal.
7. Avoid technical terms.
8. Avoid leaving the room during consultation unless definitely necessary. Avoid looking at your watch.
9. Do not discuss other patients' treatments.
10. Avoid trying to impress patient with your credentials; the family has already selected you as their physician.
11. Discuss the problem, options, and recommendations.
12. Ask the family or patient if they have questions and provide answers.
13. Try to assess the family's reaction to the discussion. Continue discussion until the family's expectations are fulfilled.
14. Offer to provide follow-up if the family appears to need continued reassurance.

B Suggestions for establishing rapport

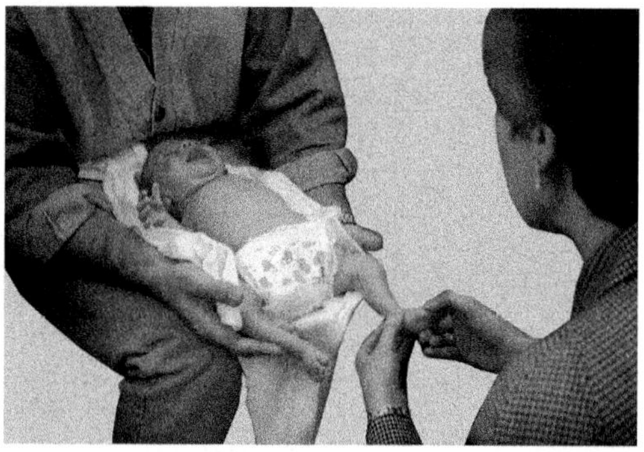

A Efficient, comfortable examination Positioned on the parent's lap, the infant or child is most secure and quiet.

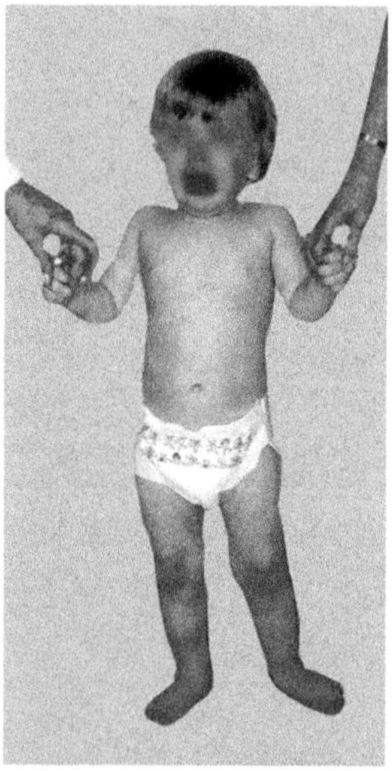

B When coaxing fails Perform the examination without the cooperation of the child.

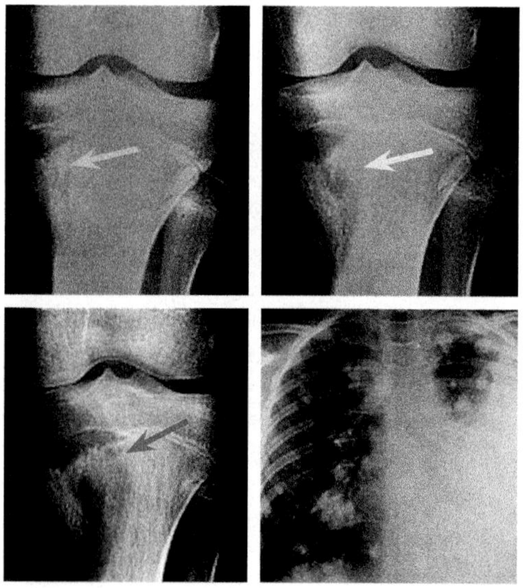

C Attributing problem to trauma A 12-year-old boy gave a history of knee trauma and pain. The initial radiograph was considered normal, but a lesion was present (orange arrow). One month later, the lesion had enlarged (yellow arrow). A diagnosis of Osgood–Schlatter disease was made. A radiograph 2 months later showed further expansion of the lesion (red arrow). A radiograph of the chest just prior to death showed multiple pulmonary metastases.

Calming the Child

Reducing the child's fear is the next objective. Consider examining the infant or younger child on the parent's lap [A]. Ask the child on whose lap he or she wishes to sit. Children will often select the family member who they believe will offer the greatest safety.

Be friendly with the child. Suggest that this will be a *game*. Make some positive statements about the child, such as "Mary, you are such a nice child." Ask some child-oriented questions, such as "What is your pet's name?"

Start gently examining the child while taking the history from the family. This first step is to convince the child that the examination will not be painful. This is the time for the screening examination, starting with the area most removed from the problem. Being gentle often results in the child becoming less threatened and more cooperative.

Sometimes, these measures fail and the infant or young child remains aggravated and uncooperative. This is the time to move to strategy two—a firm approach [B].

Present Problem

The concerns usually fall into the categories of deformity, altered function, or pain. Assessment of these complaints should take the patient's age into consideration. For example, the toddler usually manifests discitis (an intervertebral disc space infection) by altered function in the form of an unwillingness to walk. The child with discitis may primarily show a systemic illness, whereas the adolescent often complains of back pain.

A common pitfall in diagnosis is inappropriately attributing the child's problem to trauma. Although trauma is a common event in the life of a child, serious problems such as malignant tumors or infections may be mistakenly attributed to an injury [C].

In addition, graciously deal with questions and concerned by the "worried well" in an attempt to dispel unnecessary concern.

Worried Well

Is a common problem. Deal with this problem by taking their concerns seriously, seeing the source of the concern, performing a screening examination, providing reassurance and written material if available. Suggest any appropriate links to YouTube videos such as *What Parents Should Know* about common problems.

Deformity Positional deformities such as rotational problems, flatfeet, and bowlegs are common concerns but seldom significant [D and E]. More significant problems, such as congenital or neuromuscular deformities, require careful evaluation. Inquire about the onset, progression, and previous management. Are there old photographs or radiographs that document the course of the deformity? Is there associated pain or disability? Does the deformity cause a cosmetic problem and embarrass the child? Is it noticeable to others? Finally, be cautious about relying solely on the family's estimation of the time of the deformity's onset. Often a deformity originates long before it is first noticed.

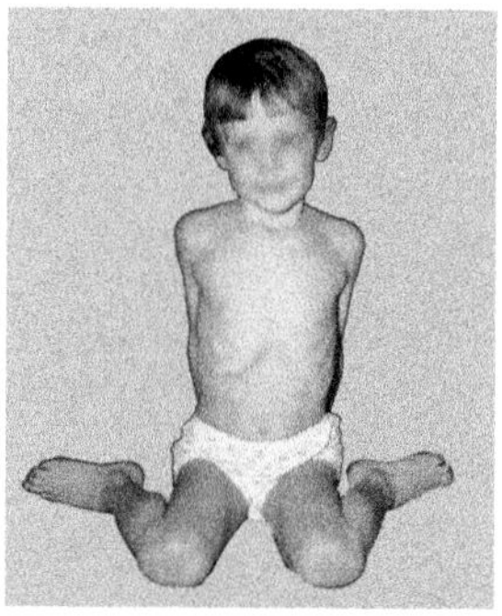

D Developmental variation This child with femoral antetorsion shows the classic sitting posture.

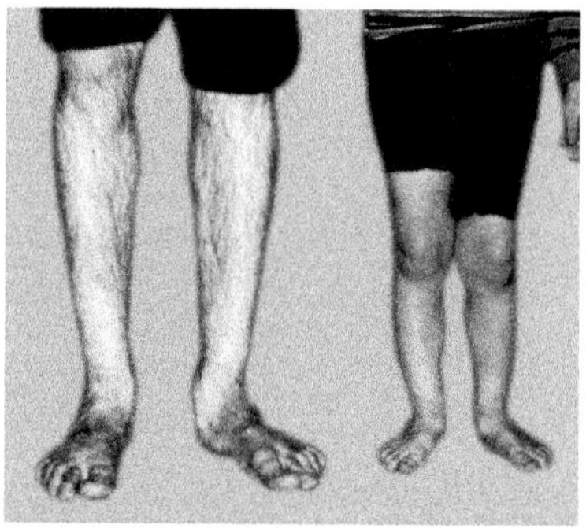

E Familial flatfeet Since the father has flatfeet, it is more likely that the child's flatfeet will persist into adult life.

Altered function Function can be altered by deformity, weakness, or pain. Pain is a common cause of altered function in the infant and child; the most common example is a limp. A toddler's fracture of the tibia may manifest itself by a limp or an unwillingness to walk. The young child with toxic synovitis may simply limp; the older child might complain of pain. The newborn whose clavicle is fractured during delivery shows a loss of arm movement on the affected side. This may be confused with a birth palsy. Altered function due to trauma, inflammation, or infection without neurologic damage is referred to as pseudoparalysis.

Pain The expression of pain is age related. The infant may simply avoid moving the painful part, may fuss and cry, or cry continuously if the pain is severe. The child may show altered function, avoid moving the affected part, or complain of discomfort [A]. The adolescent usually complains of pain.

If the pain responds to rest, it is most likely less serious and an important feature to explore while taking the history and may help with making the diagnosis.

The perception and expression of pain differs widely among individuals, particularly as adolescents grow more adult-like in their responses. A young athlete might minimize his discomfort to improve his chances of participating in the next sporting event. Others might exaggerate the problem. Some adolescents minimize pain by pain-relieving positioning. A herniated disc or an osteoid osteoma may cause scoliosis. This scoliosis results from positioning the spine in a pain-relieving posture. This secondary deformity rather than the underlying condition may be the focus of the evaluation. Unless the underlying condition is identified by the physician, a serious diagnostic error can occur.

History

The past history is essential, not only for understanding the background and general health of the child but also for gaining insight into the current problem. Important aspects of past history include the following:

Birth history Was the pregnancy and delivery normal?

Development Have the developmental milestones been met at the appropriate ages? When did the infant first sit and walk? About one-third of late walkers are pathologic. In children with conditions such as cerebral palsy, walking is always delayed, and this may be important in establishing whether the condition is progressive [B].

Mother's intuition The mother's intuition is surprisingly accurate [C]. For example, the mother's sense that something is wrong with her infant is one of the most consistent findings in infants with cerebral palsy. Take the mother's concerns seriously.

Family history Do others have problems similar to those of the patient? If so, what disability is present? A surprisingly large number of orthopedic problems run in families, and knowledge of the disability, or absence of disability, provides information regarding the patient's prognosis.

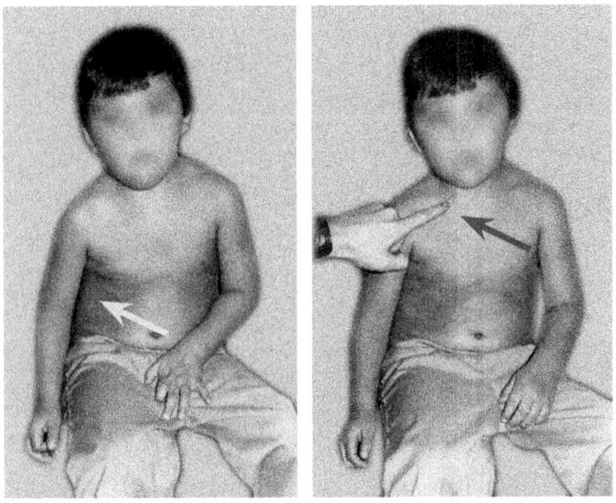

A Pseudoparalysis Use of the arm (yellow arrow) is restricted because of pain. A painful lesion of the right clavicle (red arrow) was due to a leukemic infiltrate.

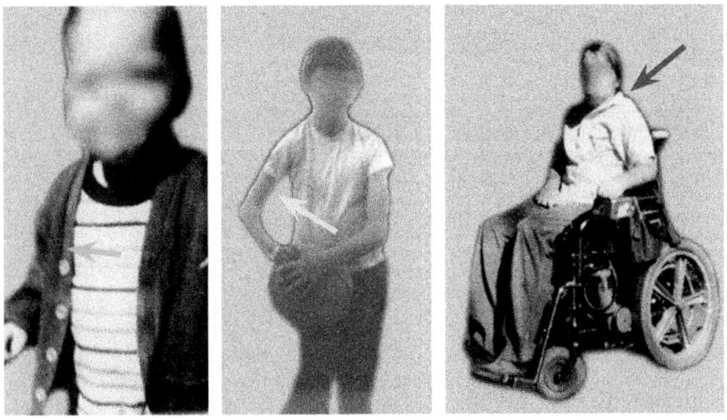

B Importance of medical history This boy had normal function of his right arm (green arrow) as an infant. During early childhood, he developed weakness of the arm (yellow arrow), and a diagnosis of cerebral palsy was made. The weakness increased, and finally during adolescence, he was found to have a tumor involving the cervical spinal cord (red arrow). He became quadriplegic. The progressive nature of the condition is inconsistent with a diagnosis of cerebral palsy. A medical history of progression would have prompted an earlier diagnosis and may have prevented this disastrous outcome.

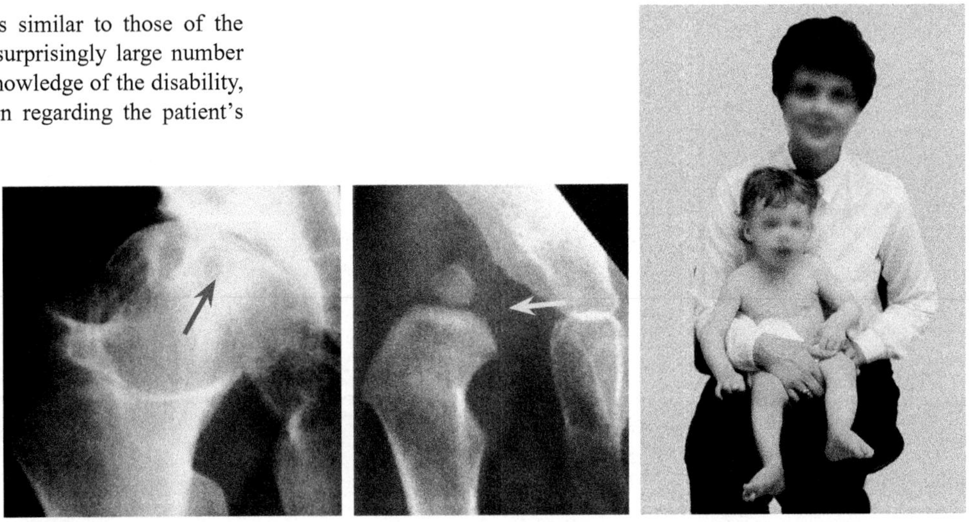

C Mother's intuition The mother with painful degenerative arthritis from developmental hip dysplasia (red arrow) sensed something was abnormal about her infant's hip. Her concern, based on intuition, was discounted by the primary physician, and the asymmetry present on examination was attributed to the child's mild hemiparesis. This resulted in a delay in diagnosis of developmental hip dysplasia until 18 months of age (yellow arrow).

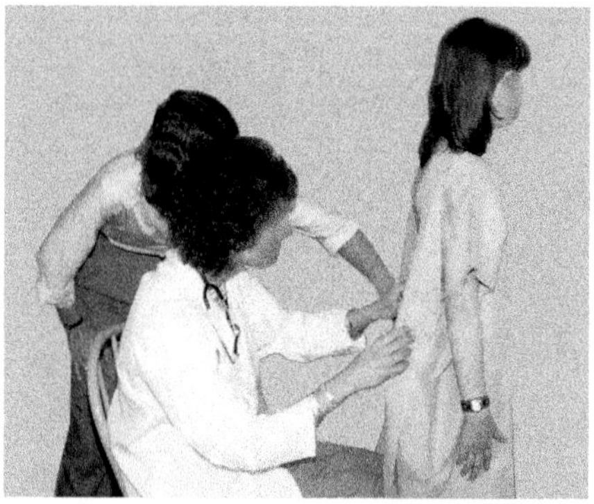

A Examination Examine the adolescent in a gown.

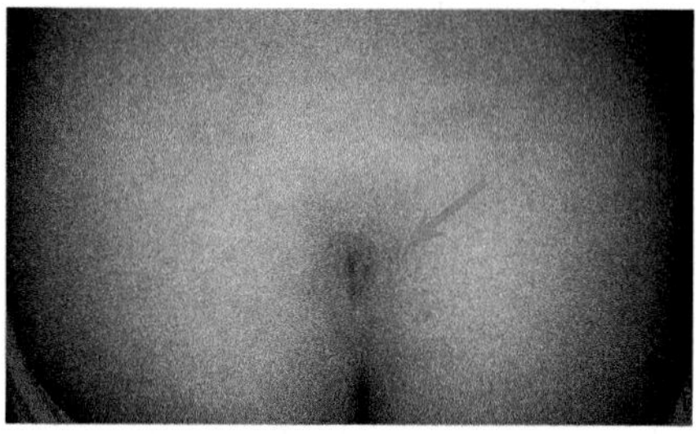

B Sacral dimple A midline skin lesion such as a sacral dimple suggests the presence of a congenital spinal dysraphism.

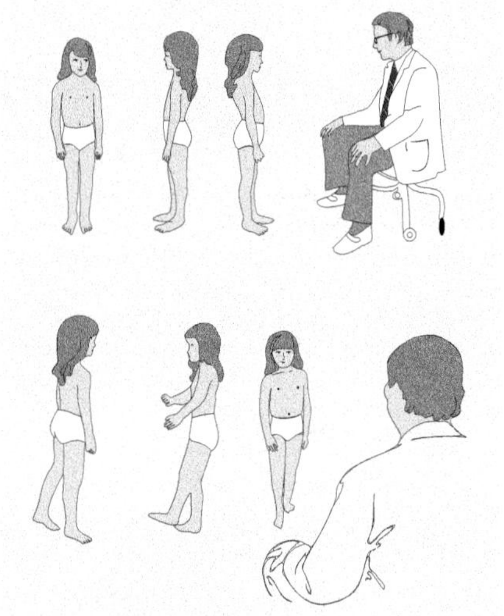

C Screening Inspect from front, side, and back. Observe the child walking normally, then on heels and toes.

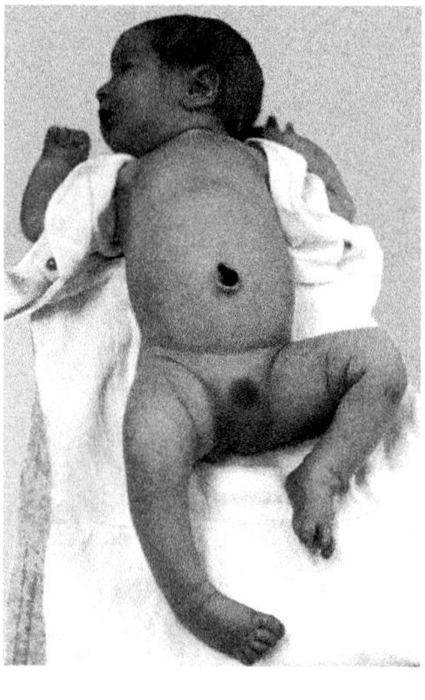

D Importance of observation This infant shows reduced spontaneous movement of the left leg and an abducted position of the left hip. The infant has septic arthritis of the left hip.

Physical Examination

Examination of the musculoskeletal system should include two steps: (1) a screening examination and (2) a complete musculoskeletal evaluation performed to assess a specific complaint. The history and physical examination provide the diagnosis in most cases. It should be thorough and carefully performed. With the proper approach, it is usually possible to perform an adequate examination even without the cooperation of the infant or child.

Approach

Approach the child in a friendly and gentle fashion. Examining the child on the mother's lap is helpful. If the child is still nervous, keep your distance while obtaining the history. Reassure the child that all you plan to do is to watch her walk or move her legs. If the child is still nervous, examine the parent or sibling first. The child may find it reassuring for you to go through the examination with the parent first. If the child will not cooperate in walking, carry her to the opposite side of the room. The child will usually walk or run back to the parents. If the child has pain, always examine the painful site last.

Screening Evaluation

Examine the adolescent in a gown [A] or, even better, in a swimsuit. It is essential to see the whole child to avoid missing important clues in diagnosis such as a skin dimple that may accompany an underlying spinal deformity [B].

Perform the screening examination [C] first before focusing on the principal complaint. This screening ensures that you do not miss any other orthopedic problems and will provide a general overview of the musculoskeletal system necessary to understand the specific problem. For example, knowledge of the degree of generalized joint laxity is valuable in assessing a flatfoot or a dysplastic hip. The examination of the back is an essential part of an evaluation of foot deformities. A cavus foot deformity is a common feature of diastematomyelia.

Infant screening Examine the infant on the mother's lap. First, observe the general body configuration. Next, observe the infant's spontaneous movement patterns for evidence of paralysis or pseudoparalysis [D]. Any reduction of spontaneous movements is an important finding. For example, the only consistent physical finding of the neonate with septic arthritis of the hip is a reduction in spontaneous movement of the affected limb. Finally, systematically examine the limbs and back for joint motion and deformity. Always perform a screening hip examination to rule out developmental hip dysplasia.

Examining the child and adolescent The examination requires several steps:

General inspection Does the child look sick [E]? With the child standing in the anatomic position, observe her from the front, side, and back. Look at body configuration, symmetry, and proportions and for specific deformities.

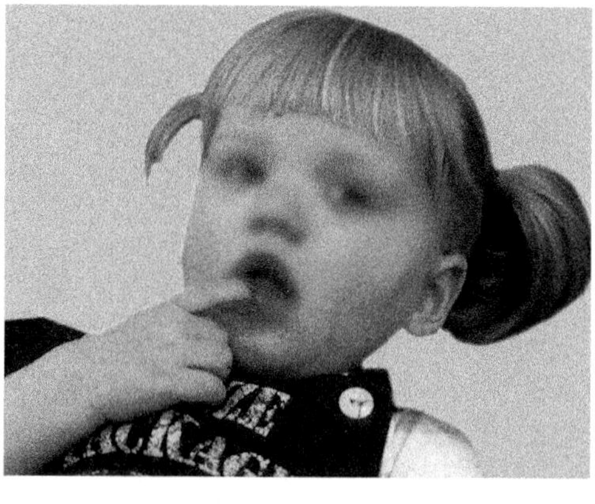

E Ill child.

Pelvis and back Place your hands on the iliac crests—are they level? A pelvic tilt usually results from a limb length difference. Next, ask the child to raise one leg at a time. A drop in the pelvis on the opposite side indicates a weakness of the hip abductors found in conditions such as hip dysplasia and cerebral palsy. With the child facing you, assess thoracic and lumbar symmetry for evidence of scoliosis by the forward-bending test. Observe the sagittal alignment of the spine [A].

Assessing gait Ask the child to walk slowly across the room and back first with normal gait and then repeated on her toes and heels. Observe the gait for evidence of asymmetry, irregularity, or weakness. Any abnormal or questionable findings discovered during the screening examination should prompt a more complete evaluation of the problem. For example, a finding of in-toeing should prompt an assessment of the rotational profile.

Specific Evaluations

The history and findings of the screening examination serve as guides to more in-depth evaluation.

Joint laxity Joint mobility is greatest in infancy and gradually declines throughout life. Joint laxity, like other traits, varies widely among individuals and is usually genetically determined [B]. Extremes in joint laxity are seen in certain disorders, such as Ehlers–Danlos and Marfan syndromes.

Assess joint laxity by testing the mobility of the ankles, knees, elbows, thumbs, and fingers [C]. Excessive laxity in four or all of the five joints tested occurs in about 7% of children. Joint laxity is a contributing factor in the pathogenesis of hip dysplasia, dislocating patellae, and flatfeet, and it increases the risk of injuries such as sprains. In general, excessive joint laxity suggests the possibility of other problems.

Range of motion (ROM) The normal values of joint motion change with age. Generally, the arc of motion is greatest in infancy and declines with age. Specific joints are affected by intrauterine position. For example, lateral hip rotation is greatest in early infancy and declines during the first 2 or 3 years of growth. In assessing ROM, a knowledge of normal values is helpful. Make certain that the position of the pelvis is determined by palpation when assessing hip abduction [D].

Contractures of diarthrodial muscles are common in children and sometimes require lengthening. For example, contracture of the gastrocnemius and gracilis occur in cerebral palsy. By proper positioning of the joints above and below the contracture, it is possible to differentiate contractures of these muscles from adjacent elements of the same muscle group.

Hip flexion motion is difficult to measure due to compensatory motion of the lumbar spine. Measure the range of motion by the Thomas or prone extension tests. The prone extension test has been found to be more reliable. ROM measurements of most joints are reproducible within about ±4°.

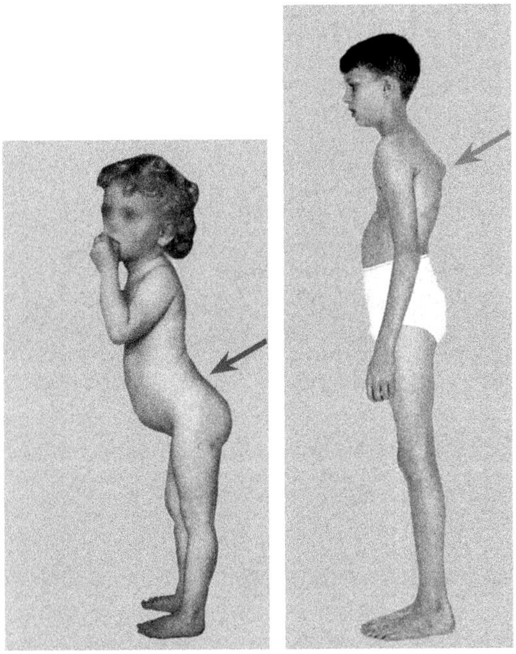

A Sagittal alignment Note the increased lordosis (red arrow) and dorsal kyphosis (blue arrow).

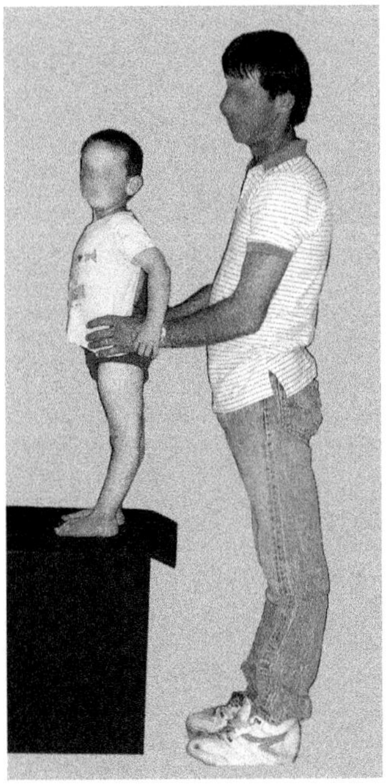

B Familial joint laxity Note hyperextension of the knee in both the child and father.

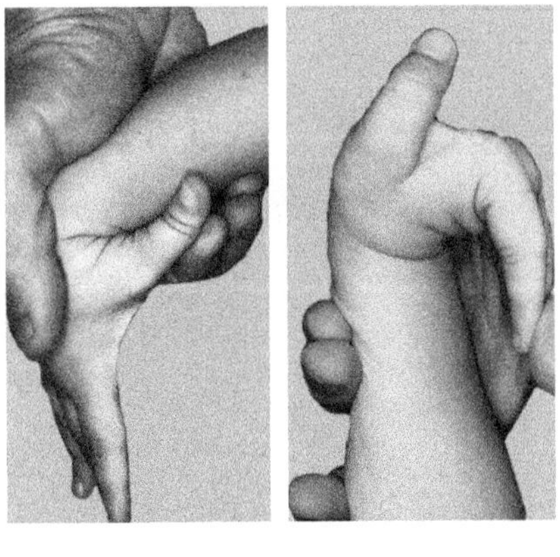

C Finger tests for joint laxity The ability to approximate the thumb and the forearm and extend the fingers to a parallel relationship with the forearm suggests an excessive degree of joint laxity.

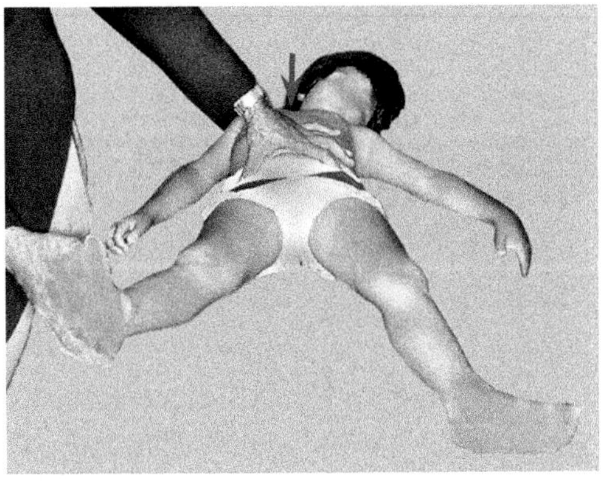

D Assessing hip abduction Stabilize the pelvis with one hand (arrow) and abduct the hip with the other. Assess abduction using the anterior iliac spines as points of reference.

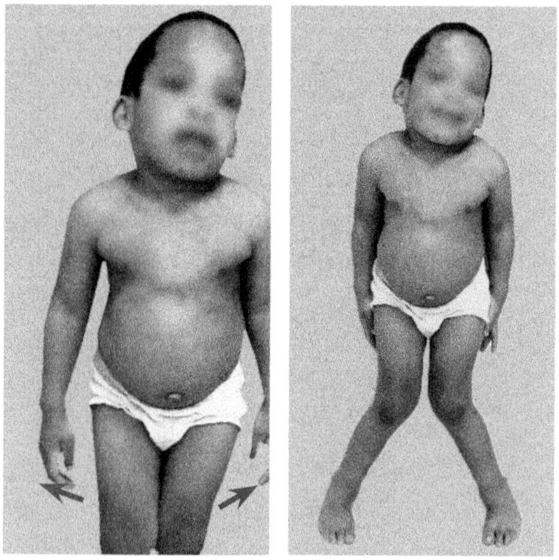

A Differentiate transverse and frontal plane deformity This child compensates a severe genu valgum deformity by walking with the feet laterally rotated (red arrows). When the legs are placed in the anatomic position, the valgus deformity of the knees becomes apparent.

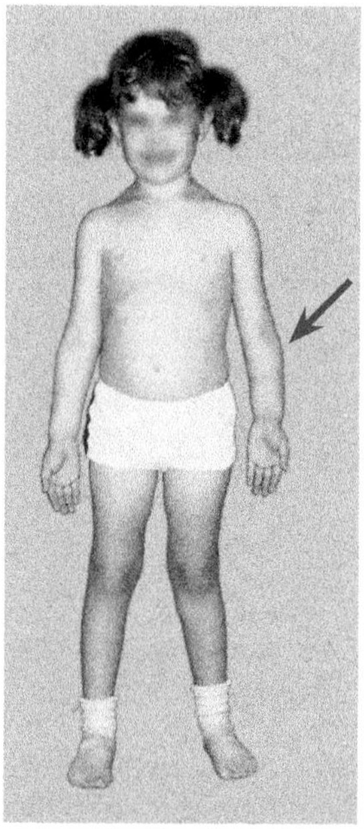

B Cubitus varus deformity This deformity is secondary to a malunited fracture. The child is unaware of any problem.

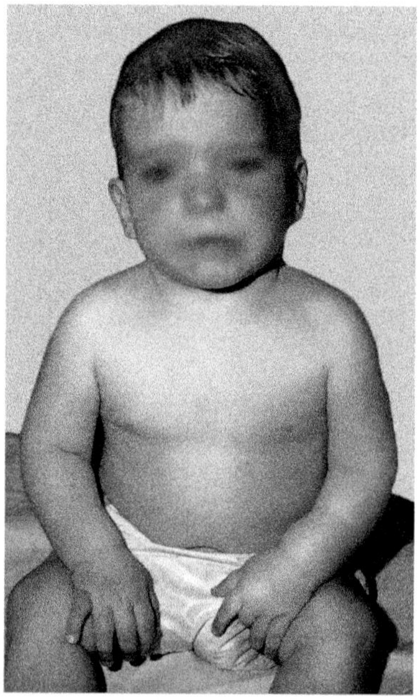

C Pseudoparalysis This child has loss of spontaneous movement of the left arm from a "pulled elbow."

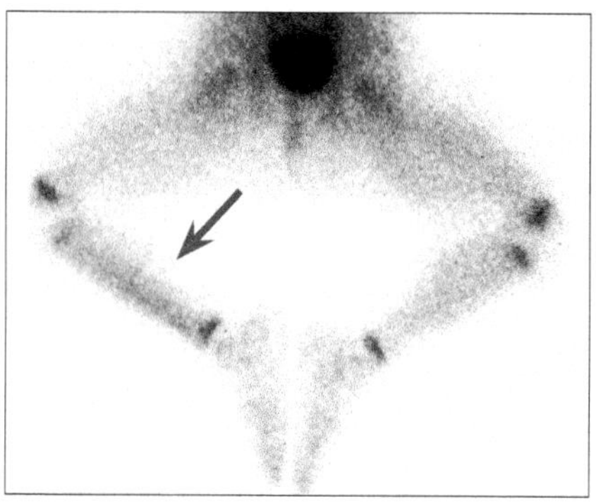

D Limp This child had an obscure limp. The bone scan demonstrated increased uptake over the tibia consistent with a toddler's fracture (arrow).

Deformity

Deformity is classified as either functional or structural. Functional deformity is secondary to muscle contracture or spasm-producing fixation of a joint in an abnormal position. For example, a fixed hip adductor contracture elevates the pelvis on the affected side, producing a functional shortening of the limb. This deformity is commonly seen in cerebral palsy and Perthes disease. In contrast, structural deformity originates within the limb. An example is the limb shortening associated with fibular hemimelia.

Assess deformity in reference to body planes with the body in the anatomic position [B]. Frontal or coronal plane deformity is most easily observed and creates the most significant cosmetic disability. Sagittal plane deformity produces problems in the plane of motion. Finally, transverse or horizontal plane deformity is most difficult to visualize and had often been overlooked in the past. Currently, CT and MRI studies allow visualization and documentation of this plane and increase the appreciation of transverse plane problems. In assessing and documenting deformity, it is essential that each plane be separated clearly and described independently [A]. For example, in tibia vara, deformity occurs in both the frontal and transverse planes. Failure to clearly separate these planes may result in serious errors if operative correction is undertaken.

Altered Function

Function may be impaired by many mechanisms. The impairment is most obvious when the onset is acute and recent. The parents are aware when the pseudoparalysis is due to their child's "pulled" or "nursemaid's" elbow [C]. Conversely, long-standing changes in function may be overlooked or just considered as an unusual characteristic of the child. A child's bilateral abductor lurch from dislocated hips may go unappreciated for years. Limping of recent origin is usually obvious to the parents. Sometimes the examination is normal, and imaging studies are necessary to establish the diagnosis [D].

Evaluate altered function of recent onset for evidence of trauma or infection. Look for deformity, swelling, or discoloration. Palpate to determine if tenderness is present. Finally, evaluate joint motion for stiffness or guarding. For example, inflammatory and traumatic hip disorders cause a loss of medial hip rotation and guarding of the joint. Evaluate chronic problems for evidence of deformity and an underlying disease. The chronic problem is much more likely to be serious and require a complete and thorough evaluation.

Functional disability is more significant than deformity. Deformity is static; function is dynamic. Deformity is most significant when it adversely affects function. This concept is becoming more universally accepted with time. In the past, handicapped children with conditions such as cerebral palsy were subjected to endless treatments to correct deformity. Often, deformity was corrected at the expense of function. The net effect was harmful.

Some alteration in function is subtle and not readily apparent. For example, a malunited bone forearm fracture may cause a permanent reduction of forearm rotation in the older child. The child compensates for the deformity by rotating the shoulder and may not be aware of any problem. This loss of motion can be detected by physical examination. Determine the degree of disability by functional tests that focus on activities requiring pronation and supination.

Pain

Pain in the child is usually significant. For example, the majority of adults experience back pain, but rarely does it require active treatment. In contrast, back pain in children is much more likely to be organic. Pain in the adolescent is more likely to have a functional basis, as is so common in adults. The most common cause of pain in children is trauma. Trauma may result from acute injury or from the so-called microtrauma or overuse syndromes. Overuse syndromes account for the majority of sports medicine problems in children and adolescents.

Point of Maximum Tenderness The most useful test in establishing the cause of pain is determining its anatomic origin by locating the *point of maximum tenderness* (*PMT*) [A]. Localization of the PMT, together with the history, often establishes the diagnosis. For example, a PMT over the tibial tubercle in a 13-year-old boy very likely means the boy has Osgood–Schlatter disease [B]. A PMT over the anterior aspect of the distal fibula [C, upper], together with a history of an ankle injury, probably points to an ankle sprain. A PMT over the tarsal navicular in a 12-year-old girl suggests the diagnosis of an accessory ossicle [C, lower].

The examination to establish the PMT should start distant from the problem. Palpate gently, moving progressively closer to the site of discomfort. Watch the child's face for signs of discomfort. Often a change in facial expression is more reliable than a verbal response. Be gentle. Ask the child to tell you where the tenderness is greatest. With gentleness, patience, and sensitivity, the PMT can usually be established accurately with minimal discomfort.

The PMT is a useful guide in ordering radiographs. A PMT over the tibial tubercle suggests the diagnosis of Osgood–Schlatter disease. If confirmation is necessary, order a lateral radiograph of the knee. Similarly, order oblique radiographs of the elbow if the PMT is over the lateral condyle and the AP and lateral views of the elbow are normal. Fracture of the lateral condyle may be demonstrated only on the oblique radiograph.

The PMT is helpful in evaluating the radiographs. For example, locating the PMT aids in differentiating an accessory ossification center from a fracture. Only a fracture will be tender. To determine if a subtle cortical irregularity in the contour of the distal radius represents a buckle fracture, locate the PMT. If the cortical irregularity represents a fracture, the PMT and the questionable radiographic change will coincide exactly in location.

Spondyloarthropathy Seronegative spondyloarthropathies in the incipient stage are associated with a PMT in specific locations. These are referred to as enthesopathies. Common sites include the metatarsal heads, plantar fascia, achilles tendon insertion, greater trochanter, and sacroiliac joints.

Leg Aches Leg aches, or *growing pains,* are discomforts of unknown cause that occur in 15–30% of otherwise normal children. Headaches, stomachaches, and leg aches, in that order, are the common pains of childhood. Leg aches characteristically occur at night, are poorly localized, have a long duration, and produce no limp or apparent disability. Spontaneous resolution occurs, without sequelae, over a period of several years.

Because the pain of leg aches is so diffuse and nondescript, the differential diagnosis includes most painful disorders of childhood. The conditions a physician must rule out include neoplastic disorders such as leukemia, hematologic problems such as sickle cell anemia, infections such as subacute osteomyelitis, and various inflammatory conditions. The diagnosis of growing pains is one of exclusion, relying primarily on the medical history and the physical examination. Rarely are a CBC and ESR or radiographs necessary. Evaluation and management of growing pains is discussed in greater detail in Chapter 8.

Muscle Testing

Muscle testing is done to determine the strength of muscle groups [D]. Testing is performed for neuromuscular problems such as poliomyelitis and muscular dystrophy. The grades can be further subdivided by a plus or minus designation.

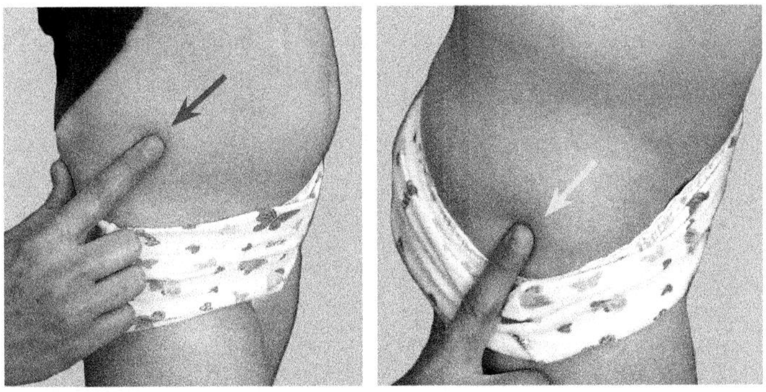

A PMT about the hip The anterior iliac spine (red arrow) and the greater trochanter (yellow arrow) are useful landmarks for determining the PMT about the hip.

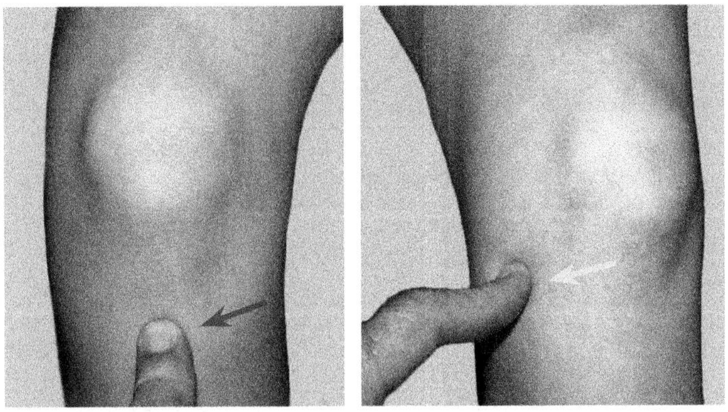

B PMT about the knee The PMT is easily determined about the knee. The tibial tubercle (red arrow) is tender in Osgood–Schlatter disease. Medial joint line tenderness (yellow arrow) is found with meniscal injuries.

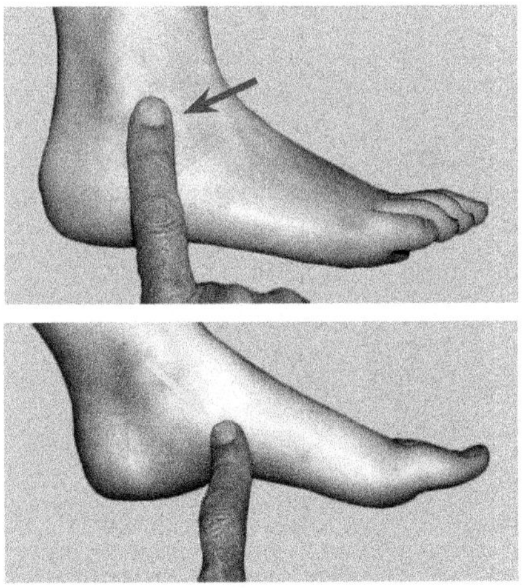

C PMT about the foot Because bone and joints of the foot are subcutaneous, the PMT is very accurate and an especially valuable sign. The PMT over the lateral malleolus (red arrow) and over the navicular (yellow arrow) are readily localized.

Grade	Strength	Physical Findings
0	None	No contraction
1	Trace	Palpable contraction only
2	Poor	Moves joint without gravity
3	Fair	Moves joint against gravity
4	Good	Moves against gravity and resistance
5	Normal	Normal strength

D Muscle grading Manual muscle testing is useful in documenting and classifying muscle strength into six categories.

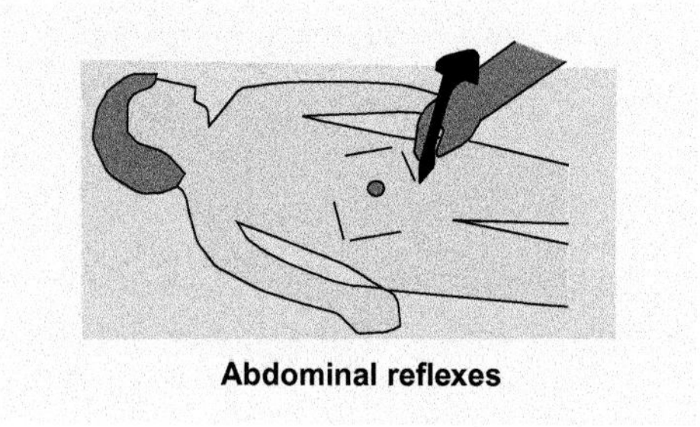

A Abdominal reflexes The abdomen is stroked in all four quadrants. This stimulation causes the umbilicus to move toward the quadrant stimulated. The absence of this response is abnormal.

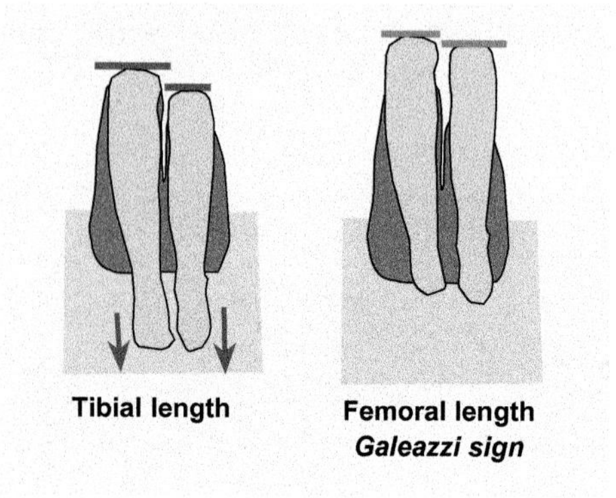

B Assessing femoral and tibial lengths Note the difference in tibial and femoral lengths as observed at the flexed knee. With the feet on the table, tibial length differences are apparent (red arrows). With the hips flexed and the feet free, note the differences in femoral lengths (blue lines).

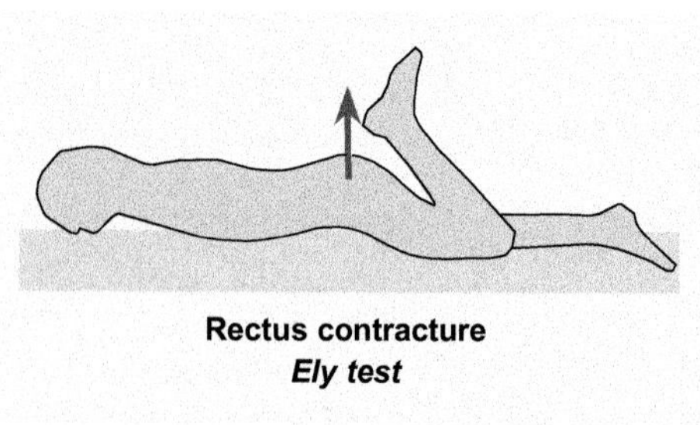

C Rectus femoris contracture evaluation With this contracture, flexion of the knee causes elevation of the pelvis (red arrow).

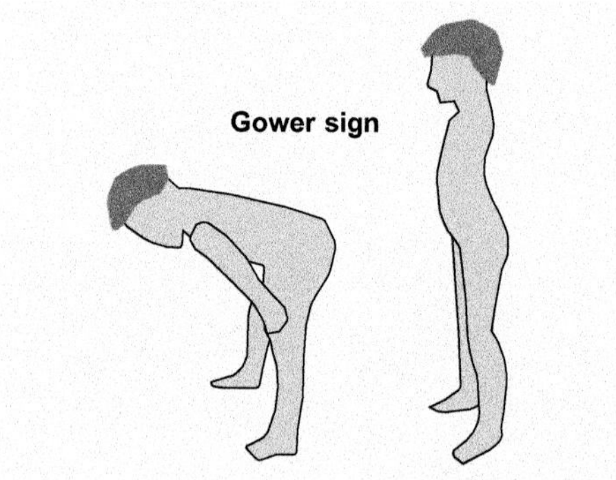

D Gower sign The Gower sign tests for generalized muscle weakness.

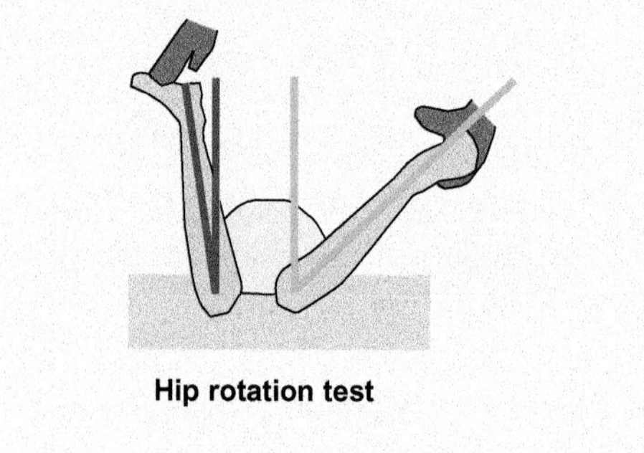

E Hip rotation test This screens for traumatic or inflammatory hip problems. A reduction of medial rotation (red angle compared with normal green angle) is significant, as hip rotation is usually symmetrical in children.

Clinical Tests

Various tests are useful to supplement the general physical examination in children. Some of the more commonly used tests are described below, presented in alphabetical order.

Abdominal Reflex

Stimulate each quadrant of the abdomen [A]. Normally the umbilicus moves toward the side being stimulated. This test is commonly used to assess a neurologic basis for spinal deformity.

Anvil Test

This tests for the localization of discitis. Percussion on top of the head causes pain at the site of discitis.

Barlow Maneuver

This maneuver is a provocative test for hip instability in developmental hip dysplasia. See Chapter 11.

Coleman Block Test

This tests for hindfoot flexibility. Ask the child to stand on a block positioned under the lateral side of the foot. With weight bearing, the failure of the heel to assume a valgus position is indicative of a fixed deformity.

Tibial Length

This test assesses the tibia–hindfoot length [B, left]. With the patient supine, flex the knees fully. The difference between the knee heights indicates the amount of shortening. This test can also be performed with the child prone. This allows the knees to be flexed to a full 90°.

Ely Test

This test assesses for rectus contracture [C]. Place the child prone and flex the knee. If the rectus is spastic or contacted, the pelvis will rise.

Foot-Progression Angle

This test assesses the degree of in-toeing or out-toeing (see Chapter 8).

Forward Bend Test

This assesses the functional and structural stiffness and deformity of the back. While observing the patient from the back and again from the side, ask the patient to bend forward as far as possible. Note asymmetry and stiffness. The normal child should show symmetrical flexion and be able to extend the fingers to at least the knee. The spine should show an even flexion of the thoracic spine and reversal of the lumbar lordosis. The thorax should be symmetrical as viewed from the back and front. Spinal cord tumors, inflammatory lesions, spinal deformity, and hamstring contractures all cause abnormal findings.

Galeazzi Sign

This tests for shortening due to developmental hip dysplasia [B, right]. Flex both hips and knees to a right angle. Note any difference in apparent length of thighs.

Goldthwaite Test

This test detects lumbar spine inflammation, as occurs with discitis. Position prone with hips extended and knees flexed. Moving the pelvis from side to side causes a synchondrous movement of the lumbar spine.

Gower Test

This tests for general muscle weakness [D]. Ask the patient to sit on the floor and then stand up without external supports. With trunk weakness, the child uses his hands to climb up his thighs for support.

Hip Rotation Test

This test screens for inflammatory or traumatic hip problems [E]. Place child in prone position, knees flexed to 90°, and medially rotate both hips. A loss of medial rotation is a positive sign.

Nélaton's Line
This test is useful in clinical assessment of hip dislocation. The tip of the trochanter should fall below a line connecting the anterior iliac spine and the ischial tuberosity.

Ober Test
This tests for tensor fascia contracture [A]. Position the patient on one side with the lower knee and hip flexed to a right angle. Abduct and fully extend the upper hip. While maintaining the hip extended, allow the leg to fall into full adduction. An abduction contracture is present if the thigh fails to fall into adduction. The degree of contracture equals the abducted position above the neutral or horizontal position.

Ortolani Maneuver
This maneuver tests for hip instability in developmental dysplasia of the hip (DDH). See Chapter 11.

Patellar Apprehension Sign
This test is for patellar instability. With the knee extended, gradually apply pressure to laterally displace the patella while observing the patient's facial expression. Apprehension indicates previous experience with patellar dislocation.

Patrick or Faber Test
This test detects sacroiliac (SI) inflammation [B]. Place the ipsilateral foot over the opposite knee. While holding down the opposite ilium, apply a downward force on the flexed knee. Pain at the SI joint is a positive finding.

Pelvic Obliquity Test
This differentiates suprapelvic from infrapelvic obliquity. Position the child prone with the pelvis on the edge of the examining table, allowing the lower limbs to flex. Windswept positioning of the legs brings the pelvis to neutral if the obliquity is infrapelvic in origin.

Phelps Gracilis Test
This test is a measure of gracilis spasticity or contracture. Position the patient prone and abduct the hip with the knee flexed. Passive knee extension causes hip adduction if the gracilis is contracted.

Popliteal Angle Measure
This measures hamstring contracture [C]. With the patient supine, flex the hip to a right angle and the knee to a comfortable maximum. The contracture equals the degree of lack of full knee extension.

Prone Extension Test
This tests for hip flexion contracture [D]. Position the patient prone with the thigh over the edge of the examining table. With one hand on the pelvis and other holding onto the leg, extend the leg until the pelvis starts to elevate. The horizontal–thigh angle demonstrates the degree of contracture.

Thigh–Foot Angle
This is a measure of tibial and hindfoot rotation. See Chapter 8.

Thomas Test
This tests for hip flexion contracture. Flex the contralateral hip fully. The ipsilateral horizontal–thigh angle equals the hip flexion contracture.

Transmalleolar Angle
This angle is a measure of tibial rotation.

Trendelenburg Test
This test assesses abductor strength [E]. While observing the pelvis from behind, ask the patient to raise one leg (without holding for support). A drop in the contralateral pelvis indicates weakness of the ipsilateral abductors.

A *delayed* Trendelenburg test is performed by determining the time necessary for the abductors to fatigue, allowing the pelvis to sag. If the elevation of the contralateral pelvis cannot be maintained for 60 seconds, the test is positive.

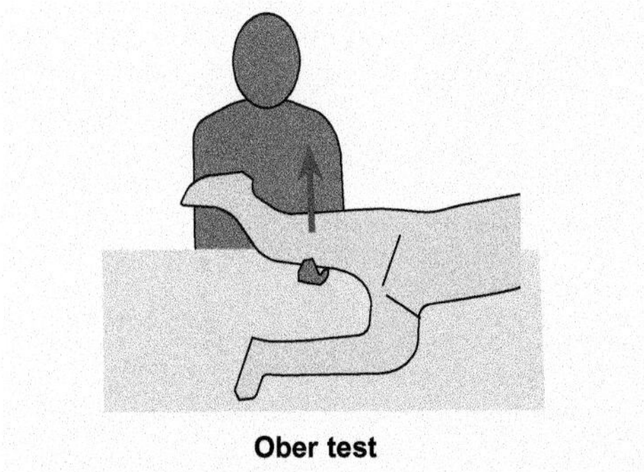

A Ober test This tests for tensor fascia contracture. Abduct and extend the leg, then allow it to fall. A failure of adduction is positive for a tensor contracture.

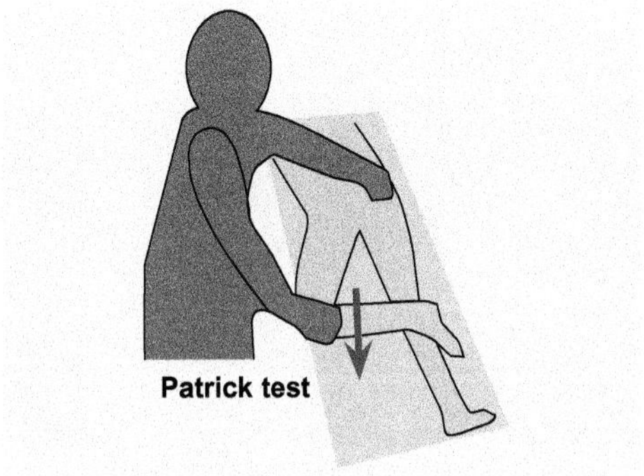

B Patrick test This test is performed by positioning the leg across the other and applying downward pressure. This elicits pain in the ipsilateral sacroiliac joint region.

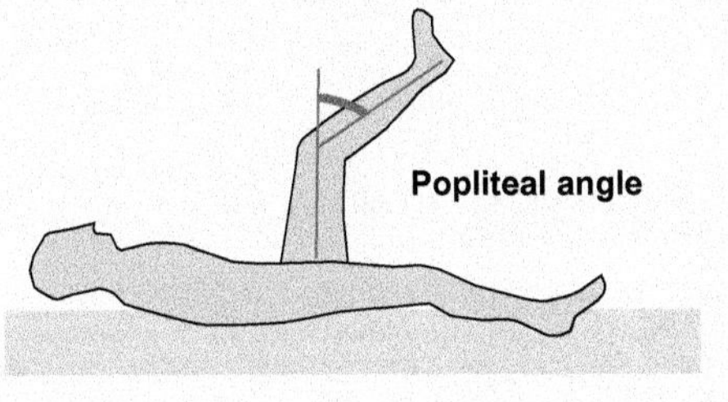

C Popliteal angle With the hip flexed, extend the knee. The degrees short of full extension equal the popliteal angle (blue arc).

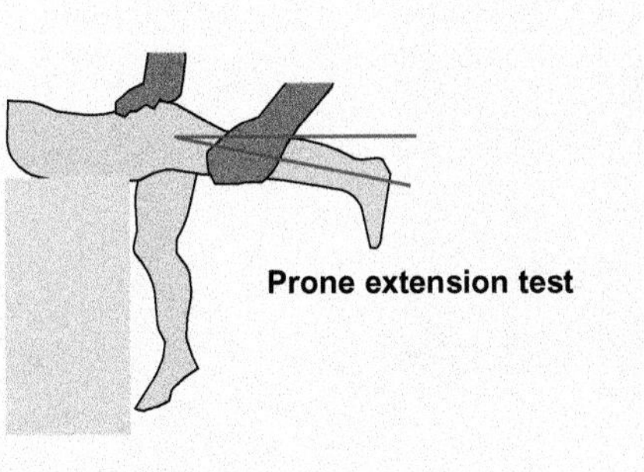

D Prone extension This test assesses hip flexion contracture. With the contralateral hip flexed, extend the ipsilateral side to the degree that causes the pelvis to elevate. The degrees short of full extension equal the degrees of contracture.

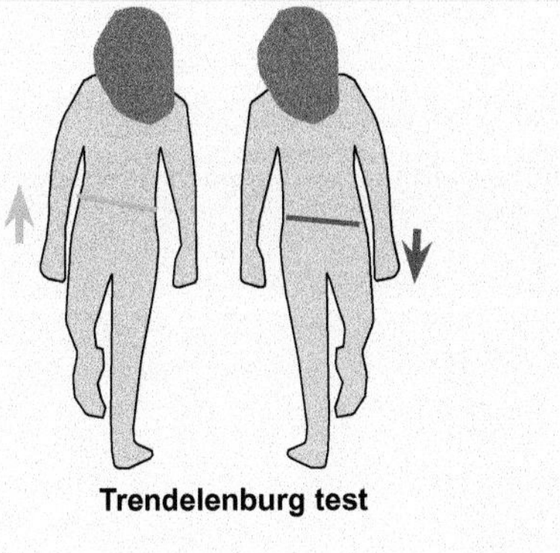

E Trendelenburg test Standing on the normal side elicits an elevation in the opposite side (green line). A drop in the opposite side (red line) indicates weakness of hip abduction.

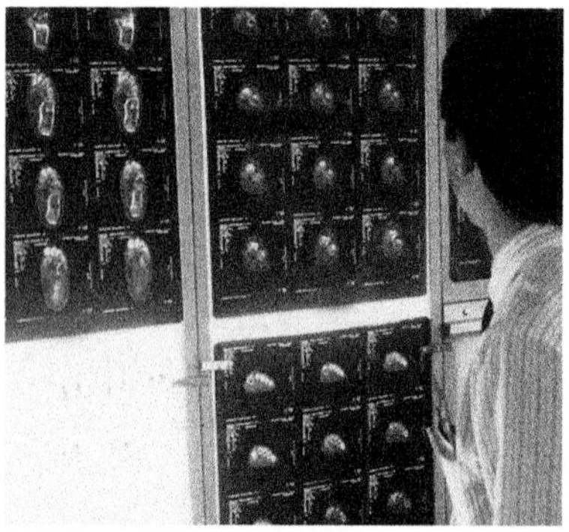

A Be cautious about over reading New imaging techniques often result in over reading, which sometimes results in over-treatment.

Imaging

New imaging methods make musculoskeletal evaluation more rapid, precise, and complete. However, new images must be interpreted with caution [A]. Even after 100 years of experience reading conventional radiographs, it is still difficult to separate disease from normal variability [B]. The lack of experience with new imaging methods makes interpretation even more difficult. Over reading imaging, such as the MRI, poses risks and may lead to over-treatment. For example, MRI studies of discitis often show extensive soft tissue changes, which might prompt operative drainage if the nature of the disease is not appreciated.

Conventional Radiography

Conventional radiographs are still the mainstay of diagnostic imaging. They are the least expensive, most readily available, and the least apt to be misread. Radiographs show bone, water, fat, and air density well. Bone density must be reduced by 30–50% to show changes on radiographs. Proper positioning of the child is essential. Therefore, sometimes the physician, rather than the technician, needs to position the child. For example, to study genu varum or genu valgum, the child must be placed in the anatomic position with the patellae directed forward. The technician may try to rotate the limbs laterally to fit the legs on the film, creating a deceptive image [C].

Limiting radiographs Try to limit radiation exposure by reducing the number of radiographs ordered. The risk of one chest x-ray is considered comparable to smoking 1.4 cigarettes or driving 30 miles. Although the risk is small, it is prudent to limit exposure when possible. Use the following principles to limit exposure to your patients:

Shield the gonads when possible except for the initial pelvic image.

Order screening radiographs first For example, if spondylolisthesis is suspected, a single lateral standing spot view of the lumbosacral junction may demonstrate the lesion. AP and oblique studies may not be necessary.

Single radiographs are often adequate. For example, a single AP view of the pelvis is usually adequate for evaluating hip dysplasia in the infant or child.

Make upright radiographs Lower extremity and spine radiographs should be taken in the upright position. These standardized views are less likely to be repeated if a referral is necessary.

Allow consultant to order imaging studies Suggest to primary care physicians that if a consultation is necessary, to have the consultant order the studies. Suggest that parents hand-carry previous radiographs for consultation, as radiographs are often mysteriously lost in the mail.

Make follow-up radiographs only when the information is likely to alter management. For example, ordering a radiograph of a wrist fracture at 3 weeks is generally useless. It is too soon to discontinue immobilization and too late to change position.

Avoid routine opposite side comparative radiographs.

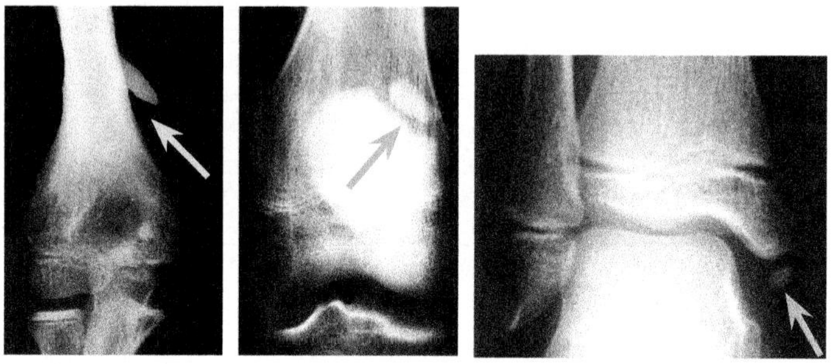

B Normal variation The supracondyloid process of the humerus (yellow arrow), a bipartite patella (green arrow), and malleolar ossicles (orange arrow) are uncommon developmental variations of normal.

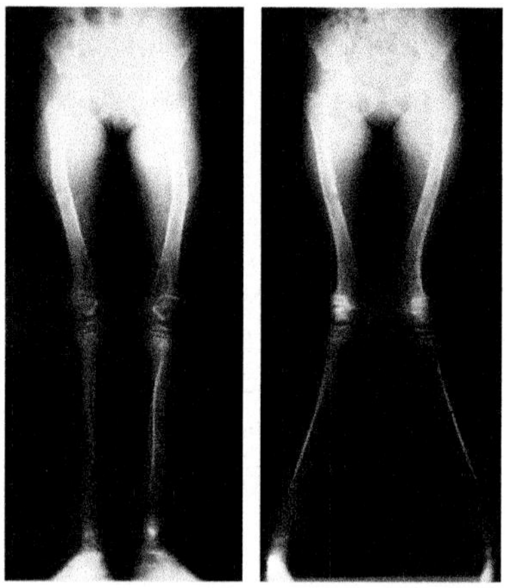

C Proper positioning for radiographs This patient had a radiograph made for measuring mechanical axis of the lower limb. The technician rotated the limbs to get the radiograph on one film (left image). A second film was necessary (right image) in which the physician positioned the child in the anatomic position necessary for an accurate measurement.

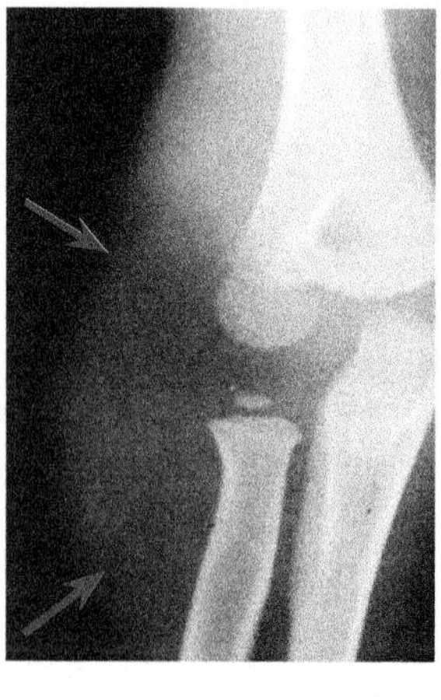

D Soft tissue swelling Soft tissue swelling is an important finding because it suggests that a significant injury has occurred. In this case, the swelling over the lateral condyle (red arrows) was consistent with a lateral condylar fracture. Additional radiographs showed the fracture.

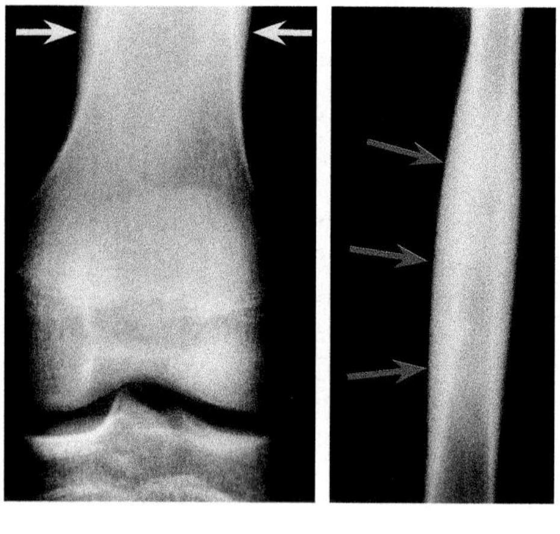

E Study the edge of the film This is the initial radiograph of an adolescent complaining of leg pain. The film was read as normal and a diagnosis made of a "conversion reaction." In a later review of the radiograph, periosteal reaction involving femoral distal diaphysis (yellow arrows) was appreciated. Additional radiographs of the whole femur showed extensive sclerosis of the diaphysis (red arrows) due to chronic sclerosing osteomyelitis.

Reading errors Here are some suggestions to avoid reading errors:

Standardize sequence to radiographs, starting with the soft tissues [D, previous page].

Study the edge of the film before concentrating on the presumed area of pathology [E, previous page].

Order additional views if the radiographic and physical findings are inconsistent. For example, order oblique radiographs of the elbow if the child has unexplained swelling over the elbow [D, previous page] and no evidence of a fracture on the initial AP and lateral views. The oblique views will often demonstrate a fracture.

Be aware that false negative studies occur in certain situations, such as in the early phase of osteomyelitis and in septic arthritis or developmental hip dysplasia in the newborn.

Variations of ossification are often misleading. The accessory ossicles of the foot may be confused with fractures; irregular ossification on the lateral femoral condyle may be misinterpreted as osteochondritis dissecans.

Computerized Tomography Imaging

Computerized tomography (CT) studies provide excellent bone and soft tissue detail [A]. The soft tissue images can be manipulated by computer to enhance tissue separations. This makes the method useful for assessing soft tissue lesions about the pelvis. CT studies can be combined with contrast material for special evaluations, such as CT myelography. Images are obtained in the transverse plane and can be reconstructed by computer with the frontal and sagittal planes or presented as 3-D images for a more graphic display [B]. These studies show relationships well, such as the concentricity of hip reduction and the detailing of dysplasia [C]. For complex deformity, plastic models can be fabricated based on the CT study [D].

The disadvantages of CT imaging include the need for sedation in the infant and young child, greater radiation exposure, and greater cost than for conventional studies.

Arthrography

Arthrographic studies provide visualization of soft tissue structures of the joints [E]. The contrast is usually provided by air, nitrogen, carbon dioxide, or an iodinated contrast solution. The procedure can be combined with CT or tomography. Arthrography is most useful in evaluating the hip [F] and knee. In septic arthritis, an arthrogram is helpful to confirm joint entry. Arthrography is useful for hip dysplasia and meniscal lesions and in identifying loose or foreign bodies in joints. Disadvantages include the need for sedating younger children and occasional reactions to the iodinated contrast material.

Uses for CT Scans

Bone detailing—when conventional radiographs are inadequate
Spine and pelvic lesions—inflammatory, neoplastic, traumatic
Complex hip deformity prior to reconstruction
DDH assessment of reduction in cast
Physeal bridge assessment
Complex fractures—such as triplane ankle fractures

A Uses of CT scans These are some typical examples of the use of CT scans in assessing musculoskeletal problems in children.

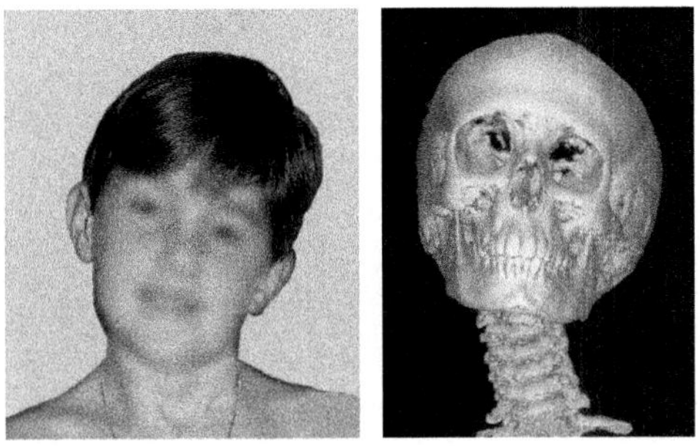

B Torticollis with plagiocephaly Asymmetry of the face and skull are demonstrated by 3-D CT reconstructions.

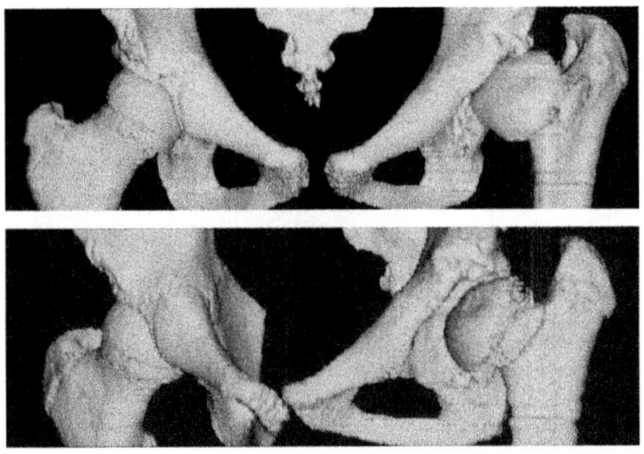

C 3-D reconstruction in hip dysplasia These reconstructions allow assessment of complex hip pathology and often facilitate operative planning.

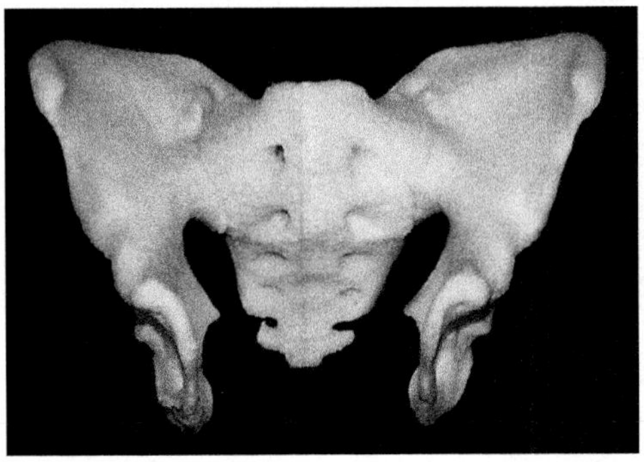

D Plastic model from CT reconstruction Models in plastic can be created that allow preoperative planning and execution of operative correction.

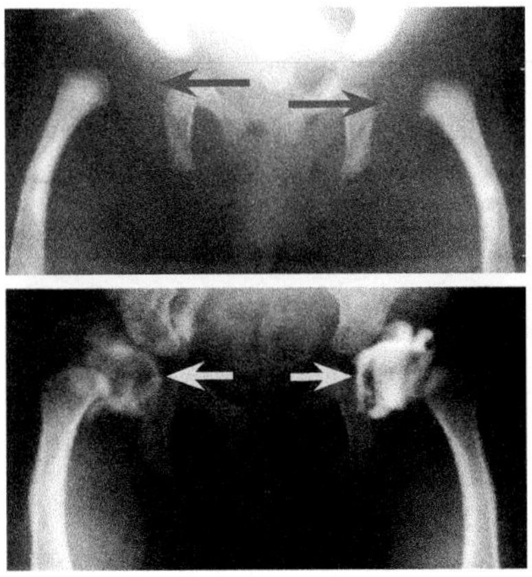

E Arthrography Initial radiograph showed a lateral displacement of the upper femoral metaphysis (red arrows), suggesting the possibility of a hip dislocation or subluxation. The arthrogram showed the femoral head to be reduced (yellow arrow) and established the diagnosis of coxa vara.

Uses for Arthrography

DDH—initial evaluation and when management uncertain
Perthes disease—to assess shape of cartilaginous femoral head
Complex trauma—such as elbow injuries in the infant
Osteochondritis dissecans

F Arthrography uses These are typical examples of the use of arthrograms for assessing musculoskeletal problems in children.

Uses for Bone Scans

Screening—for child abuse
Trauma—early stress fractures
Tumors—localizing lesions, lesion age, differentiating cyst types
Infections—localizing site or early osteomyelitis, discitis
Avascular necrosis—Legg-Calvé-Perthes (LCP) disease, osteochondritis staging

A Uses of bone scans These are some examples of the use of bone scans for assessing musculoskeletal problems in children.

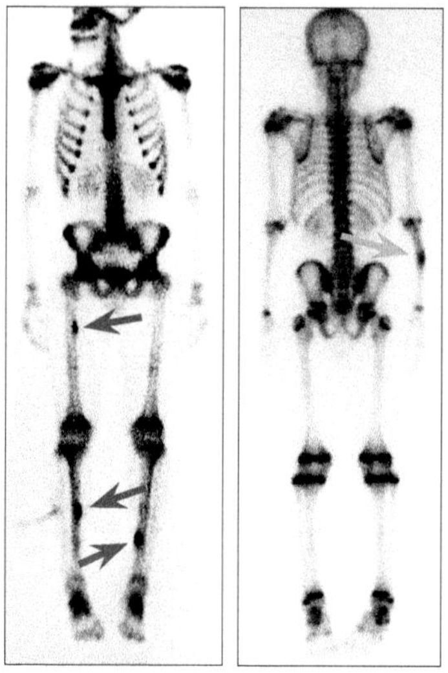

B Bone scans for screening These screening bone scans demonstrate unsuspected multiple stress reactions in an athlete (red arrows) and in another boy (right) who has osteomyelitis that is localized to the left ulna (orange arrow).

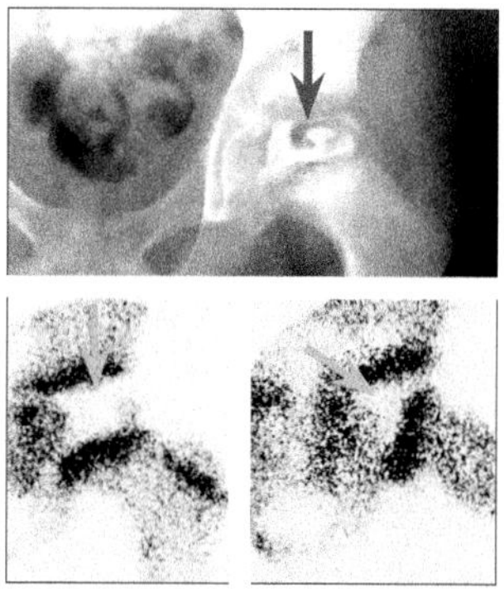

C Pinhole collimated bone scan Conventional radiograph shows avascular necrosis of the femoral head (red arrow). Pinhole collimated scans show reduced uptake in the avascular femoral head (orange arrows).

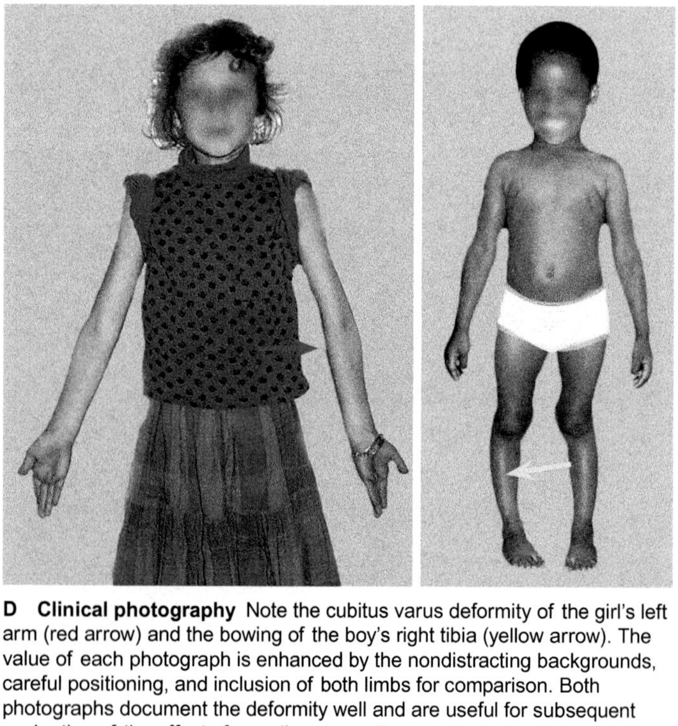

D Clinical photography Note the cubitus varus deformity of the girl's left arm (red arrow) and the bowing of the boy's right tibia (yellow arrow). The value of each photograph is enhanced by the nondistracting backgrounds, careful positioning, and inclusion of both limbs for comparison. Both photographs document the deformity well and are useful for subsequent evaluation of the effect of growth on severity.

Scintography

Scans utilizing technetium-99m, gallium-67, and indium-111 provide imaging of a variety of tissues. Scintographies are more sensitive and show abnormal uptake much earlier than radiographic imaging [A]. In addition, bone scanning has a broad scope of applications, including the evaluation of obscure skeletal pain [B]. The radiation exposure is equivalent to a skeletal survey with conventional radiographs. Useful options in scanning include a variety of agents, collimator selection, timing of scans, and the use of special techniques.

Collimation "Pinhole" collimation increases the resolution of the image. This is particularly useful for assessing avascular necrosis (AVN) of the femoral head. Order both AP and lateral views [C].

Agents The vast majority of scans use technetium-99m. This agent has a half-life of 6 hours and, combined with phosphate, is bone seeking. It is highly sensitive, and the images usually become positive in 24–48 hours. Gallium-67 and indium-111 are used primarily for localization of infections. Indium is combined with a sample of the white blood cells from the patient.

Timing Phasic bone scans show the initial perfusion immediately. The soft tissue phase or pooling occurs at 10–20 minutes, and finally, the bone phase is shown after 3–4 hours. Bone scans are not affected by joint aspiration.

Photography

Medical photography provides an excellent means of documentation [D]. Photographs are inexpensive, safe, and accurate. They are useful in documentation and parent education. The documenting value of photographs is increased by taking certain steps:

Positioning Position for photographs as for a radiograph. Make anterior, lateral, or special views. Position the patient in the anatomic position.

Background Attempt to find a neutral, nondistracting background.

Distance Take photographs as close as possible while including enough of the body to orient the viewer.

Uses for MRI Studies

Cartilage imaging—meniscal lesion, growth plate injuries
Avascular necrosis—LCP disease, AVN at hip, distal femur
Neural status—spinal cord lesions
Tumors—margins, staging
Infections—soft tissue lesions

E Uses for MRI These studies are useful in imaging soft tissue lesions. The usefulness in infants and children is limited by the cost and the need for sedation or anesthesia for immobilization.

Magnetic Resonance Imaging

MRI provides excellent images of soft tissue without exposure to ionizing radiation [E previous page]. However, it requires expensive, sophisticated equipment as well as sedation or anesthesia in the infant or younger child for necessary immobilization. Bone imaging is poor, but for soft tissues, MRI is excellent. The interpretation may be difficult because of limited experience, making over-reading a potential problem. Despite these problems, MRIs are proving useful for an increasingly wide variety of conditions [A, B, and C].

Ultrasound Imaging

Ultrasound applications for the musculoskeletal system are numerous, and the technique is underutilized [D].

Prenatal ultrasound These studies [E] have the potential of making dramatic changes in orthopedic practice. Here are some useful applications of prenatal ultrasound:

Pathogenesis Improving our understanding of disease in turn improves our ability to prevent or treat diseases.

Prenatal treatment Prenatal treatment, utilizing replacement, substitution therapies, or improving intrauterine environment may correct or improve the problem.

Family preparation Resources can be made available for early postnatal treatment as necessary and for preparing families psychologically and educationally.

Pregnancy termination For serious conditions, ultrasound can help determine the need for termination based on the family's choice.

Musculoskeletal disorders The number of these disorders that can be diagnosed by prenatal ultrasound [F] are increasing rapidly with higher resolution studies and greater user experience. False positive studies do occur, however, and may cause considerable unnecessary anxiety in the families.

Clinical uses These studies are highly dependent on operator skill and experience; in North America, they are usually performed by the radiologist [G]. Ultrasound studies could become a practical extension of the physical examination. Ultrasound is safe, potentially inexpensive, versatile, and probably underutilized in North America.

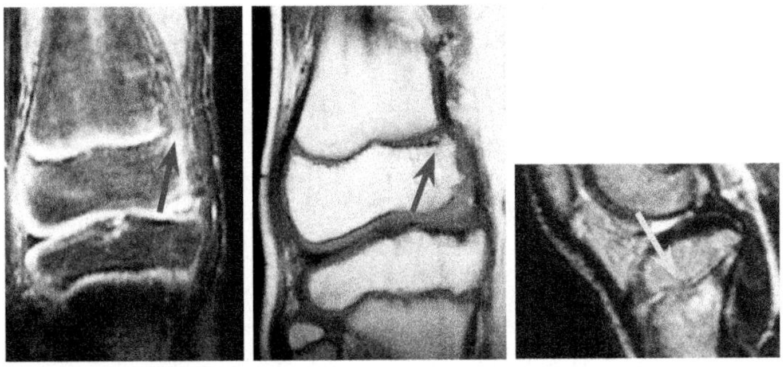

A MRI in physeal injury Note the defect in the distal femoral physis (red arrows) and the proximal tibial growth plate (yellow arrow).

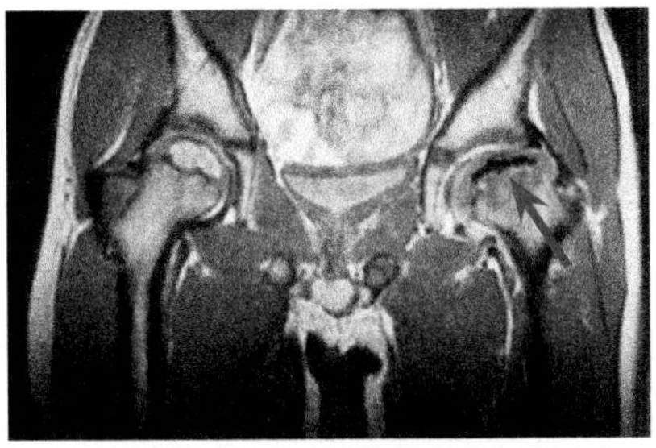

B MRI in Perthes disease The avascular necrosis is clearly demonstrated (arrow).

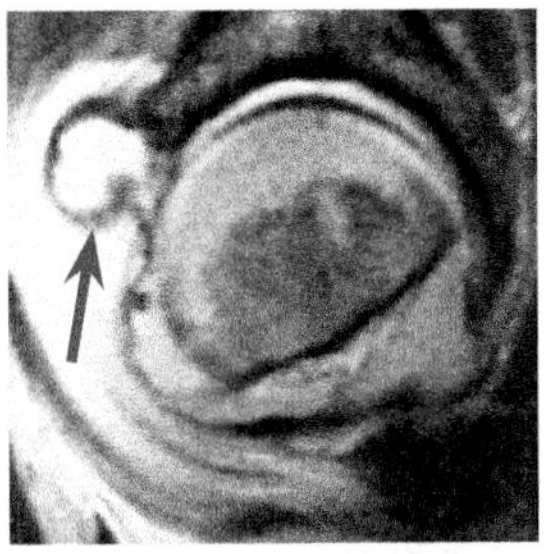

C Synovial cyst in hip The cyst (arrow) is clearly seen on this MRI study.

Uses for Postnatal Ultrasound

DDH—evaluation in the young infant
Infections—localization of abscess, joint effusions
Foreign bodies—of the foot
Tumors—especially cystic varieties
Trauma—cartilaginous injuries in young children
Research—measuring torsion, joint configuration

D Postnatal ultrasound diagnosis These are typical examples of the uses of ultrasound for assessing musculoskeletal problems in children.

Uses for Prenatal Ultrasound

Clubfeet
Skeletal dysplasias
Limb deficiencies
Spina bifida
Arthrogryposis

E Prenatal ultrasound diagnosis These musculoskeletal problems can usually be diagnosed.

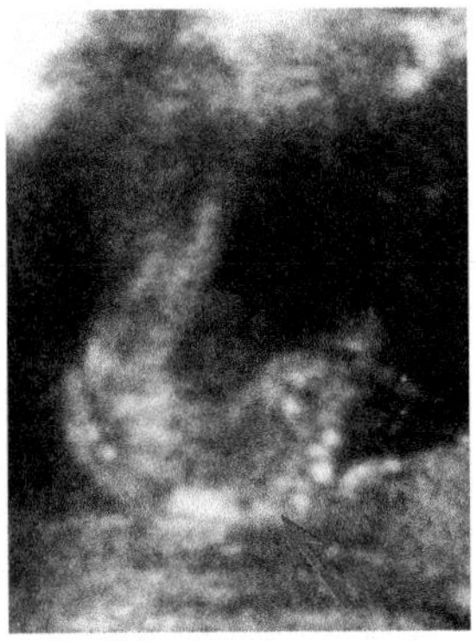

F Clubfoot This clubfoot was identified at 16 weeks of gestation by ultrasound.

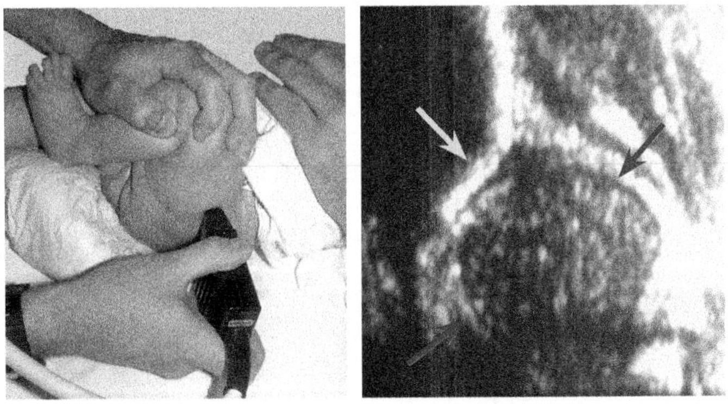

G Ultrasound hip evaluation The ultrasound evaluation (left) of the hip allows effective imaging before ossification occurs. The ultrasound image clearly shows the acetabulum (yellow arrow) and the femoral head (red arrows).

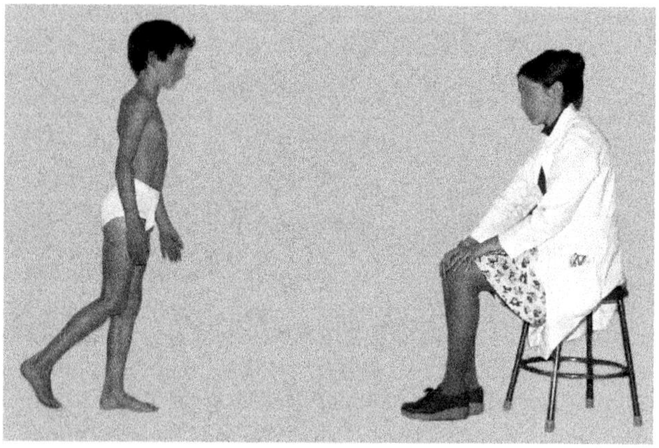

A Clinical observational gait examination Evaluation of the child's gait is best performed in an open area.

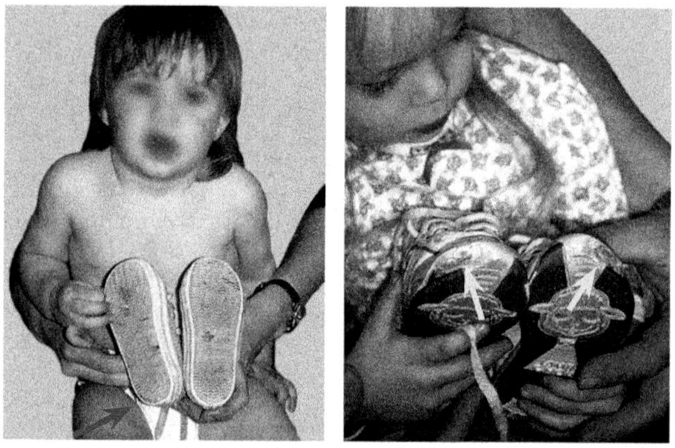

B Value of observing foot wear The lack of heel wear (red arrow, left) is evidence of an equinus gait on the left side. Excessive wear on the toes of the shoes is indicative of a more severe degree of equinus (yellow arrows, right) in a child with spastic diplegia.

Gait Evaluation

Gait can be evaluated at three levels of sophistication.

Screening Examination

Gait evaluation is part of the standard screening examination and is usually performed in the hallway of the clinic [A].

Clinical Observational Examination

This examination [C] is indicated if (1) the family has reported that the child limps, (2) an abnormality is seen during the screening examination, or (3) the physical findings point to a disease likely to affect gait. In the hallway of the clinic, observe the child walking from the front, behind, and both sides if possible. Look at the child's shoes for evidence of abnormal wear [B]. An abnormal gait often falls into readily identifiable categories:

Antalgic gait Pain with weight bearing causes shortening of the stance phase on the affected side.

In-toeing and out-toeing gaits Assess the foot–progression angle for each side. Average the estimated values and express in degrees.

Equinus gait Toe strike replaces heel strike at the beginning of the stance phase.

Abductor lurch or Trendelenburg gait Abductor weakness causes the shoulders to sway to the same side.

Instrumented Gait Analysis

Gait can be assessed by using a videocamera to record visual observations. More sophisticated techniques can also be used, including dynamic electromyography to assess muscle firing sequences, kinemetric techniques for assessing joint motion, force plate to measure ground reaction forces, and sequence and rate measurements [A, next page]. These values are usually compared with normal values.

Currently, greater attention is being focused on the efficiency of gait by analyzing oxygen consumption and heart rate changes. Over time, we become more concerned about effective and efficient mobility and less about mechanical variations.

The role of the gait laboratory is still controversial. It is clearly an important research tool, but its practicality as a clinical tool remains uncertain.

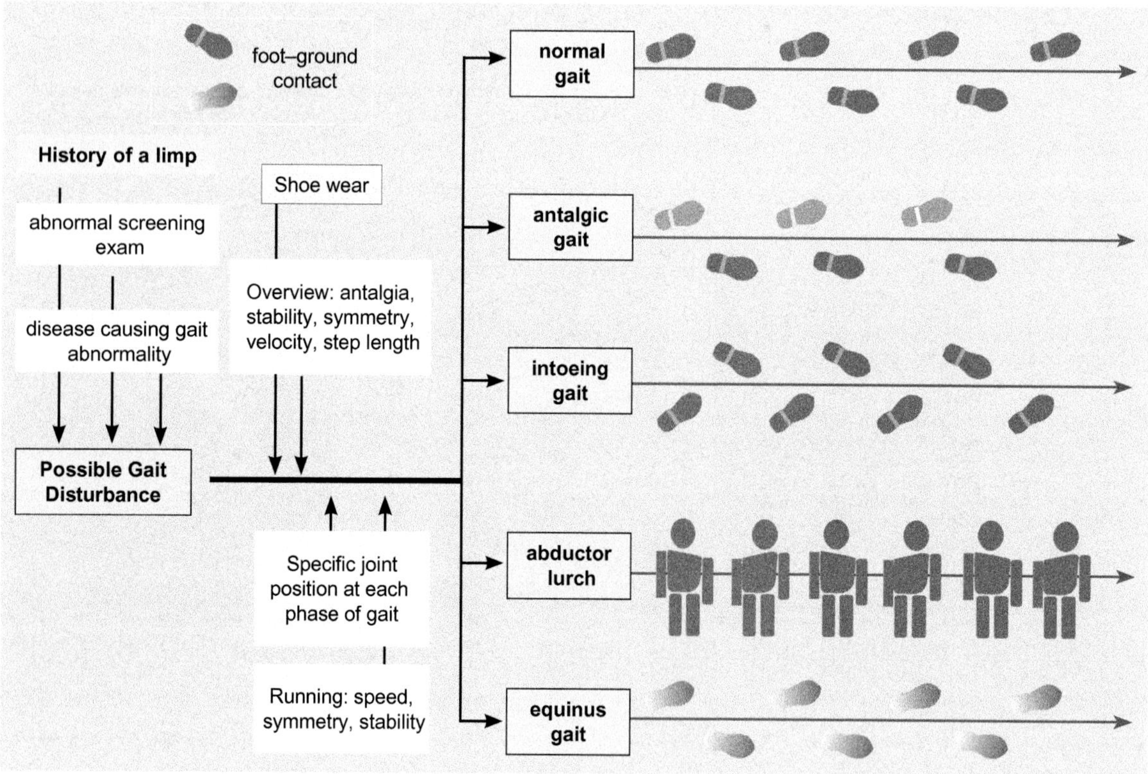

C Algorithm for gait assessment

Laboratory Studies

Laboratory studies provide a limited but useful role in orthopedics. The studies can be combined to reduce the number of needle aspirations.

Hematology

Order a complete blood count (CBC) and erythrocyte sedimentation rate (ESR) and/or C-reactive protein (CRP) as part of a screening evaluation to assess the general health of the patient [B], or when infection, neoplasm, or hematologic conditions are suspected.

The ESR is valuable in differentiating infections from inflammation and traumatic conditions. The CRP elevates more rapidly and returns to normal sooner than the ESR. The upper range of value for the ESR is 20 mm/hr. Inflammatory conditions such as toxic synovitis may raise the ESR to the 20–30 mm/hr range, but ESRs above 30 mm/hr are usually due to infection, neoplasm, or significant trauma. Except in the neonate, the CRP and ESR are usually always elevated by infections such as septic arthritis and osteomyelitis. In contrast, a leukocytosis is a less consistent finding.

Chemistry

Serum studies of calcium metabolism are occasionally useful when the possibility of conditions such as rickets is suspected. The normal range of these values is age dependent.

Enzymes

Screen for muscular dystrophy by ordering a creatinine phosphokinase (CPK) determination. Order the test if the young child appears weak, shows a clumsy gait, and has tight heel cords.

Chromosomal Studies

Chromosome studies are indicated for evaluating syndromes with features suggestive of a genetic disorder. These features include multiple system congenital malformations; mental retardation of unknown cause; abnormal hands, feet, and ears; and skin creases.

Bone Mineral Content

Mineral content of bones can be quantitated using several techniques. Cortical measurements can be made by radiography. The second metacarpal is a common standard. Single and dual photon absorptiometry are other alternatives. These studies are indicated for metabolic diseases, idiopathic osteopenia, and similar disorders.

Joint Fluid

Joint fluid should be visually examined [C] and also sent to the lab for cell counts, chemistry, culturing, and staining [D]. The joint sugar is usually about 90% serum level and is reduced in infection. In about one-third of cases of septic arthritis, cultures are negative.

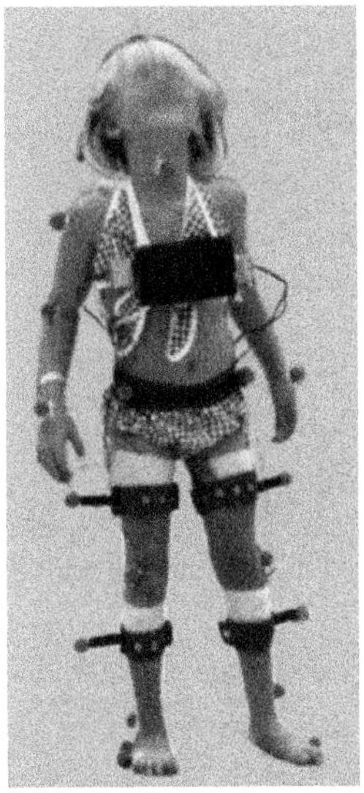

A Gait laboratory The modern gait lab has sophisticated measuring devices to analyze gait.

Condition	Indication for CBC, ESR, and/or CRP
Growing pain	Suspicious features, rule out leukemia
Bone pain	Rule out sickle cell anemia
Stress fracture	Rule out infection
Hip pain	Separate septic arthritis and toxic synovitis
Back pain	Evaluate for discitis
Infection	Follow course of infection

B Indications for CBC, ESR, and/or CRP These screening tests are helpful in evaluating a variety of clinical problems.

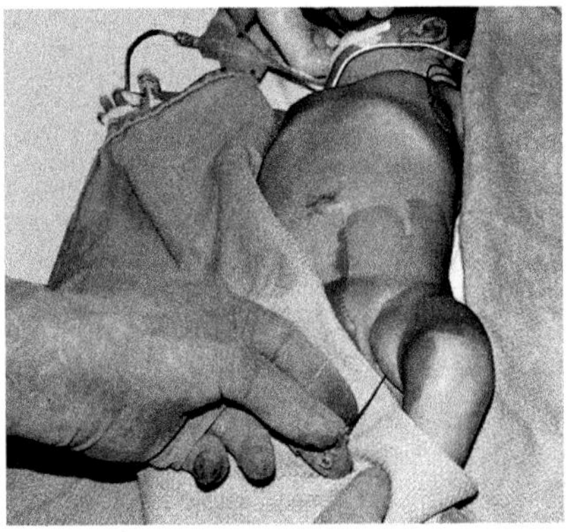

C Joint aspiration The hip joint in the infant is readily aspirated by the medial approach. Visually examine the joint fluid.

Examination	Normal	Septic arthritis	JIA	Traumatic arthritis
Appearance	Straw colored	Grayish	Straw colored	Bloody
Clarity	Clear	Turbid	Slightly cloudy	Bloody
Viscosity	Normal	Decreased	Decreased	Decreased
Total WBC	0–200	50,000–100,000	20,000–50,000	RBCs
PMNs	90+%	Mostly PMNs	Predominate	
Bacteria	None	Seen in about half	None	None
Culture	Negative	Positive 2/3	Negative	Negative
Protein	1.8 g/100 ml	4 g/100 ml	3–4 g/100 ml	4 g/100 ml
Glucose	20 mg/100 ml below serum	30–50 mg/100 ml below serum	Normal	Normal
Inspection				Fat in aspirate

D Joint fluid evaluation Joint fluid differences can be seen among common causes of joint effusions.

Diagnostic Procedures

Other studies are sometimes helpful.

Electromyography

Electromyography (EMG) is done using either surface or deep electrodes. Surface electrode studies are limited because of artifacts and poor muscle selectivity. The placement of deep electrodes is painful and thus poorly tolerated in children. Furthermore, EMG studies do not show the strength of contraction, only the electrical activity.

EMG is useful in evaluating peripheral nerve injuries, anterior horn cell degeneration, and diseases such as myotonia and myelitis. In peripheral nerve injuries, denervation causes fibrillation potentials 1–2 weeks after injury. During regeneration, the EMG will show polyphasic wave forms. In anterior horn cell degeneration, fasciculations appear.

Nerve Conduction Velocity

Nerve conduction velocity is measured by the time difference shown between the point of stimulation and the recording by EMG. Normal values change with age, from about 25 m/sec at birth to 45 m/sec at age 3 years to about 45–65 m/sec in mid-childhood. The peroneal, posterior tibial, ulnar, median, and facial nerves are usually studied. In children, perform these studies in evaluating peripheral and hereditary neuropathies.

Diagnostic Blocks

Diagnostic blocks are most useful in children for evaluating incisional neuroma and for pain of unknown cause around the foot. By this means, it is possible to localize the site of pain precisely.

Biopsy

The biopsy is an important diagnostic procedure [A], but it is not always a simple process. It is preferable for the same surgeon to perform both the biopsy and any reconstructive or ablative procedures. Planning is important. Generally, open biopsy is routine, with needle biopsy performed for lesions in inaccessible sites such as vertebral bodies. Plan ahead with the lab to coordinate tissue removal [B and C], transfer solutions, frozen sections, and electron microscopic studies. Culture the lesion if there is even the remotest possibility of an infectious etiology [D].

Arthrocentesis

Joint aspiration is diagnostic [E] and sometimes therapeutic. These studies are indicated whenever an infectious etiology is possible.

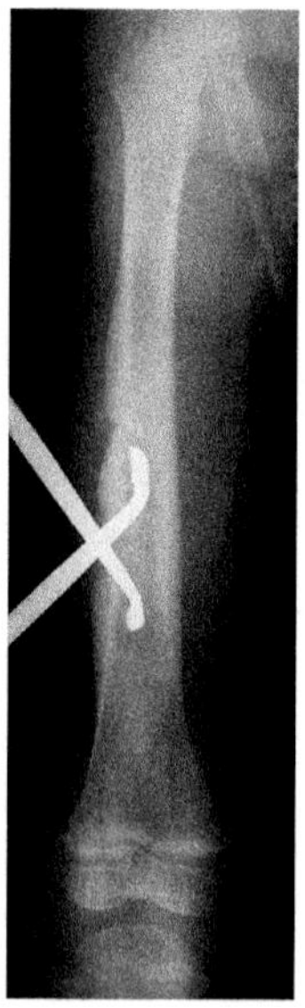

Tissue	Indication
Muscle	Muscular dystrophy Myositis
Bone	Neoplasm, infection
Skin	Osteogenesis imperfecta
Nerve	Neuropathy

A Common indications for biopsy Tissue from bone (left) or other tissues is useful to establish the diagnosis.

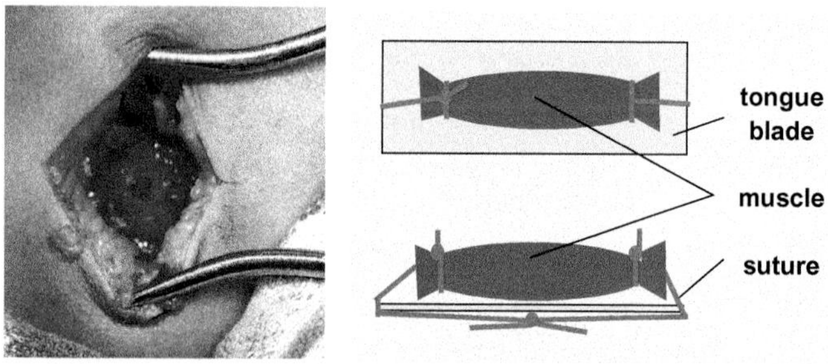

B Technique of muscle biopsy Remove a segment of muscle for biopsy (left). Secure the specimen to a segment of a tongue blade with sutures (blue lines, right) to maintain length and orientation during transport and initial fixation.

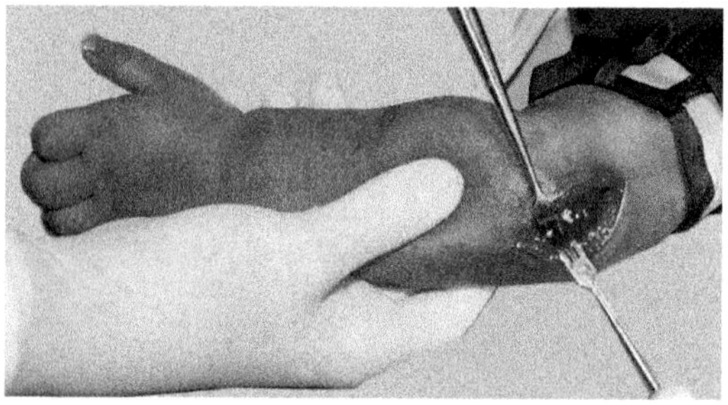

C Biopsy of bone Biopsies are important procedures that require planning, careful technique, and competent pathologic evaluation.

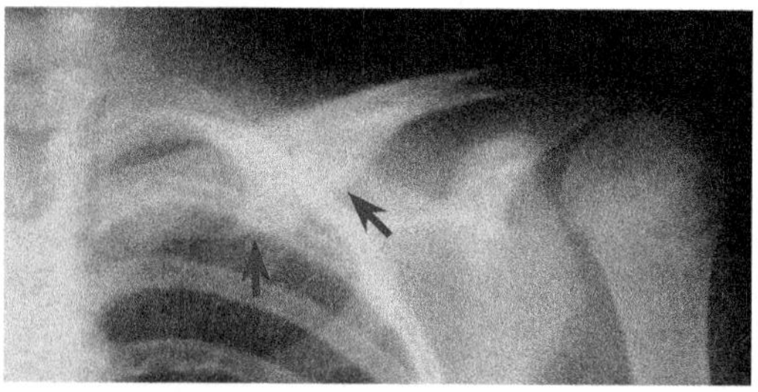

D Osteomyelitis of the clavicle This lesion is often confused with a tumor. Be certain to obtain biopsy cultures.

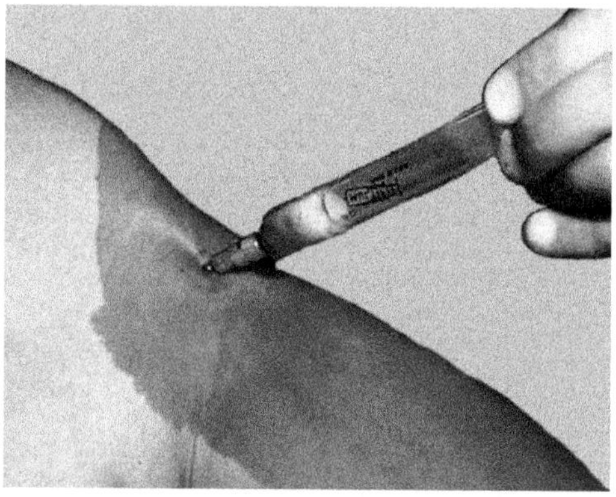

E Arthrocentesis Pus is aspirated from this septic hip.

Time Line

The effect of time and growth on a disorder is called the *time line.* This is also referred to as the *natural history,* or what would happen without treatment. The natural history of many conditions is well known. For instance, we know that nearly all rotational problems resolve with time. Unfortunately, variability from child to child makes the best predictions only estimates. In less common conditions, the course is unknown and the time line is of even greater importance. Sometimes the time line is established by chance [A], but it is usually established by serial radiographs [B, C, and D] or photographs [E]. To establish a time line, document the status of the disorder at intervals. During the first visit, obtain baseline studies. Repeat the studies at intervals, depending on the disease.

A classic example is in physeal bridge management. If a child sustains a medial malleolar Salter type III or IV injury, it is useful to obtain a baseline full-length radiograph of both tibiae on one film. The same study is made at 3-month intervals. A change in relative lengths of the tibia or a tilting of the articular surface of the ankle is early evidence of a physeal bridge.

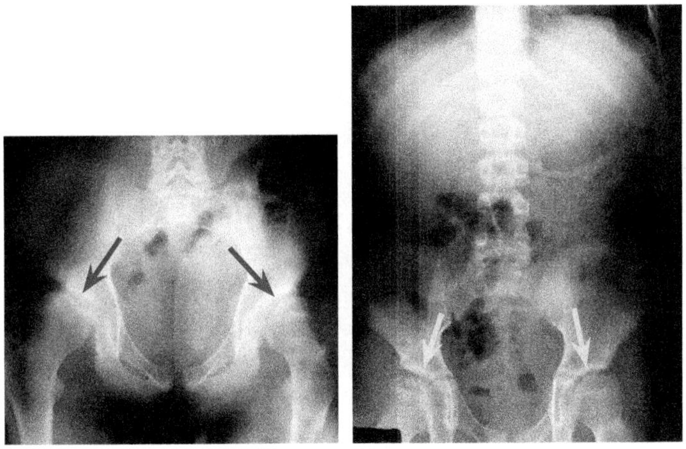

A Chance "time line" This 15-year-old boy was seen for bilateral hip pain. Radiographs demonstrated severe hip dysplasia with subluxation (red arrows). By chance, his old x-ray folder contained an abdominal study that was taken when he was 12 years old. His hips showed only mild dysplasia (yellow arrows) at that age.

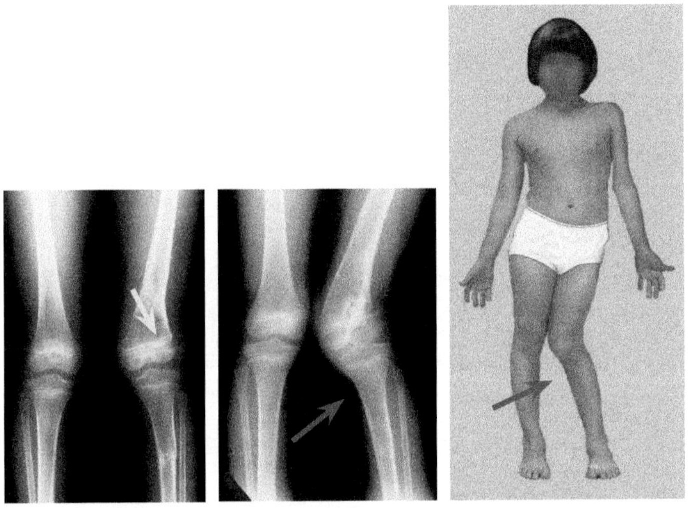

B Effect of growth These radiographs show the effect of time and growth when a physeal bridge is present (yellow arrow). Two years later, this 12-year-old boy shows a dramatic increase in valgus deformity of the knee (red arrows).

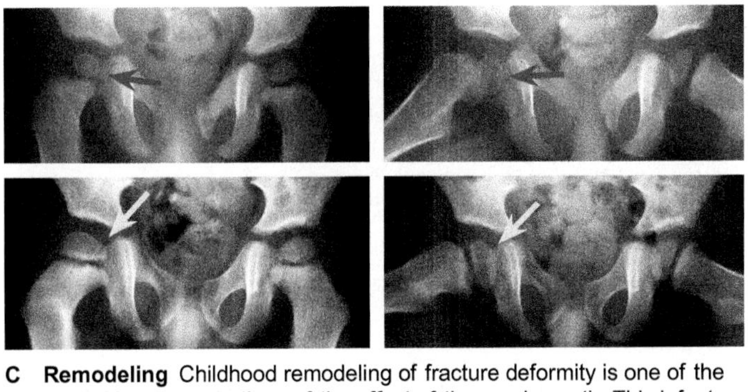

C Remodeling Childhood remodeling of fracture deformity is one of the most graphic demonstrations of the effect of time and growth. This infant sustained a physeal fracture with malunion at 12 months (red arrows). Note the extensive remodeling of the deformity by age 24 months (yellow arrows).

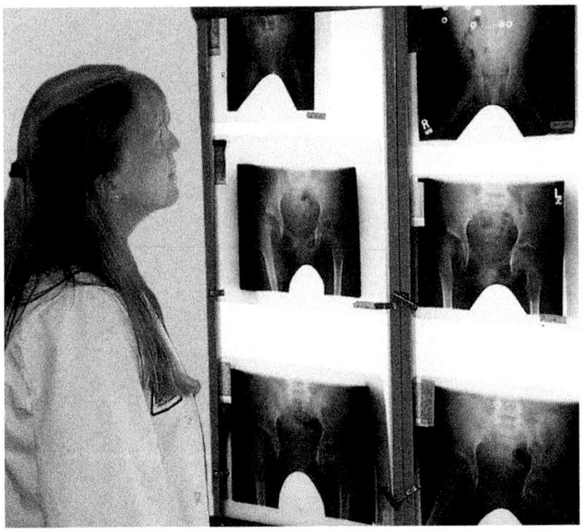

D Time line using radiographs Comparing a sequence of radiographs is a very practical method of assessing the effect of time on deformity.

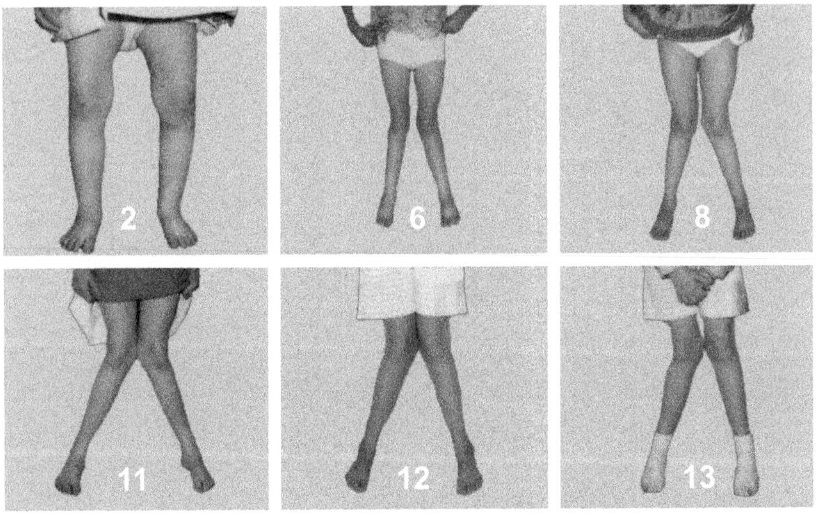

E Time line using photographs In this child with vitamin D-resistant rickets, the progression of the genu valgum deformities at ages 2, 6, 8, 11, 12, and 13 years is illustrated. The family and patient elected to delay correction until 14 years of age to avoid recurrence.

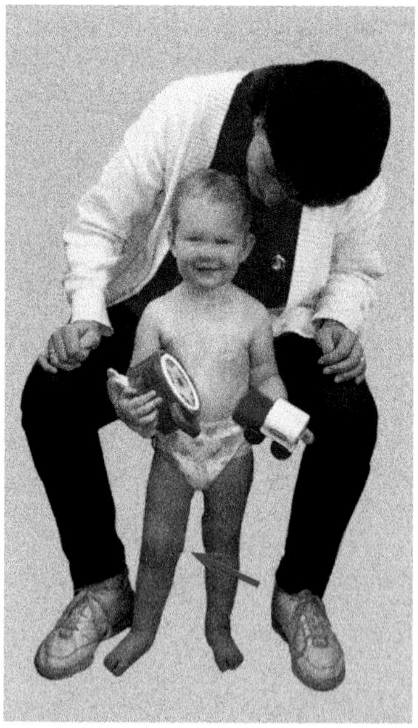

A Oligoarticular juvenile idiopathic arthritis (JIA) This young girl has little discomfort. Note the swollen right knee.

Joint Swelling

Joint inflammation is termed arthritis [A], whereas joint pain without signs of inflammation is referred to as arthralgia. Rheumatologists call pain at ligament and tendon insertions enthesopathy. Arthritis occurs in about 2 in 1000 children. The causes of swollen joints in children are numerous [B]. In most cases, the diagnosis [C] is established through the approach outlined below.

Approach

History Ask the patient and family about systemic symptoms, night pain, morning stiffness, other illnesses, family history, duration, severity, and general health.

Examination Perform a careful screening examination. Is the child systemically ill? Carefully examine all extremities to determine if any other large or small joints are involved. Note the degree of inflammation, localization of tenderness, joint range of motion, and any fixed deformities. Consider an Ophthalmology consultation as iritis is the most serious complication and can be prevented by early diagnosis and treatment.

Laboratory studies If one suspects juvenile rheumatoid arthritis, order a CBC, ESR, CRP, ANA, RF, and urinalysis. Order other studies to help separate your short-list differential diagnosis.

Imaging Start with conventional radiographs and add other studies as appropriate.

Joint aspiration Joint aspiration is indicated if an infectious etiology is included in the differential diagnosis.

Clinical Types

Polyarticular JIA occurs in two clinical patterns [C]: young girls and those in adolescence with multiple small and large joint involvement.

Differential Diagnosis of Arthritis

Primary

Traumatic
- Direct injury—dislocation, fracture
- Slipped capital femoral epiphysis
- Introduction—foreign body synovitis

Infection
- Bacterial
- Lyme disease
- Tuberculosis

Juvenile rheumatoid arthritis
- Systemic JIA
- Polyarticular JIA
- Oligoarticular JIA
- Spondyloarthropathy

Tumors
- Intraarticular hemangiomata
- Pigmented villonodular synovitis

Vascular
- Legg-Calvé-Perthes disease
- Osteochondritis dissecans

Idiopathic
- Toxic synovitis hip

Secondary

Adjacent inflammation
- Osteomyelitis
- Osteoid osteoma

Systemic disorders
- Leukemia
- Hemophilia with joint effusion
- Acute rheumatic fever
- Systemic lupus erythematosis
- Henoch-Schönlein purpura
- Sarcoidosis
- Postinfectious disorders
- Reflex sympathetic dystrophy

B Differential diagnosis of joint swelling and pain

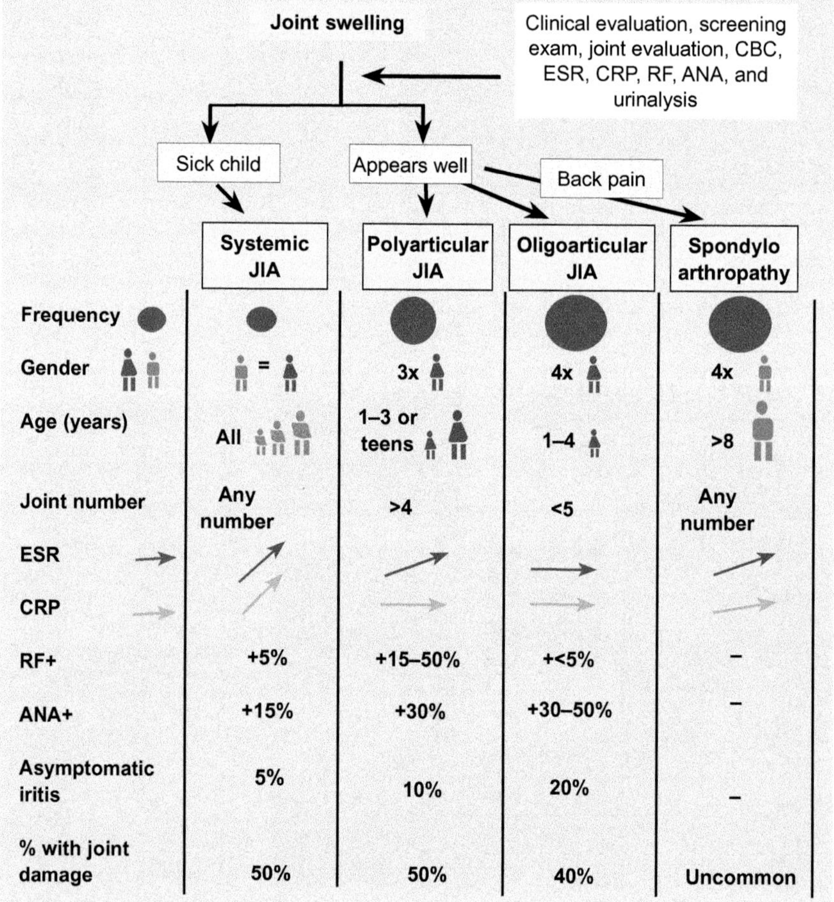

	Systemic JIA	Polyarticular JIA	Oligoarticular JIA	Spondylo arthropathy
Frequency				
Gender	=	3x	4x	4x
Age (years)	All	1–3 or teens	1–4	>8
Joint number	Any number	>4	<5	Any number
ESR	↗	↗	→	↗
CRP	↗	→	→	↗
RF+	+5%	+15–50%	+<5%	–
ANA+	+15%	+30%	+30–50%	–
Asymptomatic iritis	5%	10%	20%	–
% with joint damage	50%	50%	40%	Uncommon

C Differential diagnosis of JIA

Oligoarticular JIA is the most common form of juvenile arthritis. The patient is most likely a 1- to 4-year-old girl [A and C, previous page]. About a quarter have no pain but are seen because of a swollen joint such as the knee, ankle, and fingers. ANA is positive in 70%, RF negative. About 20% have iritis [A]. Early referral of these patients to an ophthalmologist is essential.

Systemic JIA occurs in boys and girls usually between 3 and 10 years [C, previous page]. These children are febrile, toxic; have severe myalgias, enlarged nodes, liver, and spleen; and sometimes have pericarditis, myocarditis, disseminated intravascular coagulation, and polyarthritis [B]. The course of the disease is variable. Some cases resolve in months; others persist, causing joint destruction and disability.

Seronegative spondyloarthropathies Seronegativity is an absence of a rheumatoid factor. These disorders include ankylosing spondylitis, reactive synovitis, Reiter syndrome, and those associated with inflammatory bowel disease and psoriasis. These patients are frequently HLA-B27 positive and are usually adolescent boys. These patients may have low-grade systemic signs of fever, weight loss, and malaise.

Ankylosing spondylitis This condition is most common in adults but does occur in older children. Inflammation involves the spine, SI, and large joints. Back pain and morning stiffness are common complaints. Stiffness on forward bend test is found. Laboratory findings usually include a mildly elevated ESR and CRP, a positive HLA-B27, and negative ANA and RF. Radiographic changes are late.

Reiter syndrome The triad of arthritis, urethritis, and conjunctivitis are usually found. Painful photophobic iritis can occur. The disease usually follows dysentery or a sexually transmitted disease.

Management

Intraarticular triamcinolone hexacetonide (steroid) injections are effective in reducing synovitis and sometimes preventing joint destruction [C].

Systemic agents include ibuprofen, methotrexate, and etanercept. These drugs are best administered by a pediatric rheumatologist.

Joint damage occurs in most types of JIA [D]. Oligoarticular arthritis causes damage, but the interval between onset and damage is longer.

Pitfalls

Confusion with trauma A swollen joint is frequently thought to be secondary to an injury. As injuries are a daily occurrence in the lives of children, a history of an injury is common. Swollen joints are seldom the result of an injury. They require evaluation and an accurate diagnosis.

Iritis can accompany oligoarticular and some polyarticular forms of JIA [E]. The iritis is usually asymptomatic and can lead to blindness. Children with these forms of arthritis should be referred to an ophthalmologist for evaluation. The risk of iritis makes an early diagnosis of arthritis of great importance.

Missing septic etiology Permanent joint damage is most likely to occur quickly from septic arthritis. Septic arthritis of the hip is most difficult to differentiate. Monarticular arthritis of the hip is seldom due to JIA.

Missing leukemia Bone and joint complaints are the initial symptoms in 20% of children with leukemia. Leukemia causes bone pain, systemic illness, high ESR, and anemia.

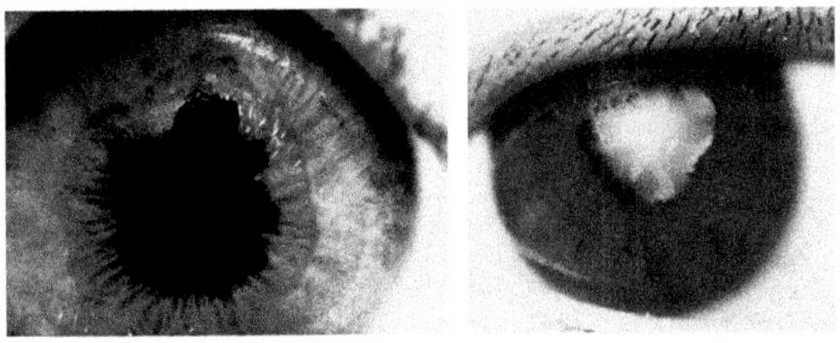

A Features of iritis These photographs show irregularity of the pupil. These are late findings that result from adhesions between the iris and lens. Courtesy DD Sherry.

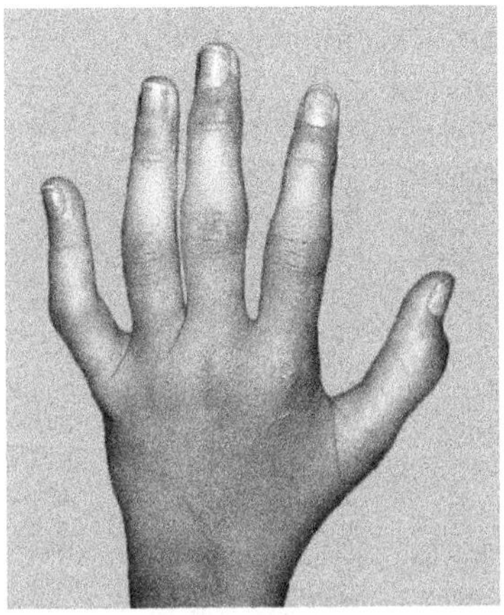

B Hand involvement in systemic JIA Note the swelling of multiple joints.

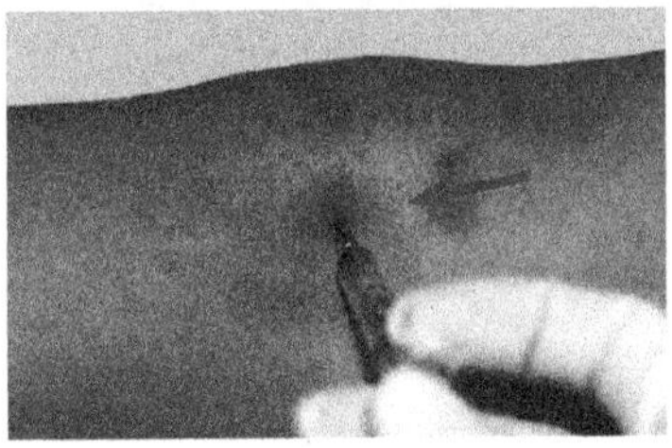

C Joint injections with steroids Injections in JIA affected joints dramatically reduce the synovitis and joint destruction.

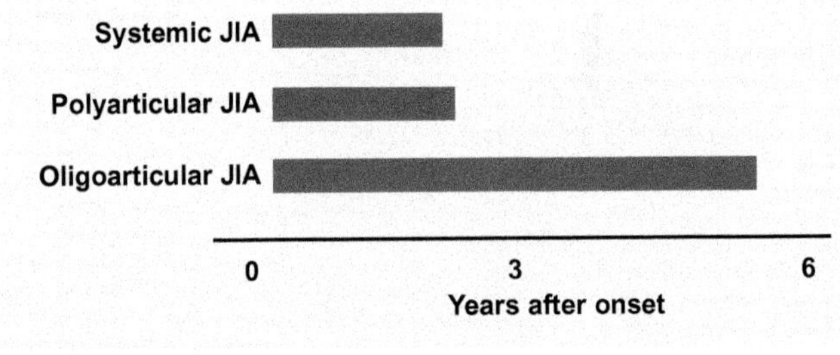

D Time between onset and joint damage Mean time between onset of different types of JIA and onset of joint damage.

Feature	Early	Late
Age	1–4 years	Adolescence
Sex	Girls	Girls
Joint involvement	Varied and symmetrical	Large and small, symmetrical
ANA	Positive	Few
Rheumatoid factor	Negative	Half are positive
Iritis	Uncommon	Half are positive

E Types of polyarticular JIA This shows two types of presentation of polyarticular JIA. From Sherry (1998).

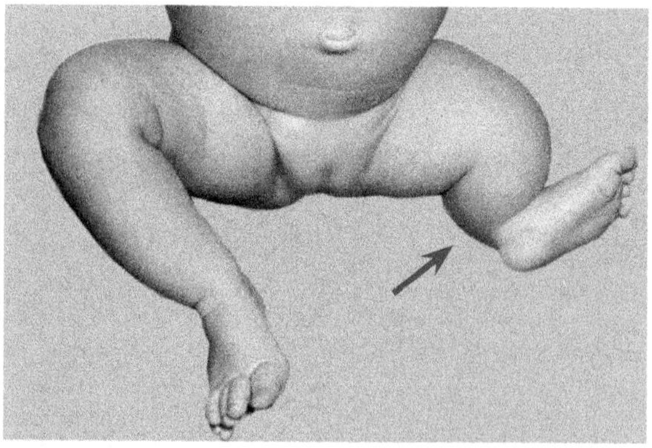

A Tibial deficiency Note the short leg with a normal foot.

Limb Deficiencies

Congenital limb deficiencies occur in about 0.1 to 0.2 in 1000 children, or about one-tenth the frequency of clubfeet or DDH.

Causes

Most deficiencies occur in children who are otherwise normal, and they have no genetic basis. Thalidomide is known to cause multi-limb deficiencies [D]. Most limb deficiencies are sporatic [B and C]. Tibial hemimelia [A] is transmitted as a dominant trait. In other cases, deficiencies are associated with various syndromes such as the radial aplasia–thrombocytopenia syndrome. Acquired amputations result from trauma or treatment of malignant tumors.

Nomenclature

The most widely accepted nomenclature is that of Frantz and O'Rahilly, which divides limb deficiencies into intercalary and terminal types [E]. Every type of deficiency is usually classified [A – F, next page]. These classifications aid in defining severity and indicating treatment methods (see Chapters 8 and 13 for details of treatment).

Prevalence

Males with limb deficiencies outnumber females 3:2, and lower extremities are twice as affected as upper. In 80% of cases, single limbs are involved. Congenital causes are three to four times more frequent than acquired amputations.

Evaluation

Most deficiencies are associated with limb shortening. Order comparative radiographs if a reduction deformity is suspected. Classify the deformity according to the radiographic appearance. Classification is more difficult early on because of lack of ossification. Consider possible associated problems, especially in children with radial deficiencies.

Refer most patients to a limb deficiency clinic. Such clinics provide several important resources for the family: (1) geneticists to evaluate for possible associations and provide family genetic counseling, (2) families to provide support groups, (3) prosthetics to provide often complex fitting problems, and (4) orthopedic surgeons to provide overall management.

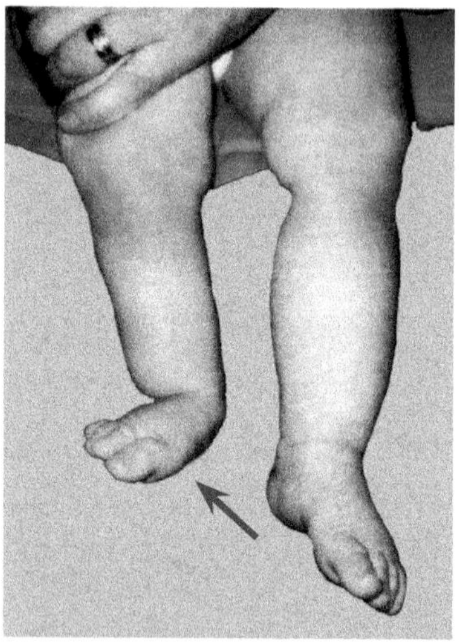

B Fibular deficiency Note the shortening, ankle valgus, and hypoplasia of the foot.

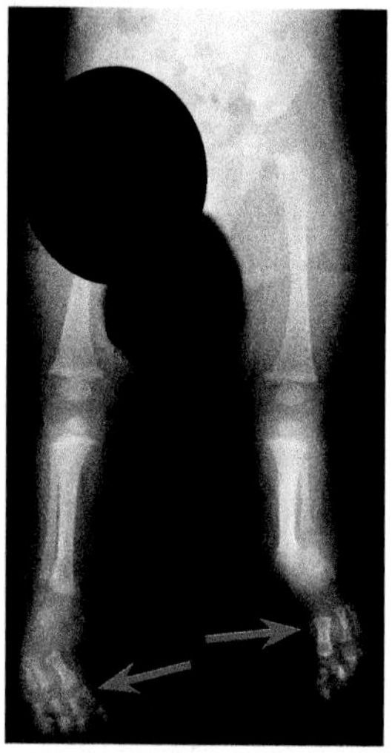

C Fibular deficiency with bilateral three-rayed feet

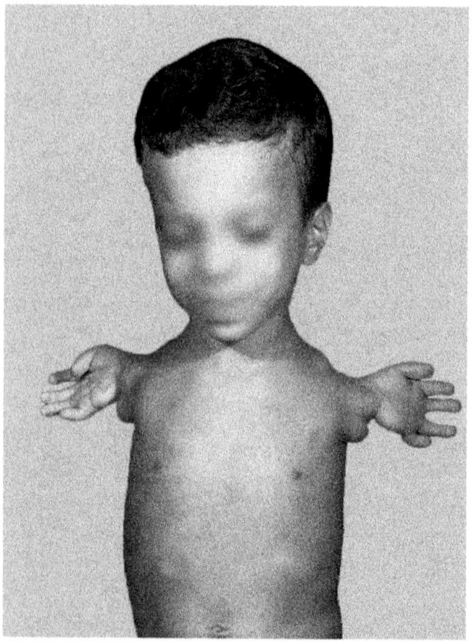

D Phocomelia

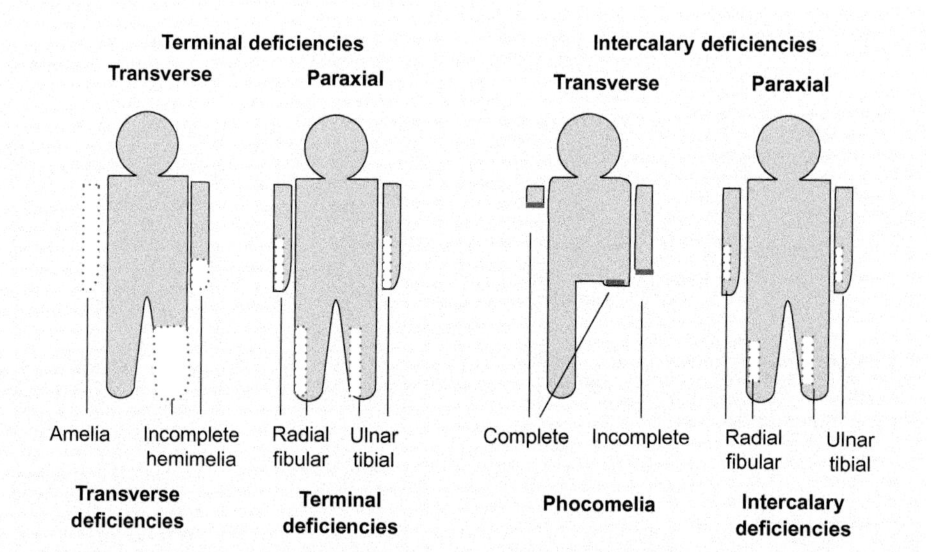

E Frantz–O'Rahilly classification of congenital limb deficiencies

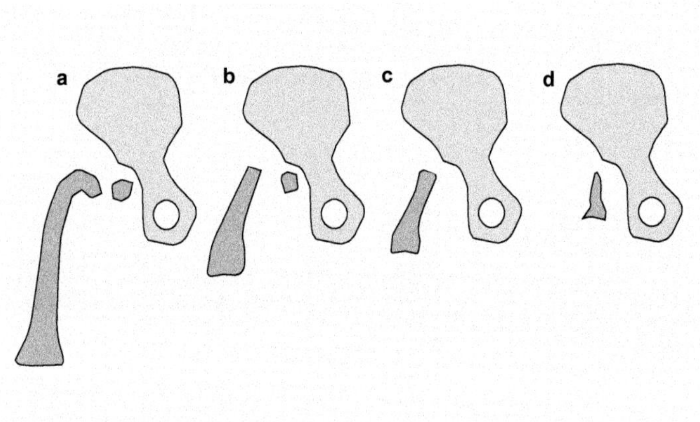

A Proximal focal femoral deficiency (a) Good acetabulum, varus deformity of femur. (b) Fair acetabulum, delayed ossification of femur. (c) Poor acetabulum, femoral head absent, femur very short. (d) No acetabulum, femur nearly absent. Based on Aitken (1968).

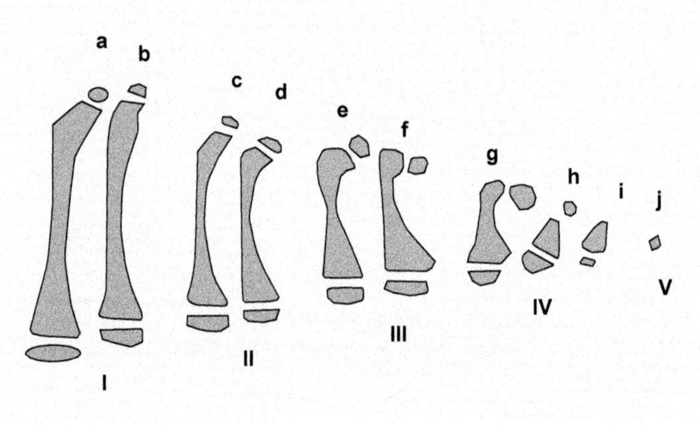

B Spectrum of the congenitally short femur This figure shows the wide variation in deformities included in this classification. Based on Hamanishi, JBJS 62B:569 (1980).

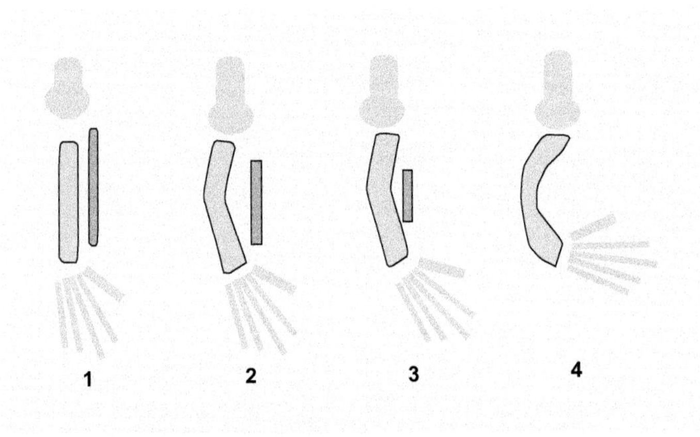

C Heikel classification of radial deficiencies (1) Hypoplasia of distal radius. (2) Distal and proximal shortening and ulnar bowing. (3) Varied ulnar shortening with carpal deviation. (4) Radial aplasia. From Heikel (1959).

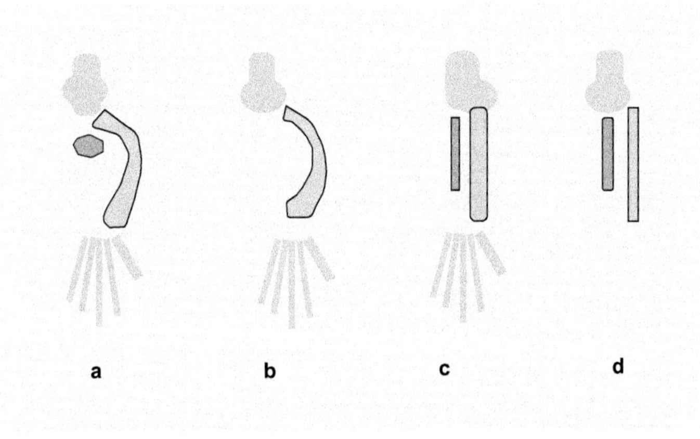

D Swanson classification of ulnar deficiencies (a) Hypoplasia of the ulna. (b) Absence of the ulna. (c) Fusion of the humerus and radius with hypoplasia of the ulna. (d) Hypoplasia of the ulna with absence of the hand. From Swanson et al. (1984).

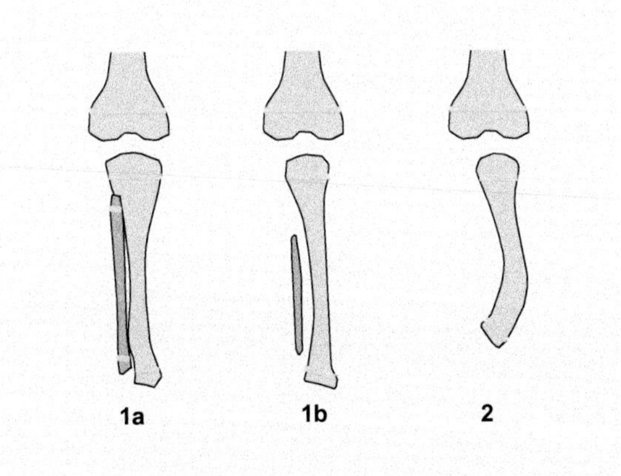

E Fibular deficiency classification Type 1 includes all cases in which some fibula is present. In type 1a, the fibula is short with the proximal fibular physes below that of the tibia and the distal physis above the ankle. In type 1b, the fibula is significantly shortened and not supporting the ankle. In type 2, no fibula is present. From Achterman and Kalamchi, JBJS 61B:133 (1979).

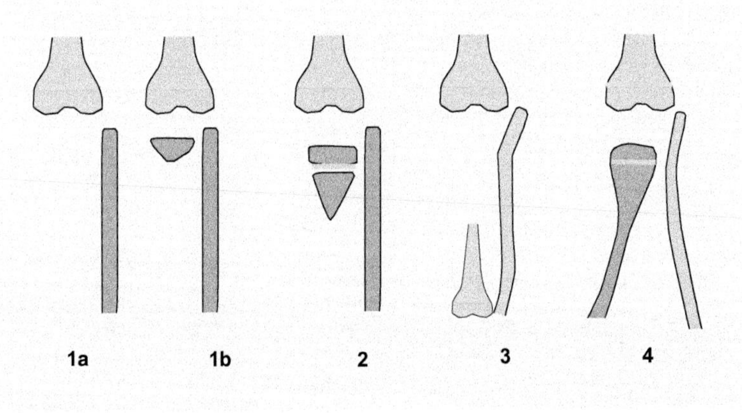

F Tibial deficiency classification (1a) The tibia is not seen. (1b) Tibia seen on MRI or ultrasound. (2) Distal tibia not seen. (3) Proximal tibia not seen. (4) Diastasis. Based on Jones et al., JBJS 60B:31 (1978).

Aboulafia AJ, Levin AM, Blum J. Prereferral evaluation of patients with suspected bone and soft tissue tumors. Clin Orthop 2002 Apr;(397): p83-8.

Aitken GT, Proximal femoral focal deficiency–definition, classification, and management. In: Symposium Washington DC June 13, 1968. pp 1-22, National Academy of Sciences, Washington DC.

Aktas S, Aiona MD, Orendurff M. Evaluation of rotational gait abnormality in patients with cerebral palsy. J Pediatr Orthop 2000 Mar-Apr;20(2): p217-20.

Bartlett MD, Wolf LS, Shurtleff DB, et al. Hip flexion contractures: A comparison of measurement methods. Arch Phys Med Rehabil 1985;66:620-625.

Belmont PJ, Kuklo TR, Taylor KF, Freedman BA, Prahinski JR, Kruse RW. Intraspinal anomalies associated with isolated congenital hemivertebra: the role of routine magnetic resonance imaging. J Bone Joint Surg Am 2004 Aug;86-A(8): p1704-10.

Breugem CC, Maas M, Breugem SJ, Schaap GR, van der Horst CM. Vascular malformations of the lower limb with osseous involvement. J Bone Joint Surg Br 2003 Apr;85(3): p399-405.

Caskey PM, Lester EL. Association of fibular hemimelia and clubfoot. J Pediatr Orthop 2002 Jul-Aug;22(4): p522-5.

Choi IH, Lipton GE, Mackenzie W, Bowen JR, Kumar SJ. Wedge-shaped distal tibial epiphysis in the pathogenesis of equinovalgus deformity of the foot and ankle in tibial lengthening for fibular hemimelia. J Pediatr Orthop 2000 Jul-Aug;20(4): p428-36.

Christensen CP, Ferguson RL. Lower extremity deformities associated with thrombocytopenia and absent radius syndrome. Clin Orthop 2000 Jun;(375): p202-6.

Coleman SS, Chesnut WJ. A simple test for hindfoot flexibility in cavovarus foot. CO 123:60 1977.

Devitt AT, O'Donnell T, Fogarty EE, Dowling FE, Moore DP. Tibial hemimelia of a different class. J Pediatr Orthop 2000 Sep-Oct;20(5): p616-22.

Erlich MG, Zaleske DJ. Pediatric orthopedic pain of unknown origin. J Pediatr Orthop 1986;460-468.

Farley FA, Kuhns L, Jacobson JA, Di Pietro M. Ultrasound examination of ankle injuries in children. J Pediatr Orthop 2001 Sep-Oct;21(5): p604-7.

Fixsen JA. Major lower limb congenital shortening: a mini review. J Pediatr Orthop B 2003 Jan;12(1): p1-12.

Flynn JM, Closkey RF, Mahboubi S, Dormans JP. Role of magnetic resonance imaging in the assessment of pediatric cervical spine injuries. J Pediatr Orthop 2002 Sep-Oct;22(5): p573-7.

Flynn JM, Mackenzie W, Kolstad K, Sandifer E, Jawad AF, Galinat B. Objective evaluation of knee laxity in children. J Pediatr Orthop 2000 Mar-Apr;20(2): p259-63.

Fujii H, Doi K, Baliarsing AS. Transtibial amputation with plantar flap for congenital deficiency of the tibia. Clin Orthop 2002 Oct;(403): p186-90.

Graham HK, Harvey A, Rodda J, Nattrass GR, Pirpiris M. The Functional Mobility Scale (FMS). J Pediatr Orthop 2004 Sep-Oct;24(5): p514-20.

Greulich WW, Pyle SI. Radiographic atlas of skeletal development of the hand and wrist. 2nd ed. Stanford, CA, Stanford University Press, 1959:50.

Hempfing A, Placzek R, Gottsche T, Meiss AL. Primary subacute epiphyseal and metaepiphyseal osteomyelitis in children. diagnosis and treatment guided by MRI. J Bone Joint Surg Br 2003 May;85(4): p559-64.

Hubner U, Schlicht W, Outzen S, Barthel M, Halsband H. Ultrasound in the diagnosis of fractures in children. J Bone Joint Surg Br 2000 Nov;82(8): p1170-3.

James MA, Green HD, McCarroll HR, Manske PR. The association of radial deficiency with thumb hypoplasia. J Bone Joint Surg Am 2004 Oct;86-A(10): p2196-205.

Kara CS, Toros T. Congenital deficiency of the tibia: a report of 22 cases. J Pediatr Orthop B 2001 Apr;10(2): p161-3.

Kawaguchi AT, Otsuka NY, Delgado ED, Genant HK, Lang P. Magnetic resonance arthrography in children with developmental hip dysplasia. Clin Orthop 2000 May;(374): p235-46.

Kevern L; Warwick D; Wellesley D; Senbaga R; Clarke NM. Prenatal ultrasound: detection and diagnosis of limb abnormalities. J Pediatr Orthop 2003 Mar-Apr;23(2): p251-3.

Kokavec M, Makai F, Maresch P. Present status of screening and prevention of developmental dysplasia of the hip in the Slovak Republic. J Pediatr Orthop B 2003 Mar;12(2): p106-8.

Kozin SH. Correlation between external rotation of the glenohumeral joint and deformity after brachial plexus birth palsy. J Pediatr Orthop 2004 Mar-Apr;24(2): p189-93.

Loder RT, Greenfield ML. Clinical characteristics of children with atypical and idiopathic slipped capital femoral epiphysis: description of the age-weight test and implications for further diagnostic investigation. J Pediatr Orthop 2001 Jul-Aug;21(4): p481-7.

Maenpaa H, Kuusela P, Lehtinen J, Savolainen A, Kautiainen H, Belt E. Elbow synovectomy on patients with juvenile rheumatoid arthritis. Clin Orthop 2003 Jul;(412): p65-70.

Mazur JM, et al. Usefulness of magnetic resonance imaging for the diagnosis of acute musculoskeletal infections in children. JPO 1995;15:144.

McCarthy JJ, Glancy GL, Chnag FM, Eilert RE. Fibular hemimelia: comparison of outcome measurements after amputation and lengthening. J Bone Joint Surg Am 2000 Dec;82-A(12): p1732-5.

McMulkin ML, Gulliford JJ, Williamson RV, Ferguson R. Correlation of static to dynamic measures of lower extremity range of motion in cerebral palsy and control populations. J Pediatr Orthop 2000 May-Jun;20(3): p366-9.

Mirovsky Y, Jakim I, Halperin N, Lev L. Non-specific back pain in children and adolescents: a prospective study until maturity. J Pediatr Orthop Br 2002 Oct;11(4): p275-8.

Nnadi C, Chawla T, Redfern A, Argent J, Fairhurst J, Clarke N. Radiograph evaluation in children with acute hip pain. J Pediatr Orthop 2002 May-Jun;22(3): p342-4.

Noonan KJ, Halliday S, Browne R, O'Brien S, Kayes K, Feinberg J. Interobserver variability of gait analysis in patients with cerebral palsy. J Pediatr Orthop 2003 May-Jun;23(3): p279-87; discussion 288-91.

Parvizi J, Lajam CM, Trousdale RT, Shaughnessy WJ, Cabanela ME. Total knee arthroplasty in young patients with juvenile rheumatoid arthritis. J Bone Joint Surg Am 2003 Jun;85-A(6): p1090-4.

Patel M, Paley D, Herzenberg JE. Limb-lengthening versus amputation for fibular hemimelia. J Bone Joint Surg Am 2002 Feb;84-A(2): p317-9.

Pearl ML, Edgerton BW, Kon DS, Darakjian AB, Kosco AE, Kazimiroff PB, Burchette RJ. Comparison of arthroscopic findings with magnetic resonance imaging and arthrography in children with glenohumeral deformities secondary to brachial plexus birth palsy. J Bone Joint Surg Am 2003 May;85-A(5): p890-8.

Pill SG, Ganley TJ, Milam RA, Lou JE, Meyer JS, Flynn JM. Role of magnetic resonance imaging and clinical criteria in predicting successful nonoperative treatment of osteochondritis dissecans in children. J Pediatr Orthop 2003 Jan-Feb;23(1): p102-8.

Prahinski JR, Polly DW, McHale KA, Ellenbogen RG. Occult intraspinal anomalies in congenital scoliosis. J Pediatr Orthop 2000 Jan-Feb;20(1): p59-63.

Rao KN, Joseph B. Value of measurement of hip movements in childhood hip disorders. J Pediatr Orthop 2001 Jul-Aug;21(4): p495-501.

Saraph V, Zwick EB, Zwick G, Steinwender C, Steinwender G, Linhart W. Multilevel surgery in spastic diplegia: evaluation by physical examination and gait analysis in 25 children. J Pediatr Orthop 2002 Mar-Apr;22(2): p150-7.

Sauer ST, Farrell E, Geller E, Pizzutillo PD. Septic arthritis in a patient with juvenile rheumatoid arthritis. Clin Orthop 2004 Jan;(418): p219-21.

Searle CP, Hildebrand RK, Lester EL, Caskey PM. Findings of fibular hemimelia syndrome with radiographically normal fibulae. J Pediatr Orthop Br 2004 May;13(3): p184-8.

Sherry DD. What's new in the diagnosis and treatment of juvenile rheumatoid arthritis. J Pediatr Orthop 2000 Jul-Aug;20(4): p419-20.

Skytta E, Savolainen A, Kautiainen H, Lehtinen J, Belt EA. Treatment of leg length discrepancy with temporary epiphyseal stapling in children with juvenile idiopathic arthritis during 1957-99. Pediatr Orthop 2003 May-Jun;23(3): p378-80.

Staheli LT. Fever following trauma in childhood. JAMA 1967;199:503-504.

Staheli LT. Strontium 87m scanning. Early diagnosis of bone and joint infections in children. JAMA 1972;221:1159.

Staheli LT. The prone hip extension test: a method of measuring hip flexion deformity. Clin Orthop 1977;123:12-15.

Stanitski DF, Stanitski CL. Fibular hemimelia: a new classification system. J Pediatr Orthop 2003 Jan-Feb;23(1): p30-4.

Stansfield BW, Hillman SJ, Hazlewood ME, Lawson AA, Mann AM, Loudon IR, Robb JE. Normalized speed, not age, characterizes ground reaction force patterns in 5-to 12-year-old children walking at self-selected speeds. J Pediatr Orthop 2001 May-Jun;21(3): p395-402.

Stevens PM, Arms D. Postaxial hypoplasia of the lower extremity. J Pediatr Orthop 2000 Mar-Apr;20(2): p166-72.

Straw R, Chell J, Dhar S. Adduction sign in pediatric hip arthrography. J Pediatr Orthop 2002 May-Jun;22(3): p350-1.

Sutherland DH, Olshen R, Cooper L, et al. The development of mature gait. J Bone Joint Surg 1980;62A:336.

Sutherland DH, Olshen R, Cooper L, et al. The pathomechanics of gait in Duchenne muscular dystrophy. Dev Med Child Neurol 1982;23:3.

Sutherland DH. Gait disorders in childhood and adolescence. Baltimore: Williams & Wilkins, 1984:631.

Takagi T, Mitani S, Aoki K, Miyake A, Inoue H. Three-dimensional assessment of the hip joint by two-directional arthrography. J Pediatr Orthop 2002 Mar-Apr;22(2): p232-8.

Treadwell MC, Stanitski CL, King M. Prenatal sonographic diagnosis of clubfoot: implications for patient counseling. JPO 1999;19:8.

Vocke-Hell AK, Schmid A. Sonographic differentiation of stable and unstable lateral condyle fractures of the humerus in children. J Pediatr Orthop Br 2001 Apr;10(2): p138-41.

Wientroub S, et al. Prenatal sonographic diagnosis of musculoskeletal disorders. JPO 1999;19:1.

Wong-Chung J, Bagali M, Kaneker S. Physical signs in pyomyositis presenting as a painful hip in children: a case report and review of the literature. J Pediatr Orthop Br 2004 May;13(3): p211-3.

Woods D, Macnicol M. The flexion-adduction test: an early sign of hip disease. J Pediatr Orthop B 2001 Jul;10(3): p180-5.

Zwick EB, Saraph V, Linhart WE, Steinwender G. Propulsive function during gait in diplegic children: evaluation after surgery for gait improvement. J Pediatr Orthop B 2001 Jul;10(3): p226-33.

Management

CHAPTER 3

This chapter covers the principles of management. Details for each topic are provided in later chapters.

When to Refer

The decision when to refer is a critical decision facing primary care providers. As cost containment is an increasingly important challenge, making this decision is important and sometimes difficult [A].

Managing the Family

Skill in dealing with the parents and family is essential in providing optimum care for the child. This requires professional competence, patience, and empathy for child and family. Dealing with parents is often the area of greatest difficulty for the orthopedic resident. Developing appreciation, sensitivity, and skill in communicating with parents and the ability to calm their anxieties are essential skills in dealing effectively with the child's problem.

Child

The child's overall well-being is the primary objective of management. Doing what is best for the child requires respect for the inherent value of childhood as an important time of life. Childhood is more than just a preparatory period of life; it has intrinsic value [B]. Moreover, unnecessary interference with the child's life deprives the child of important life experiences. This concept is especially important in pediatric orthopedics, where the physician often deals with chronic disease; "medicalization" of childhood is a serious risk. We may create what is referred to as the vulnerable child syndrome. These children are often harmed by unnecessary restrictions. Some philosophical and practical guidelines are given here:

Resist the pressure to treat the child simply to satisfy the parents or just to "do something." This is harmful to the child, disruptive to the family, expensive for society, and poor medical practice.

Order treatment only when intervention is both necessary and effective In the past, treatment was commonly prescribed for conditions that resolve spontaneously, such as intoeing, flexible flatfeet, and physiological bowlegs. Observational management, a policy of monitoring the child's condition with minimum intervention, provides optimum care for a large percentage of pediatric orthopedic problems. It is least disruptive to the child's and family's life and generates a reputation of honesty and competence for the physician.

Emergent Conditions	Urgent Conditions
Trauma	**Trauma**
Any dislocation	Any epiphyseal fracture
Open fracture	Nondisplaced elbow fracture
Vascular compromise	Reduced patellar dislocation
Fracture base of distal phalanx	Possible malignant tumor
Any compartment syndrome	**Cast complication**
Infection	Wet
Any possible bone and joint infection	Breakage
Necrotizing soft tissue infection	Painful (possible pressure area)
Other	**Postoperative concern**
Possible slipped capital femoral epiphysis	Excessive pain
	Wound dehiscence

A Guidelines on when to refer These tables were created by Brenda Eng, ARNP (see page ii) to help with these important decisions (2014).

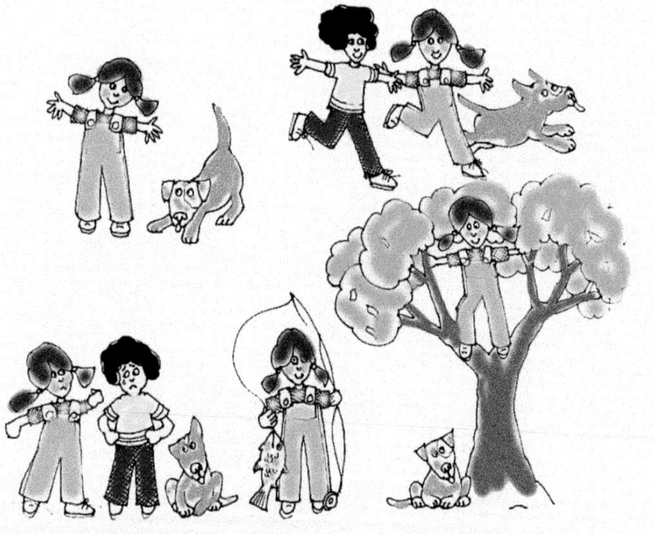

B Play is the occupation of the child Childhood is the time for varied experiences and has intrinsic value.

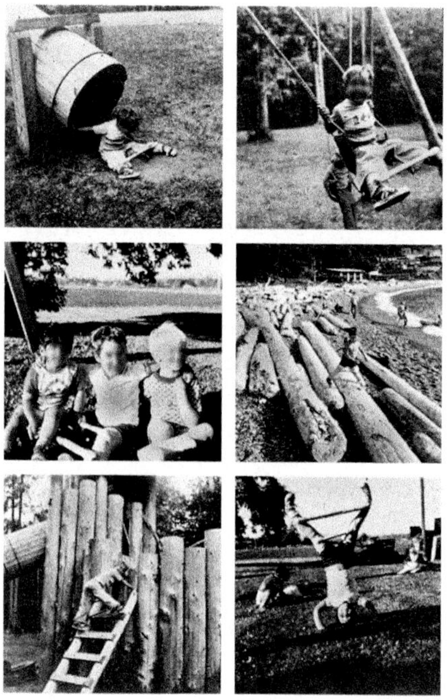

A Integrate treatment with play Encourage families to have their children participate in physically active play during treatment. These pictures were taken by a mother who achieved this goal.

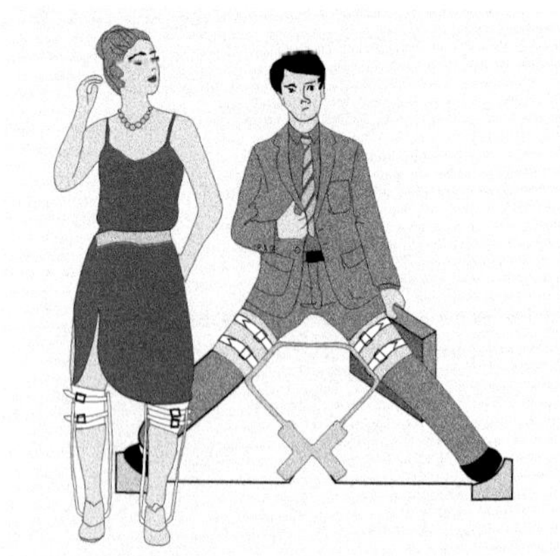

B Child's treatment may be unacceptable for adults Treatment that has been commonly prescribed for children, such as twister cables for intoeing girls or Perthes disease braces for boys, would never be accepted by an adult patient.

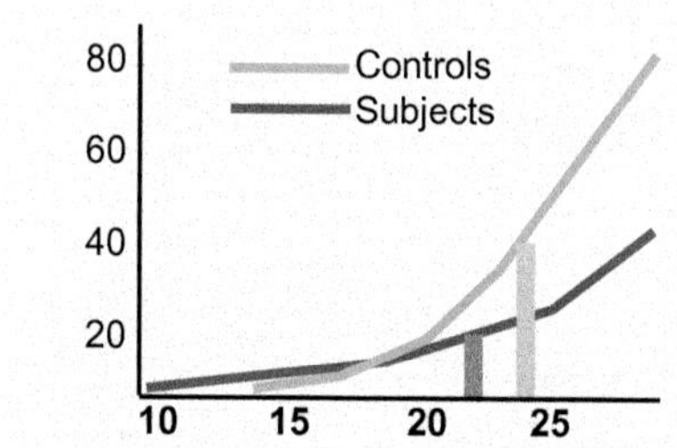

C Orthopedic treatments and self-image Adults who wore corrective devices as children (red) showed a significantly lowered self-image compared to controls (green). From Driano, Staheli, and Staheli (1988).

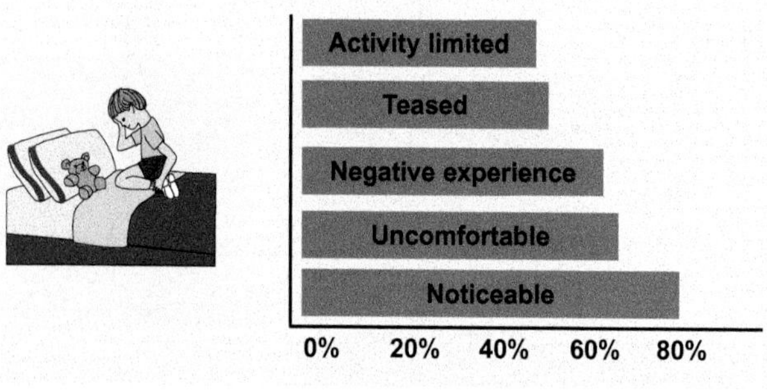

D Recollections Percentage of adults recalling experience about wearing orthopedic devices during childhood. From Driano, Staheli, and Staheli (1998).

Limit the child's activity only after thoughtful consideration Play is the primary occupation of the child. Unnecessary restriction denies the child play experiences vital to enjoying childhood and developing critical skills. In some situations, the physician may need to curb the parents' tendency to overprotect the child. It may be in the child's best interest to risk injury rather than to have long-term constraints on natural activity [A].

Avoid medicalization of the handicapped child Overtreatment can further limit the child and overwhelm the family. Excessive numbers of physician's visits, operations, therapies, braces, and other treatments will result in a large share of the child's life being expended on treatment that may provide little or no benefit.

Before considering any treatment, consider the child as a whole Treatment methods readily prescribed for children would never be accepted by an adult [B]. Orthopedic treatment can be damaging to the individual's self-image [C] and be uncomfortable or embarrassing for the child [D]. Make certain that the anticipated benefits of treatment exceed the harmful psychological, social, and physical effects on the child.

Care of the child requires the highest medical standard The results of treating a child, whether good or bad, may remain with the patient for 70 years or more.

Parents

Dealing with parents is an essential part of a pediatric practice [E]. Each family has certain rights, such as privacy, that must be respected, as well as differing needs and values.

Family coping ability should be respected. Respect the family's resources concerning time, energy, and money. A handicapped child adds stress and complexity for any family. Balance the treatment plan and the family's resources. Consider the well-being of the other children and the health of the marriage; if these are marginal, it may be prudent to order only essential treatment. At different times during management, encourage questions and discuss progress with the family. Being sensitive to the coping ability of the family is part of the physician's responsibility. Demanding more than the family can handle results in noncompliance that may be more the fault of the physician than the family.

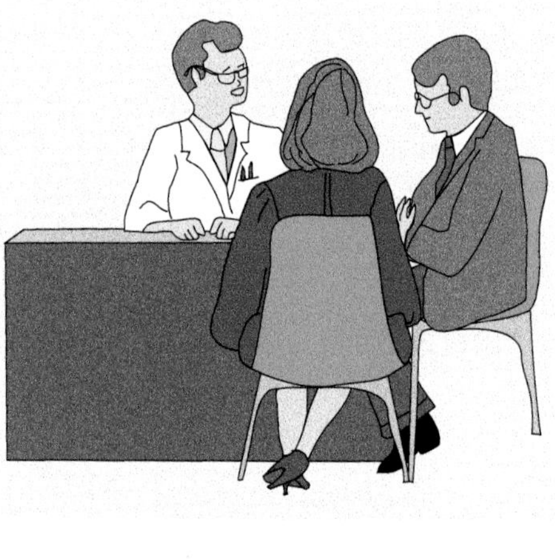

E Parent discussions Take the families' concerns seriously. Allow enough time to explain the disease and treatment options thoroughly.

Informed consent should be part of all management, whether surgical or not. The family has the right to know the pros and cons of the management alternatives. The physician's influence is greater with adults as parents than as patients. Most parents are very sensitive to the possibility that the child's current condition may cause some disability in adult life. Certain words, such as "arthritis," "crippled," and "pain," have a powerful effect on parents and should be used with caution. For example, in the past, many rotational osteotomies were performed to correct femoral antetorsion under the assumption that the procedure would prevent arthritis of the hip. Although the prophylactic value of the procedure was uncertain, parents readily gave their consent under the presumed threat of arthritis [A]. Several recent studies have shown no relationship between femoral antetorsion and arthritis.

Support and reassurance should be provided for patients and parents. In managing common resolving problems such as intoeing [B], reassurance is the main treatment. With more serious problems, reassurance may take the form of providing information that dispels the parents' fears about the future. In critical conditions, reassurance consists of assuring the family that you will support them throughout the disease. The process of providing effective support and reassurance involves several steps:

Make certain that you understand the family's concerns and take these concerns seriously.

Conduct a thorough evaluation of the child Pay attention to the family's specific concerns. For example, if they are anxious about the way the child runs, be certain that you observe the child running in the hallway.

Provide information about the condition, especially the natural history. Make copies of appropriate pages of what families should know for the family to take home and show other family members.

Offer to follow the problem in the future Not all positional deformities resolve with time. Offer to see the child again if the family has additional concerns. If the family is obviously apprehensive, or there is someone in the family who is the major source of concerns, such as the grandmother, it may be necessary to provide reassurance repeatedly. For example, suggest that the grandmother accompany the child during the next visit.

If the family is still unconvinced, suggest a consultation An offer to refer the child usually increases the family's confidence in the physician. Be certain to communicate to the consultant the family's need for reassurance and not that you are recommending some treatment.

Avoid submitting to family pressure for treatment that is not medically indicated Performing unnecessary or ineffective procedures because of family pressure is never appropriate.

Procedures are a source of family stress. Whether the family should be present during procedures, such as joint aspiration, should be managed individually. Some parents prefer not to be present; others insist on being with the child. Whenever possible, give the family a choice. Be aware that if the parents are present, one of them (usually the father) may feel ill or dizzy and need to lie down. More often, a parent can help calm the child [C and D]. Moreover, the presence of parents helps to prevent feelings of abandonment in the child. In summary, even though the parents' presence may add a complicating factor for the physician, it may be of benefit to the child.

Litigious problems are fortunately less common in pediatrics compared with other orthopedic subspecialities. However, the legal exposure period for the physician is much longer, because the statute of limitations usually starts at the age of majority. Medical competence, attention to detail, and good rapport with the family are the best protective measures. Additional measures include complete records, generous use of consultants, and avoidance of nonstandard treatments. If an unusual or tragic incident occurs, document the circumstances honestly and thoroughly. Be especially attentive to the family at this time and respond quickly to their concerns.

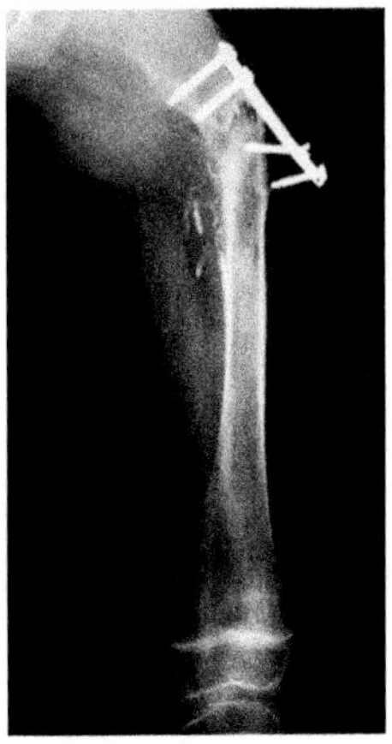

A Complications of rotational osteotomy This patient underwent an osteotomy for correction of femoral antetorsion. He developed a streptococcal wound infection. This was further complicated by failure of the fixation, nonunion, osteomyelitis, and limb shortening. He had 13 operations to manage complications.

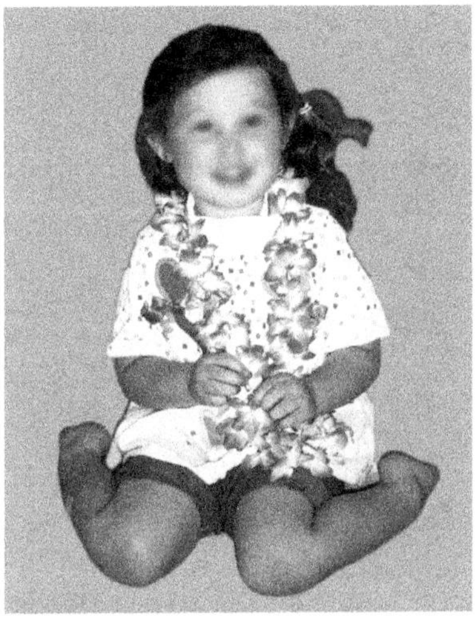

B Femoral antetorsion improves with growth This is considered a variation of normal that requires no treatment.

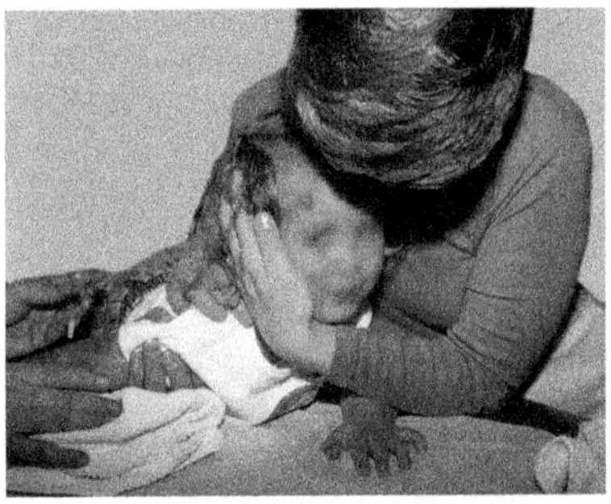

C Procedures are less stressful in a supportive environment Often the mother is best able to comfort the child.

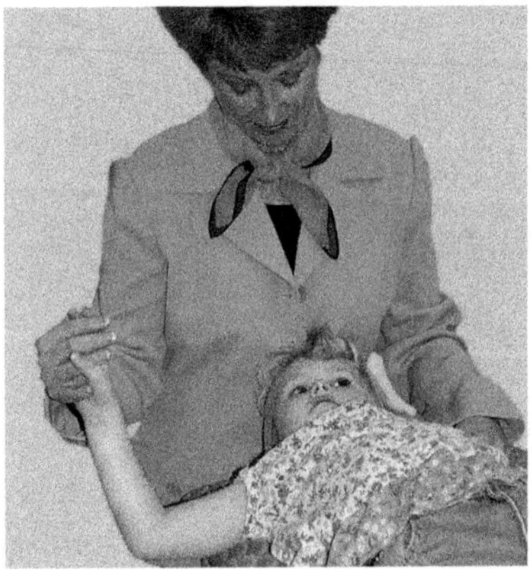

D Supportive measures during casting Ongoing support of the child during simple procedures calms and quiets the child.

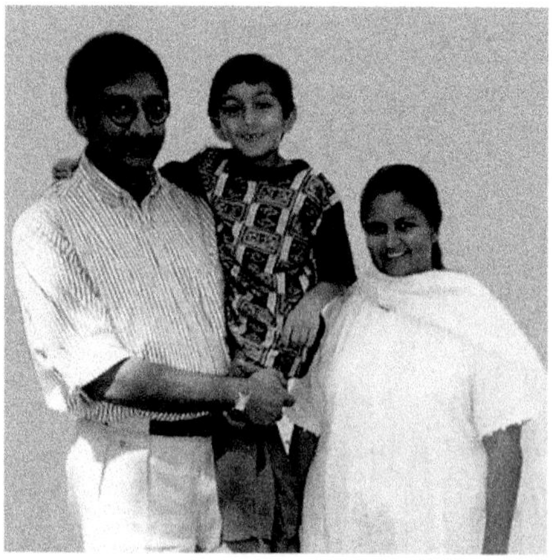

A Religious beliefs Respect the family's right to make or at least influence medical decisions that do not compromise the child's treatment.

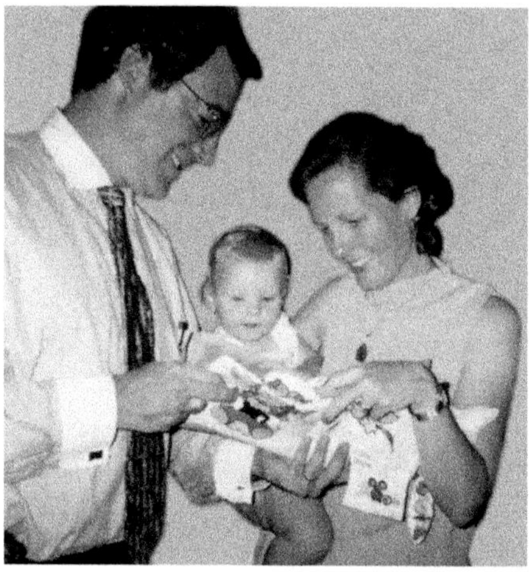

B Family's values Incorporate these values in planning management.

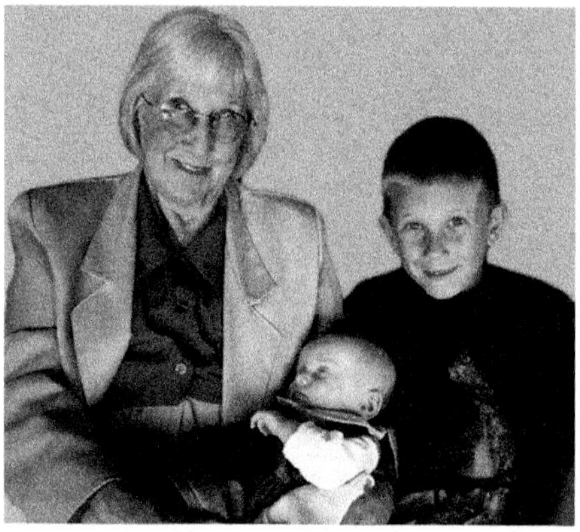

C Grandparents in the clinic This grandmother is very well informed and an asset in helping the parents deal with their children's problems.

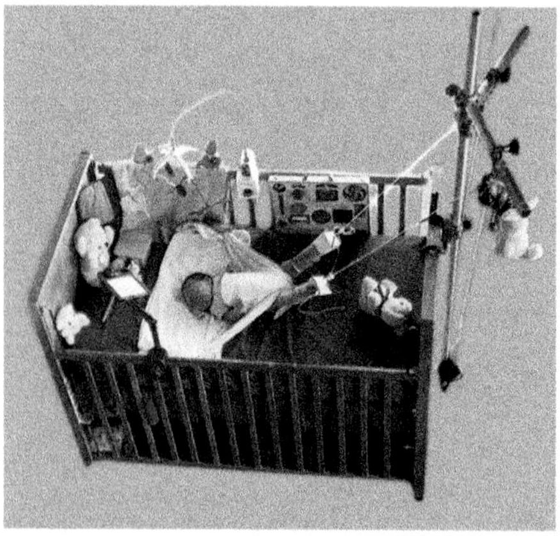

D Home traction Home treatment programs provide cost-effective and convenient management.

Religious beliefs may affect the physician's management. Religious beliefs should be respected to the extent that they do not compromise the child's treatment [A]. Discuss the parents' beliefs and concerns openly. Issues regarding blood replacement are common. Alternatives are possible, so do not victimize the child by taking a rigid position against the family. With planning, careful technique, hypotensive anesthesia, and staging if necessary, nearly all orthopedic procedures can be managed without blood replacement. Some families will want a period of time for prayer before giving consent for an operative procedure. Unless time is critical, a negotiated delay is appropriate. Establish a time limit and determine some objective outcome measures in advance.

Family values should be incorporated into the management plan. For some medical conditions, management indications are unclear or controversial. Inform the family of the situation and discuss the choices openly so that the management is consistent with the family's values [B]. Family feelings about operative procedures, bracing, therapy, and other treatment methods vary considerably. The family's feelings and values should be respected but should not supersede the delivery of optimal medical care. Performing an operation that is medically not indicated because of family insistence is not appropriate.

Difficult families may tax the physician's ability to deal with the parents' reaction to their child's illness. The parents may become overprotective or, conversely, may abandon the child. Some parents become abusive toward the physician and staff. Be sure that the parents' behavior does not adversely affect your management of the child. Be understanding but firm, and when appropriate, support abused staff members. Write a note in the chart summarizing the parents' behavior.

Grandparents often accompany the child to the clinic [C]. Grandmothers are often concerned about infants' flatfeet, intoeing, or bowlegs. In the grandmother's child-rearing era, positional problems were poorly understood and routinely treated. Overcoming such misconceptions requires a willingness to respectfully explain the reasons for current management.

Unorthodox methods of care by nonphysician practitioners are often considered by parents. Such practitioners usually prescribe treatment, and the treatment often continues over a long period of time. By current standards, such treatments are generally unnecessary and ineffective. Moreover, the treatment may delay necessary treatment. Avoid criticism when discussing these "treatments" with the family; instead, focus on parent education. This is much more effective than criticism. If the parents insist on unorthodox treatment, suggest an objective outcome measure and reevaluate the child later. If appropriate management cannot wait, use a more aggressive approach. Start with the basic facts, obtaining consultations for reinforcement if necessary.

Society

The physician's responsibility to society is seldom addressed. Physicians do have the responsibility to keep health care costs to a minimum by avoiding inappropriate management. Physicians can also choose the least expensive alternatives among equivalent management methods [D].

Shoes

For a long time, shoe modifications were a traditional treatment for infants and children for a wide variety of pathological and physiological problems. Because shoe modifications were usually prescribed for otherwise spontaneously resolving conditions, resolution was falsely attributed to the shoe. This led to the concept of the "corrective shoe." Recently, database studies have consistently shown that natural history, rather than shoe modification, was responsible for the improvement [A]. We now know that the term "corrective shoe" is a misnomer. Barefooted people have been shown to have feet that are stronger, more flexible, and less deformed than those wearing shoes [B and D]. The feet of infants and children do not require support and do best with freedom of movement without shoes.

Shoe Selection

The selection of shoes should be the same as for other clothing. The shoe should protect the foot from injury and cold and be acceptable in appearance. The best shoes are those that interfere least with function and simulate the barefoot state [E]. High-top shoes are necessary in the toddler to keep the shoes on the feet. Proper fit is desirable, not to promote support but to avoid falls and compression of the toes. Falls are more common if the shoes are too long or have sole material that is slippery or sticky.

Useful Modifications

Shock-absorbing footwear may be helpful for the adolescent in reducing the incidence of overuse syndromes [C]. Some shoe modifications are helpful [F]. These are not for correction but to improve function or provide comfort. Shoe lifts may be useful if leg length difference exceeds 2.5 cm. Orthotics are effective in evenly distributing loading on the sole of the foot.

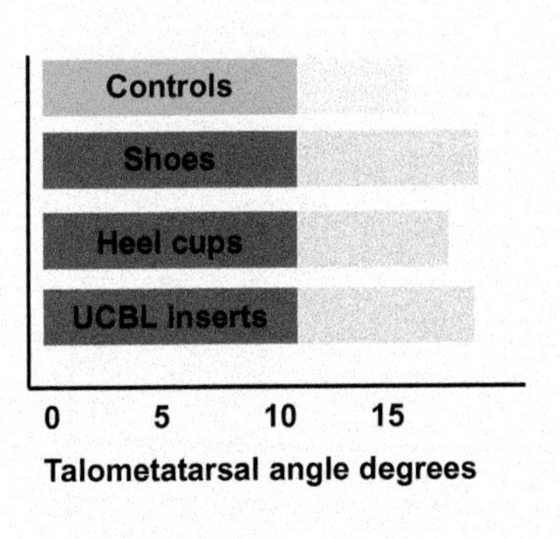

A Effect of shoe modifications in flatfeet This prospective, controlled study compared arch development with various treatments. No difference was found. Talometatarsal angles before (light shade) and after treatment (dark shade). From Wenger et al. (1989).

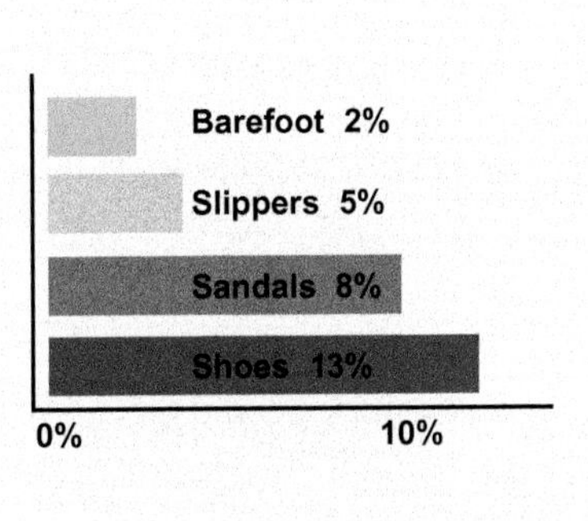

B Correlation of shoe wearing on incidence of flatfoot in adults In a survey of adults, the percentage with flatfeet was related to shoewear during childhood. Note that flatfeet were least common among barefoot children. From Roe and Joseph (1992).

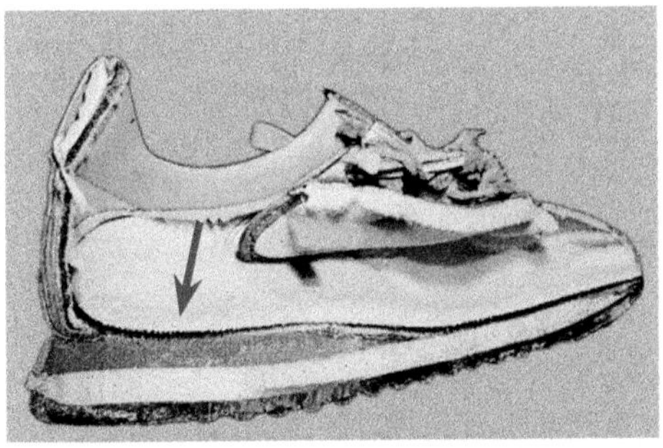

C Cushioned shoes Shoes have cushioned heels and soles (arrow) that may reduce the incidence of overuse syndromes.

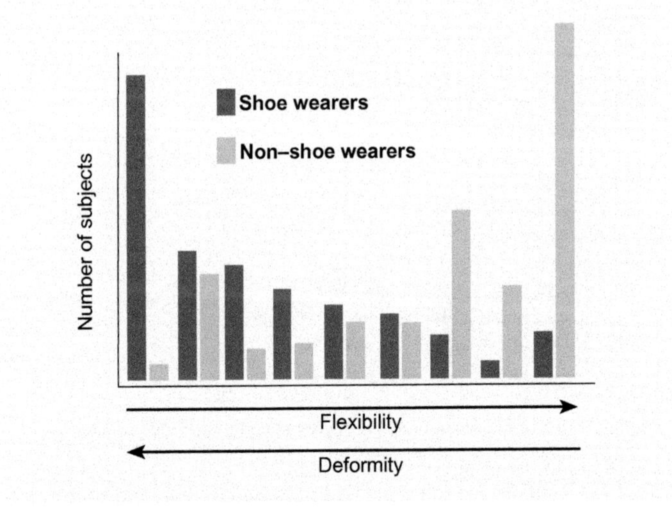

D Effect of shoe wearing on the incidence of deformity and flexibility in adults In a survey of Chinese adults, those who wore shoes had more deformity and less flexibility than nonshoe wearers. From Simfook and Hodgson (1958).

Feature	Purpose
Flexible	Improves mobility and strength
Flat	Distributes weight evenly
Foot Shaped	Noncompressive
Friction	Prevents slipping & sticking
Appearance	Acceptable for the child
Cost	Acceptable for the parent

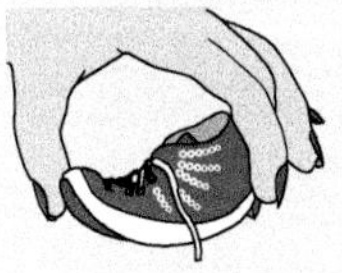

E Characteristics of a good shoe The best shoes are those that allow normal function of the foot.

Problem	Modification
Short Leg	Shoe lift for differences >1"
Rigid Deformity	Orthotic to equalize loading
Heel Pain	Elevate heel
Overuse Syn.	Shock-absorbing features
Bunions	Stretch shoe over bunion

F Useful shoe modifications These modifications are useful to improve the mechanics of load bearing.

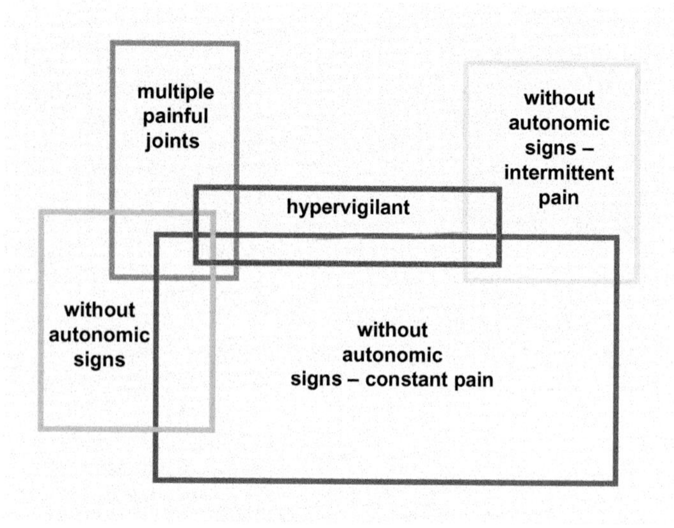

A Overlap of chronic regional pain syndromes Note the varied patterns. From Sherry (2000).

Chronic Regional Pain Syndromes

Included in this category of syndromes are reflex sympathetic dystrophy (RSD) or reflex neurovascular dystrophy (RND), idiopathic pain syndrome, and fibromyalgia.

Scope

These pain syndromes are varied and may be associated with autonomic signs [A]. The patients typically present features of disability out of proportion to the trauma history or clinical findings. These patients are often seen first by the orthopedist because the pain is musculoskeletal and frequently follows minor injury.

Diagnosis

The patients present with a wide variety of clinical features [B]. Usually the evaluation elicits a sense of disparity. The pain or disability is exaggerated beyond any signs of underlying disease. The findings may show dynamic or fixed deformity [C], considerable variations from autonomic features [D].

Management

These patients are difficult to manage. The psychological or functional underlying problem is often clear, but the family will likely be offended if that possibility is presented as the primary problem.

Referral When available, consider referring the child to a pediatric rheumatologist to manage care.

Active treatment is usually successful. Order functional aerobic training using the involved limbs, such as drills, running, play activities, and swimming for a period of 5 hours daily. Desensitize the skin with towel rubbing. Refer for psychological evaluation and provide psychotherapy as appropriate. This intensive treatment may require inpatient care with a follow-up home program for another month.

Outcome 80% cured, 15% improved, 5% unimproved; relapse 15%; 90% doing well at five years.

Common Features of Chronic Regional Pain Syndrome

Most common in preadolescent or adolescent girls
Increasing pain after minimal or no trauma
Significant disability
Crawls around house or on stairs
Discomfort with light touch—clothing, bed sheets, etc.
Autonomic changes—cold, color, clammy, edema
Worse or not better with cast immobilization
Unsuccessful previous treatment
High-level athletes or dancers
Personality features—mature, excels at school, perfectionistic, etc.
Recent major life change—move, school, friends, divorce, etc.
Mother speaks for the child
Incongruent affect for degree of pain or disability
La belle indifference about pain
Compliant when asked to use the limb
Autonomic signs, especially after use
Pain not restricted to dermatome or peripheral nerve distribution
Negative neurological examination

B Common features of chronic regional pain syndrome Based on Sherry (2000).

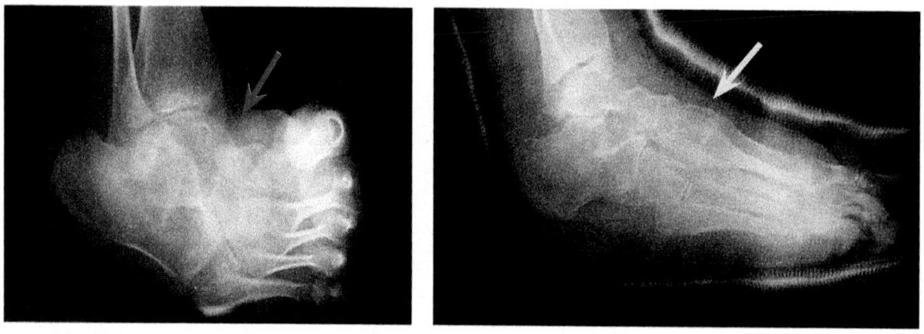

C Severe fixed deformity from RSD This 15-year-old girl developed a fixed equinovarus deformity of the foot (red arrow) over a period of many months. Correction required soft tissue releases and casting (yellow arrow).

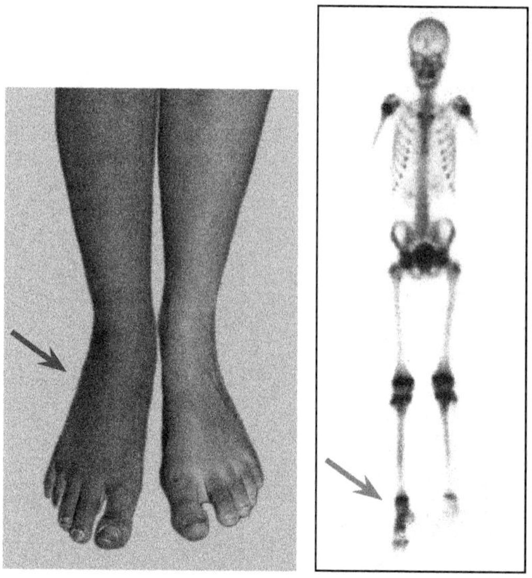

D Autonomic features of right foot Note the discoloration and swelling of the leg and foot (red arrow) and increased uptake on bone scan (blue arrow).

Traction

Traction still has a role in management. Although less than in the past, specific indications have replaced standard management.

Common Indications for Traction

Temporary stabilization Skin traction is commonly used for femoral shaft fractures before cast immobilization or operative fixation and for preoperative management of unstable proximal femoral epiphyseal slips.

Home traction Home traction programs have been used for preliminary traction in DDH management [A] and in home management of femoral shaft fractures in young children.

Fracture management The common uses of traction include supracondylar humeral fractures, femoral shaft [B] fractures, and subtrochanteric fractures.

Overcoming contracture Traction is sometimes used to improve motion in Perthes disease or chondrolysis of the hip. Whether the improvement is due to the traction or simply the enforced bed rest and immobilization is unclear.

Spine problems Complex spine problems, such as congenital and neuromuscular deformities, are sometimes managed by a combination of traction and surgery.

Traction Cautions

Inflammatory hip disorders Avoid traction in inflammatory hip disorders such as toxic synovitis or septic arthritis. Traction often positions the limb in less flexion, external rotation, and abduction, resulting in increased intraarticular pressure and possible avascular necrosis.

Overhead leg position Avoid Bryant traction in patients weighing more than 25 pounds because the vertical positioning may result in limb ischemia. This traction is seldom used today. It is preferable to reduce the flexion of the hips from 90° to about 45° to reduce the risk of ischemia.

Proximal tibial pin traction Avoid proximal tibial skeletal traction, as distal femoral traction [B] provides greater safety. Reports of recurvatum deformity and knee ligamentous laxity make proximal tibial pin traction risky.

Complications of Traction

Skin irritation This is common under skin traction [C]. Prevent this problem by avoiding excessive traction or compression. Frequent inspection of the skin reduces this risk.

Nerve compression This most commonly involves the peroneal nerve [D] from skin traction. Avoid excessive pressure over the upper fibula.

Vascular compromise This complication is most commonly associated with overhead traction for femoral fractures in infants more than 25 pounds.

Physeal damage from pins This complication has been most common from upper tibial pin traction.

Cranial penetration of halo pins The thin calvarium in children makes inadvertent penetration a risk [E]. The risks are reduced by using more pins with less compression. Preapplication CT studies may be helpful in determining proper sites for pin placement.

Superior mesenteric artery syndrome This serious complication may result from long periods of supine positioning in poorly nourished individuals.

Hypertension The mechanism is unknown.

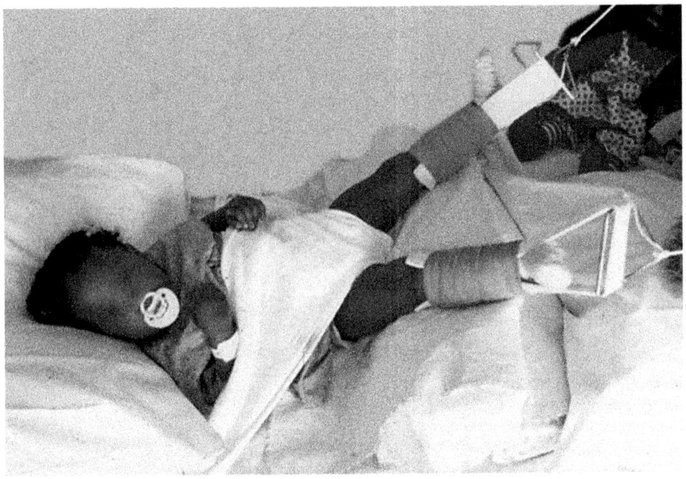

A Skin traction for DDH Sometimes prereduction skin traction is used to overcome contractures to facilitate reduction and possibly reduce the risk of AVN.

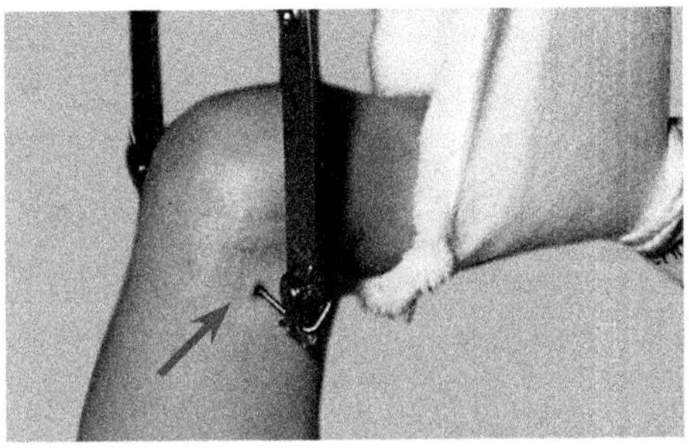

B Distal femoral traction This is the preferable site for traction when treating femoral shaft fractures.

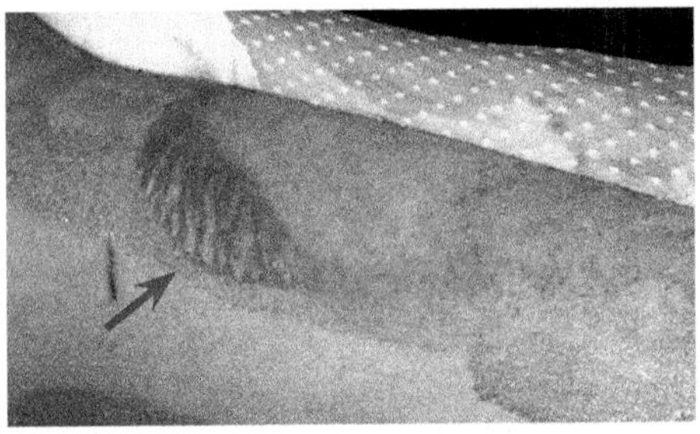

C Skin irritation under traction tapes This skin blister is due to excessive pressure and traction.

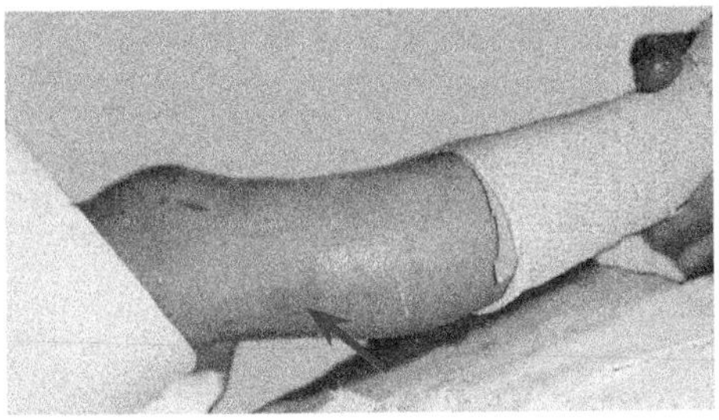

D Peroneal nerve palsy The excessive pressure resulted in a loss of function.

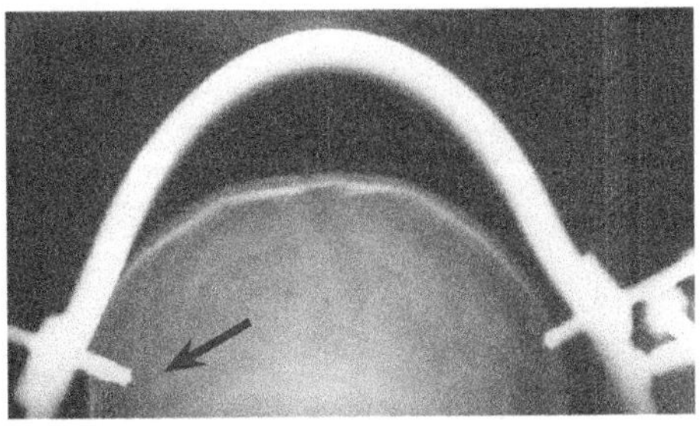

E Halo pin penetration This is prevented by using multiple pins and limiting penetration pressure during application.

Casting

Casting is useful for immobilization, control of position, correction of deformity, and sometimes to ensure compliance with treatment. Cast treatment is relatively safe, inexpensive, and well tolerated by children. Casts may be made of plaster or fiberglass. Plaster casts are least expensive and readily molded. Fiberglass casts are expensive, lightweight, water-resistant, radiographically transparent, and less messy, and provide many color and decorating options [A]. Sometimes the materials are combined in treating deformities such as clubfeet.

Categories of Casts

Casts are remarkably versatile and take many forms. They may be circumferential or applied as splints.

Cast Problems for Children

When applying casts for children, keep in mind the unique problems that may be encountered.

Compliance Children are less compliant than adults. They may not hold still for cast application, may allow the cast to become wet, or damage the cast in play.

Communication Infants or young children may not be able to communicate the pain that precedes the development of pressure sores over bony prominences.

Sensation The child with myelodysplasia or cerebral palsy has poor sensation and is at risk for pressure sores.

Cast Application

Positioning First, make certain the child is comfortable, and hold the limb in the position desired after the cast is completed. For cylinder casts or body jackets, the child should be standing. For long-leg casts, it is helpful to apply the short-leg section first; after it has hardened, extend it to the thigh. Include the toes in children's casts to provide protection. Apply the cast only when the patient is comfortable and the limb immobile. Make certain the assistant holding the limb maintains the proper position until the cast has hardened.

Padding Apply at least two layers of padding [B]. The first is the tubular stockinette that allows a neat trim for the cast edges. The material is usually cotton or dacron. The second layer is the actual padding. Apply extra padding over bony prominences if the child is likely to move during cast application or if the child is at risk for pressure sores.

In applying the cast [C], start at one end and proceed in an orderly fashion to the other end of the cast. Apply with a 50% overlap by rolling rather than pulling on the material. The techniques for application of plaster versus fiberglass are different. Tucks are taken in plaster casts to make a neat application.

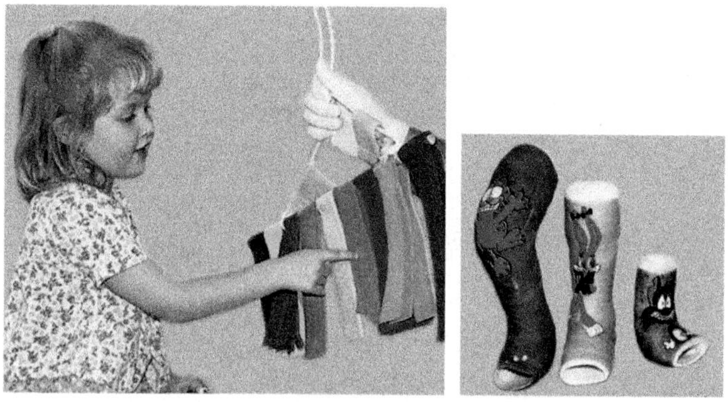

A Colorful casts Allowing the child to choose the color makes the experience less threatening. Casts can be decorated.

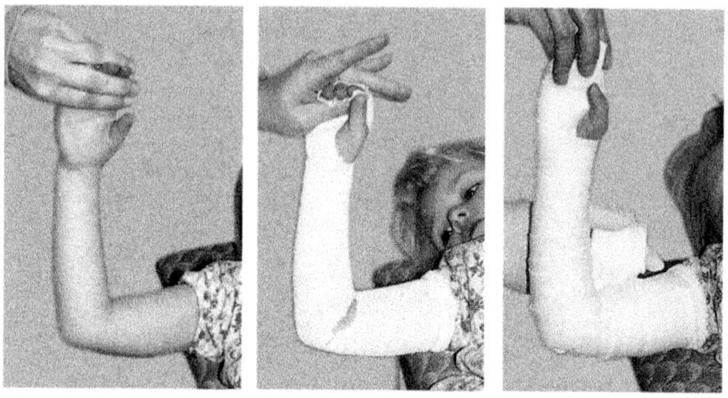

B Padding Hold the desired position the same throughout the casting process. Apply the stockinette then the padding.

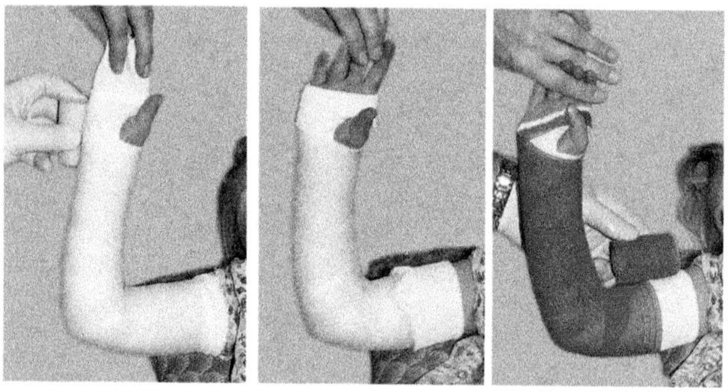

C Cast application Apply the first layers, then turn the stockinette back for trim. Apply the final layer to trim the cast and add the desired color.

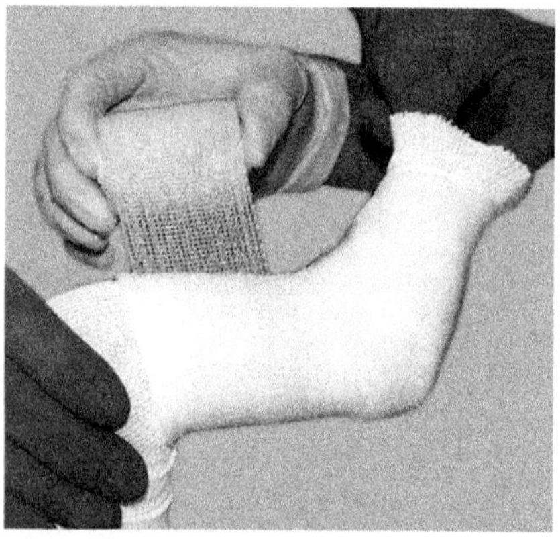

D Cast technique with fiberglass Unroll a length and then lay the material down without tension.

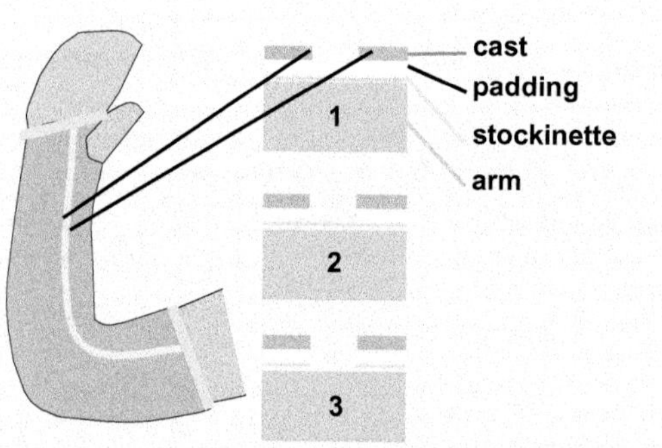

E Stages of cast splitting Casts can be split to different levels. Note that in cross section only the cast is divided (1); cast and padding are divided (2); or all layers are divided (3).

Fiberglass application Fiberglass rolls must be guided to maintain control of direction. *When applying fiberglass, free a segment of material from the roll, then apply it smoothly and without tension* [D, previous page]. Whereas plaster has a definite time of crystallization and hardens rather abruptly, fiberglass hardens slowly. The ideal thickness of most casts is three layers. Apply extra layers over sites of greater stress, such as the hip in spica casts or the knee and ankle in long-leg casts.

Early Cast Care

Bivalving Bivalving or splitting casts may be by degree [E, previous page]. Be aware that padding is often not elastic and may create as much compression as cast material. For complete relief of pressure, it is necessary to divide all layers of the cast on both sides.

Pressure relief If sensation is poor or communication limited, consider relieving pressure over bony prominences. Cut a rectangle of cast or cut an *X* over the site for relief. Elevate the cast edges and leave the padding intact. To make the child in a spica cast more comfortable, consider flaring the thoracic edges and creating a *stomach hole* [A].

Trim cast edges To save operating room time, consider trimming the cast in the recovery room or on the ward. Provide a generous amount of space around the perineum.

Cast Care

When the child bathes or plays in the rain, have the parent cover the cast with a plastic bag to keep it dry. Even fiberglass casts are uncomfortable when wet. In infants, spica casts pose a special problem. Instruct staff and parents to change the infant's diapers frequently and to avoid tucking the diaper under the cast. Skin irritation is best managed by exposure to air and light. Avoid criticizing the child for the appearance of the cast. Often a worn cast is evidence of success in incorporating the treatment in the play activity of the child [B].

Cast Removal

Cast removal is often the most risky phase of cast treatment. Cast saws can cut the skin if contact is made under pressure. Cast saw lacerations are most likely over bony prominences such as the malleoli. Plaster casts may be soaked off by the parents prior to the clinic visit. The crying, struggling child is at special risk.

Reassurance Try to reassure the child by placing the moving blade gently against your arm to show that it only vibrates and normally does not cut skin [C]. Compare the saw noise to an airplane. Have the parent comfort the child as well.

Technique Use consecutive in-and-out movements to cut the cast [D]. Try to avoid cutting directly over the bony prominences. Insist that the inexperienced assistant learn to remove casts on adolescents or adults and not infants or children.

Hair grows more rapidly under casts. The adolescent girl is often shocked by the amount of hair on her leg following cast removal. Reassure her that in a month or so the hair growth will return to normal.

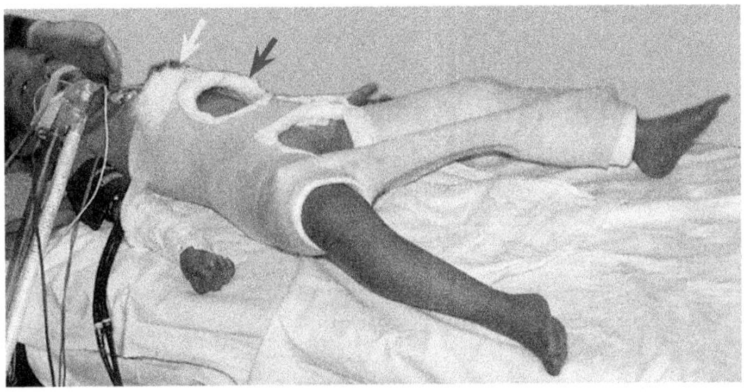

A Spica cast Note the large abdominal window (red arrow) and extra space around the thorax (yellow arrow).

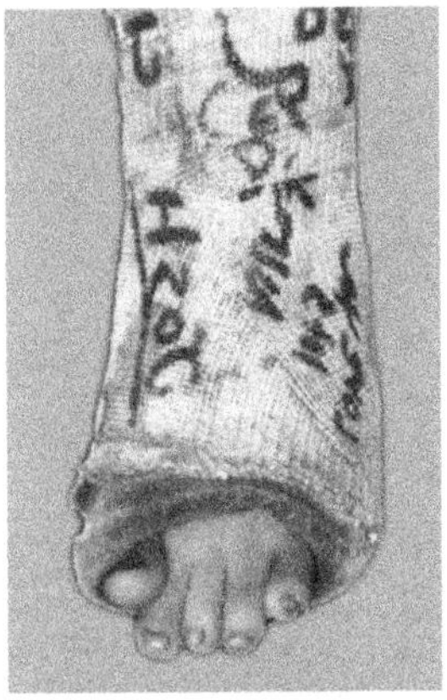

B "Well-used" cast Ideally, the child will be very active in the cast.

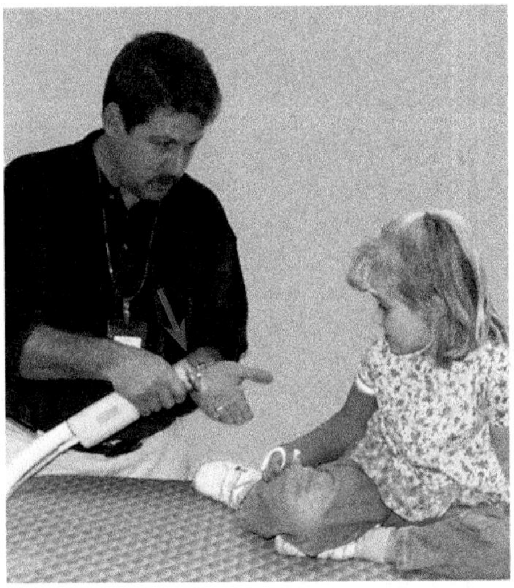

C Reassurance Show the child that the cast saw can touch the skin without cutting.

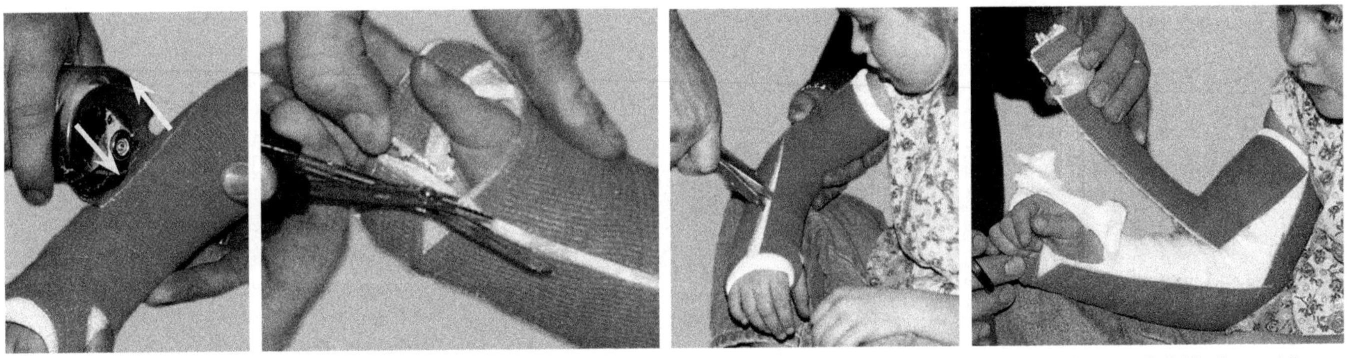

D Cast removal Cut the cast with in-and-out movements (yellow arrows). Cut both sides of the cast, spread the cut edges, and divide the padding with a scissors. This allows the cast to be removed.

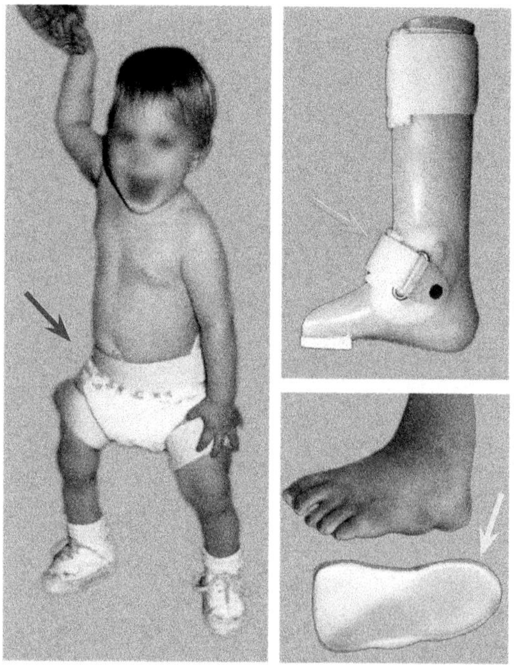

A Common orthotics Hip abduction (red arrow), foot orthosis (yellow arrow), and ankle–foot orthosis (orange arrow) are the most common braces.

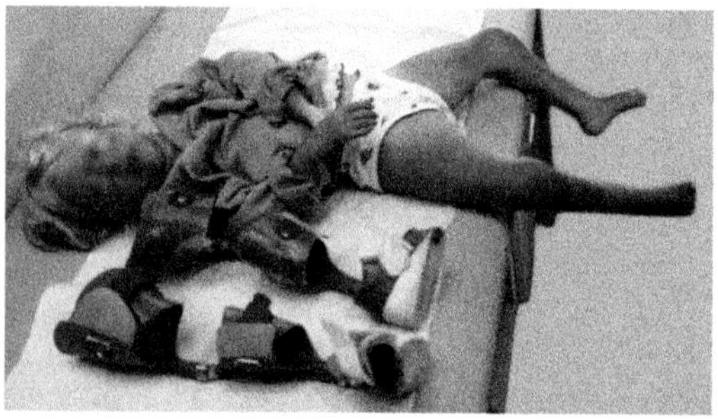

B Functional bracing This child with arthrogryposis has special braces that incorporate light weight, heel elevations, knee flexion, and internal rotation components.

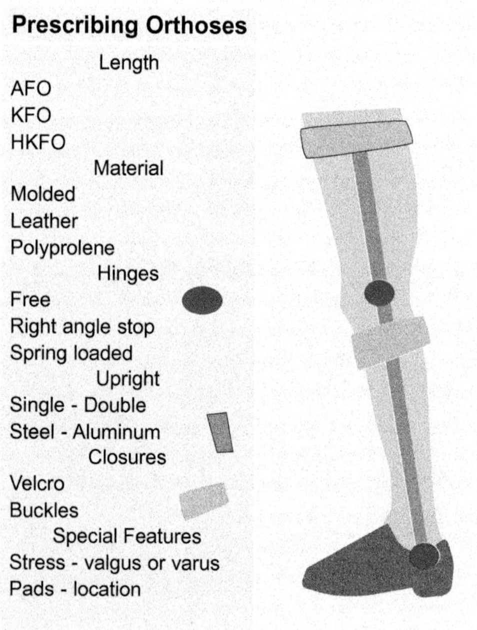

C Orthosis prescription Specify each element of the brace.

Orthotics

Orthoses are used to control alignment, facilitate function, and provide protection. They include braces and splints [A].

Splints provide static support or positioning and often encompass only half of the limb. They are often worn only part-time.

Braces are usually more elaborate and worn while the child is active [B]. Braces are sometimes divided into passive and active types.

Passive braces are those that simply provide support, such as some scoliosis braces in children with neuromuscular disorders.

Active braces are those that facilitate function. Such braces may promote active correction, as seen in scoliosis braces that incorporate pads.

Goals

Be realistic about the goals of bracing. Bracing will not correct static deformity or scoliosis. At best, braces prevent progression. Orthotics do not correct physiologic flatfeet or torsional deformity. Although radiographs taken with the orthotics in place may show improvement, this correction is not maintained after the brace is removed. Unbraced radiographs can be made to assess real correction.

Naming Orthoses

The name of the device is determined by which joints are involved. An AFO includes the ankle and foot; a KFO adds the knee; an HKFO includes the hip, knee, and ankle. Special braces are often named by city of origin.

Ordering Orthoses

The prescription should include several components: the extent, material, joint characteristics, and closure types [C]. Order orthoses thoughtfully, as any orthosis is a burden for the child.

Minimizing the Orthotic Burden

Attempt to reduce the burden to the child.

Effectiveness Many orthoses are ineffective and should not be used. Examples include all orthoses for developmental deformities that occur in normal children. These include orthoses for flatfeet, twister cables for torsional problems, or wedges for bowlegs.

Perform the child test For children with neuromuscular problems, orthoses such as AFOs are frequently ordered to improve function. If the brace truly improves function, the child will usually prefer to use the brace. If the brace causes more trouble than benefit, the child will prefer to go without. Make certain the brace is comfortable and fits properly. If the child prefers to go without a comfortable, well-fitting orthosis, it generally means that the brace is a functional liability. In most cases, the unwanted brace should be discontinued.

Minimum duration Duration of bracing is critical to success and acceptance. The effectiveness of bracing to arrest progression of a deformity depends upon two factors: the amount of corrective force applied and the duration this force is applied (based on a 24-hour day). The effectiveness of bracing increases with duration. The psychological and physiological costs also increase with duration. Balancing the benefit and cost is a challenge. Nighttime bracing is least "costly" for the patient because bracing does not interfere with play, is convenient to use, and causes little effect on the child's self-image. The duration of bracing can vary from full-time (allow an hour free), to nighttime, or part-time. Part-time bracing is commonly ordered for 4-, 8-, or 12-hour periods per day. Negotiate with the child to make certain that the precious free hours coincide with the child's priorities, such as school or specific athletic or social activities. This will improve compliance.

Minimal length The longer the brace the greater the disability. Extending braces to the pelvis is seldom necessary. Likewise, shoe lifts for leg length inequality may be prescribed that are less than needed to completely level the pelvis. Usually allowing up to 2 cm undercorrection is acceptable to reduce the weight, instability, and unsightly appearance of a higher lift.

Prosthetics

Prostheses are artificial substitutes for body parts. Most prostheses for children are designed to replace limb deficiencies secondary to congenital, traumatic, or neoplastic problems.

Naming Prostheses

Name the prosthesis based on the level of the deficiency or type of amputation [A].

Prescribing Prostheses

Detail each element of the limb [B].

Special Needs of Children

Children have special prosthetic needs. Children grow, making prosthetic adjustments necessary 3–4 times a year. The prosthesis must be rugged and simple in design. Because multiple limb deficiencies occur in up to 30% of congenital losses and 15% of acquired losses, customized prosthetic management is often necessary.

Age for Fitting

Lower limb Fit lower limb prosthetics when the child first pulls up to stand, about 10 months of age. Initially, the knee may be omitted to keep the limb simple, light, and stable [C]. Delay bilateral amputee fitting a few months.

Upper limb The timing of fitting upper limb deficiencies is controversial. Some fit at about 6 months of age. Others prefer to wait until a need is recognized by the child, which usually occurs in mid-childhood.

Acceptance

Lower limb prostheses are well accepted as they clearly enhance function and appearance [D]. Stability and symmetry required for walking are readily provided by the prosthesis.

Upper limb prostheses are less well accepted. Some find the artificial limb to be a burden without sufficient compensation in improved function to justify the trouble. The lack of sensibility limits function. Children learn to function well with one hand. Children seldom use the prehensile function of upper limb terminal devices. Cosmetic hands are useful in adolescence.

Myoelectric Power

Powered limbs have the advantage of slightly improving appearance but the disadvantages of being more complex, heavier, and slower. The results are mixed.

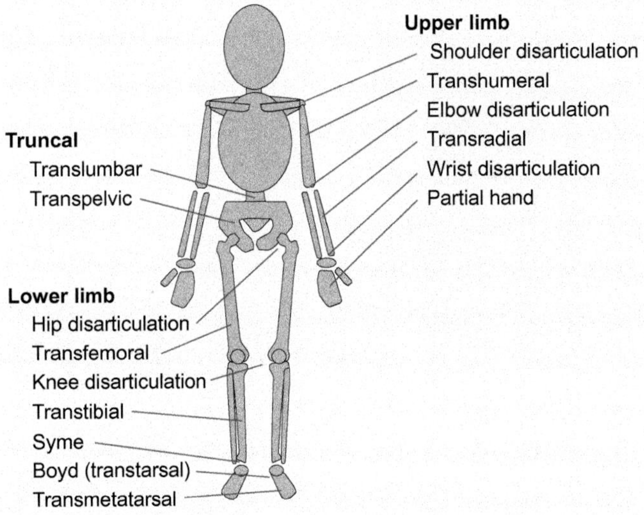

A Amputation levels

Lower Limb Prostheses

Type
Immediate
Early
Preparatory
Definitive

Design
Endoskeletal
Exoskeletal

Suspension
Transfemoral
Transtibial

Socket Liners

Components
Knee
Ankle
Foot

Special Features
Compensate deformity
Include foot

Upper Limb Prostheses

Type
Infant
Child

Harnessing

Control Motion

Terminal Device

Components
Wrist
Elbow
Shoulder

Motor
Body
Myoelectric

Special Features
Partial amputations

B Prostheses prescription When ordering prostheses, describe each of these features.

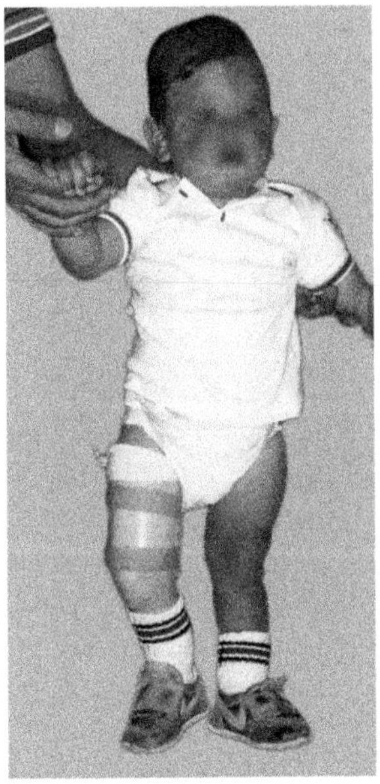

C Toddler with nonarticulated prosthesis This is his first prosthesis.

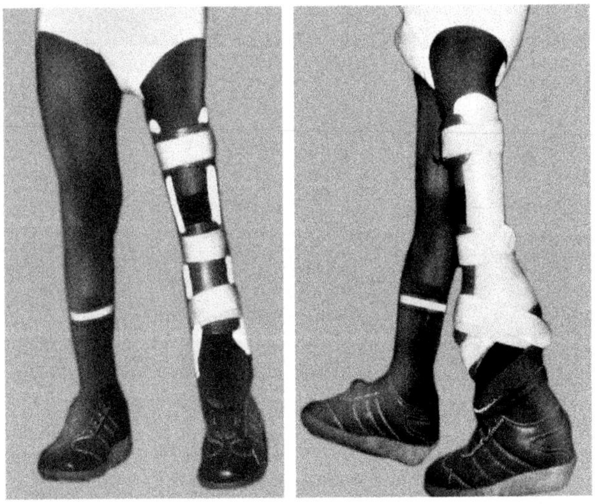

D High below-knee prosthesis This boy with tibial deficiency has a short stump with strong quads. He is fully active in sports.

Therapy

Therapy utilizes the treatment methods of physical medicine, including manipulations, exercises [A], positioning, stimulation, massage, and application of cold and heat. The role of the pediatric therapist is much broader than that of the general therapist, requiring knowledge of growth and development [B].

The current emphasis on function has improved the effectiveness of therapy programs. Emphasis on effective mobility, independence skills, and communication focuses therapeutic energy and resources on an outcome that optimizes the child's quality of life.

Physical Therapy

In pediatric orthopedics, the primary focus of physical therapy is on lower limb function and mobility.

Effective mobility A child needs independent and efficient mobility [C]. Without this capability, the child's psychosocial and educational experiences are significantly limited. The level of mobility should be appropriate to the child's mental age. The method of mobility is not critical.

Whether mobility is provided by walking or by the use of adaptive equipment [D], the method of mobility should be manageable by the child himself, conserve the child's energy, and be functionally practical. Options range from the use of an electric wheelchair [E] to unassisted walking. The objective of management is to provide effective mobility by whatever means necessary while helping the child progress toward a realistic mobility objective. The objective should be an optimistic target within a realistic range. The therapist's accurate appraisal of the child, knowledge of mobility potential for the disease, and periodic assessments of progress help protect the child from disappointment, frustration, and wasted efforts. With time, objectives may change, depending upon the rate of progress.

A major objective of therapy is support and education of the family. Often, the family has unrealistic expectations that create an additional burden for the child. The family's major concern often is "Will my child walk?" A better objective would be "Will my child be independent and happy?" Assisting the family and guiding their concepts and expectations is an important role for the therapist.

Infant stimulation programs Helping the parents to interact positively with the child is a vital role of therapy. Parents may be uncomfortable with the infant, and this strained relationship further limits the child. Interactive play therapy, taught to the parents [F] by the therapist, provides the positive physical contact infants need for optimal emotional and intellectual growth. Infant stimulation programs are effective in promoting cognitive, motor, language, and emotional development.

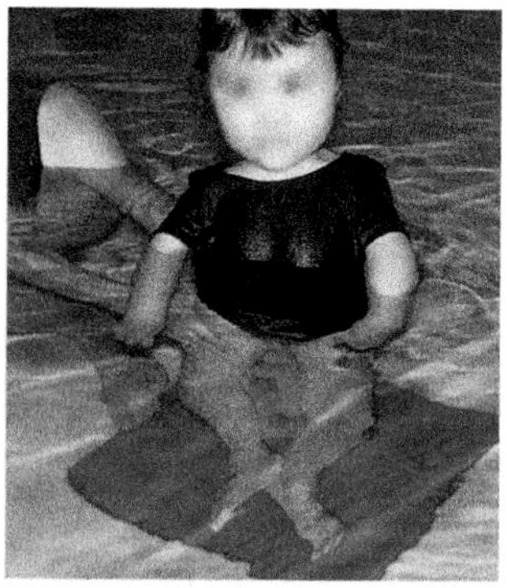

A Hydrotherapy This child with arthrogryposis with knee flexion contractures is given her first walking experience.

Expanded role of the pediatric therapist
Assesses function
Educates family
Provides psychological support for the family
Explores uses of adaptive equipment
Documents management and research

B Role of pediatric therapist The therapist's role is considerably broader than simply providing exercises and manipulation.

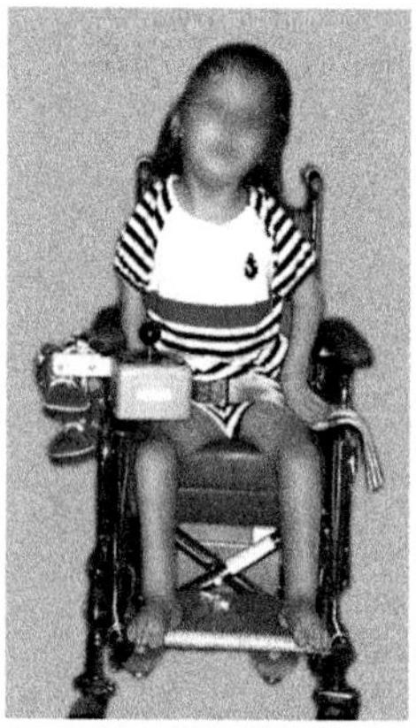

Objective	Device
Mobility	Walkers Wheelchairs Motorized vehicles
Self-Care	Lifts Ramps Special toilets
Communication	Communication boards Computers

C Effective mobility The mobility of this bright child with severe arthrogryposis is provided by an electric wheelchair.

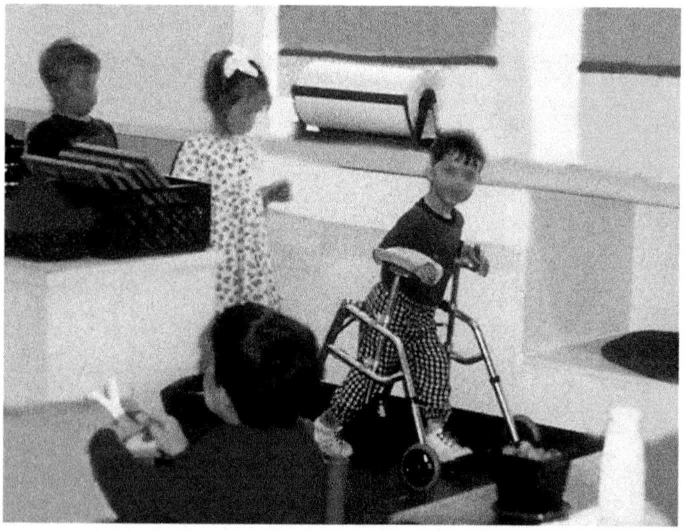

D Integration Mainstreaming or integration into a normal environment is very helpful for social development.

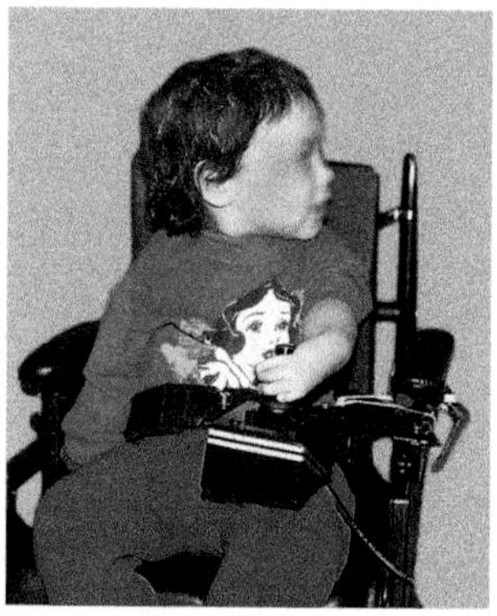

E Effective mobility This electric wheelchair allows this child self-determined mobility.

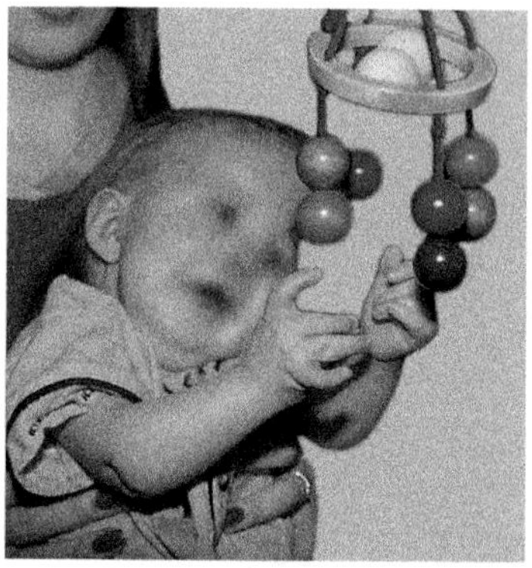

F Infant stimulation This infant is provided play experience, that is necessary for intellectual development.

Neurodevelopmental therapy Neurodevelopment therapy (NDT) focuses on motor development. NDT is more effective than the original passive treatment methods but is being replaced by therapy with a broader focus.

Accepting disability Accepting the disability and working around it, using adaptive equipment, is often the most effective management strategy for the child. Usually the physician or therapist cannot cure the disease, but can minimize the disability.

Adaptive equipment is useful to help the child become more independent and functional. Adaptive equipment is useful for the child's mobility, self-care skills, and communication, and often enhances care of the child by the caregiver.

Exercises are not very useful for the young child because the child lacks the interest and discipline to perform the exercises. Fortunately, children have little need for exercises, as muscle strength and function usually recover spontaneously. Moreover, assistive or stretching exercises can be harmful. In posttraumatic stiffness, stretching often increases stiffness by adding new injury and scarring. Exercise should not be painful. Exercises take on a variety of forms [A]. Chronic passive motion is a new technique for maintaining joint motion following operative release or injury. The joint is moved slowly and continuously through a range of motion during healing.

Stretching is a traditional treatment for contracture [B]. Flaccid contractures respond best to stretching. The prolonged effects of spasticity, as in cerebral palsy, cannot be controlled by intermittent stretching. To prevent contracture, the elongated or stretched position must be maintained for about 4 hours in each 24-hour day. This requires bracing or splinting. Stretching beyond the child's pain threshold is not advisable; overstretching causes further injury and scar formation.

Therapy at home, with a parent acting as therapist and the therapist as a consultant, is effective and practical when the family is willing and able. Home therapy programs reduce stress on the family by making the treatment more convenient and less expensive. The therapy can often be incorporated into the daily routines, increasing frequency and improving outcomes. Home therapy may also have a bonding effect on the family. This requires parent education and periodic visits to the therapist to assess technique and progress.

Treatments of doubtful value include massage, thermotherapy, injections, and diathermy. These "treatments" are not helpful in pediatric orthopedics.

Occupational Therapy

Occupational therapy focuses on upper extremity function [C] and activities of daily living [D], including independence skills and correction of deformity [E]. This aspect of therapy plays a broad role in managing childhood disabilities because modern management places greater emphasis on assessment and self-care skills. Physical and occupational therapists often work together, especially for children with long-term disabilities, as part of a management team.

Self-care skills are taught to increase independence in feeding, dressing, and toileting. Self-care can be achieved by learning special techniques from the therapist, using adaptive equipment, or making the environment more easily livable for the child. Independence learned in childhood enhances the individual's self-respect and happiness and reduces the burden for the family and the costs for society.

Form	Indication
Isotonic	Contraction through an arc
Isometric	Static contraction
Active Range of Motion	Maximum range of motion by patient unassisted
Assistive Range	Therapist-assisted maximum range of motion

A Forms of exercises for children Several forms of exercise are available. Passive exercise that causes pain is contraindicated in children, as it often increases stiffness by injuring the joint.

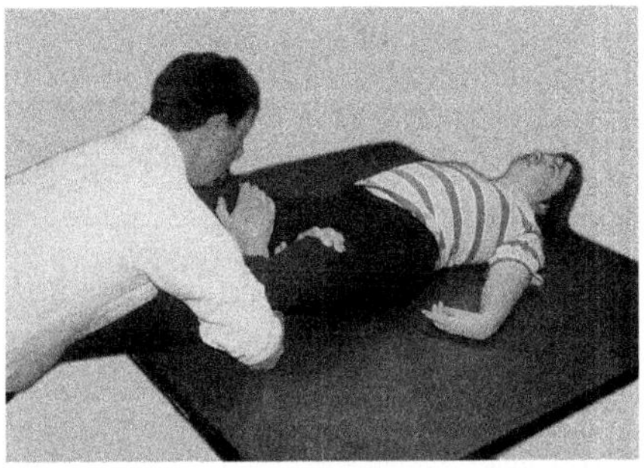

B Stretching Stretching exercises should be done carefully to avoid fractures and causing pain.

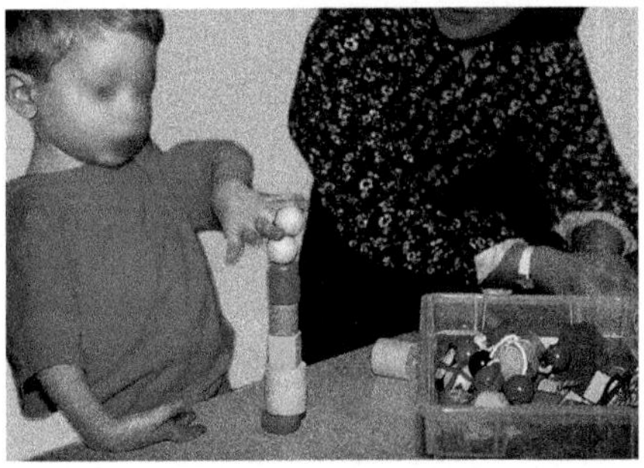

C Occupational therapy Teaching families how to provide play activities for each child is essential for development.

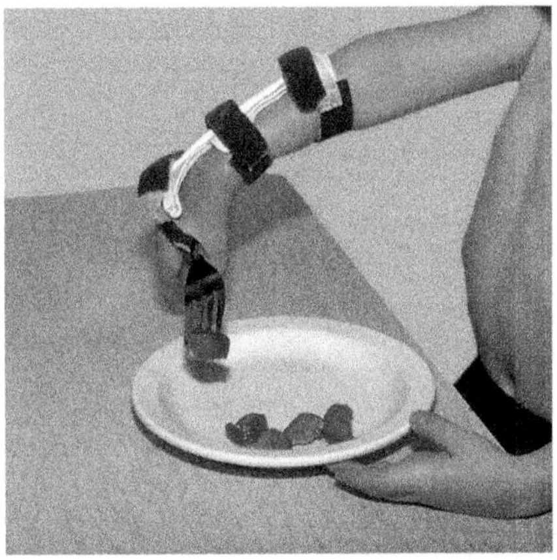

D Adaptive equipment Selection or development of special devices to facilitate activities of daily living is very valuable in developing independence.

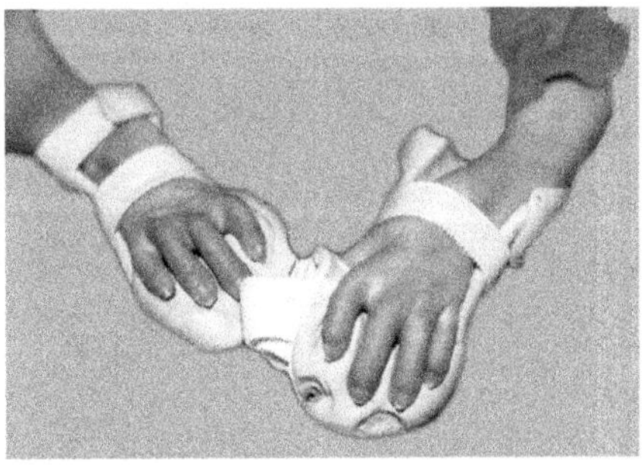

E Hand splints These resting splints are invaluable in preventing recurrence of deformity in children with muscle imbalance, burns, or following surgery.

Abraham E. Remodeling potential of long bones following angular osteotomies. J Pediatr Orthop 1989;9:37-43.

Agus H, Kalenderer O, Eryanilmaz G, Omeroglu H. Biological internal fixation of comminuted femur shaft fractures by bridge plating in children. J Pediatr Orthop 2003 Mar-Apr;23(2): p184-9.

Agus H, Kalenderer O, Kayali C, Eryanilmaz G. Skeletal traction and delayed percutaneous fixation of complicated supracondylar humerus fractures due to delayed or unsuccessful reductions and extensive swelling in children. J Pediatr Orthop B 2002 Apr;11(2): p150-4.

American Academy of Orthopaedic Surgeons. Sports and recreational programs for the child and young adult with physical disability. Proceedings of the Winter Park Seminar, Winter Park, Clin Orthop 11-13 1983 Apr: p 883-993.

American Academy of Pediatrics. The Dorman-Delacato treatment of neurologically handicapped children: Policy statement. Pediatrics 1982;70:810-812.

Angel JD, Blasier RD, Allison R. Postoperative fever in pediatric orthopaedic patients. J Pediatr Orthop 1994;14:799.

Armstrong PF, Brighton CT. Failure of the rabbit tibial growth plate to respond to long-term application of a capacitively coupled electrical field. J Orthop Res 1986;4:446.

Bailey R, Dubow H. Evolution of the concept of an extensible nail accommodating to normal longitudinal bone growth: Clinical considerations and implications. Clin Orthop 1981: 159:157-171.

Barry M, Paterson JM, A flexible intramedullary nails for fractures in children. J Bone Joint Surg Br 2004 Sep;86(7): p947-53.

Birmingham PK, RM Dsida, JJ Grayhack, J Han, M Wheeler, JA Pongracic, CJ Cote and SC Hall Do latex precautions in children with myelodysplasia reduce intraoperative allergic reactions? J Pediatr Orthop 1996: 16:799-802.

Bleck EE. Severe orthopedic disability in childhood: Solutions provided by rehabilitation engineering. Orthop Clin North Am 1978: 9:509-28.

Crandall RC, Tomhave W. Pediatric unilateral below-elbow amputees: retrospective analysis of 34 patients given multiple prosthetic options. J Pediatr Orthop 2002 May-Jun;22(3): p380-3.

Crenshaw S, Herzog R, Castagno P, Richards J, Miller F, Michaloski G, Moran E. The efficacy of tone-reducing features in orthotics on the gait of children with spastic diplegic cerebral palsy. J Pediatr Orthop 2000 Mar-Apr;20(2): p210-6.

Dietz FR, Weinstein SL. Spike osteotomy for angular deformities of the long bones in children. J Bone Joint Surg 1988; 70:848.

Dominkus M, Krepler P, Schwameis E, Windhager R, Kotz R. Growth prediction in extendable tumor prostheses in children. Clin Orthop 2001 Sep;(390): p212-20.

Driano AN, Staheli LR, Staheli LT. Psychosocial development and corrective shoewear use in children. J. Pediatr Ortho 1998: 18:346.

Duffy CM, Graham HK, Cosgrove AP. The influence of ankle-foot orthoses on gait and energy expenditure in spina bifida. J Pediatr Orthop 2000 May-Jun;20(3): p356-61.

El Hayek T, Daher AA, Meouchy W, Ley P, Chammas N, Griffet J. External fixators in the treatment of fractures in children. J Pediatr Orthop B 2004 Mar;13(2): p103-9.

Fischer AQ, Strasburger J. Footdrop in the neonate secondary to use of footboards. J Pediatr Orthop 1982: 101:1033.

Foulk DA, Boakes J, Rab GT, Schulman S. The use of caudal epidural anesthesia in clubfoot surgery. J Pediatr Orthop 1995 Sep-Oct; 15 (5):604-7.

Frimodt-Moller N, Riegels-Nielson P. Antibiotic penetration into the infected knee: A rabbit experiment. Acta Orthop Scand 1987;58:256.

Gordon JE, Kelly-Hahn J, Carpenter CJ, Schoenecker PL. Pin site care during external fixation in children: results of a nihilistic approach. J Pediatr Orthop 2000 Mar-Apr;20(2): p163-5.

Gould N. Shoes versus sneakers in toddler ambulation. Foot Ankle 1985;6:105.

Greene WB. Use of continuous passive slow motion in the postoperative rehabilitation of difficult pediatric knee and elbow problems. J Pediatr Orthop 1983:3:419-423.

Guidera KJ, Hontas R, Ogden JA. Use of continuous passive motion in pediatric orthopedics. J Pediatr Orthop 1990:10:120-123.

Hamdan JA, Taleb YA, Ahmed MS. Traction-induced hypertension in children. Clin Orthop 1984;185:87.

Herrera JA, Wall EJ, Foad SL. Hematoma block reduces narcotic pain medication after femoral elastic nailing in children. J Pediatr Orthop 2004 May-Jun;24(3): p254-6.

Hoffer MM, Feiwell E, Perry LR, et al. Functional ambulation in patients with myelomeningocele. J Bone Joint Surg 1973;55A:137-148.

Hoffer MM, Koffman M. Cerebral palsy: The first three years. Clin Orthop 1980:151:222-227.

Holzman RS. Clinical management of latex-allergic children. Anesth Analg 1997: 85:529-33.

Iobst CA, Hresko MT, Karlin LI, Hall JE. Postoperative shoulder-spine spica cast for young children. J Pediatr Orthop 2004 Mar-Apr;24(2): p227-30.

Ito H, Minami A, Suzuki K, Matsuno T. Three-dimensionally corrective external fixator system for proximal femoral osteotomy. J Pediatr Orthop 2001 Sep-Oct;21(5): p652-6.

Johnston TE, Finson RL, McCarthy JJ, Smith BT, Betz RR, Mulcahey MJ. Use of functional electrical stimulation to augment traditional orthopaedic surgery in children with cerebral palsy. J Pediatr Orthop 2004 May-Jun;24(3): p283-91.

Jones KL, Robinson LK. An approach to the child with structural defects. J Pediatr Orthop 1983;3:238-244.

Jones S, Chell J, Davies G. Broomstick plaster with a removable abduction bar: a simple technique that facilitates early postoperative physical therapy and handling. J Pediatr Orthop 2000 Sep-Oct;20(5): p640-1.

Kanda T, Yuge M, Yamori Y, et al. Early physiotherapy in the treatment of spastic diplegia. Dev Med Child Neurol 1984:26:438-444.

Kay RM, Dennis S, Rethlefsen S, Skaggs DL, Tolo VT. Impact of postoperative gait analysis on orthopaedic care. Clin Orthop 2000 May;(374): p259-64.

Knittel G, Staheli LT. The effectiveness of shoe modifications for intoeing. Orthop Clin North Am 1976;7:1019-1025.

McCann HL, Stanitski DF. Pediatric orthopaedic surgery pain management. J Pediatr Orthop 2004 Sep-Oct;24(5): p581-6.

McGill SM, Dainty DA. Computer analysis of energy transfers in children walking with crutches. Arch Phys Med Rehabil 1984;65:115.

McGrath PJ, et al. Assistive devices: Utilization by children. Arch Phys Med Rehabil 1985;66:430.

Meyer S, Gordon RL, Robin GC. The pathogenesis of neurovascular complications following penicillin injection. J Pediatr Orthop 1981;1:215-218.

Nather A, Balasubramaniam P, Bose K. A comparative study of different methods of tendon lengthening: An experimental study in rabbits. J Pediatr Orthop 1986:6:456-459.

O'Hara M, McGrath PJ, D'Astous J, et al. Oral morphine versus injected meperidine (Demerol) for pain relief in children after orthopedic surgery. J Pediatr Orthop 1987:7:78-82.

Palmer FB, Shapiro BK, Wachtel RC, et al. The effects of physical therapy on cerebral palsy: A controlled trial in infants with spastic diplegia. N Engl J Med 1988:318:803-808.

Parette HP Jr, Houcade JJ. A review of therapeutic intervention research on gross and fine motor progress in young children with cerebral palsy. Am J Occup Ther 1984:38:462-468.

Rang M, Douglas G, Bennet GC, et al. Seating for children with cerebral palsy. J Pediatr Orthop 1981;1:279-287.

Rebello G, Joseph B, Chincholkar A. Connecting bar for hip spica reinforcement: does it help?. J Pediatr Orthop B 2004 Sep;13(5): p345-6.

Respet PJ, Kleinman PG, Meinhard BP. Pin tract infections: A canine model. J Orthop Res 1987;5:600.

Rose GK, Sankarankutty M, Stallar J. A clinical review of the orthotic treatment of myelomeningocele patients. J Bone Joint Surg 1983;65B:242-246.

Rose J, Gamble JG, Medeiros J, et al. Energy cost of walking in normal children and in those with cerebral palsy: Comparison of heart rate and oxygen uptake. J Pediatr Orthop 1989:71A:276-279.

Rose J, Medeiros JM, Parker R. Energy cost index as an estimate of energy expenditure of cerebral-palsied children during assisted ambulation. Dev Med Child Neurol 1985;27:485-490.

Rosenthal RK. The use of orthotics in foot and ankle problems in cerebral palsy. Foot Ankle 1984;4:195-200.

Safavi FZ. Chapter 14 Anesthesia in Pediatric Orthopedic Secrets 1998 Hanley & Belfus, Staheli LT, editor.

Salter RB et al. Clinical application of basic research on continuous passive motion for disorders and injuries of synovial joints: A preliminary report of a feasibility study. J Orthop Res 1984:1:325.

Salter RB. The biologic concept of continuous passive motion of synovial joints. The first 18 years of basic research and its clinical application. Clin Orthop 1989:242:12.

Seibert JJ, et al. Acquired bone dysplasia secondary to catheter-related complications in the neonate. Pediatr Radiol 1986:16:43.

Short DL, Schade JK, Herring JA. Parent involvement in physical therapy: A controversial issue. J Pediatr Orthop 1989:9:444-446.

Simmons DJ, et al. The effect of protracted tetracycline treatment on bone growth and maturation. Clin Orthop 1983:180:253.

Sink EL, Karol LA, Sanders J, Birch JG, Johnston CE, Herring JA. Efficacy of perioperative halo-gravity traction in the treatment of severe scoliosis in children. J Pediatr Orthop 2001 Jul-Aug;21(4): p519-24.

Spencer GE Jr, Vignos PJ Jr. Bracing for ambulation in childhood progressive muscular dystrophy. J Bone Joint Surg 1962:44A:234-242.

Staheli LT. Lower positional deformity in infants and children: A review. J Pediatr Orthop 1990;10:559-563.

Staheli LT. Philosophy of care. Pediatr Clin North Am 1986;33:1269-1275.

Staheli LT. Shoes for children: A review. Pediatrics 1991;88:371-375.

Vankoski SJ, Michaud S, Dias L. External tibial torsion and the effectiveness of the solid ankle-foot orthoses. J Pediatr Orthop 2000 May-Jun;20(3): p349-55.

Wong J, Boyd R, Keenan NW, Baker R, Selber P, Wright JG, Nattrass GR, Graham HK. Gait patterns after fracture of the femoral shaft in children, managed by external fixation or early hip spica cast. J Pediatr Orthop 2004 Sep-Oct;24(5): p463-71.

TRAUMA

CHAPTER 4

Trauma is the leading cause of death of children and second to infection as a cause of morbidity. Fractures account for about 15% of all injuries in children [A].

Children's injuries not only differ from those of adults, they also vary depending on the age of the child. Infants, children, and adolescents experience different injuries. Appreciating these differences is essential to optimal management.

Statistics

Boys are injured more often than girls. Injuries increase in frequency with advancing age during childhood, and the percentage of fractures that occur through the physis increases with age as well [B].

About half of boys and one-fourth of girls can expect to experience a fracture during childhood. Fractures are becoming more common as sports activities increase. The wrist is the most frequent site of injury [C]. Age affects the pattern of injury.

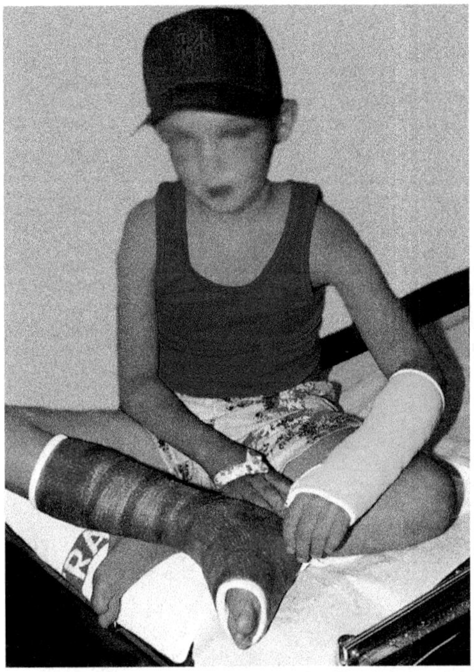

A Trauma is part of a child's life This boy sustained a fracture of his forearm and ankle during play.

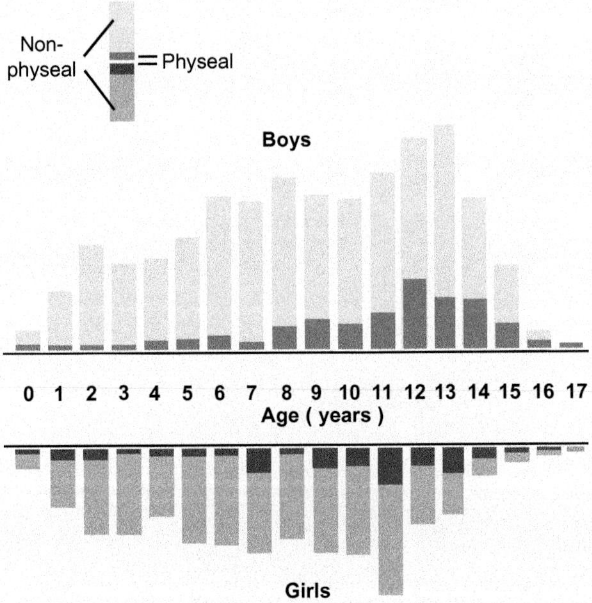

B Age distribution of physeal and nonphyseal injuries Note the differences between boys (blue) and girls (red). From Mizuta et al. (1987).

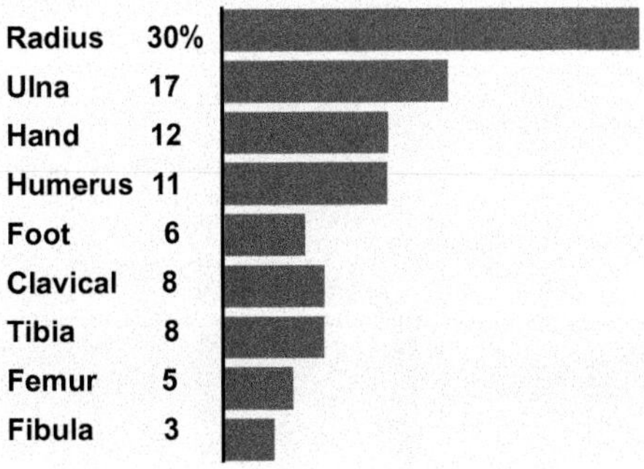

C Fracture frequency in infants and children Frequency of fractures in a sample of 923 children's fractures. From Mizuta (1987).

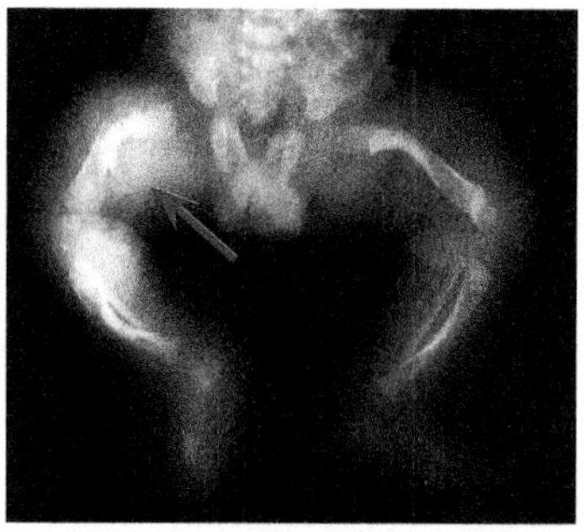

A Multiple fractures in osteogenesis imperfecta This newborn's fragile bones resulted in paranatal fractures.

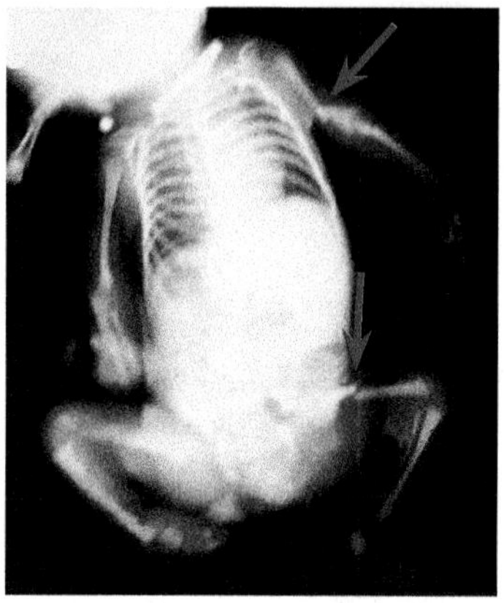

B Fractures due to joint stiffness in arthrogryposis These birth fractures resulted from trauma at delivery due to joint contractures.

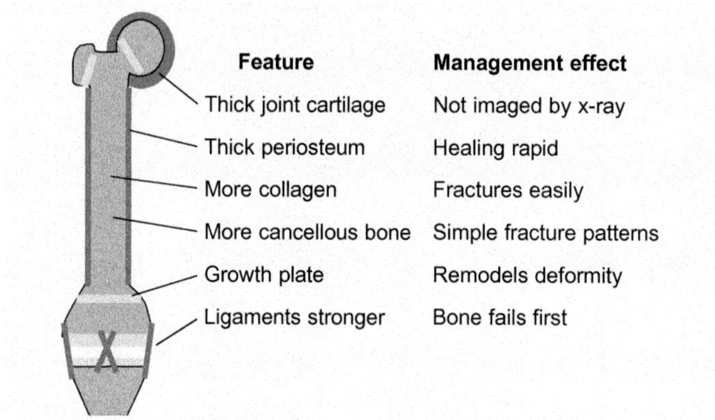

C Bone structural features affecting management The child's musculoskeletal system is different from the adult's in several important ways. These differences significantly affect management.

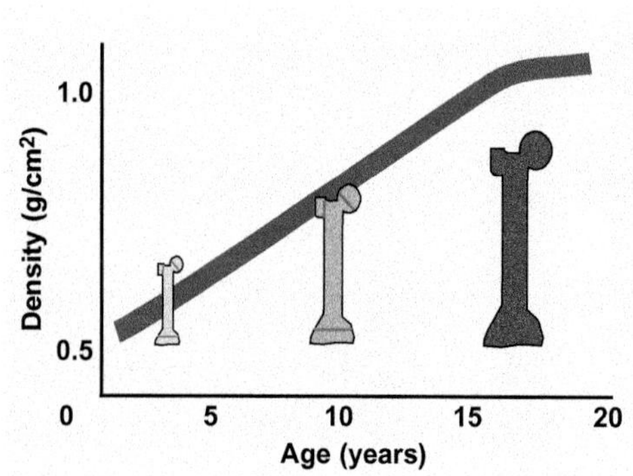

D Bone mineral density This graph shows bone mineral density in the femoral neck in normal subjects. From Thomas (1991).

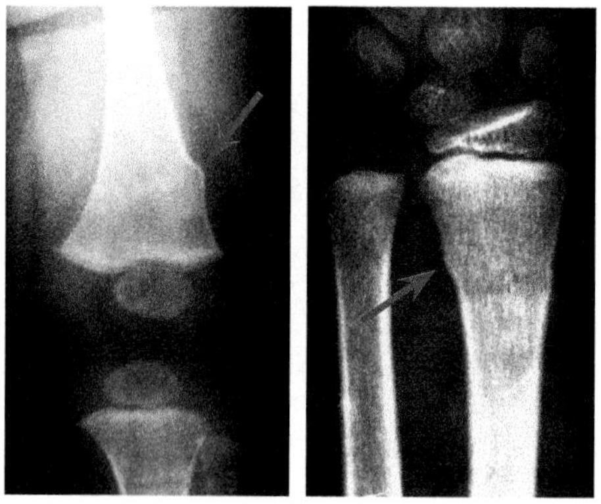

E Buckle fractures These fractures are common in children because the bone fails in both tension and compression and because of the high collagen content.

Children Prone to Injury

Low bone mineral content Children with generalized disorders such as osteogenesis imperfecta [A], renal diseases, cystic fibrosis, diabetes mellitus, and growth hormone deficiencies are at risk.

Neuromuscular disorders Children with cerebral palsy, spina bifida, and arthrogryposis [B] are fracture prone because of the combination of poor mineralization and joint stiffness.

Fracture personality Children in general are at greater risk due to their higher activity levels, and some children in particular who have risk-prone behaviors are at even greater risk.

Physiology

The musculoskeletal system of children is different from that of adults, which explains why children's fractures are different [C]. These differences gradually diminish with age, so that fractures in the adolescent are similar to those in the adult.

Growth Plate

The most obvious musculoskeletal difference is that the child has a growth plate [C]. The relative strength of the growth plate compared to adjacent bone changes with age. For example, the physis in infants is stronger than the adjacent bone, so diaphyseal fractures are most common.

Helps fracture management The growth plate usually helps in managing fractures. Growth facilitates remodeling that corrects residual angulation. The potential for remodeling depends on the growth rate of the adjacent physis and on the remaining growth of the child.

Injured growth plate causes deformity Just as the physis can resolve deformity, asymmetrical physical growth causes deformity.

Bone

Higher collagen-to-bone ratio This lowers the modulus of elasticity and reduces the tensile strength of the bone [D].

Higher cellular and porous bone This reduces tensile strength and reduces the tendency of fractures to propagate and explains why comminuted fractures are uncommon in children.

Bone fails in both tension and compression This explains the mechanism of the common buckle fracture in children [E].

Bone transitions between metaphysis and diaphysis cause a mechanical discontinuity, leading to certain fracture types.

Periosteum

Metabolically active The periosteum is more metabolically active in the child than in the adult. This explains the exuberant callus seen in the infant [A and B] and the rapid union and increased potential for remodeling seen throughout childhood. Bone forms with the periosteal sleeve to create bone continuity. This active periosteum also contributes appositional bone, which facilitates remodeling.

Thickness and strength Children have increased thickness and strength of the periosteum. Fractures within the intact periosteal sleeve may have little displacement and be difficult to diagnose [C]. The intact periosteal hinge affects the fracture pattern [D] and may be helpful in reduction of fractures.

Age-Related Fracture Patterns

These changes in bone result in changing fracture patterns throughout growth [E]. The infant with the diaphyseal fracture, the child with a fracture through the metaphysis, and the adolescent with an epiphyseal injury are examples of this effect.

Ligaments

Ligaments are relatively stronger than bone. Usually bone fails before ligaments, which explains various injury patterns. Avulsion injuries are common in children [F and G]. The distal femoral physis fails before the collateral ligaments [H].

Cartilage

The increased ratio of cartilage to bone in children improves resilience but makes evaluation by radiography more difficult. The size of the articular fragment is often underestimated.

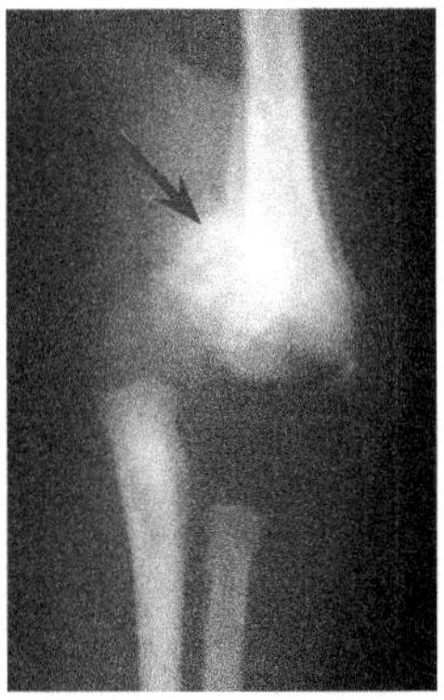

A Exuberant callus formation in the newborn fracture This physeal separation resulted from birth trauma.

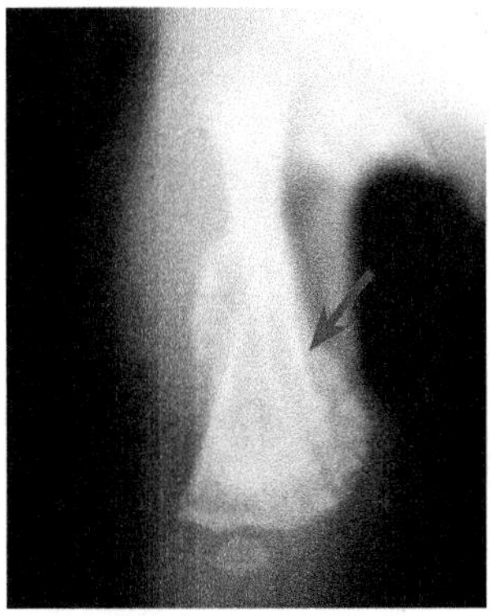

B Callus from femur fracture in an infant Note the extensive callus formation.

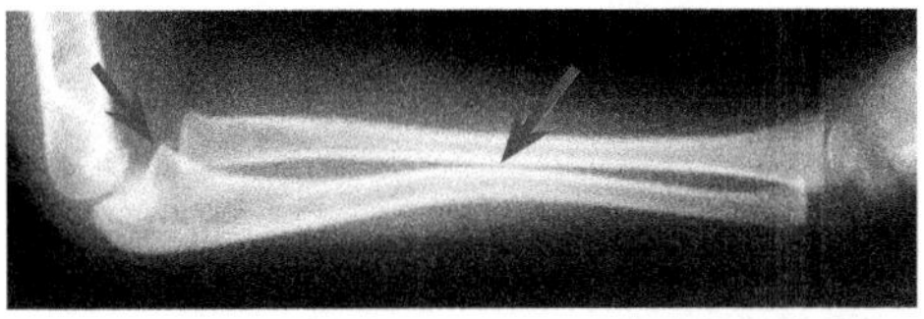

C Plastic bowing of the ulna This child has a dislocation of the radial head with plastic bowing of the ulna.

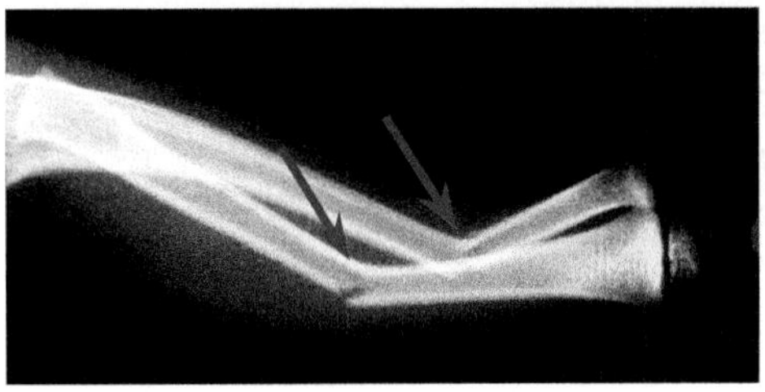

D Greenstick fracture of the forearm Greenstick fractures are common in the forearm, as bone bends before it fractures and the periosteal sleeve maintains apposition.

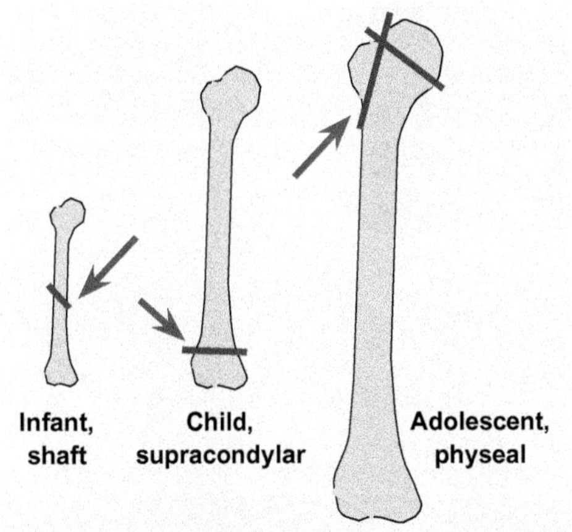

E Age-related injury types of the humerus This injury pattern is present in other long bones, with diaphyseal fractures in infants, metaphyseal fractures in children, and epiphyseal fractures in adolescents.

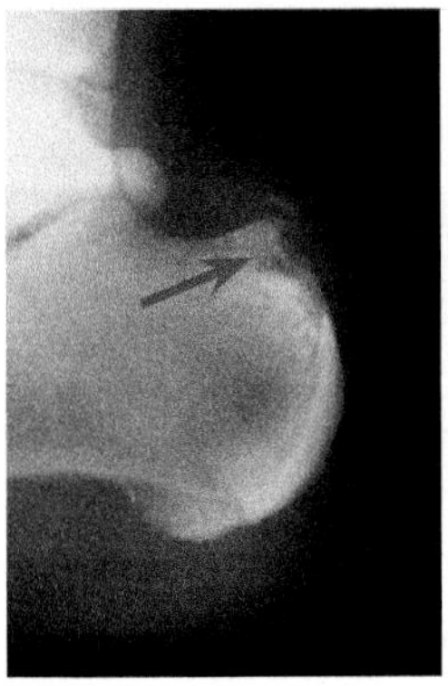

F Avulsion injury of the triceps Avulsion of the tendo-Achilles insertion is due to the greater tensile strength of the triceps tendon than calcaneal bone in the adolescent.

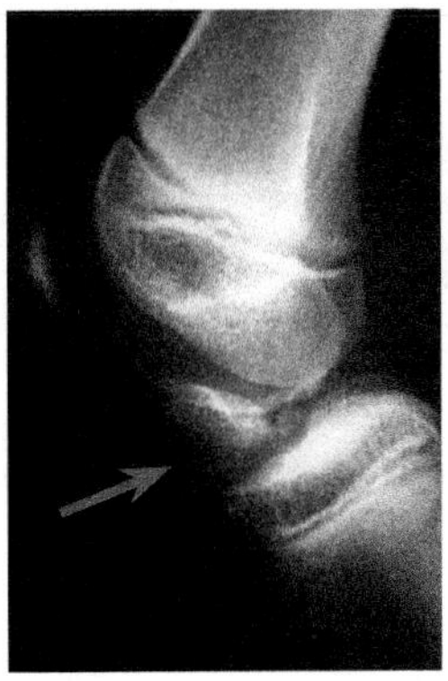

G Avulsion of the tibial spine The bone fails before the anterior cruciate ligament (ACL), resulting in a fracture of the tibial spine.

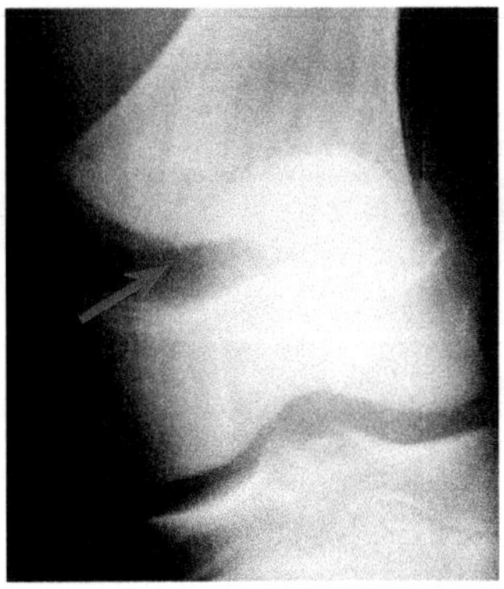

H Fracture of distal femoral epiphysis The physis fails before the adjacent bone or collateral ligaments. This is a common injury type in adolescents.

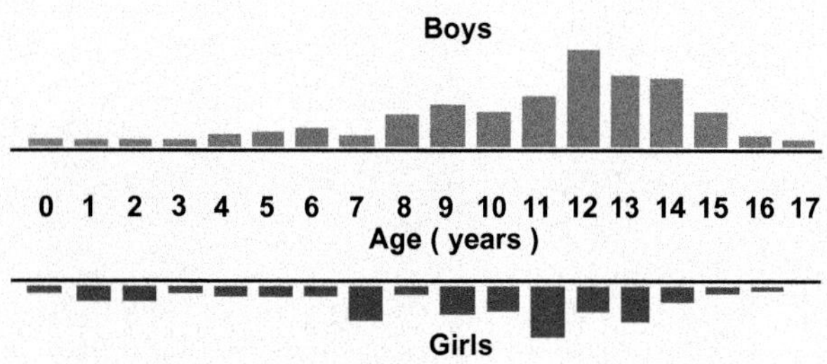

A Age distribution of physeal injuries in boys (blue) and girls (red) From Mizuta (1987).

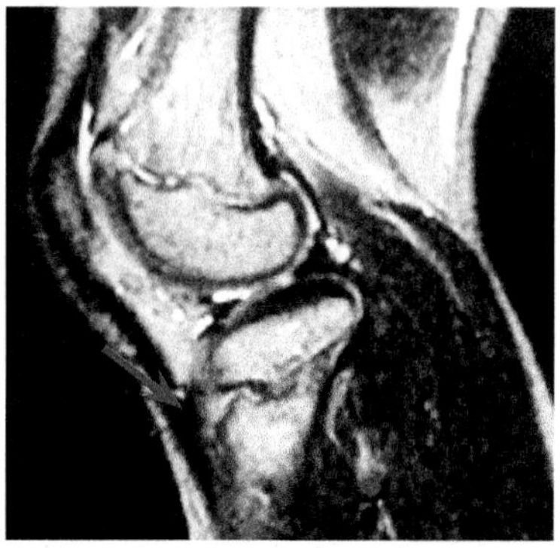

B Recurvatum deformity due to anterior tibial physeal arrest This physis is very vulnerable to arrest.

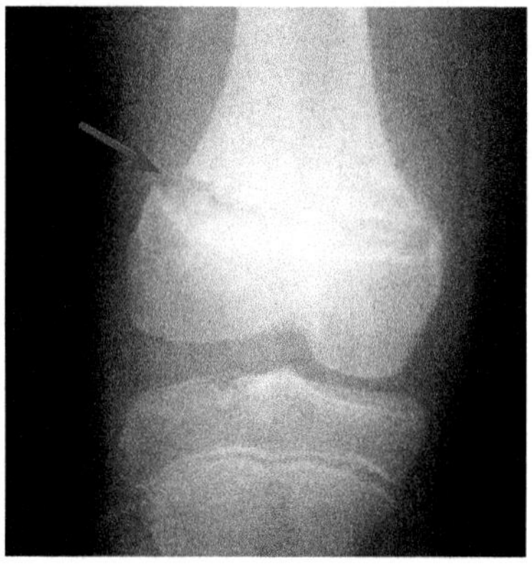

C Physeal injury in myelodysplasia Note the physeal widening.

Physeal Injuries

Physeal injuries account for about one-fourth of all childhood fractures. They are most common in boys, in the upper limb, and in childhood [A]. Physeal injuries may also occur from infection, tumors, or ischemia. Physeal fractures are of great importance, as these injuries can affect subsequent growth and remodeling potential.

Anatomy

The physeal anatomy is varied but the pattern is similar.

Physes can be classified into three main categories:

Long bones The femur is one of the long bones.

Ring epiphyses occur in round bones (cuboid) and around secondary ossification centers.

Apophyses occur at the site of muscle or tendon insertions (e.g., greater trochanteric apophysis).

Growth disturbances of long bone physes are most likely to be damaged and create the greatest deformity.

Long-bone physes often show an undulating pattern with *mamallary processes.* This provides greater sheer strength but may lead to an increased risk of physeal damage from high-impact injuries. An example is the greater likelihood of growth arrest from simple physeal fractures of the distal femoral physis.

Injury

The physis usually fractures through the zone of provisional calcification, sparing the germinal cells so growth is unaffected. Less common injuries that damage the germinal zone or create a tethering bridge across the physis may slow or arrest growth.

Physeal susceptibility to arrest varies. The most sensitive long-bone physis is the anterior portion of the proximal tibial epiphysis. Recurvatum deformity may occur from trivial injury [B].

Stress injuries to the physis are most commonly observed in athletes and children with myelodysplasia [C]. The gymnast may develop a stress fracture of the distal radial physis. Such physeal injuries often cause growth arrest.

Physeal arrest is most common in injuries that allow the bone to bridge the growth plate. The location and percentage of the cross-sectional area occupied by the bony bridge determines the extent of the secondary deformity.

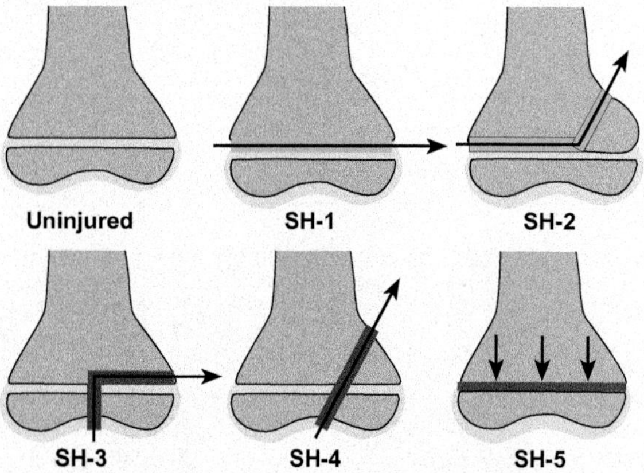

D Salter–Harris (SH) classification of growth plate injuries These are classified as types 1 through 5 based on the fracture pattern. Types 1 and 2 (green lines) do not traverse the epiphysis and usually do not cause growth problems. Types 3 to 5 (red lines) may cause growth arrest and progressive deformity.

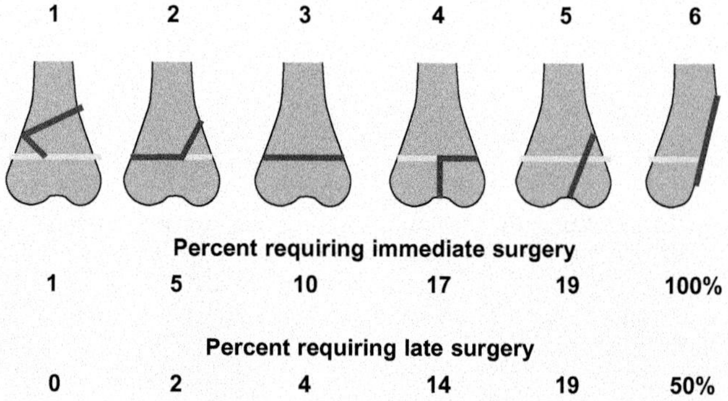

E Peterson classification The frequency of injuries of each type requiring immediate and late surgery are shown. From Peterson (1994).

Classification

Several classification systems for physeal injuries exist. The most simple and widely used is that originated by Salter and Harris (SH). Fractures are divided into five categories based on pattern [D, previous page]. SH-5 injuries are very rare. More comprehensive classifications include those devised by Peterson [E, previous page] and by Ogden. For complex injuries, use a more comprehensive classification.

Classification of injury type is usually done by radiography. Imaging by CT scans may clarify complex fracture patterns such as those in triplane fractures of the ankle. MRI studies [A] often show considerably more physeal damage than was suspected from radiographs, and may change the SH category. Because experience is based on radiographic imaging, prognosis and management based on the more sensitive MRI may lead to overtreatment.

Natural History

Most acute physeal injuries heal rapidly; any deformity remodels completely, and growth proceeds normally. About 1% of physeal injuries cause physeal bridging and altered growth [B]. Small bridges (<10%) may lyse spontaneously. Central bridges are more likely to lyse and less likely to cause deformity than peripheral ones. Central bridges may cause a fishtail deformity, which only slows rather than arrests growth [D].

Physeal Bridge Management

Physeal bridge formation usually follows SH-3, SH-4, or SH-5 injuries. The mechanism is either a crush injury to the germinal layer or a displaced fracture that allows bone to form across the physis. The prognostic significance of the type is not always consistent. For example, physeal arrest also occurs in about half of SH-1 and SH-2 injuries of the distal femur in the older child or adolescent [C]. Physeal injury may also follow fracture of the diaphysis. The mechanism is unclear.

Avoid physeal injury when placing fixation devices in children. Reaming of the upper femur for fixation of femoral shaft fractures is a common cause of physeal damage. Use alternative ways of fixation before the end of growth.

Prevention of physeal bridge formation is best achieved by an anatomic reduction of SH-3 and SH-4 fractures. Open reduction and internal fixation that does not traverse the physis is best. If fixation is necessary across the growth plate, use small, smooth K wires.

Monitor growth for detection of a physeal bridge. If a bridge is found, make a radiograph of the involved bone and the contralateral side on the same film every 4–6 months. Note changes in relative overall length or angulation of the adjacent joint surface.

Imaging physeal bars may be done by CT scans or MRI studies. Order frontal and sagittal computer reconstruction of 1-mm CT scans. MRIs tend to show more soft tissue information but may be more difficult to interpret. Assess the location of the percentage of the cross-sectional area of the physis that the bridge occupies.

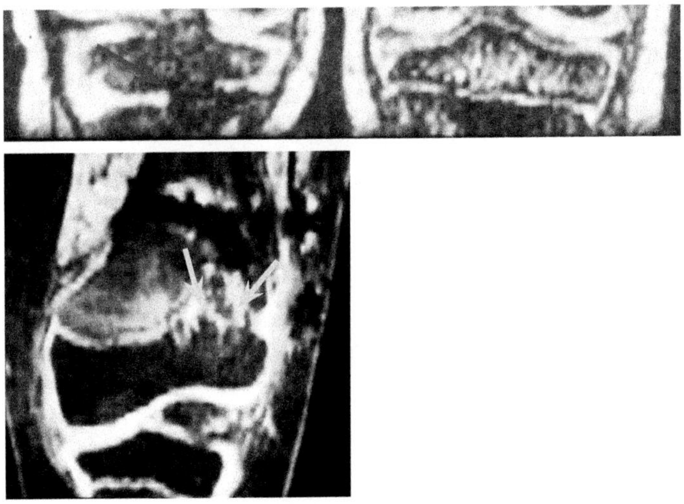

A MRI evaluation of physeal bars The bar may appear as a bridging bone (red arrow) or as an irregularity of the physis (yellow arrows).

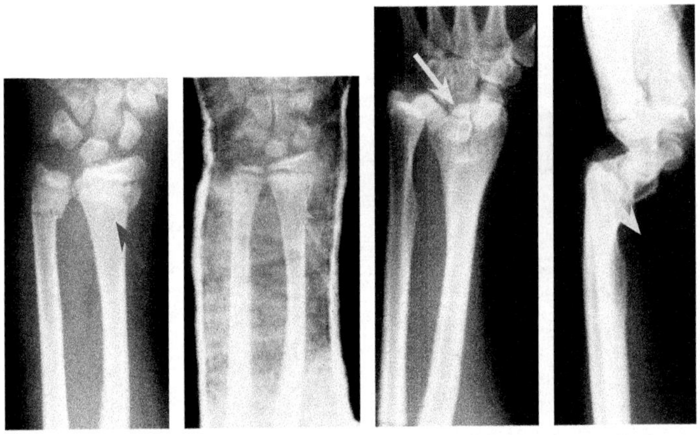

B Natural history of physeal injuries of the distal radius This fracture occurred at age 10 years (red arrow). The reduction looks anatomic (orange arrow). The girl was not seen until age 20, when she complained of a wrist deformity. Note the effect of a volar bridge on the distal radius (yellow arrows).

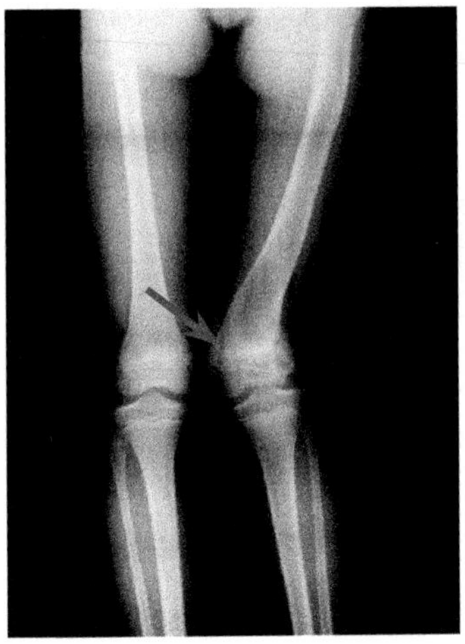

C Physeal bridge of distal femur This bar from a SH-2 fracture caused severe valgus deformity.

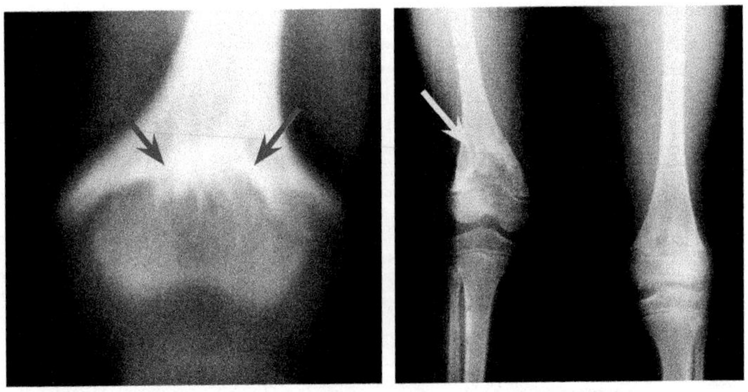

D Central bridge resection in an infant This central bridge (red arrows) resulted from a birth fracture. The bridge was resected (yellow arrow), and growth resumed.

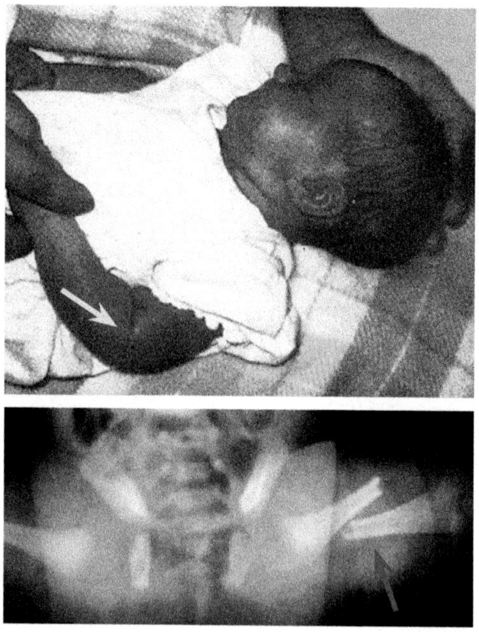

A Birth fractures Joint injuries (yellow arrow) and diaphyseal fractures (red arrow) are examples of the spectrum of these injuries.

Birth and Neonatal Injuries

Birth Injuries

Birth injuries often occur in some unusual obstetrical situations such as large birth weight, shoulder dystocia, mechanically assisted delivery, or prolonged gestational age. It also occurs in infants with some underlying problem such as osteogenesis imperfecta or arthrogryposis.

The most common injuries include brachial plexus injuries and fractures of the clavicle. Other injuries include femoral shaft fractures [A] and neurologic injuries at the intracranial and spinal cord level.

Manage these fractures by simple splinting. Manage clavicular fractures by simply strapping the arm to the thorax for comfort. Manage femoral shaft fractures in a Pavlik harness. Remodeling will correct any remaining deformity.

Fractures in Early Infancy

Neonatal fractures are most common in very low birth weight premature infants who have developmental nutritional rickets. Fractures most commonly involve the ribs, radius, humerus, and femur. Manage by metabolic therapy and splinting. Avoid casts.

Child Abuse

Because child abuse or nonaccidental trauma is a potentially lethal condition, consider this possibility in every infant or young child with a fracture. When the diagnosis of child abuse is missed, recurrent injuries occur in about half, and it is lethal in 10% of infants and children.

Evaluation

Be suspicious of any long-bone fractures in an otherwise normal infant in the first year. Many femoral shaft fractures in early infancy are due to abuse. Be concerned if the caregiver reports only a change in behavior without a history of injury or a trivial injury. Remember that abuse can occur at any socioeconomic level.

Examination Look at the whole child. Other than the current problem, does the infant appear normal? Note any evidence of swelling, pseudoparalysis, or soft tissue trauma [B]. Bruising is more common than fractures.

Imaging If you are suspicious, order an AP radiograph of the chest, all four limbs, and a lateral of the skull. Order a bone scan to show recent fractures if further evaluation is indicated.

Fracture patterns in abuse Fractures that have a high degree of specificity for abuse are metaphyseal fractures and fractures of the humeral shaft, ribs [C], scapula, outer end of the clavicle, and vertebra. Bilateral fractures, complex skull fractures, and those of different ages are suspect. Fractures of varying ages occur in only about 13% of cases. Try to date the fractures by radiographic appearance [C, and A, next page].

If abuse is a possibility Personally call a social worker or case worker if abuse is suspected. Communicate the concern and index of suspicion. Consult pediatric colleagues for their opinions. Carefully document any findings and efforts. Parents of infants with accidental injuries usually accept consultations with a simple explanation of the reason. Objection should raise suspicion.

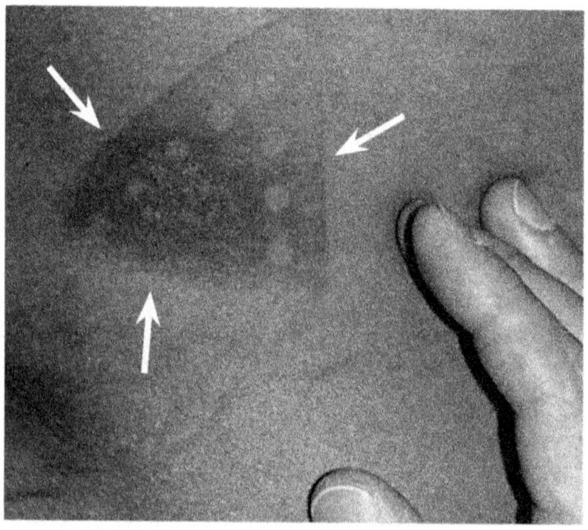

B Child abuse This hot iron burn scar is permanent and unmistakable (white arrows).

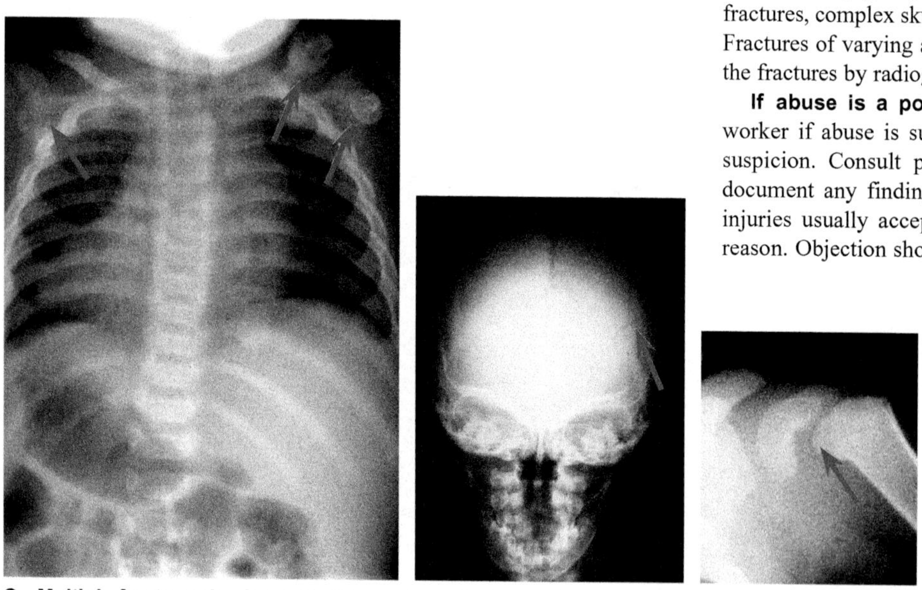

C Multiple fractures in abuse Multiple fractures (red arrows) at varying stages of development are common in abuse.

Remodeling

The capacity of bone to remodel significantly influences the management of fractures in children. One of the great challenges in pediatric orthopedics is to predict accurately which fractures require reduction and which will remodel sufficiently on their own.

Mechanism

Remodeling results from a combination of appositional bone deposition on the concavity of the deformity, resorption on the convexity, and asymmetrical physeal growth [A and B]. Remodeling requires a functional physis and intact periosteum.

Factors Affecting Remodeling Potential

Some generalizations are possible to predict whether a specific malunion will remodel without reduction [C].

Years of remaining growth This is possibly the most important factor.

Position in the bone The best examples are forearm fractures. Midshaft fracture remodeling is substantially less than fractures near the wrist [D].

Growth potential of adjacent physis As an example, fractures of the upper humerus show spectacular remodeling [F] as compared with distal humeral fractures.

Plane of motion Remodeling is generally greatest for sagittal plane, then frontal, and least for transverse plane malunions.

Physeal status Any damage to the adjacent physis reduces growth and the potential for remodeling.

Examples of Remodeling

Remodeling is one of the most forgiving features of childhood fracture management. Examples are useful to show the potential for correction to the clinician and for reassuring families. (See pages 294–295 to show families the potential for remodeling.)

Wrist Note that the wrist has extensive remodeling potential [D].

Femoral shaft Femoral shaft fractures in the child remodel completely [E].

Proximal humerus Because the shoulder joint is multiaxial with rapid growth, remodeling is often spectacular [F].

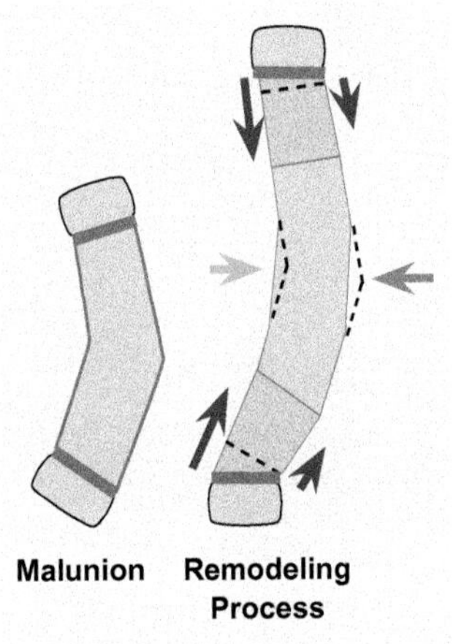

A Mechanism for remodeling Remodeling occurs from appositional periosteal formation (green arrow), resorption (blue arrow), and asymmetrical physeal growth (red arrows). Redrawn from Gasco (1997).

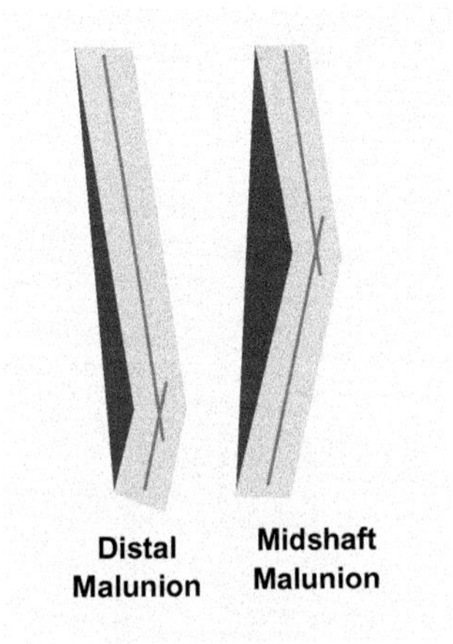

B Greater remodeling for mid shaft deformity For the same angular deformity, more correction (area in red) is required for midshaft than distal deformity.

Greatest Remodeling Potential

- Years of remaining growth
- Position in the bone
- Growth potential of adjacent physis
- Plane of motion
- Physeal status

C Factors affecting remodeling potential These are the significant factors to consider in management.

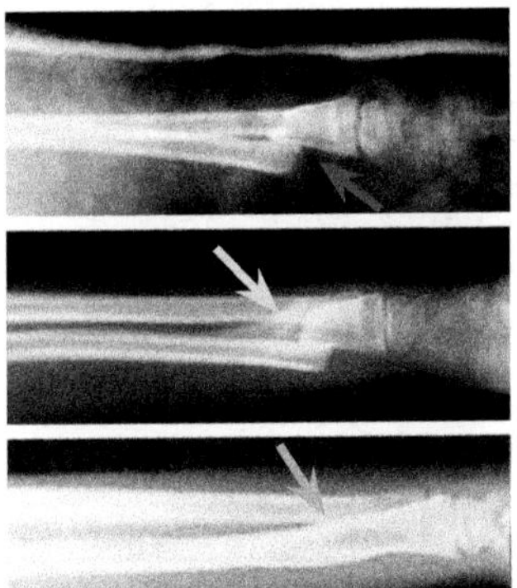

D Remodeling of forearm The fracture fragments were in bayonet apposition (red arrow). Three months later, remodeling was in progress (yellow arrow). At 2 years (orange arrow), remodeling was nearly complete.

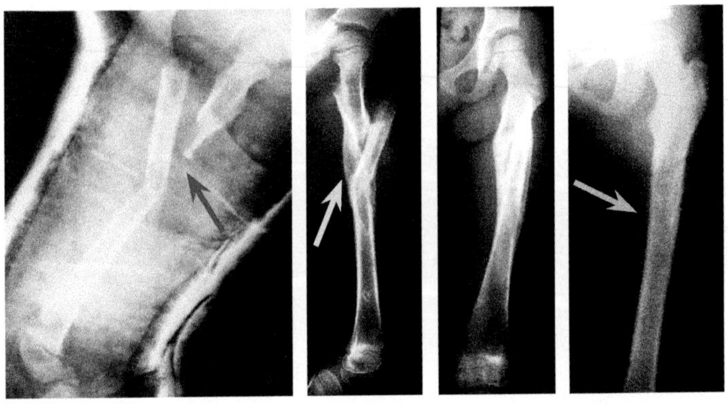

E Remodeling of femoral shaft fracture This segmental fracture in an 8-year-old girl was managed in traction and in a cast (red arrow). Note the filling in of the periosteal sheath at 6 months (yellow arrow) and restoration of normal femoral shape at age 13 years (orange arrow).

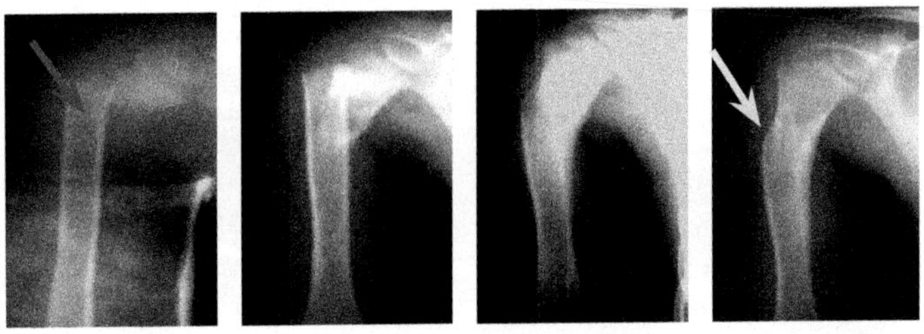

F Remodeling of the humerus This 8-year-old boy shows a complete loss of apposition (red arrow). Note the remodeling over the next 2 years (yellow arrow).

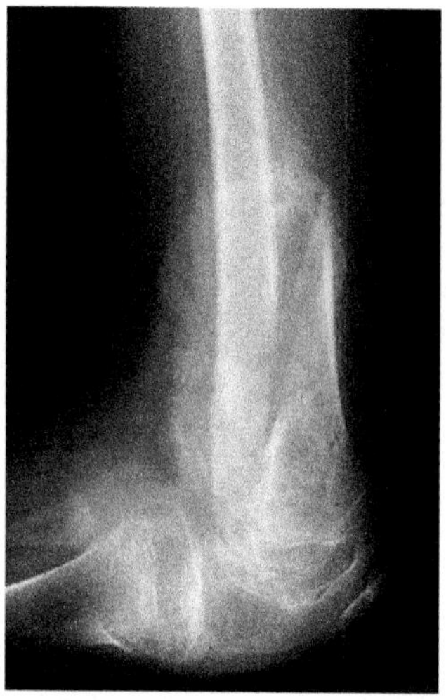

A Fracture in child with cerebral palsy The bone easily fractures, and abundant callus occurs during healing.

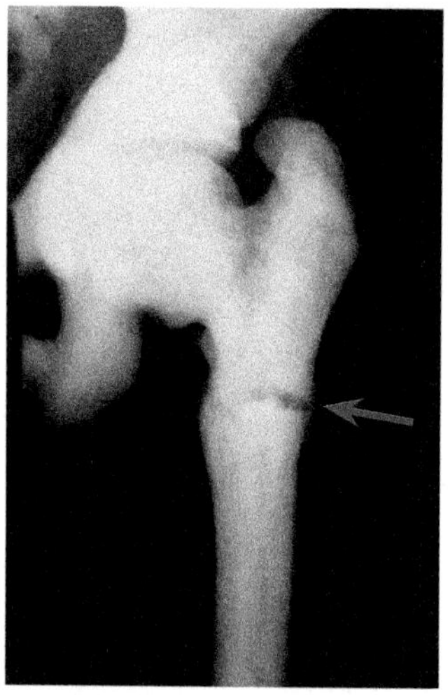

B Fracture in osteopetrosis These bones fracture easily and are difficult to fix internally.

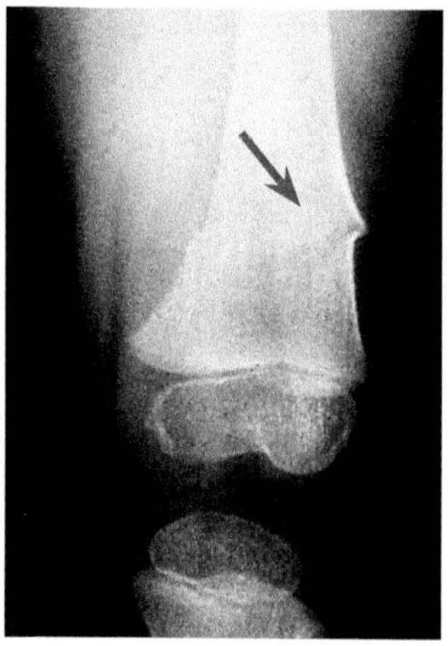

C Fracture following DDH treatment in a spica cast

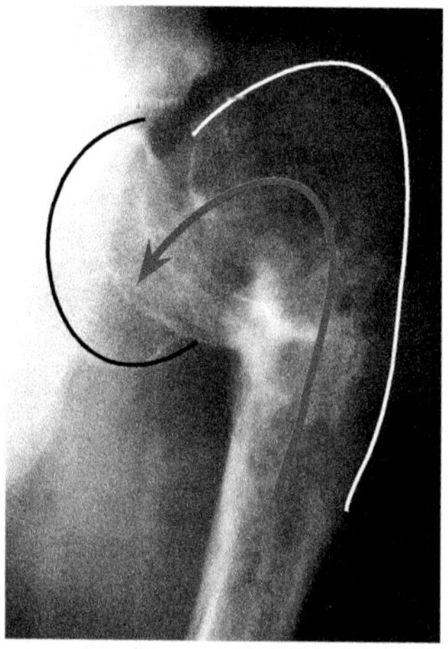

D Multiple fractures in fibrous dysplasia This child has developed a shepherd crook deformity from repeated fractures.

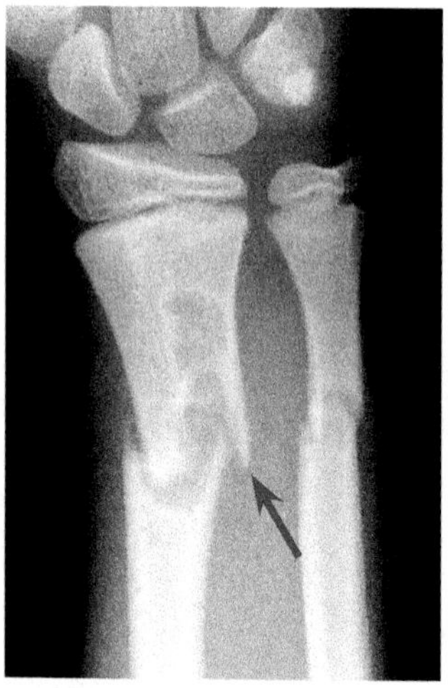

E Fracture through a nonossifying fibroma

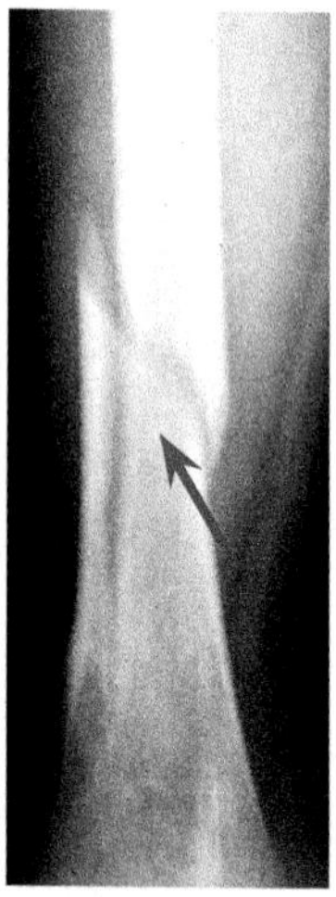

F Fracture through malignant osteogenic sarcoma This is the most worrisome fracture to miss.

Pathologic Fractures

Pathologic fractures are relatively common in children. Fractures frequently occur through osteopenic bone in children with neuromuscular disorders and through bone weakened by tumors.

Evaluation

Be concerned if the trauma required for fracture is less than normal. Normal infants and young children's bones can fracture with simple falls. Usually a history and screening examination will separate normal children from those with underlying osteopenic problems.

Management

Generalized disorders include those that decrease or increase bone density. Manage fractures through osteopenic bone in children with conditions such as cerebral palsy [A], spina bifida, and osteogenesis imperfecta with a minimum period of immobilization because mobilization increases deossification and increases the risk of additional fractures. Dysplasias increase bone density and may also be prone to fracture [B].

Cast treatment for conditions such as developmental hip dysplasia increase the risk of fracture. The period of greatest vulnerability is shortly after cast removal, as joints are stiff and bone is weakened by immobilization [C].

Benign bone lesions are often the sites of fracture.

Small localized tumors If the lesion is small and the trauma significant, immobilize in a cast until union has occurred. Usually, it is best to allow the fracture to heal and then deal with the lesion. For larger lesions, especially those involving the upper femur, stabilization and bone grafting may be necessary.

Fibrous dysplasia Consider early augmentation with a flexible intramedullary rod [D] to increase bone strength and reduce the risk of fracture. This treatment usually shortens the period of convalescence.

Unicameral bone cysts Most cysts should be allowed to heal and then be managed as described in Chapter 7. Those of the upper femur require special consideration. Most require internal fixation to prevent malunion. Graft and fix during the same operative session. Avoid threaded or large fixation across any growth plate in the child under age 8–10 years. Smooth K wires may be applied across the proximal femoral physis. Bend the pins over to avoid migration.

Nonossifying fibromas are common sites of fractures [E]. If they involve more than 50% of the transverse bone area, they may require grafting.

Malignant tumors Be most concerned about missing a fracture through a malignant tumor such as an osteogenic sarcoma [F]. Ask if the child or adolescent had night pain before the fracture. Night pain is often an indicator of a malignant tumor. Carefully review the radiograph with attention to the character of the bone. Early identification of the pathologic aspect of the fracture is the primary concern.

Open Fractures

Open fractures in children most commonly involve the tibia, but they may also complicate supracondylar fractures and fractures of the forearm, femur, and other bones.

Classification

The classification of open injuries is basically the same as for adults [A]. Overall, the prognosis for a given grade is better in children, especially infants and young children. Adolescents behave more like adults.

Management

Sequence Manage acute injuries in the same sequence as done for adults. This involves antibiotic prophylaxis, tetanus update, debridement [B and C], and immobilization. Limb salvage is usually feasible. Open fractures in younger children can be managed less aggressively than those of the adolescent.

Different management for the child Managing the child differs from managing the adult in several ways: (1) soft tissue healing is much more rapid and complete, (2) devitalized bone that is not contaminated can be left in place and will incorporate, (3) the periosteum will generate new bone when bone is lost [D], (4) delayed union or nonunion is uncommon, and (5) external fixators may be left in place for prolonged periods to be certain bony union is solid.

Type	Soft tissue	Bone
Type 1	Clean wound	< 1 cm laceration
Type 2	Soft tissue injury	> 1 cm laceration not extensive
Type 3	Extensive soft tissue injury	Includes segmental fractures

A Gustilo classification of open fractures in children

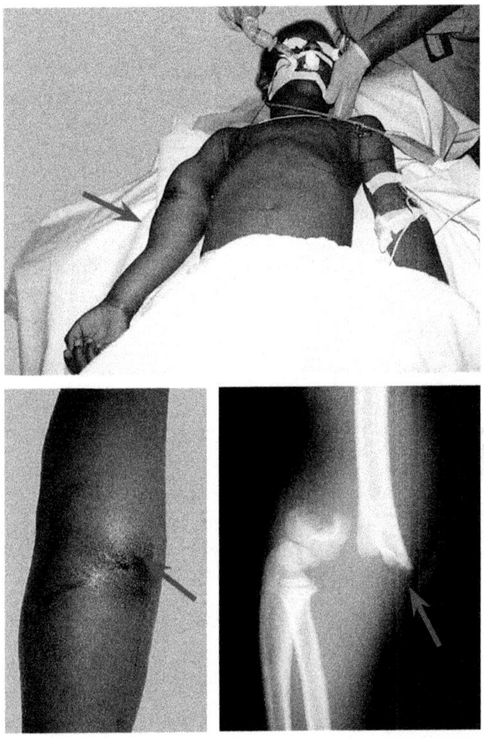

B Open supracondylar fracture This type 1 open fracture (arrows) produced only a puncture wound above the elbow. The wound was irrigated and edges debrided.

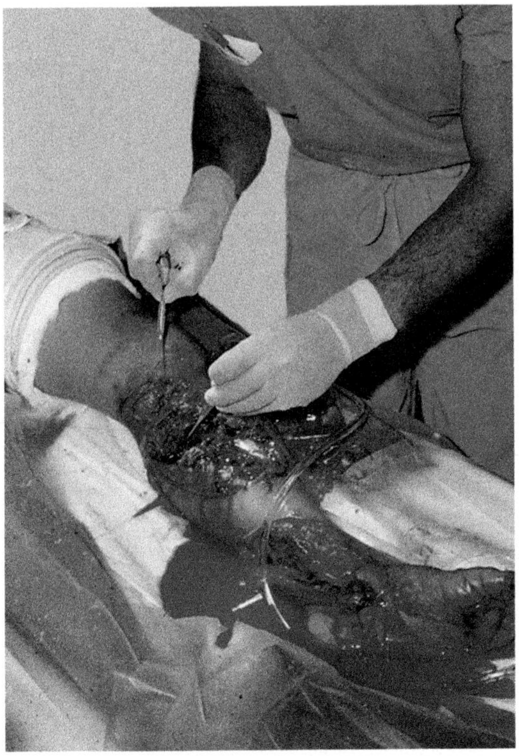

C Fracture debridement While swimming, this boy sustained an open tibial fracture from a boat propeller. This debridement was carefully performed to remove all devitalized and foreign material. An external fixator was placed, and the bone healed without infection.

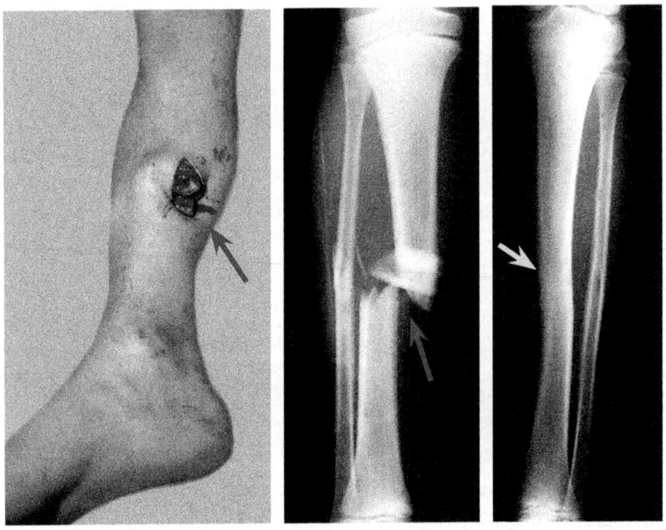

D Open segmental fracture of the tibia This fracture (red arrows) was managed by debridement and removal of the loose contaminated segment. Note that the bone regenerated within the periosteum (yellow arrow).

Evaluation

Establishing an accurate diagnosis is the most important step in managing childhood injuries. Most major management errors are due to an inaccurate diagnosis. The evaluation of the injured child is difficult because injuries are sometimes multiple, the child is frequently uncooperative, and the emergency situation makes a thorough evaluation difficult.

Diagnostic errors are most significant in the child sustaining polytrauma, as subtle fractures are easily overlooked and musculoskeletal injuries are the most common cause of residual disability. In the polytraumatized child, musculoskeletal injuries seldom cause death but are a common cause of residual disability [A].

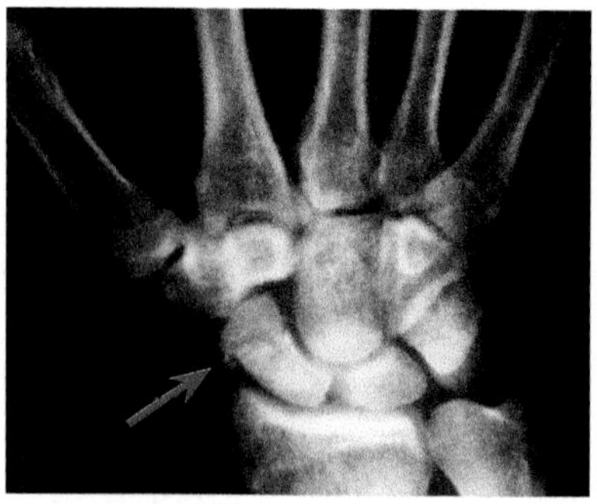

A Missed navicular fracture This 14-year-old boy sustained polytrauma. During rehabilitation, he complained of wrist pain. A radiograph demonstrated this navicular fracture.

Priorities

Make the first priority the evaluation of the pulmonary, cardiovascular, and neurologic status. Musculoskeletal priorities include cervical spine injury, joint dislocations (especially the hip), and unstable and open fractures.

History

The history should include the situation, velocity, mechanism, and any unique features of the accident. Be aware that a history of trauma may cloud the diagnosis of a more serious problem [B].

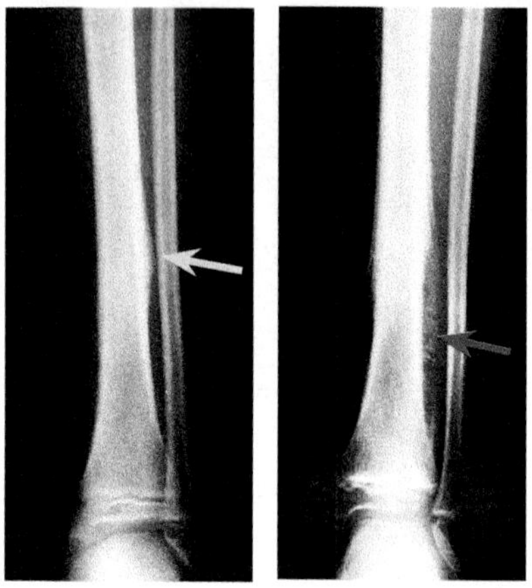

B Misleading history of trauma This 12-year-old girl was initially seen with a history of injury to her leg. The radiographs showed periosteal new bone (yellow arrow) that was thought to be due to trauma. The pain increased gradually, and 2 months later, the lesion was larger (red arrow). A biopsy demonstrated Ewing sarcoma.

Physical Examination

Most diagnostic errors are due to an incomplete physical examination. Perform a screening examination first. Look at the whole child. Look for obvious deformity and spontaneous movement. Pseudoparalysis in the child or infant is commonly due to trauma [D].

Remove any splints [C] or bandages so the examination can be complete. Look for deformity and swelling, and localize the point of maximum tenderness (PMT) [E]. Identifying the site of injury by physical examination is very important because much of the immature skeleton is unossified and difficult to image (see Chapter 2). Determining the PMT is one of the most important steps in diagnosing occult injuries in children.

Evaluate the vascular status [F]. Be aware that the pulse is inadequate as a test of circulation. Observe the capillary refill rate and observe the child's reaction while extending the fingers or toes. Pain on passive stretching is an early sign of ischemia. Compartment syndromes may be silent in children.

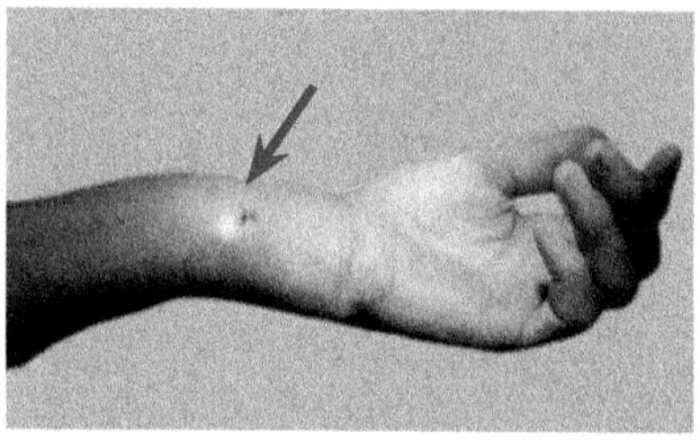

C Arm splint hiding puncture from an open fracture The open nature of the forearm fracture was not initially appreciated due to an arm splint.

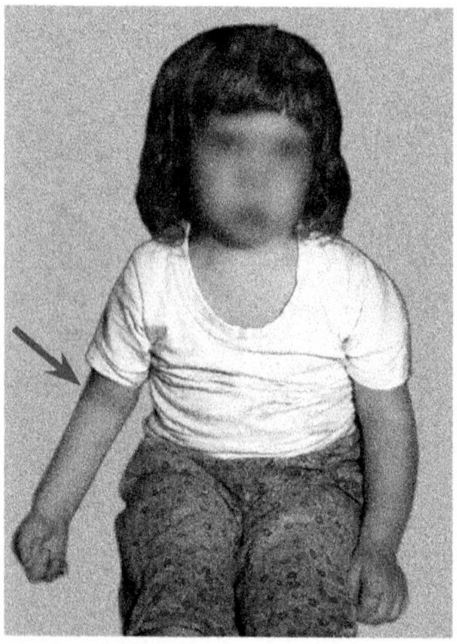

D Pseudoparalysis This child has a pulled elbow and will not use the arm. The loss of spontaneous or volitional movement is a common sign of trauma in infants and young children.

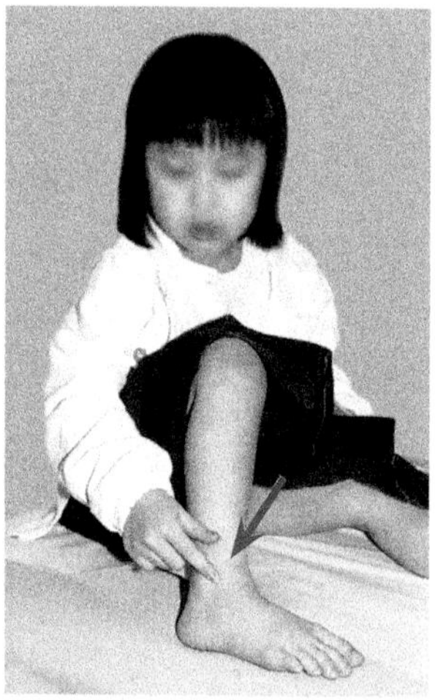

E Localization of the point of maximum tenderness The exact PMT is a valuable finding that is sometimes diagnostic, as in this child with an anterior leaf collateral ligament sprain.

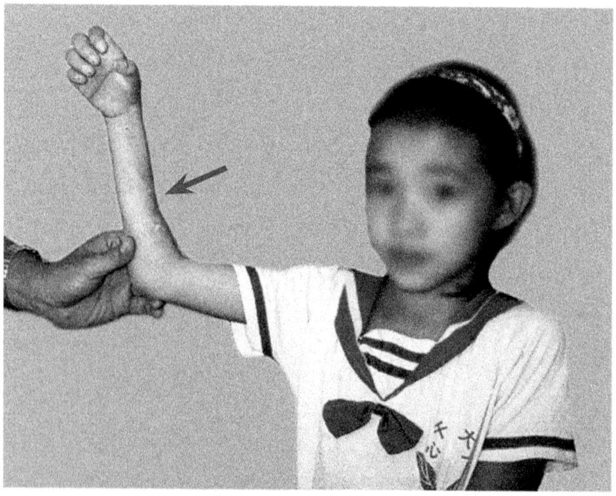

F Ischemic contracture of the forearm This child has a contracture complicating a supracondylar fracture treated in a cast.

Imaging for Trauma

The vast majority of trauma problems can be satisfactorily imaged by conventional radiographs. Comparative radiographs of the opposite side are rarely necessary in evaluating injuries in the child. Order comparative views only for special needs, such as assessing ossification irregularities. Subtle fractures are often identified by an unexpected change in the cortical contour [A]. Soft tissue swelling [B] may indicate the presence of a fracture that may not otherwise be apparent.

Ordering special imaging First consider additional radiographic views. Oblique radiographs may show a fracture that is suspected from the physical findings but not seen in the standard AP and lateral screening radiographs [C]. Displacement of articular or physeal fractures must be determined. Additional oblique projections may provide further information that may be helpful in deciding whether to accept the current reduction. Special imaging studies are indicated in certain situations when conventional radiographs provide insufficient information. The selection of the type of imaging is based on the physical examination findings and on a knowledge of common injury types typical in the child's age group.

Arthrography may be useful in assessing cartilagenous injuries [D].

Bone scans are useful in screening for injuries [E]. Order a high-resolution study to pinpoint the exact location of a suspected fracture. For example, if "snuff-box" tenderness is found on physical examination and the radiographs are negative, order a high-resolution scan to determine if the scaphoid is fractured.

MRI studies require deep sedation of the infant and younger child and therefore have limited indications. Order these studies when suspecting such serious problems [F] as spinal or nonaccidental injury.

Ultrasound studies are underutilized. Consider ultrasonography when evaluating such conditions as a possible physeal separation of the distal humeral epiphyseal complex in the newborn.

Arthroscopy may be helpful for evaluation of articular injuries when radiographic studies are negative [G].

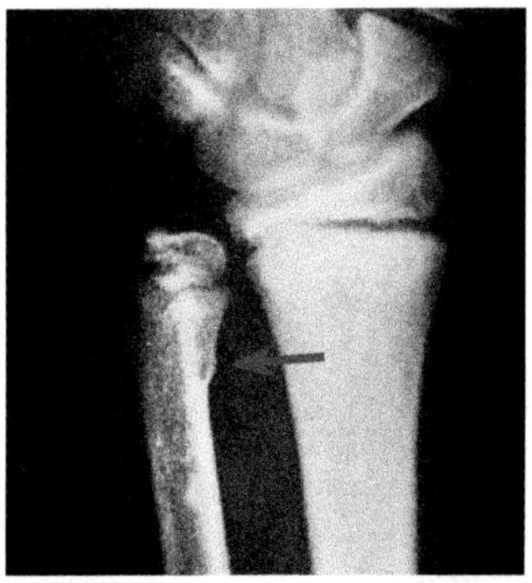

A Cortical irregularity due to a fracture A change in contour when associated with tenderness over the same site is diagnostic of a fracture.

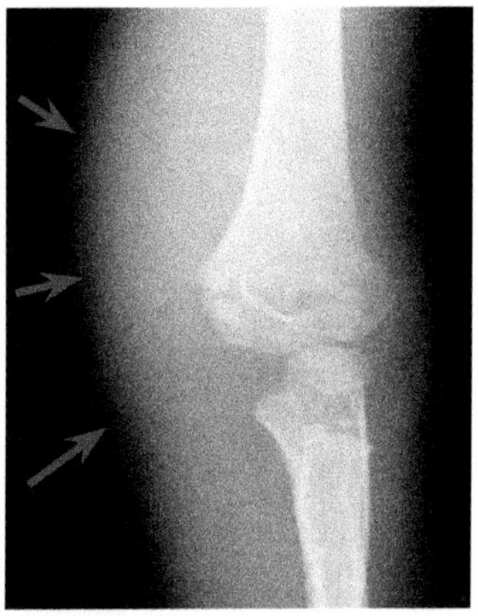

B Soft tissue swelling This extensive soft tissue swelling is evidence of a fracture.

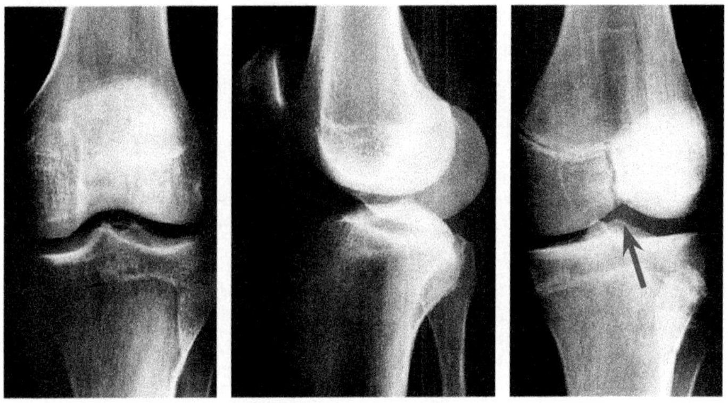

C Value of oblique radiograph This intracondylar fracture (arrow) was not seen in the AP or lateral radiographs.

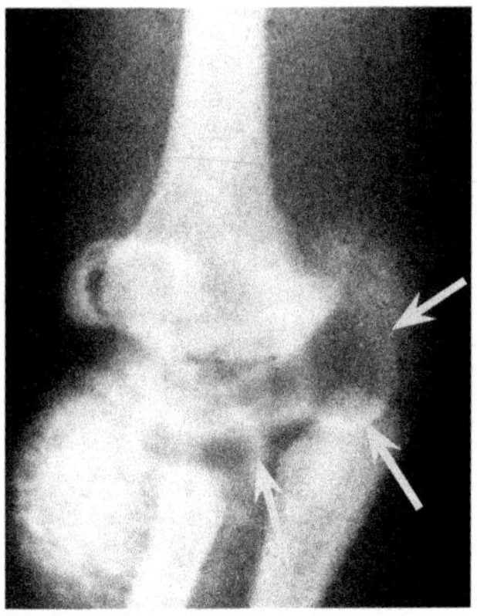

D Arthrogram An arthrogram of an infant shows a physeal fracture not apparent on radiographs (yellow arrows).

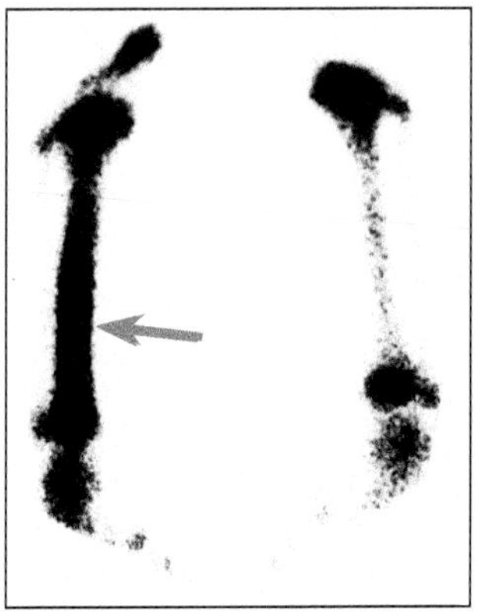

E Bone scan A toddler's fracture (blue arrow) is demonstrated that was not visible on radiographs.

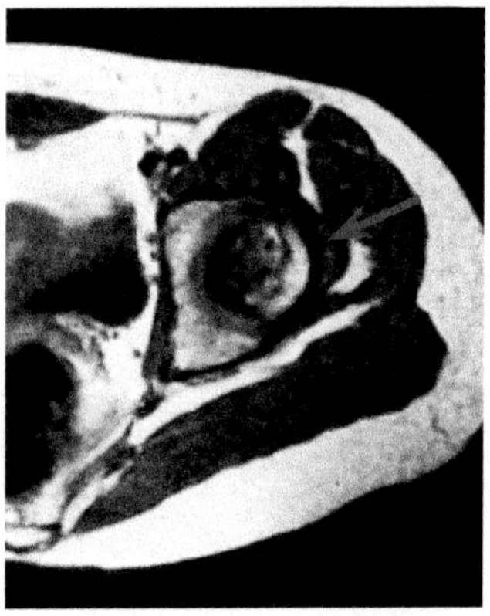

F MRI AVN is demonstrated in this child following a femoral neck fracture (red arrow) prior to radiographic changes.

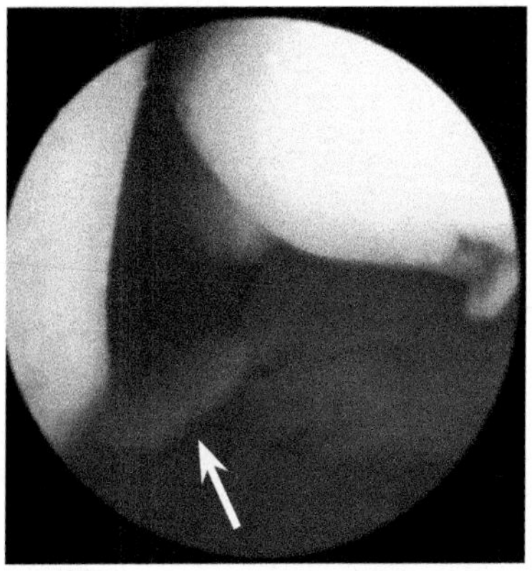

G Arthroscopy This articular fracture (white arrow) was not visible by radiography.

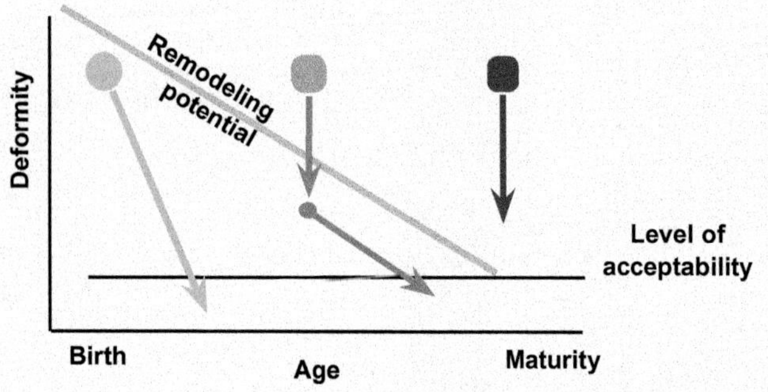

A Age-determined changes affecting reduction With increasing age, the potential for remodeling declines (orange line). For a given angulation, the age determines the required degree of reduction. In infancy (green arrow), reduction is not necessary, as remodeling is rapid and complete. The same angulation in a child (blue arrows) requires partial reduction, with remodeling correcting the remaining deformity. In the adolescent (red arrow), anatomic reduction is required.

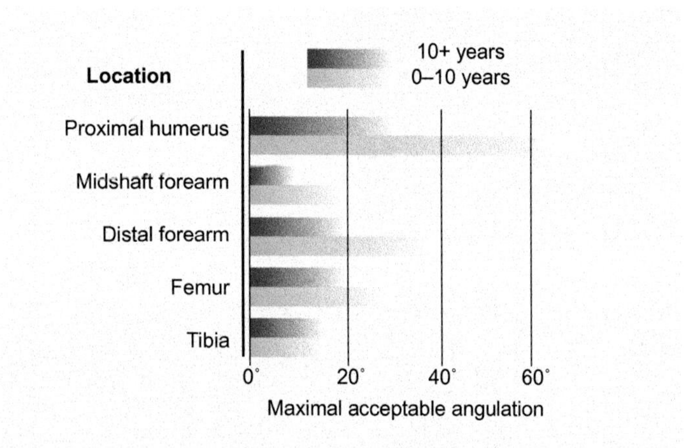

B Potential for remodeling This graph suggests limits of acceptable, angular deformity following long-bone fractures in children. From Casco and de Pablos (1997).

Principles of Reduction

Indications for the need and accuracy of fracture reduction in children are often complex and require good judgment. Base these decisions on underlying principles whenever possible. Unfortunately, data on which to base these principles is limited. Some generally accepted principles can be outlined for different types of fractures. A flowchart is often helpful [C].

Metaphyseal–Diaphyseal Fractures

Several principles are helpful in deciding whether a fracture requires reduction in the child.

Age The younger the child, the greater the potential for remodeling [A and B]. This is possibly the most important factor. Generally, children under age 10 years can be expected to remodel significant deformity.

Bone position Remodeling is greatest near the ends of bones. The amount of remodeling necessary to correct a deformity is proportional to the distance from the adjacent joint. For example, distal forearm fractures remodel much better than midshaft deformities.

Plane of deformity Remodeling is usually greater in the sagittal than the frontal planes. Rotational or transverse plane deformity can remodel, but the amount is controversial. One reason for this controversy is the difficulty in assessing and imaging rotational remodeling.

Also, the plane of deformity is related to the axis of motion of the adjacent joints. Deformity that lies in the plane of motion of the adjacent joint will resolve or is better tolerated. For example, an anterior or posterior bow of the femur is more accepted than varus or valgus deformity.

Growth rate of adjacent physis Accept more deformity close to a physis with a great growth rate and potential. For example, the rapid growth rate of the upper humeral epiphysis contributes to its spectacular remodeling potential. In contrast, growth at the elbow is limited and varus–valgus deformities remodel poorly.

Completion of remodeling Remodeling is completed in about 5–6 years. Most occurs in the first 1 or 2 years.

Unique features Some malunions remodel poorly. The classic example is the cubitus varus deformity, resulting from malunion of supracondylar humeral fractures. Lateral condylar fractures are prone to nonunion [A, next page]. The reason is unclear.

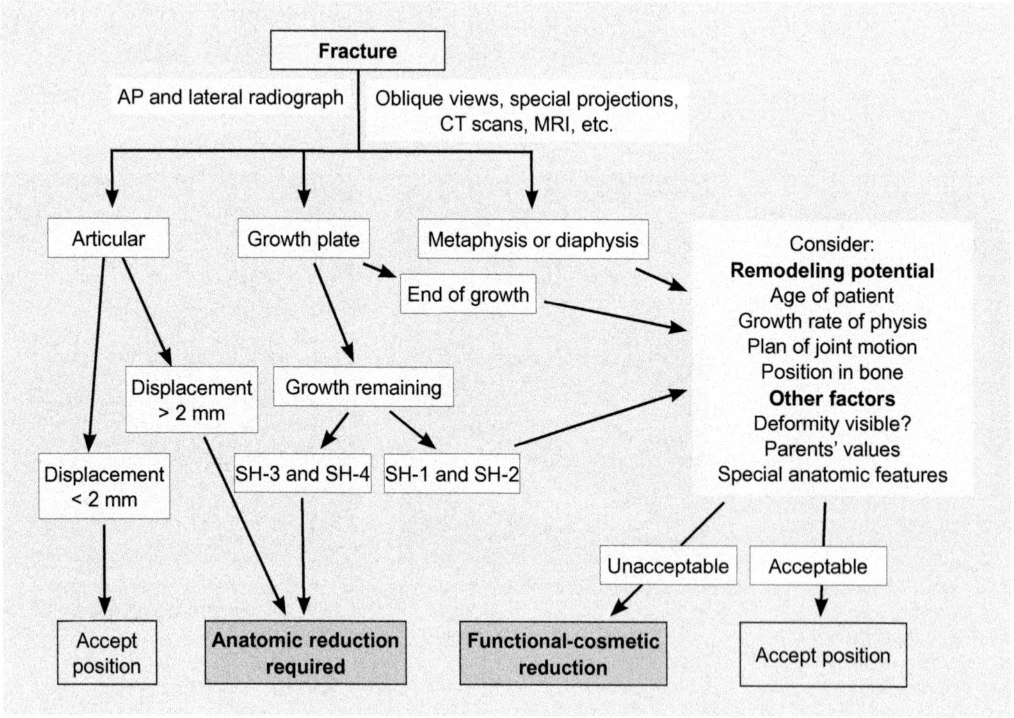

C Reduction flowchart This flowchart may help in determining the need for reduction.

Physeal Fractures

Physeal fracture reduction is well established. SH-3 and SH-4 fractures should be anatomically reduced to prevent physeal bridge formation and reduce the risk of bar formation [C, previous page]. Consider SH-1 and SH-2 fractures like metaphyseal injuries and apply the same principles to make decisions about management.

Articular Fractures

Articular fractures [B and C] are less common in children than in adults, as the cartilage is more resilient and less readily injured. Some generalizations can be made.

Remodeling may correct some deformity Accept more articular deformity in the infant or young child than in older children or adolescents. Consider adolescents like adults.

Accept more horizontal than longitudinal displacement A step-off deformity that increases the articular loading may be less acceptable than one that widens the joint.

Apply the 2-mm rule Generally, we accept displacement of less than 2 mm. This rule was established based on clinical experience. Be aware that MRI or CT studies will usually show more displacement than conventional radiographs [B].

Indications for Open Reduction

Indications for open reduction change with time. These indications are affected by social, medical, and economic factors with considerable variation. Some generalizations can be made [D and E].

Polytrauma suggests multisystem injury, not simply a child with several fractures. Many children with multiple fractures are best managed by cast immobilization, traction, or other noninvasive methods.

Economic indications The financial cost of management should be a factor only when deciding between options that are all medically acceptable.

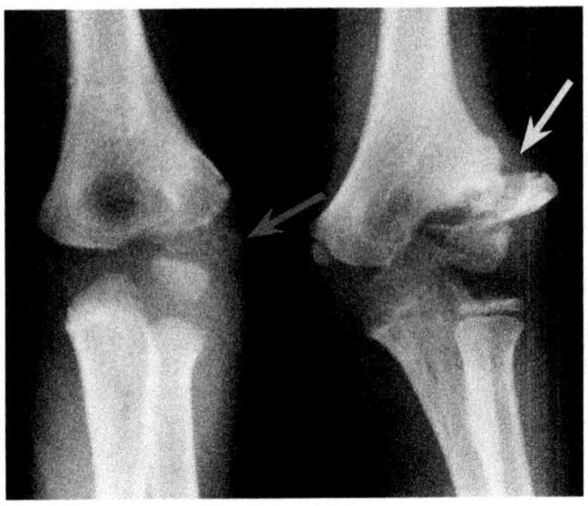

A Displaced lateral condylar fractures require anatomic reduction This unique fracture (red arrow) is not only an articular injury but also an SH-4 fracture that is prone to nonunion. These are all indications for an anatomic reduction and internal fixation. Note that the unfixed fracture developed a nonunion (yellow arrow).

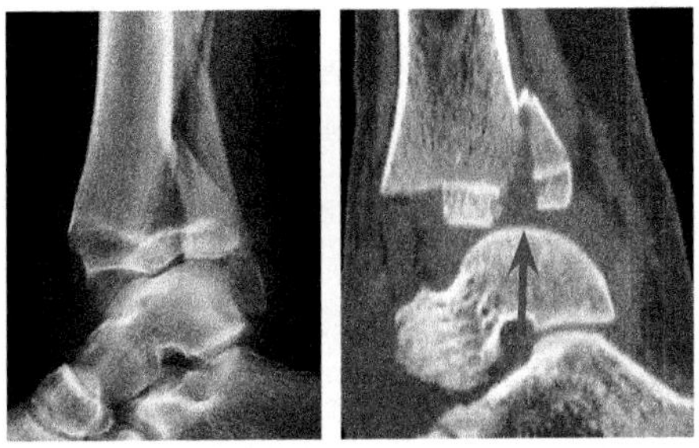

B CT imaging more accurate The fracture is readily apparent on the lateral radiograph, but the CT scan (red arrow) best shows the extent of displacement and the need for reduction.

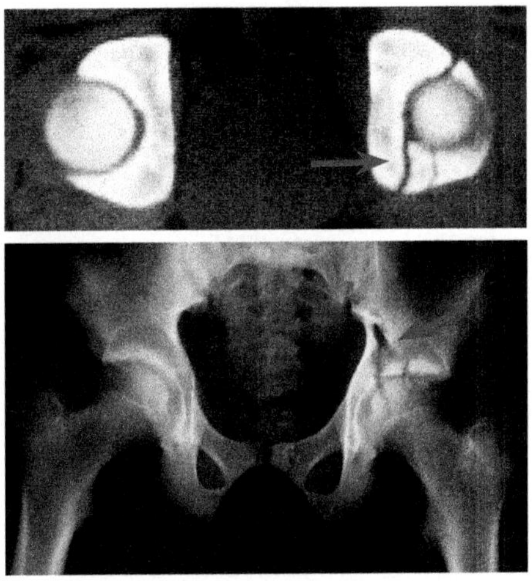

C Acetabular fractures Anatomic reduction of most displaced acetabular fractures in adolescents is usually indicated, as the hip joint poorly tolerates deformity.

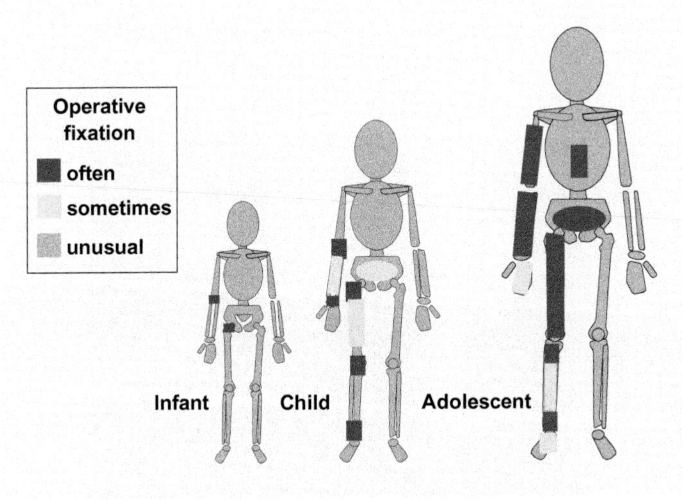

D Need for operative reduction and fixation The need for open procedures in managing childhood fractures increases with age.

Open Reduction Indications
All ages
Lateral condylar fracture, humerus SH-3 and SH-4 fractures Polytrauma Displaced articular fractures
End of growth
Tibial triplane fractures
Age 10+ years
Femoral shaft fractures Displaced midshaft forearm fracture

E Common indications for open reduction These are also indications for internal fixation of displaced fractures.

Management in Primary Care

A large percentage of traumatic problems can be safely managed in primary care. These include many common fractures and sprains. Treating such injuries in the primary care setting is convenient, inexpensive, and effective for the child and family, and is satisfying for the physician. The injuries listed in the section can usually safely and effectively managed in the primary care setting.

Suggestions for Management

Some guidelines in trauma management.

Perform a careful physical examination This should include a general assessment of the child as well an evaluation of the injured part.

Examine for bony tenderness Tenderness over bone is a common feature of a fracture [A]. If tenderness is absent, the bone is nearly always intact. A classic example is the toddler's fracture. Swelling may be absent but the child is more tender over the shaft of the tibia.

Beware of elbow and knee injuries These are most difficult to assess. The elbow and knee are the most likely site of misdiagnoses and adverse outcomes [B, C, and D]. An exception is the pulled elbow.

Limit imaging to radiographs As MR, CT, bone scans, and other imaging are expensive and sometimes difficult to interpret, delegate ordering of special imaging to the orthopedist. This practice will save the family unnecessary expense and the child the possibility of the wrong diagnosis.

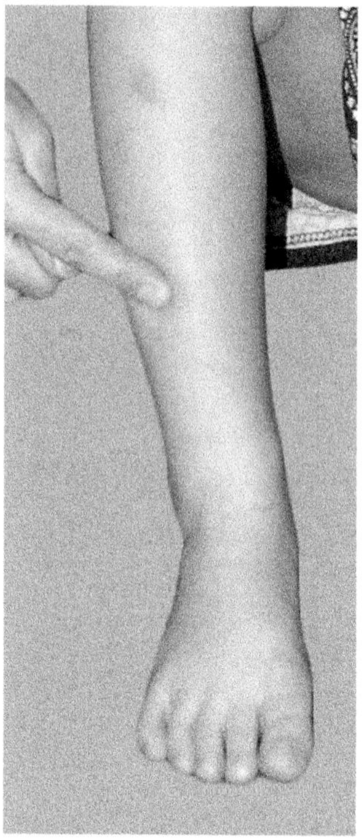

A Bony tenderness Tenderness localized over bone is highly diagnostic of a fracture.

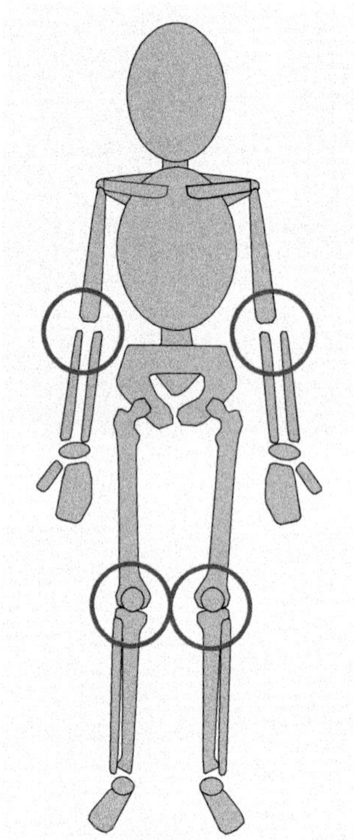

B Problem regions The knee and the elbow are common locations of diagnostic errors.

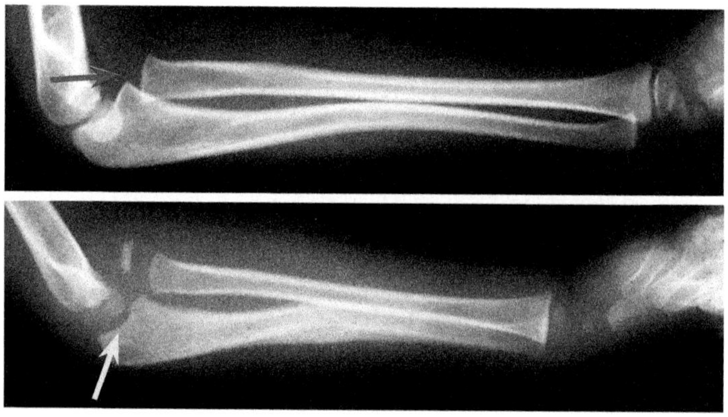

C Monteggia equivalents A variant is the dislocation of the radial head (red arrow) with plastic deformation of the ulna. A chronic lesion is present in this 5-year-old child (bottom). The ulna fracture was treated with a cast, but the dislocated radial head (yellow arrow) was not diagnosed for 6 months.

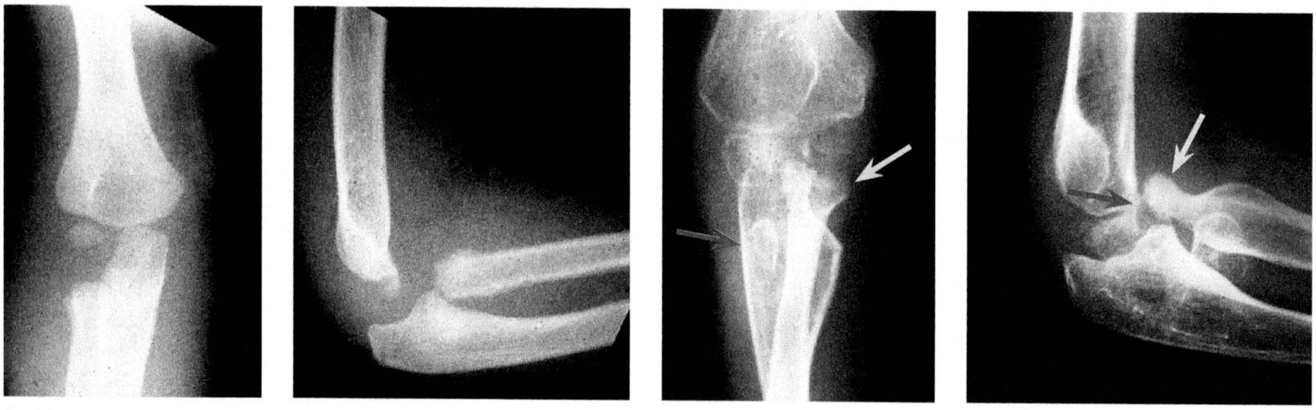

D Unrecognized fracture of the radial neck A toddler sustained an elbow injury, and the radiographs were thought to be negative (left). He was next seen at age 7 years with a severe elbow deformity. Radiographs showed the radial head (red arrows) to be a separate fragment. The proximal radius (yellow arrows) was partly regenerated and lying anterior to the capitellum.

Trauma Pitfalls

The pitfalls of management are numerous but these are the most common.

Radial head dislocation This dislocation is usually but not always associated with fracture of the ulna [C, previous page]. It may also be missed by the radiologist.

Osteoarticular fracture of femoral condyle Dislocation of the patella may cause this fracture [A]. It causes a knee effusion but may be difficult to identify on radiographs as most of the fragment is cartilage.

Child abuse Nonaccidental trauma may be difficult to diagnose [B]. This is the most serious occult injury and is detailed on page 62.

Slipped capital femoral epiphysis This gradual slip may direct attention to the knee where the pain is common referred [C]. The condition usually occurs in late childhood or at puberty.

Lateral humeral condylar fracture This fracture causes tenderness over the lateral condyle at the elbow. Because the fracture is minimally displaced, the fracture line may be difficult to identify on the radiographs. The fracture may displace and end with a nonunion and disability.

Tillaux fracture of ankle This is an articular fracture of the anterolateral aspect of the tibia. It occurs in juveniles and produces ankle pain and bony tenderness. It may be confused with a sprain. Because it involves the articular surfaces, it often requires internal fixation to restore the anatomy and provide fixation.

Common Treatment Mistakes

A number of less than ideal treatments are commonly administered.

Figure 8 immobilization This strap is uncomfortable for the child and ineffective in providing discomfort [D]. The child is better managed in a sling.

Overtreatment Seldom do children require physical therapy in managing common trauma problems. In some centers, such therapy is never prescribed and the outcomes are equivalent. Therapy may be useful in uncommon conditions such as children with reflex dystrophy. As Bount summarized: "Left to their own devices, children recover at the most optimal rate." Passive range of motion manipulation is practically never appropriate in children.

Excessive immobilization Prolonged casting for sprains or long arm casting for a buckle fracture is unnecessary. For undisplaced fractures, once the fracture has become nontender, immobilization is no longer required.

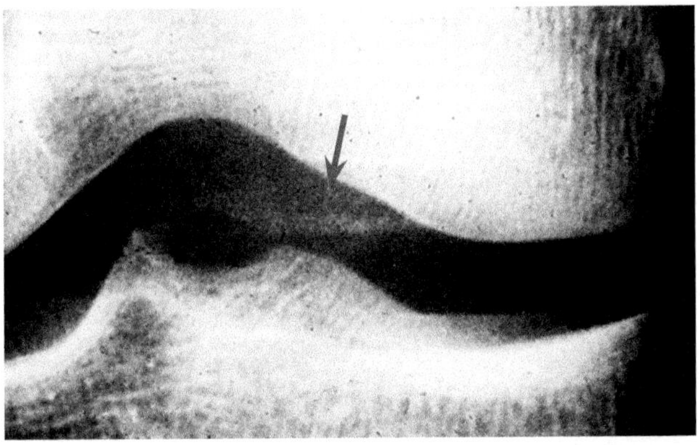

A Osteochondral fracture This adolescent sustained an acute patellar dislocation with an osteochondral fracture. The bony rim is difficult to see on radiographs (red arrow).

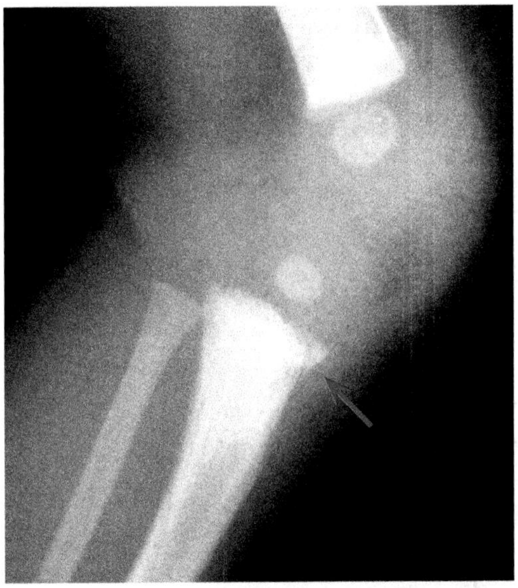

B Nonaccidental trauma This subtle fracture of the tibial metaphysis was found to be due to child abuse.

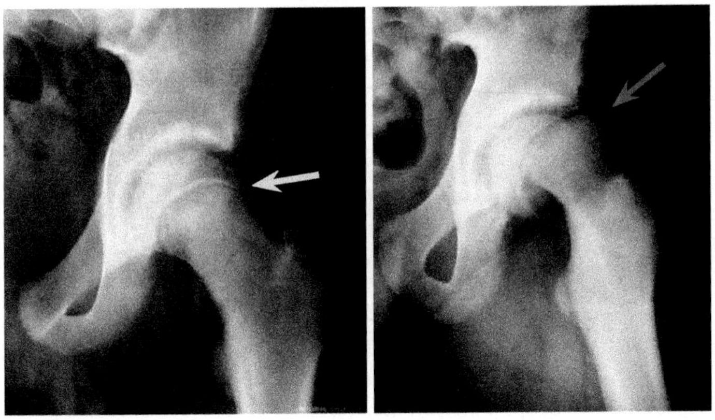

C Slipped capital femoral epiphysis The left radiograph shows the signs of a preslip with rarefaction of the metaphysis (yellow arrow). An acute slip (red arrow) occurred before operative stabilization was performed.

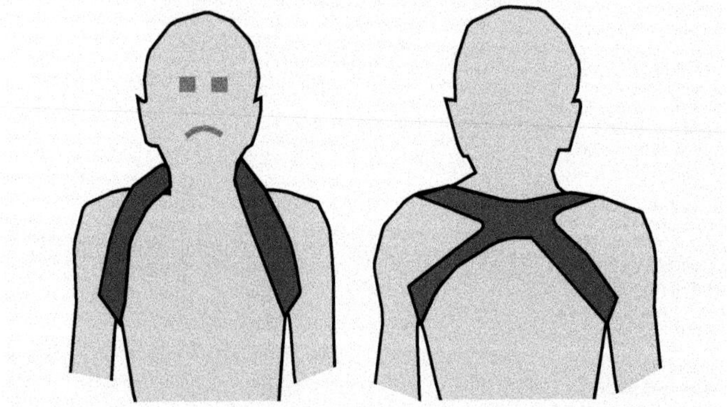

D Figure 8 splint This attempted form of immobilization is uncomfortable and ineffective.

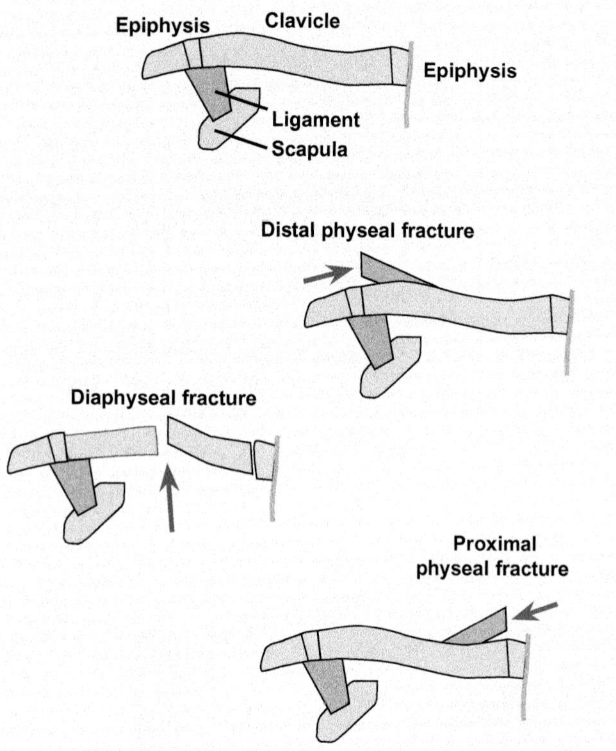

A Clavicular fracture types Fractures may occur at numerous sites along the clavicle. Note that the physeal fractures usually tear through the periosteum. These physeal fractures through the proximal and distal physis can be easily confused with dislocations.

Clavicle Fractures

Clavicle fractures may occur through bone or through proximal or distal growth plates [A].

Diaphyseal fractures are most common in the midclavicle. Unless open or with neurovascular compromise, manage closed. Less is best. Place the affected arm in a sling [B] until the pain has subsided. The common figure-eight strapping is uncomfortable and unnecessary. Shortening and malunion are rarely problems.

Physeal fractures are sometimes difficult to differentiate from dislocation of the sternoclavicular or acromioclavicular joints. Physeal fractures usually occur in younger children and show tenderness over the physis rather than the joint. Physeal fractures are less serious, requiring only sling mobilization and no reduction. Remodeling and recovery of normal function occur with time.

Upper Humeral Fractures

Undisplaced fractures of the upper humeral shaft may be treated simply by applying a sling for comfort [C]. Continue the immobilization for about 3 weeks or until bony tenderness is no longer present. Consider the possibility of nonaccidental trauma in the infant or young child.

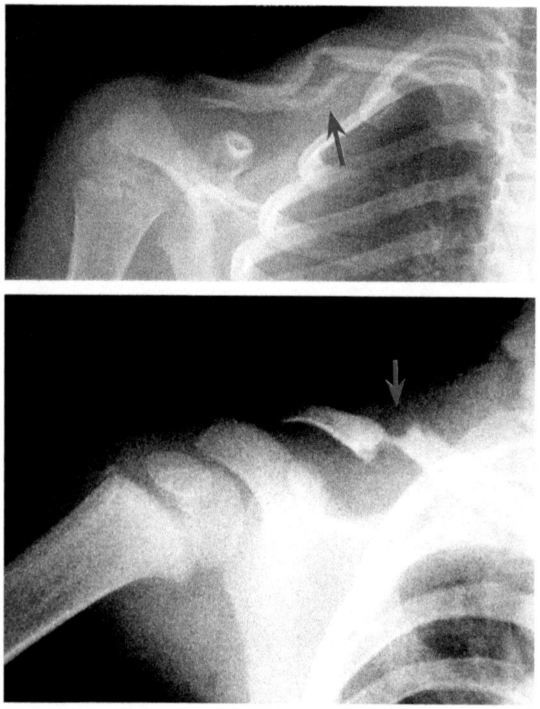

B Clavicle fractures Fracture patterns vary but healing is complete and nearly always incomplicated.

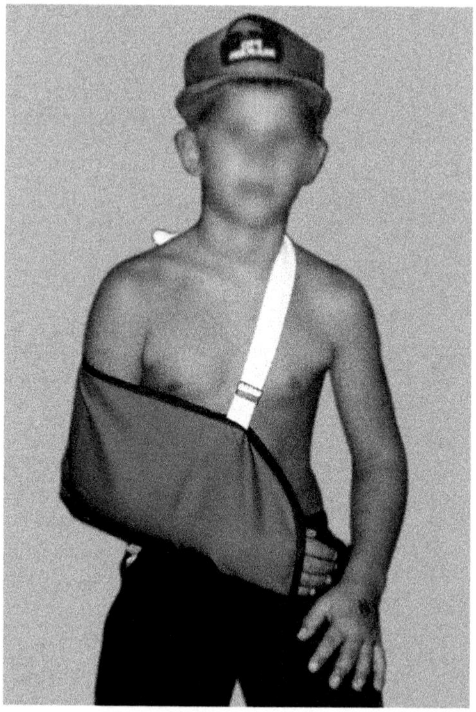

C Immobilizing shoulder injuries These simple slings are usually adequate for managing most shoulder injuries in children.

Pulled Elbow

Pulled elbow, or nursemaids elbow, occurs in about 1% of children each year. Half have no history of a pull. Whether it is more common in hypermobile children is controversial. Girls are more commonly affected. The pathology is uncertain, although capsular interposition is the most favored theory [A].

Clinical Features The arm is held in slight flexion and the forearm pronated; the child resists moving the elbow or extremity. Swelling and tenderness are absent. The diagnosis is clinical, and radiographs are necessary only if the situation or findings are atypical.

Management Rotate the forearm through 180° to free the interposed soft tissue [B]. Often a snap is felt. Repeat in 15 minutes if the first attempt is unsuccessful. Return of function is usually immediate but may be delayed, especially in infants. If function does not immediately return, apply a sling, and reevaluate after several days. If function is still limited, manipulate a second time.

Recurrence is not uncommon. Inability to free the interposition with manipulation may occur. In such cases, place the arm in a sling [C] and repeat the manipulation the next day.

Buckle Fracture of Distal Radius

These fractures are very common.

Evaluation These fractures are identified by localized tenderness over the distal radius and radiographs demonstration of a buckle [D] in the cortex of the distal radius.

Management Place in a wrist splint [D] or a short arm cast or slab splint. See the next day to confirm the diagnosis if necessary. Instruct the family to continue the splint for about 3 weeks. No clinical or additional radiographic follow-up is usually required unless a cast was applied that requires removal.

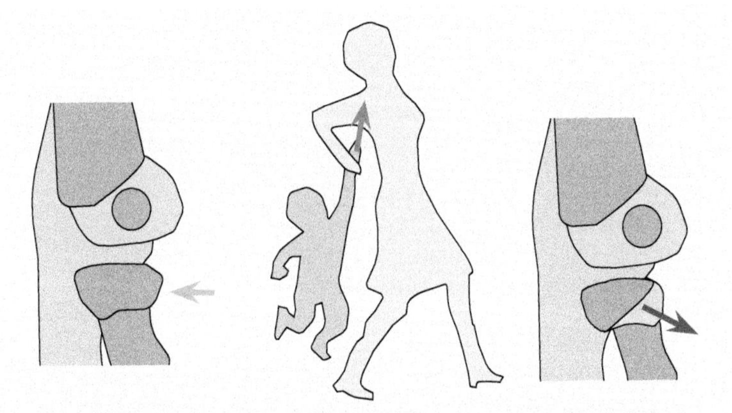

A Pulled elbow pathology The annular ligament (gray) normally extends around the radial head (green arrow). With a pull on the elbow (blue arrow), the radial head may subluxate partially out from under the ligament (red arrow). With forearm rotation or normal use, the head slips back to its original position.

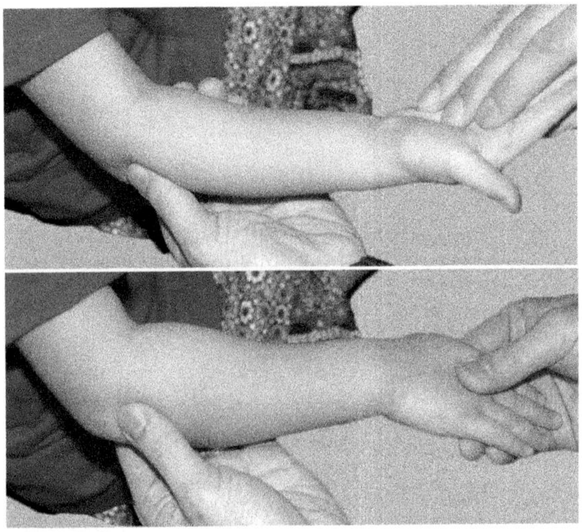

B Pulled elbow reduction Reduce by quickly supinating (upper) and pronating (lower) the forearm. Usually a click is felt and the child immediately becomes comfortable.

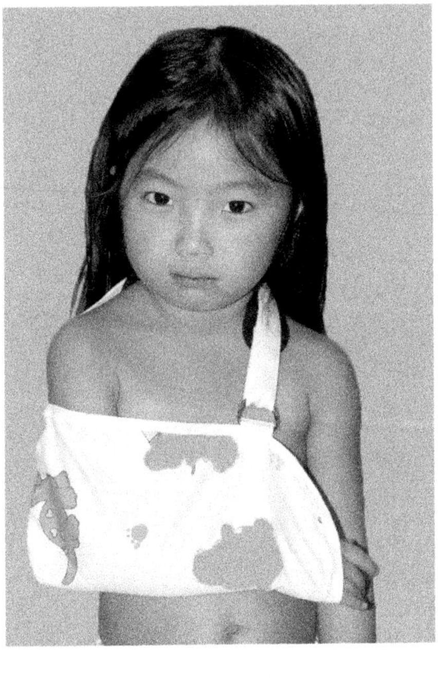

C Immobilizing shoulder injuries These simple slings are usually adequate for managing most shoulder injuries in children.

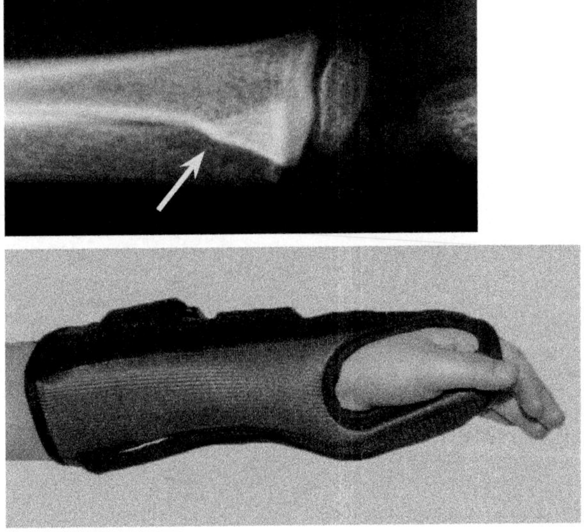

D Forearm fracture Note the change in contour of the cortex showing a buckle fracture (yellow arrow). This forearm splint is appropriate.

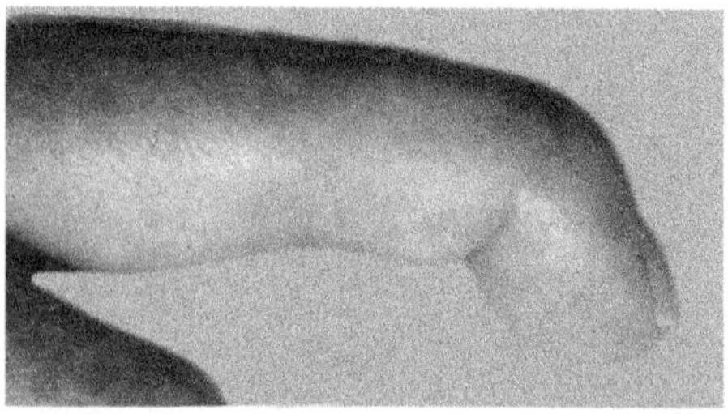

A Mallet finger The distal phalanx remains flexed. These flexion is more severely than most.

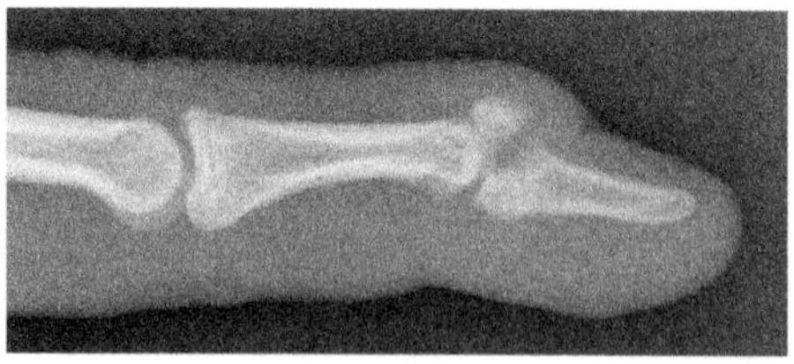

B Mallet finger Radiograph shows an articular fracture. Operative reduction and fixation is necessary.

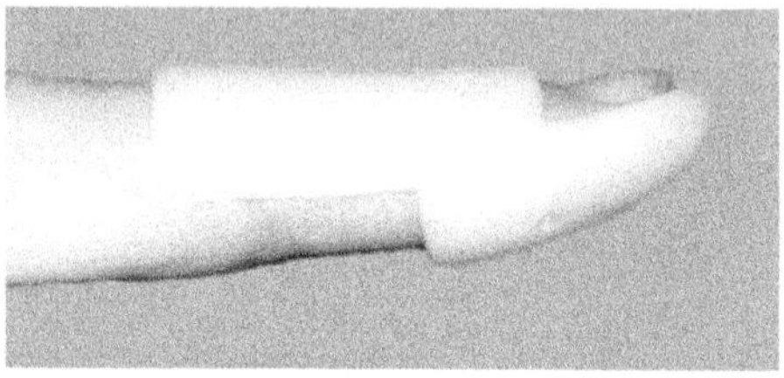

C Treatment of mallet finger If radiograph is negative, splint finger in extension.

Mallet Finger

The finger shows flexion of the distal interphalangeal joint [A]. Make a lateral radiograph of the finger to rule out a fracture [B]. Fractures in children are rare. If no fracture is seen, splint in extension with a finger splint [C] for 6 weeks.

Toddlers' Fracture

Toddlers' fractures typically occur in children 1–4 years old from minimal trauma [D]. Bony tenderness is found. Radiographs usually show a faint fracture line is corresponding in location to the bony tenderness. Sometimes the fracture line cannot be seen on radiographs. Midshaft fractures should raise suspicion of child abuse. Manage by immobilization in a splint or walking cast for 2–3 weeks.

Ankle Sprains

Ankle sprains become increasingly common with advancing age. Sprains are common in adolescents. Lateral sprains are most common.

Evaluation Careful assessment is necessary.

Weight bearing If the sprain is severe or if a fracture is present, the child usually will be unwilling to walk on the leg.

Appearance Note the extent of swelling and presence of ecchymoses. This is helpful in determining the severity of the injury.

Localization of tenderness Determine tenderness over ligaments [F]. This is useful in assessing the severity of the sprain. If tenderness is present over the lateral malleolus [E] and the child cannot bear weight, order radiographs.

Radiographs If appropriate, make AP, oblique, and lateral radiographs of the ankle. Interpret radiographs with consideration given to physical findings.

Sprains often show soft tissue swelling.

Physeal fracture of the distal tibia may not be apparent on the radiographs.

Tillaux fracture involves the distal lateral aspect of the tibial physis. This fracture occurs at the end of growth. Tenderness is usually present on the anterolateral aspect of the ankle.

Child's pain response determines how the child responds to the injury. This is a subjective assessment but often of great importance in assessing the severity of the sprain and planning management.

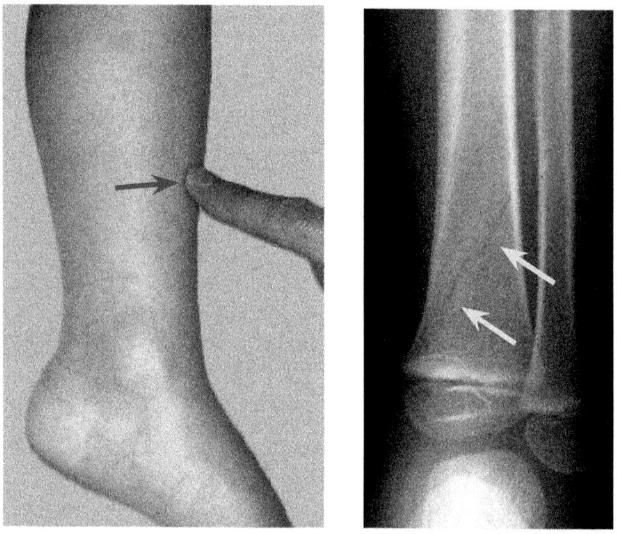

D Toddler's fractures These fractures create tenderness over the shaft of the tibia (red arrow), often with little or no swelling. Radiographs show linear defects (yellow arrows) that are sometimes difficult to identify.

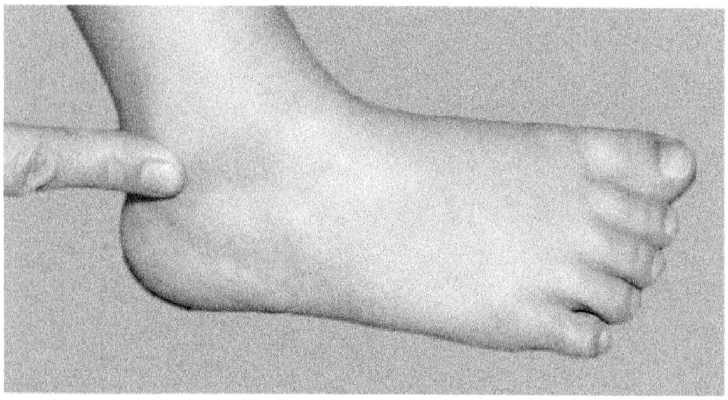

E Palpation of lateral malleolus Tenderness at this site suggests a fracture of the distal radius or commonly of the physis.

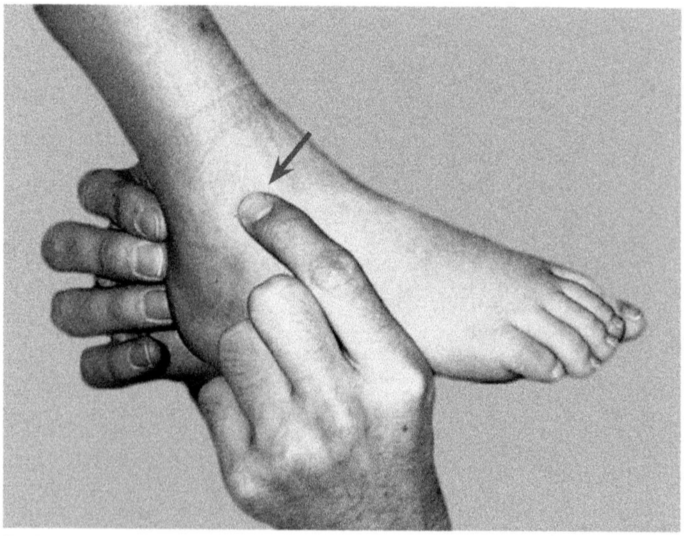

F Ligament tenderness The lateral ligaments of the ankle are most vulnerable to injury. Of these ligaments, the anterior ligament is the least strong and most vulnerable (red arrow). It may be localized just anterior to the prominence of the fibula.

Management is based on the severity of the sprain [A] by considering the ability to bear weight, degree of swelling, location of tenderness, and the child's response to the injury [D]. A variety of convenient methods of immobilization and support are available [B].

Mild sprains cause mild swelling, usually have tenderness just anterior to the lateral malleolus. Manage with an elastic bandage, elevation, and cold application. Limit activity until tenderness is no longer present.

Moderate sprains cause moderate swelling, tenderness is present just in front of or below the malleolus. Manage with cold, compression, elevation, and protection. Protect with a splint or a short leg cast for 2 weeks.

Severe sprains can be difficult to manage. In addition to the measures for moderate sprains, protection may be required for a longer period, possibly for a few months. Provide a strengthening exercise program. Some believe that special training may help in preventing future injuries.

Refer In several situations, referral is wise.

Uncertain diagnosis when unclear about the diagnosis.

Sprains in obese children are especially likely to create months of disability. Consider an early referral.

Recurrent sprains may occur if ligament injury is severe and fails to heal.

Pitfalls Several conditions may be confused with sprains [C].

Physeal fracture Although the diagnosis may be missed, the condition heals well and problems are uncommon.

Tillaux fracture involves the growth plate and articular surface. Often open reduction and screw fixation are necessary.

Osteochondritis dissecans of the talus may be confused with a sprain. If the pain fails to resolve, consider this possibility.

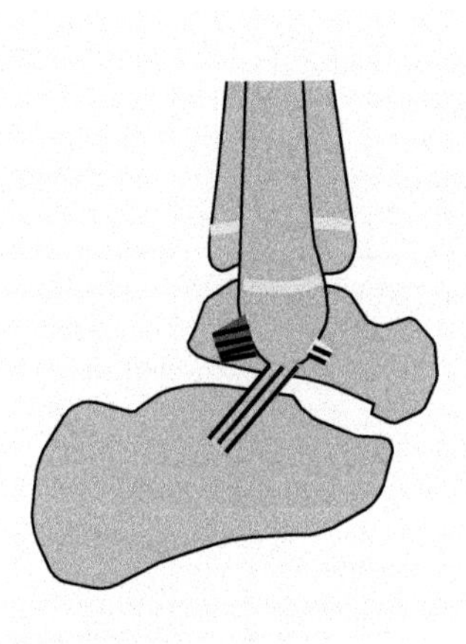

A Ankle ligaments The lateral ligaments of the ankle are most vulnerable to injury. The frequency and severity of the sprain increase (mildest, yellow; moderate, orange; and most severe, red.

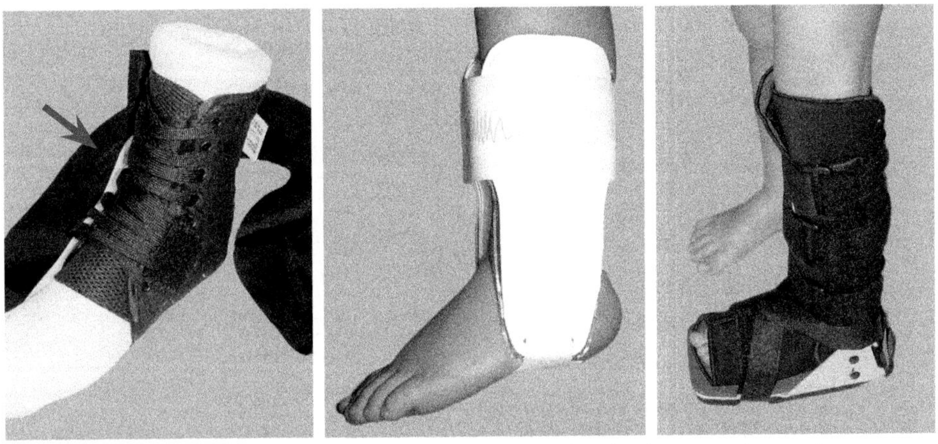

B Ankle support options These options are graded. Increasing size increases degree of immobilization but makes walking more difficult. Ankle support (red arrow) may be worn during activity. It is suitable for use while participating in sports and is appropriate for long-term use.

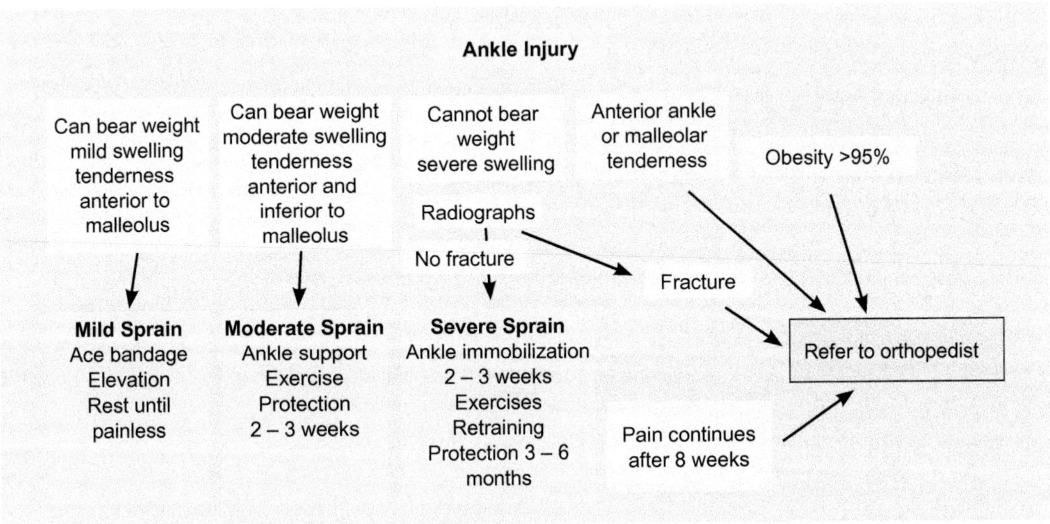

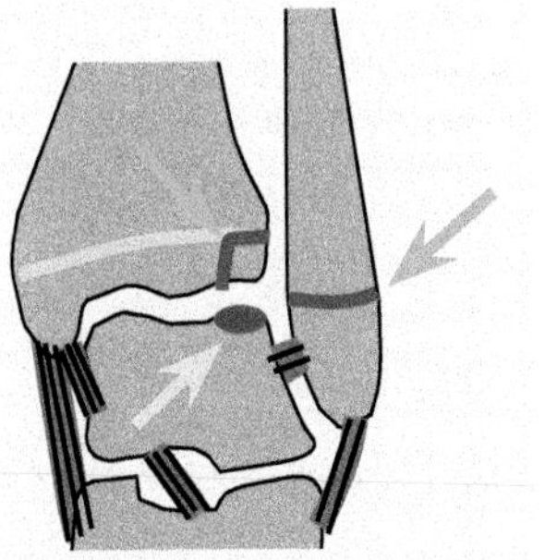

C Pitfalls The Tillaux fracture (green arrow) and the undisplaced fibular physeal fracture (orange arrow) and osteochondritis dissecans (yellow arrow) may be confused with a sprain.

D Sprain flowchart This chart outlines the steps in diagnosis and need for referral.

Leung AG, Peterson HA. Fractures of the proximal radial head and neck in children with emphasis on those that involve the articular cartilage. J Pediatr Orthop 2000 Jan-Feb;20(1): p7-14.

Liow RY, Montgomery RJ. Treatment of established and anticipated nonunion of the tibia in childhood. J Pediatr Orthop 2002 Nov-Dec;22(6): p754-60.

Loder RT. Demographics of traumatic amputations in children. Implications for prevention strategies. J Bone Joint Surg Am 2004 May;86-A(5): p923-8.

Luhmann SJ, Schootman M, Schoenecker PL, Dobbs MB, Gordon JE. Complications and outcomes of open pediatric forearm fractures. J Pediatr Orthop 2004 Jan-Feb;24(1): p1-6.

Malmvik J, Herbertsson P, Josefsson PO, Hasserius R, Besjakov J, Karlsson MK. Fracture of the radial head and neck of Mason types II and III during growth: a 14-25 year follow-up. J Pediatr Orthop B 2003 Jan;12(1): p63-8.

Mayr JM, Pierer GR, Linhart WE. Reconstruction of part of the distal tibial growth plate with an autologous graft from the iliac crest. J Bone Joint Surg Br 2000 May;82(4): p558-60.

Mazda K, Boggione C, Fitoussi F, Pennecot GF. Systematic pinning of displaced extension-type supracondylar fractures of the humerus in children. A prospective study of 116 consecutive patients. J Bone Joint Surg Br 2001 Aug;83(6): p888-93.

McLauchlan GJ, Cowan B, Annan IH, Robb JE. Management of completely displaced metaphyseal fractures of the distal radius in children. A prospective, randomised controlled trial. J Bone Joint Surg Br 2002 Apr;84(3): p413-7.

Mendelson SA, Dominick TS, Tyler-Kabara E, Moreland MS, Adelson PD. Early versus late femoral fracture stabilization in multiply injured pediatric patients with closed head injury. J Pediatr Orthop 2001 Sep-Oct;21(5): p594-9.

Miner T, Carroll KL. Outcomes of external fixation of pediatric femoral shaft fractures. J Pediatr Orthop 2000 May-Jun;20(3): p405-10.

Mohammad S, Port A, Montgomery RJ. Transepiphyseal fracture of the femoral neck with dislocation of the femoral head and fracture of the posterior column of the acetabulum in a child. J Bone Joint Surg Br 2002 Jan;84(1): p113-5.

Moulton SL. Early management of the child with multiple injuries. Clin Orthop 2000 Jul;(376): p6-14.

Mubarak SJ. Extensor retinaculum syndrome of the ankle after injury to the distal tibial physis. J Bone Joint Surg Br 2002 Jan;84(1): p11-4.

Ng A, Morley JR, Prasad RN, Giannoudis PV, Smith RM. The paediatric floating knee: a case report of ipsilateral epiphyseal injury to the distal femur and proximal tibia. J Pediatr Orthop B 2004 Mar;13(2): p110-3.

Nwakama AC, Peterson HA, Shaughnessy WJ. Fishtail deformity following fracture of the distal humerus in children: historical review, case presentations, discussion of etiology, and thoughts on treatment. J Pediatr Orthop B 2000 Oct;9(4): p309-18.

O'Hara LJ, Barlow JW, Clarke NM. Displaced supracondylar fractures of the humerus in children. Audit changes practice. J Bone Joint Surg Br 2000 Mar;82(2): p204-10.

Ogden JA, Ganey TM, Hill JD, Jaakkola JI. Sever's injury: a stress fracture of the immature calcaneal metaphysis. J Pediatr Orthop 2004 Sep-Oct;24(5): p488-92.

Ogonda L, Wong-Chung J, Wray R, Canavan B. Delayed union and non-union of the ulna following intramedullary nailing in children. J Pediatr Orthop B 2004 Sep;13(5): p330-3.

Oh CW, Park BC, Ihn JC, Kyung HS. Fracture separation of the distal humeral epiphysis in children younger than three years old. J Pediatr Orthop 2000 Mar-Apr;20(2): p173-6.

Patari SK, Lee FY, Behrens FF. Coronal split fracture of the proximal tibia epiphysis through a partially closed physis: a new fracture pattern. J Pediatr Orthop 2001 Jul-Aug;21(4): p451-5.

Peterson HA, Wood MB. Physeal arrest due to laser beam damage in a growing child. J Pediatr Orthop 2001 May-Jun;21(3): p335-7.

Pickle A, Benaroch TE, Guy P; Harvey EJ. Clinical outcome of pediatric calcaneal fractures treated with open reduction and internal fixation. J Pediatr Orthop 2004 Mar-Apr;24(2): p178-80.

Prahinski JR, Polly DW, McHale KA, Ellenbogen RG. Occult intraspinal anomalies in congenital scoliosis. J Pediatr Orthop 2000 Jan-Feb;20(1): p59-63.

Pugh DM, Galpin RD, Carey TP. Intramedullary Steinmann pin fixation of forearm fractures in children. Long-term results. Clin Orthop 2000 Jul;(376): p39-48.

Qidwai SA. Intramedullary Kirschner wiring for tibia fractures in children. J Pediatr Orthop 2001 May-Jun;21(3): p294-7.

Rasool MN. Dislocations of the elbow in children. J Bone Joint Surg Br 2004 Sep;86(7): p1050-8.

Reitman RD, Waters P, Millis M. Open reduction and internal fixation for supracondylar humerus fractures in children. J Pediatr Orthop 2001 Mar-Apr;21(2): p157-61.

Rex C, Kay PR. Features of femoral fractures in nonaccidental injury. J Pediatr Orthop 2000 May-Jun;20(3): p411-3.

Ring D, Waters PM, Hotchkiss RN, Kasser JR. Pediatric floating elbow. J Pediatr Orthop 2001 Jul-Aug;21(4): p456-9.

Robertson WW. Power lawnmower injuries. Clin Orthop 2003 Apr;(409): p37-42.

Ruiz AL, Kealey WD, Cowie HG. Percutaneous pin fixation of intercondylar fractures in young children. J Pediatr Orthop B 2001 Jul;10(3): p211-3.

Sato T, Shinozaki T, Fukuda T, Watanabe H, Aoki J, Yanagawa T, Takagishi K. Atypical growth plate closure: a possible chronic Salter and Harris Type V injury. J Pediatr Orthop B 2002 Apr;11(2): p155-8.

Sawyer JR, Flynn JM, Dormans JP, Catalano J, Drummond DS. Fracture patterns in children and young adults who fall from significant heights. J Pediatr Orthop 2000 Mar-Apr;20(2): p197-202.

Schwend RM, Werth C, Johnston A. Femur shaft fractures in toddlers and young children: rarely from child abuse. J Pediatr Orthop 2000 Jul-Aug;20(4): p475-81.

Shannon FJ, Mohan P, Chacko J, D'Souza LG. "Dorgan's" percutaneous lateral cross-wiring of supracondylar fractures of the humerus in children. J Pediatr Orthop 2004 Jul-Aug;24(4): p376-9.

Shilt JS, Yoder JS, Manuck TA, Jacks L, Rushing J, Smith BP. Role of vacuum-assisted closure in the treatment of pediatric lawnmower injuries. J Pediatr Orthop 2004 Sep-Oct;24(5): p482-7.

Silber JS, Flynn JM, Koffler KM, Dormans JP, Drummond DS. Analysis of the cause, classification, and associated injuries of 166 consecutive pediatric pelvic fractures. J Pediatr Orthop 2001 Jul-Aug;21(4): p446-50.

Silber JS, Flynn JM. Changing patterns of pediatric pelvic fractures with skeletal maturation: implications for classification and management. J Pediatr Orthop 2002 Jan-Feb;22(1): p22-6.

Skaggs DL, Kautz SM, Kay RM, Tolo VT. Effect of delay of surgical treatment on rate of infection in open fractures in children. J Pediatr Orthop 2000 Jan-Feb;20(1): p19-22.

Skaggs DL, Roy AK, Vitale MG, Pfiefer C, Baird G, Femino D, Kay RM. Quality of evaluation and management of children requiring timely orthopaedic surgery before admission to a tertiary pediatric facility. J Pediatr Orthop 2002 Mar-Apr;22(2): p265-7.

Skak SV, Olsen SD, Smaabrekke A. Deformity after fracture of the lateral humeral condyle in children. J Pediatr Orthop B 2001 Apr;10(2): p142-52.

Sledge JB, Allred D, Hyman J. Use of magnetic resonance imaging in evaluating injuries to the pediatric thoracolumbar spine. J Pediatr Orthop 2001 May-Jun;21(3): p288-93.

Song HR, Oh CW, Shin HD, Kim SJ, Kyung HS, Baek SH, Park BC, Ihn JC. Treatment of femoral shaft fractures in young children: comparison between conservative treatment and retrograde flexible nailing. J Pediatr Orthop B 2004 Jul;13(4): p275-80.

Song KS, Kim YS, Sohn SW, Ogden JA. Arthrotomy and open reduction of the displaced fracture of the femoral neck in children. J Pediatr Orthop B 2001 Jul;10(3): p205-10.

Tabrizi P, McIntyre WM, Quesnel MB, Howard AW. Limited dorsiflexion predisposes to injuries of the ankle in children. J Bone Joint Surg Br 2000 Nov;82(8): p1103-6.

Thomas DP, Howard AW, Cole WG, Hedden DM. Three weeks of Kirschner wire fixation for displaced lateral condylar fractures of the humerus in children. J Pediatr Orthop 2001 Sep-Oct;21(5): p565-9.

Thomas KC, Lalonde F, O'Neil J, Letts RM. Multiple-level thoracolumbar burst fractures in teenaged patients. J Pediatr Orthop 2003 Jan-Feb;23(1): p119-23.

Townsend DR, Hoffinger S. Intramedullary nailing of femoral shaft fractures in children via the trochanter tip. Clin Orthop 2000 Jul;(376): p113-8.

Trumble T, Verheyden J. Remodeling of articular defects in an animal model. Clin Orthop 2004 Jun;(423): p59-63.

Vocke-Hell AK, von Laer L, Slongo T, Stankovic P. Secondary radial head dislocation and dysplasia of the lateral condyle after elbow trauma in children. J Pediatr Orthop 2001 May-Jun;21(3): p319-23.

Vorlat P, De Boeck H. Bowing fractures of the forearm in children: a long-term followup. Clin Orthop 2003 Aug;(413): p233-7.

Waters PM, Bae DS, Kadiyala RK. Short-term outcomes after surgical treatment of traumatic posterior sternoclavicular fracture-dislocations in children and adolescents. J Pediatr Orthop 2003 Jul-Aug;23(4): p464-9.

Waters PM, Stewart SL. Radial neck fracture nonunion in children. J Pediatr Orthop 2001 Sep-Oct;21(5): p570-6.

Wattenbarger JM, Gerardi J, Johnston CE. Late open reduction internal fixation of lateral condyle fractures. J Pediatr Orthop 2002 May-Jun;22(3): p394-8.

Wattenbarger JM, Gruber HE, Phieffer LS. Physeal fractures, part I: histologic features of bone, cartilage, and bar formation in a small animal model. J Pediatr Orthop 2002 Nov-Dec;22(6): p703-9.

Wessel LM, Scholz S, Rusch M, Kopke J, Loff S, Duchene W, Waag KL. Hemarthrosis after trauma to the pediatric knee joint: what is the value of magnetic resonance imaging in the diagnostic algorithm?. J Pediatr Orthop 2001 May-Jun;21(3): p338-42.

Wessel LM, Scholz S, Rusch M. Characteristic pattern and management of intra-articular knee lesions in different pediatric age groups. J Pediatr Orthop 2001 Jan-Feb;21(1): p14-9.

Wong J, Boyd R, Keenan NW, Baker R, Selber P, Wright JG, Nattrass GR, Graham HK. Gait patterns after fracture of the femoral shaft in children, managed by external fixation or early hip spica cast. J Pediatr Orthop 2004 Sep-Oct;24(5): p463-71.

Yian EH, Gullahorn LJ, Loder RT. Scoring of pediatric orthopaedic polytrauma: correlations of different injury scoring systems and prognosis for hospital course. J Pediatr Orthop 2000 Mar-Apr;20(2): p203-9.

Yuan PS, Pring ME, Gaynor TP, Mubarak SJ, Newton PO. Compartment syndrome following intramedullary fixation of pediatric forearm fractures. J Pediatr Orthop 2004 Jul-Aug;24(4): p370-5.

Yung PS, Lam CY, Ng BK, Lam TP, Cheng JC. Percutaneous transphyseal intramedullary Kirschner wire pinning: a safe and effective procedure for treatment of displaced diaphyseal forearm fracture in children. J Pediatr Orthop 2004 Jan-Feb;24(1): p7-12.

Zionts LE, Moon CN. Olecranon apophysis fractures in children with osteogenesis imperfecta revisited. J Pediatr Orthop 2002 Nov-Dec;22(6): p745-50.

Sports

CHAPTER 5

Involvement in sports is increasing [A]. Over half of students in high school participate in sports. There is also a large increase in nonteam, individual sports, such as skateboarding and roller sports. A large drop-off in participation in sports occurs during middle and high school, especially in girls.

Sport participation has positive and some negative aspects. The benefits of sports are well documented and clearly exceed the negative aspects. The downside of athletic participation need to be identified and addressed [B]. In addition, the recently recognized problems of concussions, repetitive head trauma, and the increased risk of degenerative arthritis in late adult life troubling.

The role of primary care provider is expanding, requiring a need to understand the problems and management of the musculoskeletal system in children.

Advantages of Participation in Sports

Cost-effective

Adding sports adds only about 3% to a school's budget. Consider sports as just not a *diversion,* but an important component of education. Sports teaches teamwork, sportsmanship, provides experience with the joy of winning, and coping with losing. It teaches the rewards of hard work, self-discipline, enhances self-confidence, and develop skills in handling competitive situations. These skills learned through sports participation increase the likelihood of success in adult life increasing and becoming a contributing member of society.

Academic

In 1992, a Colorado study showed that sports participation was associated with significantly higher grade-point average, better attendance, a lower dropout rate, and a greater likelihood of going to college.

Social

The demands of sports motivate kids to avoid using drugs, smoking, or becoming pregnant.

Career success

In a 1987 survey of Executives (Vice President level or above) in 75 Fortune 500 companies, 95% had participated in sports during high school. This exceeds the participation in student government (54%), national honor societies (43%), scouting (35%), and school-sponsored publications (18%).

Obesity

Overweight frequency is increasing in most countries, especially in USA [C]. Researchers estimated that if all adolescents played on two or more sport teams per year, the obesity prevalence rate would decrease by about 25%. A New Hampshire/Vermont study found that adolescents who played three sports were 27% less likely to be overweight and 39% less likely to be obese as compared with those not in sport teams. Basically the same findings occurred in children who walked or biked to school.

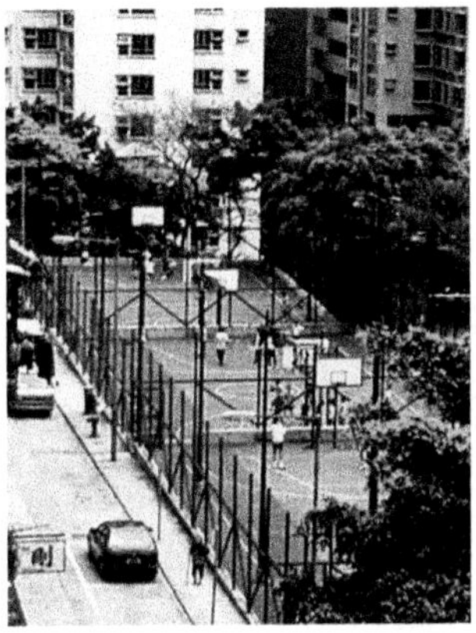

A Sports participation a priority Even in densely populated areas, providing room for sports is an important community priority (Hong Kong).

Positives	Negatives
Higher academic performance	**Overuse injures**
Less dropout	**Burnout**
Better college options	**Sleep deprivation**
Less smoking	**Single sport pressure**
Less drugs	**Enhanced aggressiveness**
Fewer pregnancies	**Loss of self-esteem**
Less obesity	**Increased adult arthritis**
Better integration	**Excessive treatments**
Enhanced leadership skills	**Focus on team sports**
Career advantages	**Lifetime sports undervalued**

B Participation in sports These tables list the positive and negative aspects of sport participation.

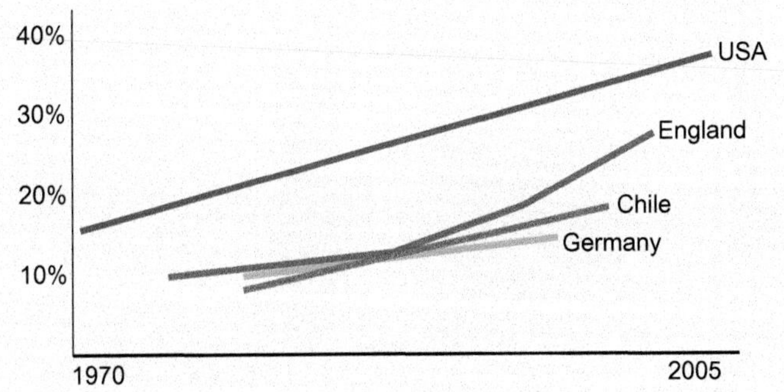

C Overweight children in different countries From Government Office of Science.

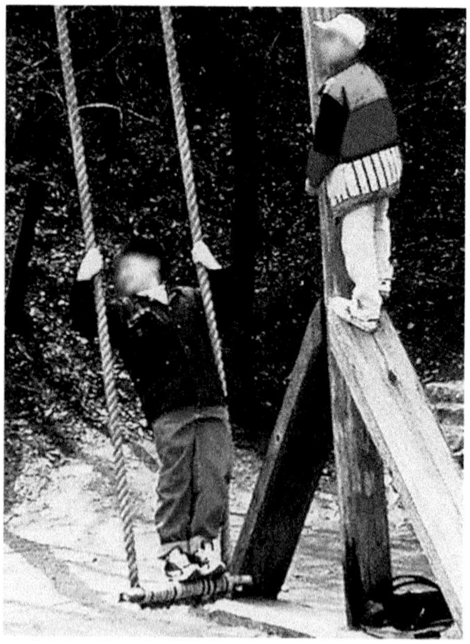

A Play, the occupation of the child Play, whether individual or in teams, is a vital part of a child's life.

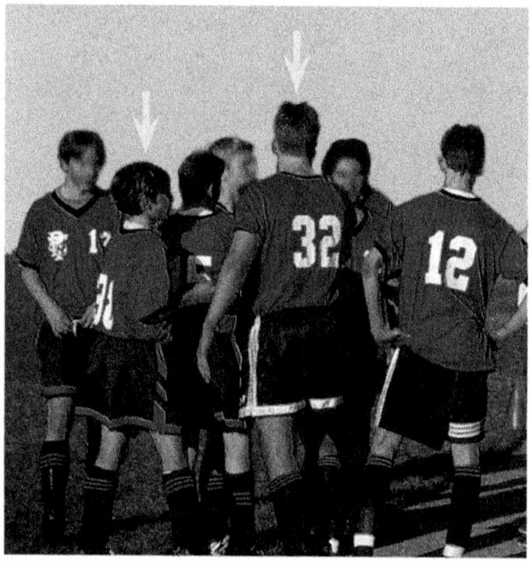

B Size differences in same-age children The largest boy is nearly double the weight of the smallest boy in the team (yellow arrows).

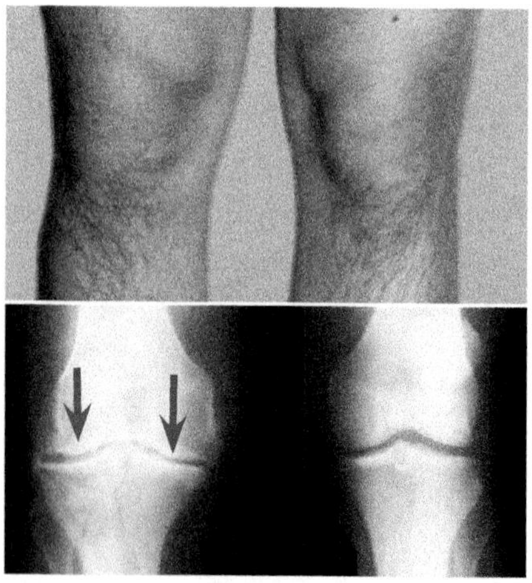

C Effect of meniscectomy during childhood At age 13, this patient sustained a torn medial meniscus while playing football. An arthroscopic meniscectomy was performed. At age 29, the man has disabling pain and significant disability. The radiograph shows severe osteoarthritis (arrows).

Goals

Make sports fun

The child's sports experience is often diminished by pushy parents, aggressive coaches, and limited options. When the major emphasis is on winning, the chances of a child continuing long-term on the team diminish with time. Most kids eventually get "cut" from the varsity team, most are not lifetime sports. Play is the *occupation* of the child [A].

Place for small, not athletic children

On the downside, the child may be pressured into a sport for which he or she has little ability. The child performs poorly, is embarrassed, and ends up with a damaged self-image. The smaller child often has a disadvantage [B].

Problems

Overuse Injuries

Overuse injuries are increasing and now account for about half of all childhood injuries. They are best prevented. Most resolve with rest. However, some injuries, like osteochondritis cause joint damage with the potential of long-term disability.

Burnout

The child may experience a conflict between the demands of athletics, their social life and education. Too much sports results in excessive pressure, loss of time for sleep, socialization, and school work. This limitation creates some long-term problems that may result in a withdrawal from sports altogether, an excessive focus on electronic games, etc.

Concussion and traumatic brain injury (TBI)

About 50,000 high school American football players are diagnosed with a concussion per year, representing about 5% of the population of high school football players. Once concussed, athletes are about five times more likely to experience a second, rare, but often lethal injury: Second Impact Syndrome (SIS) that results from relatively minor injury.

Chronic traumatic encephalopathy (CTE) is linked to American football and boxing. Its features include memory impairment, depression, aggression, and dementia that occur in mid to late adult life. In these cases, the brain shows degenerative changes with the accumulation of abnormal proteins.

Degenerative arthritis

Evidence shows that those who sustain significant joint injuries during adolescence have an increased likelihood of developing degenerative arthritis during adult life [C].

Excessive surgery

Some indications for surgery are lowered if the parents are determined to make their child as perfect as possible in preparation for a scholarship and a career as a professional athlete. Examples include open reduction of clavicular fractures, correction of rotational problems in the lower limb, etc.

Injury Statistics

Parents and children are often unaware of the potential of injury from sports. It is useful to educate them with data. Fortunately, most sports injuries are minor and heal rapidly, but some are serious. Injuries (sports-related and not) are the leading cause of childhood death. Significant injuries can cause long-term disability. Most deaths in sports are due to cardiovascular disease or head injuries. Most trauma deaths are the result of high-speed injuries beyond the velocities of childhood sports. Few injuries lead to permanent disability. The most common serious injuries occur in collision sports such as American football [A], which causes ligamentous or meniscal tears in the knee.

Sport

Injury rates vary considerably among sports [B]. Football and wrestling cause acute injuries, whereas running, throwing, and field events tend to produce overuse problems.

Age

Injury rates and severity increase with age [C]. The small child simply does not have the speed or mass to cause serious injury. In young children, fractures occur more commonly through bone and less commonly through growth plates, reducing the risk of altering growth.

Gender

Boys are injured more frequently than girls [C] because they play the highest risk games, American football and wrestling. When these two sports are removed from the injury profile, overall injury rates between boys and girls are comparable, except for the 2–3 times greater incidence of ACL injuries in girls playing basketball and soccer.

Disability

Disability may occur early from the acute injury or appear later from osteoarthritis due to articular damage.

Short-term disability from injuries is usually temporary because the majority of injuries are minor [C] and are disabling only during the period required for healing and rehabilitation.

Long-term disability is most serious and usually due to osteoarthritis in a site that has sustained more than one injury. Twenty years after playing high school football, radiographic changes showed osteoarthritis of the knee [E]. In midadult life, osteoarthritis of the hip severe enough to require total hip replacement is quadrupled in men who had moderate to high exposure to sports [C]. When these men had physically demanding work, their risk increased eightfold above the control group [F]. The majority of college football players who sustained major knee injuries had previously sustained injury to the same knee during high school. Whether modern techniques of meniscal and ACL repair will alter these statistics remains to be determined. However, without such repairs, poor outcomes are inevitable. Studies suggest that injuries from high-impact sports during adolescence are likely to have significant adverse consequences in adult life. These risks should be balanced against the substantial benefits of high school team sports participation.

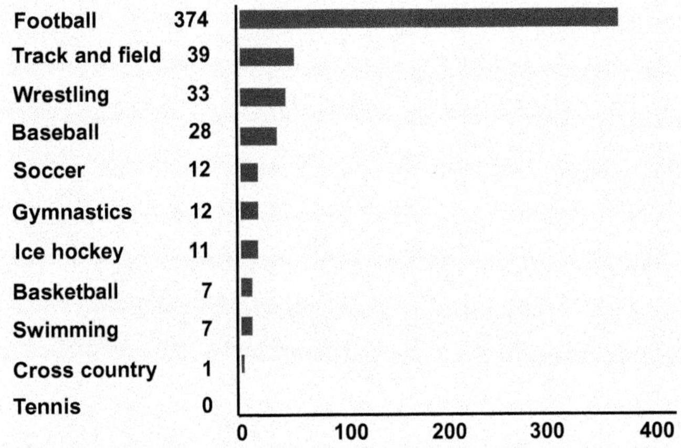

A Fatal and catastrophic injuries in high school sports Based on rates per 100,000 participants. From Cantu and Mueller (1999).

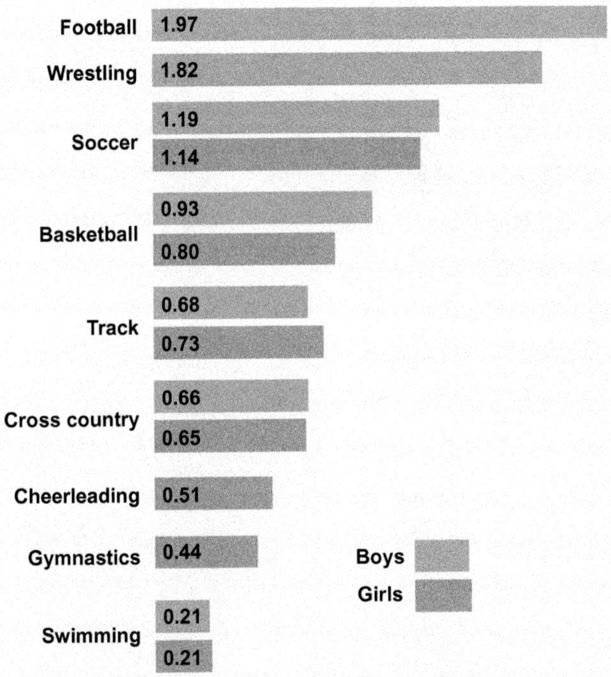

B Injuries in high school athletics per athlete per year in the United States From Beachy et al. (1997).

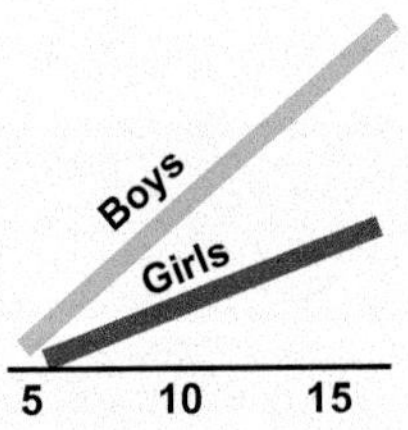

C Injuries by age groups in years From Beachy et al. (1997).

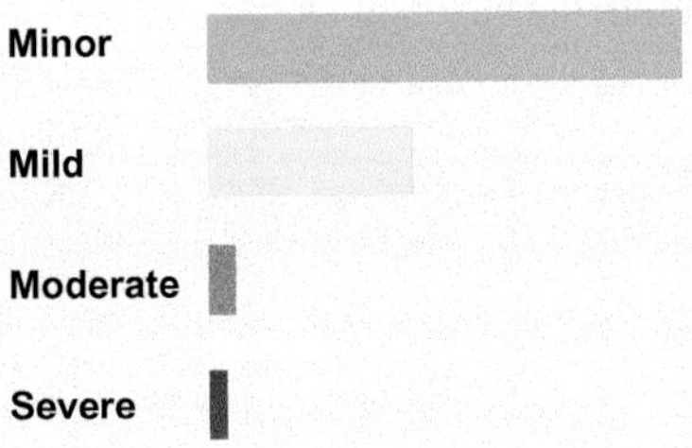

D Injury severity Proportion of injuries by severity. From Beachy et al. (1997).

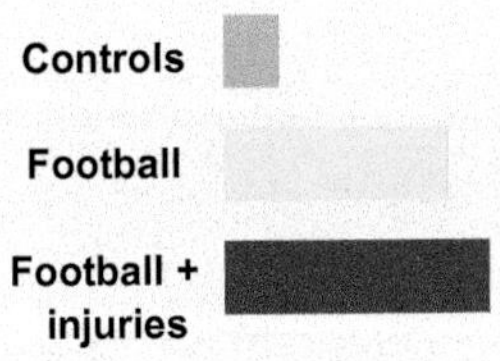

E Relative percentage with osteoarthritis 20 years after high school football From Moretz (1984).

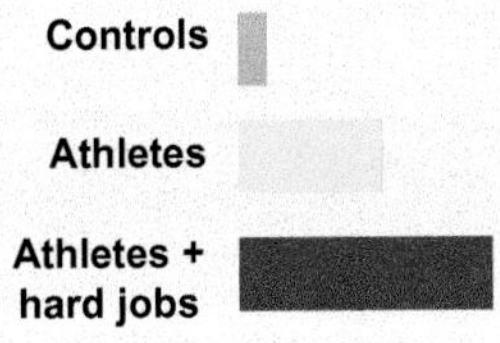

F Relative frequency of total hip replacement by history of activity From Vingard (1993).

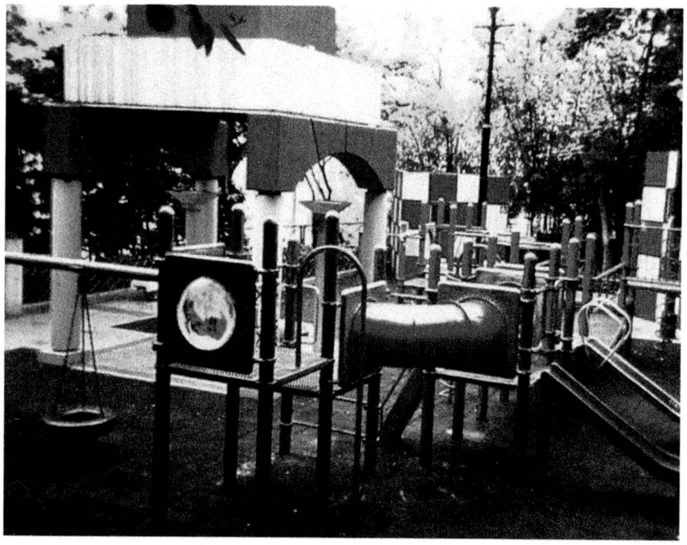

A Hard surface This attractive play area for children has a serious flaw: a concrete surface. The children may stay cleaner but are much more likely to sustain injuries with falls.

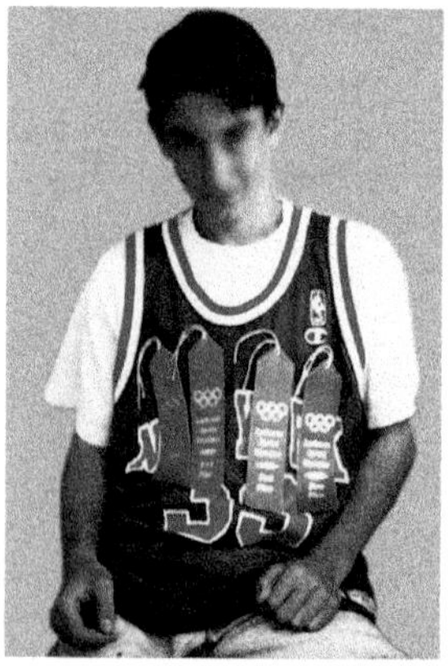

B Outstanding athlete with childhood orthopedic problem This boy had a clubfoot deformity and became an excellent athlete in many sports.

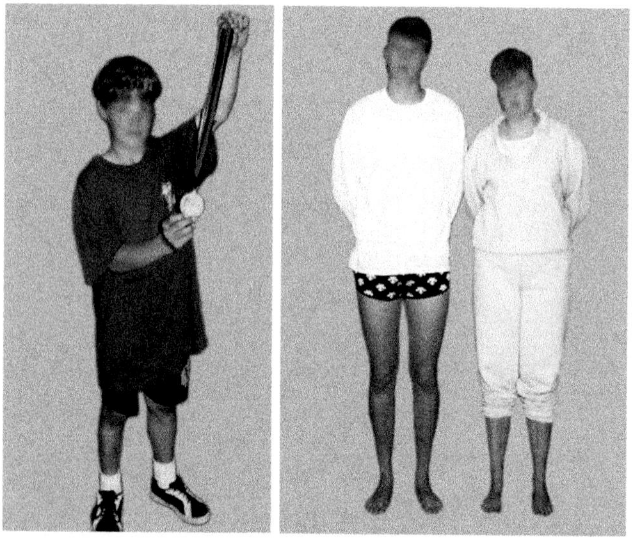

C Elite athletes These patients are excellent athletes. The boy (left) had DDH as an infant and underwent a pelvic osteotomy for correction of residual acetabular dysplasia. He is an outstanding soccer player. The brother and sister (right) have contracture of the heel-cords and secondary overuse syndromes but are still outstanding runners.

Prevention

It is estimated that about half of sports injuries are preventable. Because sports account for about one-third of all childhood injuries, the potential impact on childhood is enormous. Environmental and personal factors are both important.

Environmental Factors

Thermal regulation is of critical importance in children. Select a cool environment when possible. Avoid excessive clothing and prolonged exposure to sunlight. Insist on adequate fluid intake. Check weight before and after participation to monitor hydration status.

Playing surface should be as shock absorbing as possible [A]. Avoid running on hard surfaces. Insist on padded surfaces for playgrounds and for field events where falls are common.

Motor vehicles are dangerous in areas of play, especially for sledding and biking.

Encourage adults to focus more on safety than winning. Emphasize the importance of learning sport skills, the value of team participation, and having an enjoyable experience. Point out that participation sometimes involves losing. Learning to accept and handle losing teaches an important lesson that will be valuable throughout life.

Maintain equipment in good working condition and be certain the equipment is size appropriate and properly fitted.

Provide medical care for preparticipation evaluation and early intervention.

Individual Factors

Wear protective devices Make sure they are appropriate in size and fit. Be sure the children wear protection, such as helmets, face and mouth guards, and body protection in vulnerable sites. Also, they should remove helmets when not involved in a risk of collision.

Proper conditioning started preseason improves strength, flexibility, and endurance.

Limit rate of increase in loading or repetitions to about 10% per week (10% rule).

Proper footwear provides good shock absorption and traction.

Adequate sleep Those who sleep at least eight hours a night are about 70% less likely to be injured than those who sleep less.

Sporting Environment Control

Preseason medical evaluation should identify which conditions could be worsened by sports participation and identify musculoskeletal problems that could be improved by rehabilitation before returning to sports.

Provide medical coverage at high-risk events to provide prompt professional diagnoses and management.

Improved coaching skill is an important factor. Encourage coaches to avoid coaching by the approach used in their own childhood experience. Help them understand that the primary source of overuse injuries is too much, too soon—not just too much. Coaches should advance progression in sports participation appropriately to avoid placing the young athlete at risk. Too rapid advancement increases risk of injury.

Children with Orthopedic Disabilities

Children with hip dysplasia, clubfeet, and other orthopedic deformities may become outstanding athletes [B]. This is important information to give parents while treating these children.

Elite Athletes

Elite or outstanding athletes can have musculoskeletal problems [C]. It is commonly believed that to become elite athletes, children must start training during their first decade; however, this has not been documented.

Studies have demonstrated that the injury rate in elite juvenile athletes is lower than that of average-ability athletes. Elite athletes are stronger and more flexible than their peers. Because many will progress to participate in impact sports in late adolescence and adulthood, they risk long-term disability from osteoarthritis later in life. The risk of osteoarthritis is sport specific, and greater for those participating in collision sports.

Focused juvenile athletes are preoccupied with their sports. This is beneficial in enhancing self-esteem; promotes a healthy lifestyle by discouraging the use of drugs, smoking, and obesity; and possibly provides scholarships or other sport-generated income. On the downside, academic achievement, socialization, interpersonal skills, and other broadening experiences may be limited. The cost to girls may be greater. Menstrual irregularities, possibly shortened stature, and eating disorders may occur. The preoccupation with thinness in gymnasts and dancers creates special problems for girls.

Special Children

Children at both ends of the spectrum of ability have special needs. They are vulnerable to over- or underparticipation. Each has its unique problems. These children are in special need of the Bill of Rights for Young Athletes, as detailed by Sullivan [A].

Children with Disabilities

Children with disabilities need physical activity as much as or more than other children. An objective of management is the normalization of these children's lives [B]. This often requires special efforts by the family, sponsoring organizations, and medical providers.

Skiing programs are useful for children with limb deficiencies and mild cerebral palsy.

Wheelchair sports, such as basketball and racing [C], are excellent choices for providing exercise with little risk.

Organized sports participation requires a supportive system by the adults as well as other children to succeed. An integrated play environment is healthy not only for the disabled child but also for the teammates. The teammates gain understanding and are more likely to befriend the child with a disability.

Special summer camps are effective in providing supervised programs [D] with medical support.

Horseback riding programs are popular, but they require close adult supervision to prevent falls. Therapeutic riding associations offer this experience at reduced costs. When done appropriately, this experience is worthwhile.

Family programs are most important. Encourage the family to include the special child in their normal activities [E]. Unfortunately, families often overprotect the child, limiting the child's experiences and thereby harming the child. Encourage families to go ahead with the travel and physical activities that they would normally undertake and to include the whole family.

Bill of Rights for Young Athletes

1. The right to participate in sports
2. The right to participate on a level commensurate with each child's maturity and ability
3. The right to have qualified adult leadership
4. The right to play as a child and not as an adult
5. The right of children to share in the leadership and decision-making of their sport participation
6. The right to participate in safe and healthy environments
7. The right to proper preparation for participation in sport
8. The right to an equal opportunity to strive for success
9. The right to be treated with dignity
10. The right to have fun in sports

A Bill of rights From *The Pediatric Athlete*, Sullivan (1988).

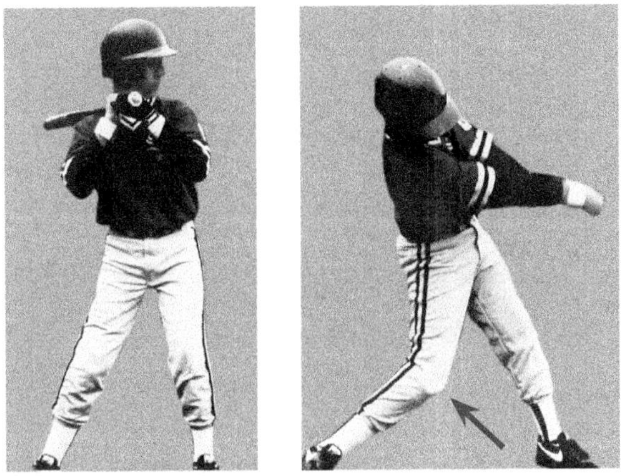

B Limb deficient child This child with a right lower limb amputation is an excellent baseball player. The only sign is the upper rim of the prosthesis visible in unusual positions (arrow).

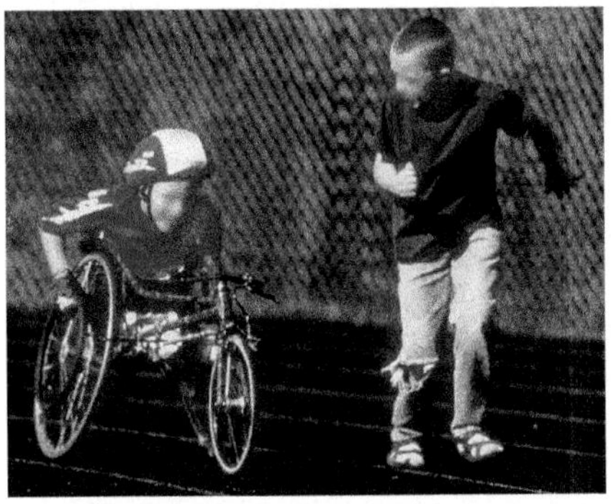

C Wheelchair sports This child has paraplegia and is an outstanding athlete.

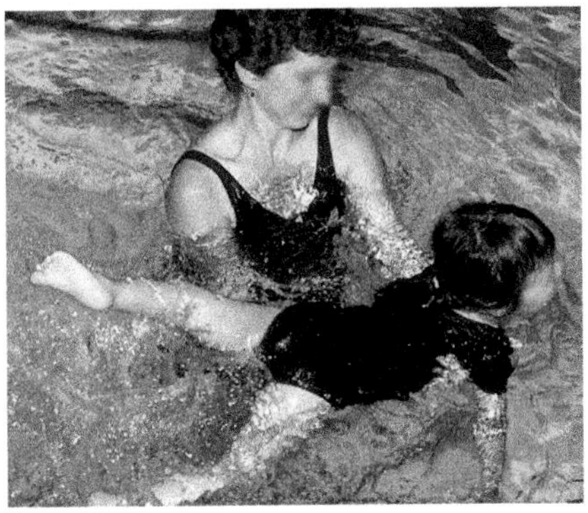

D Swimming This child with arthrogryposis is learning to swim. This can be a lifetime sport.

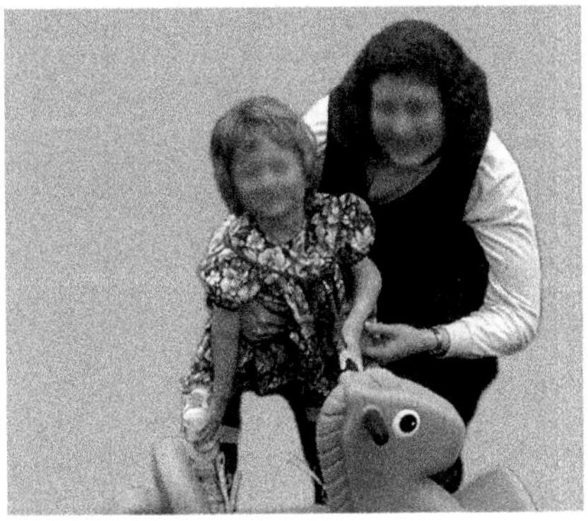

E Playing Selecting play equipment that is stable, rounded, and lightweight increases safety.

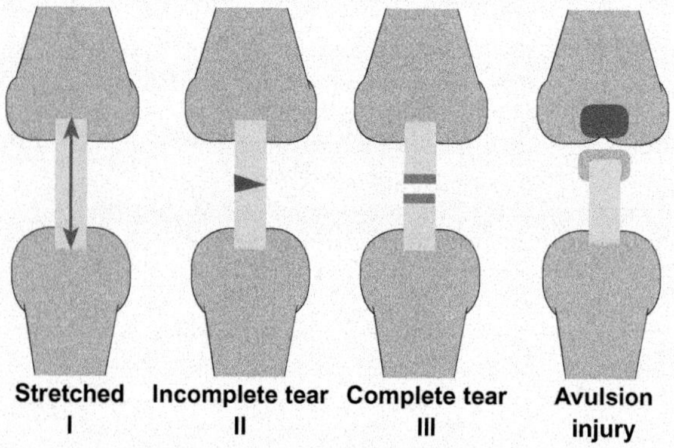

A Grading of ligamentous injury These may be graded into three categories. Avulsion with a bone fragment (right) is common in children and does not fall into the numerical classification.

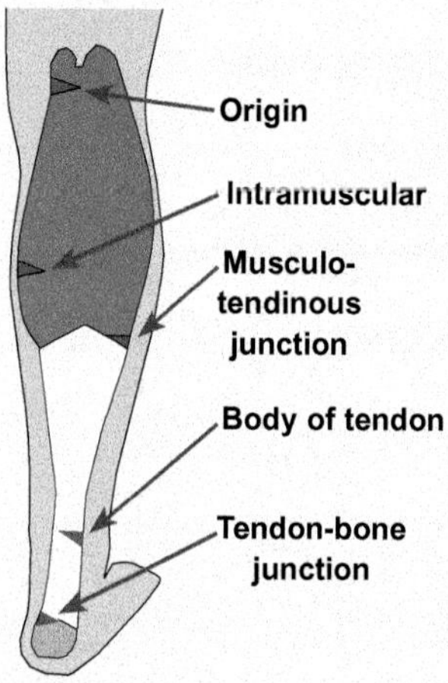

B Musculotendon injuries Injuries of this complex may occur at different locations.

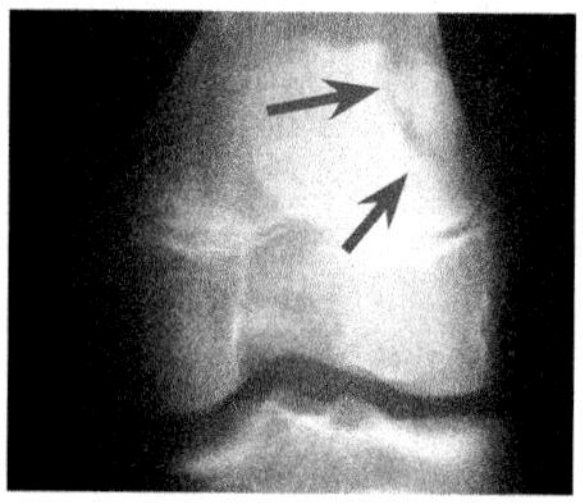

C Bipartite patella Stress injuries can disrupt the chondral junction between the patella and the ossicle, causing a synchondrosis disruption.

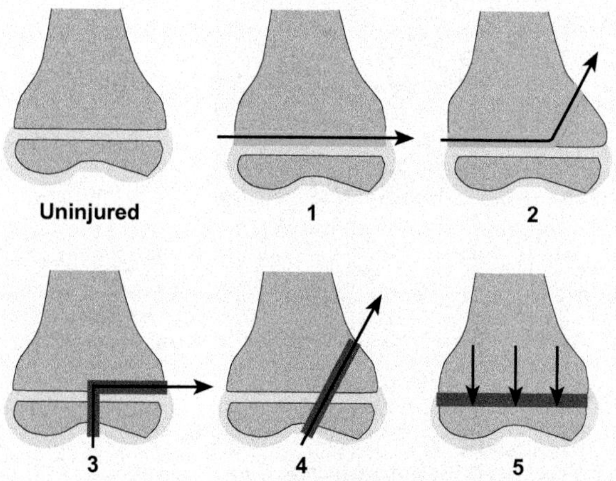

D Salter-Harris classification of growth plate injuries These are classified as types 1 through 5, based on the fracture pattern. Types 1 and 2 (green lines) do not traverse the epiphysis and usually do not cause growth problems. Types 3 to 5 (red lines) may cause growth arrest and progressive deformity.

Injury Types

Injury types from athletic participation include acute and overuse injuries. *Acute injuries* are the same as those that occur in nonsporting accidents. S*tress injuries* result from repetitive microtrauma and are unique to sports medicine. These injuries are the focus in this chapter.

Acute Injuries

Contusions are common injuries and usually heal quickly and completely. Secondary hematomas are less common in children, presumably due to enhanced hemostatic control in children. Rarely do contusions lead to formation of myositis ossificans. This is most common in the quadriceps. Avoid prolonged immobilization. These lesions mature over time. They may be confused with osteogenic sarcoma.

Ligament injuries Because ligaments are two to three times stronger than bone in children, avulsion fractures are common during growth. Ligaments tend to fail suddenly, in contrast to physeal injuries, which occur with more slowly applied loads. Ligamentous injuries can be graded [A] as follows:

Grade I represent stretch injuries without disruption of fibers that cause tenderness and swelling but without detectable instability.

Grade II are partial tears that allow greater mobility but with a definite endpoint.

Grade III are complete tears involving greater soft tissue injury, including the joint capsule and leading to joint instability.

Ligament injuries are most common around the ankle and knee and, when associated with capsular disruption, cause joint instability. They may coexist with bony injuries, as seen in tibial spine fractures. When the tibial spine is avulsed, the anterior cruciate ligament is stretched, leading to residual laxity following bony union.

Bone injuries Acute bony injuries can fall into the same patterns as those occurring from accidental trauma in nonathletic situations (they are covered in Chapter 4).

Musculotendon injuries can occur at many sites [B]. Complete separations are rare, and healing usually occurs spontaneously because no discontinuity occurs.

Synchondrosis disruptions Accessory ossification centers may become separated from their parent bone. The classic examples are the bipartite patella [C], accessory tarsal navicular, and accessory ossicles below the ankle malleoli.

Physeal injuries are classified by the fracture patterns [D]. Repetitive stress injury may damage the growth plate in a unique fashion. These stress-induced physeal injuries are most common about the wrist and upper humerus in the child. Stress results in a disruption of the growth plate, as seen in type 5 injuries. Unlike the usual simple physeal fracture, the growth plate becomes widened, irregular, and tender but not grossly unstable. Such injuries may result in physeal damage and altered growth. Type 5 injuries occur in the distal radial epiphysis in gymnasts and in the proximal humeral epiphysis in pitchers.

Common Sites	Sport
Medial epicondyle	Throwing sports, especially baseball
Iliac apophysis	Running and dancing
Ischial apophysis	Track and cheerleading
Inferior pole patella	Basketball, jumping sports, running
Tibial tubercle	Jumping sports, mainly basketball
Calcaneal apophysis	Soccer, hockey, basketball, running
Tibial spine	Bicycling

E Sites of traction injuries These are common sites and activities leading to the injury.

Traction and compression bone injuries Traction injuries may be acute or chronic and cause bony failure or inflammation at the tendon-bone junction [E, previous page]. Compression injuries are usually chronic, with the classic example being the lateral compartment of the elbow in "little league elbow." Throwing causes compression of both the capitellum and radial head, which may cause vascular damage and bone necrosis.

Juvenile Osteochondroses

This is a term describing a heterogeneous group of conditions that are characterized by sclerosis and fragmentation of the epiphysis or apophysis in the immature body. Irregular ossification may be a normal variation of ossification or represent a disorder. Classic descriptions include many sites [A]. More details are found in Chapter 1.

Osteochondritis Dissecans

Osteochondritis dissecans (OCD) is a segmental avascular necrosis of articular subchondral bone. These OCD lesions are most common at the end of growth and during early adult life and are more common in joints subjected to repetitive microtrauma. OCD lesions may be familial and may occur in several locations in the same individual.

These are lesions that affect the subchondral bone and cartilage of a joint. These lesions are discussed in chapters on their various anatomic locations, but some general features are appropriately discussed under sports because the lesions are often seen in the immature athlete and pose questions in management and athletic participation.

Etiology The causes of OCD are probably multiple. The predisposing factors include marginal vascularity, possible constitutional factors such as a coagulopathy, and repetitive microtrauma.

Classification Lesions may be classified anatomically [B] and based on radiographic or MR imaging. Assess activity and healing potential by dynamic bone scan in younger patients.

Location of lesions Lesions occur in the knee [C], talus, capitellum, patella, radial head, and femoral head. Femoral head OCD may be idiopathic but usually complicates LCP disease and avascular necrosis secondary to trauma and infection.

Natural history OCD has the potential to cause permanent disability [E] and is one of the more serious sports-related problems for the young athlete. The prognosis is better for smaller lesions, early onset, and a favorable location. Most small lesions in children heal spontaneously. Disability is more likely for large lesions in load-bearing areas of joints, such as the lateral femoral condyle, that progress to separation [D].

Management Treatment depends upon the age of the patient and the location, size, and stage of the lesion. In younger patients, small lesions that are stable may require only nonoperative management, primarily rest. Larger unstable lesions, especially in weight-bearing locations, are best managed more aggressively [D]. See Chapters 9 and 10, respectively, for the foot and knee.

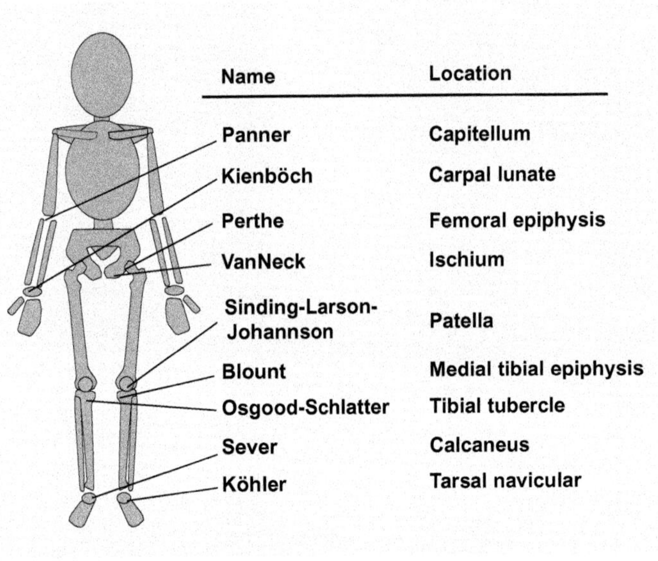

A Classic list of osteochondroses Name and location are shown.

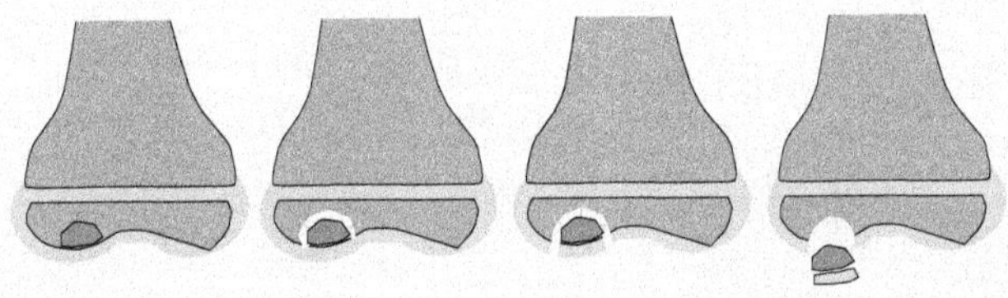

B Osteochondritis dissecans These are the stages of this disease. Over time the lesion may become unstable and finally separate into the joint and become a loose body.

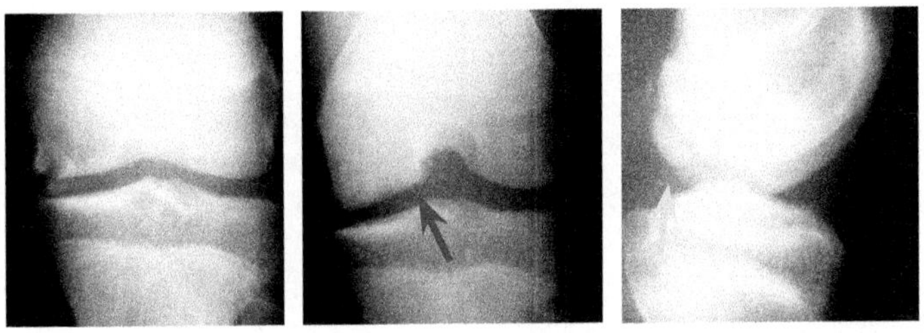

C Osteochondritis dissecans Lesion not seen on AP radiograph, but shown on notch (red arrow) and lateral (yellow arrow) views.

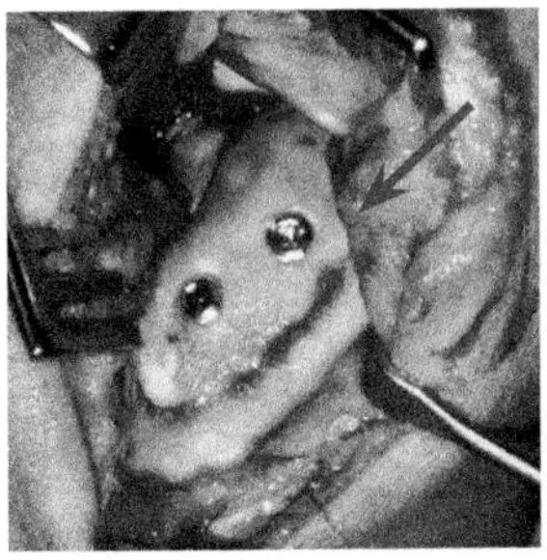

D Replaced large osteochondritic fragment This large lesion was replaced and fixed with two screws.

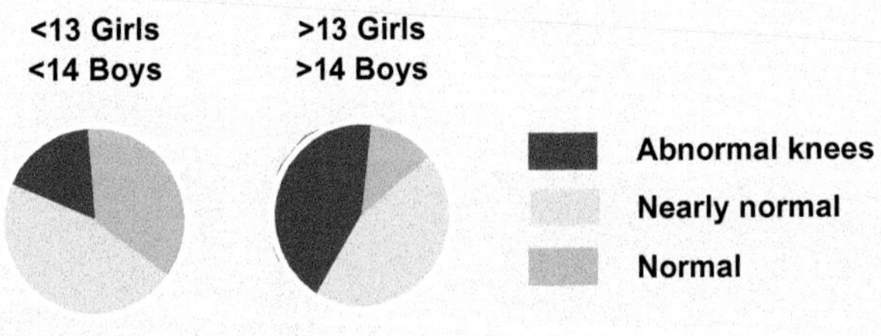

E Age and outcome for OCD lesion of the knee Based on 509 OCD lesions from Hefti (1999).

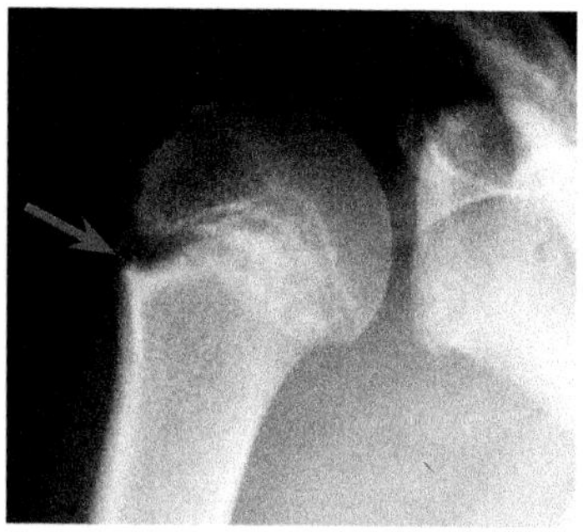

A Physeal stress injuries This adolescent pitcher developed a stress reaction causing widening of the proximal humeral physis (red arrow).

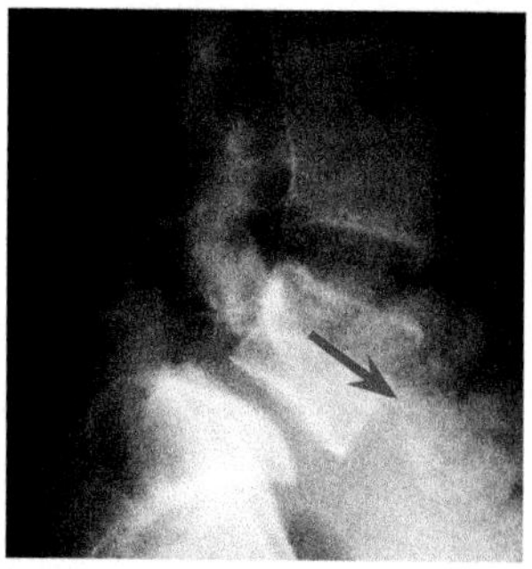

B Spondylolisthesis This gymnast had back pain and a grade I spondylolisthesis. This is due to a stress fracture through the pars.

Overuse Injuries

Between 30% and 50% of injuries of immature athletes are due to overuse. This varies from about 15% in soccer to 60% in swimmers. Sports that require repetitive acts are most likely to cause overuse problems. As compared with acute injuries, overuse injuries take longer to heal and result in more time away from competition.

Most injuries are the result of excessive demands on an unprepared system. Extremity malalignment, limited flexibility, excessive demands, and improper equipment and playing surfaces increase the risks.

Overuse injury seldom occurs in the normal play of children. The protective mechanism of pain limits overuse and promotes recovery. This protective mechanism is often repressed during regimented childhood sports. Addition risk factors are the long seasons and single sport participation. A large portion of sports medicine in children deals with the care of these overuse conditions.

Mechanism

Overuse injuries result from repetitive submaximal loading. The injuries from this *microtrauma* are usually reversed by rest. Repetitive microtrauma without intervals of rest is cumulative and causes stress injuries.

Stress injury to bone creates a progression of inflammation, periosteal swelling, and endosteal and cortical disruption. Stress injuries in children include fractures through the growth plate [A] or bone [B] and disruption of bone to tendon or muscle junctions. They may also affect the vascularity of bone, resulting in bone necrosis, as seen in osteochondritis dissecans. Before an overt fracture occurs, the injuries are referred to as *stress reactions*.

Sites of Overuse Injuries

The location of the injury depends upon the stresses created during specific activities of each sport. For example, wrist and back pain from overuse are common among gymnasts, swimmers have shoulder pain, whereas runners' injuries occur in the lower limbs [C].

Diagnosis

Make an accurate diagnosis to be certain that some more serious problem is not the cause of pain.

History should include the type of sporting activity associated with the onset, training (including frequency and duration), previous injuries, new techniques or equipment, and whether the patient is in a period of rapid growth. Detail the onset, character, location, and pain relationships with activity and time of day. Beware of night pain, as this can be a sign of a tumor.

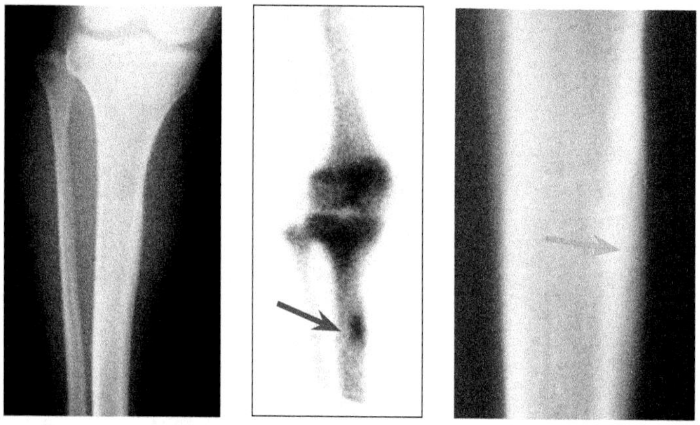

C Tibial stress fracture A 17-year-old female cross country runner has had "shin splints" for 3 months. The proximal tibia is tender. A plain radiograph (left) is negative, whereas the bone scan shows an area of increased uptake over the upper tibia (red arrow), and the CT scan shows sclerosis (orange arrow).

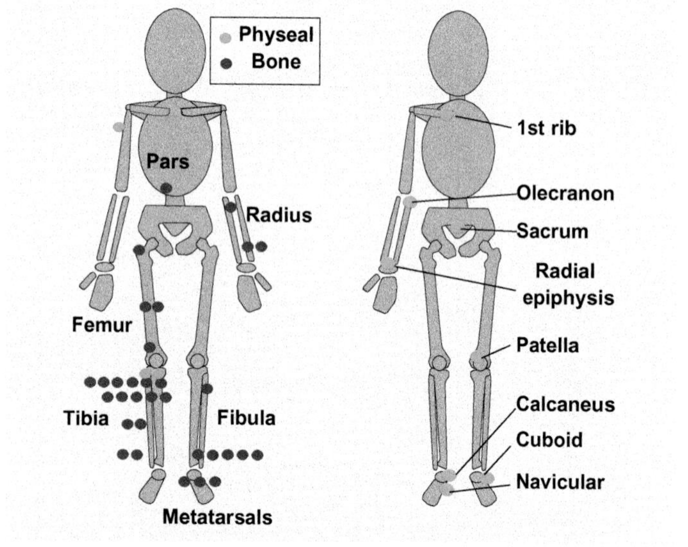

D Common and rare sites of stress fractures in children Common sites (red and blue dots) include both physeal and bony fractures. Rare sites of stress fractures (green dots) are shown on the right. Each dot represents a case in the series. From Walker (1996).

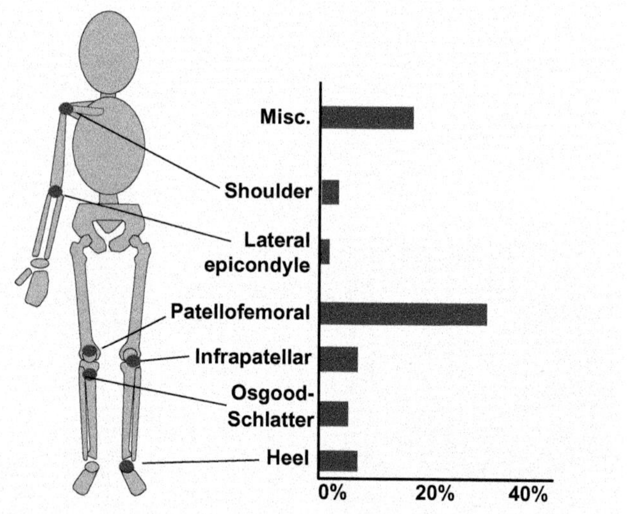

E Sites of overuse injuries Based on 139 athletes aged 9–16 years, from Dalton (1992).

Pain severity Based on the history, it is often useful to grade pain severity.

Grade I pain with excessive activity.

Grade II pain with moderate activity.

Grade III pain with routine daily activities.

Examination Localize the pain and determine the site of maximum tenderness. This will often help to establish the diagnosis [D and E, previous page]. Localized tenderness to the tibial tubercle is classic for Osgood-Schlatter disease, and tenderness over the origin of the plantar fascia and insertion of the Achilles tendon are classic findings for the common heel pain in children. Look for evidence of malalignment problems in lower limbs, such as the combination of femoral antetorsion and external tibial torsion or malalignment of the quadriceps mechanism.

Assess the interaction of the parent(s) and patient. Overzealous and controlling parents may aggravate the problem. Be concerned if the parent talks more than the child and makes comments that do not fit the appearance of the child. Such comments as "best athlete on the team," "tough minded," or "plays with pain" may be used to describe a child who is detached and unathletic appearing.

Attempt to assess the patient's attitude regarding physical education: Is participation a positive or negative experience for the patient? Does the patient exaggerate the disability in an attempt to get a *PE excuse,* or is the injury being minimized to reduce the risk of being *benched,* or is the injury overplayed to avoid unwanted participation forced on the patient in the first place?

Differentiating stress fractures from neoplasm or infection This is usually not difficult. Stress fractures occur in specific locations and show typical clinical and imaging features [A and B]. Assess the effect of rest. *With rest,* the *pain and tenderness of stress fractures resolve or improve over a period of days.* If the clinical features are atypical and the early differentiation important, image with CT scans to show the fracture line, bone scans to exactly localize the lesion, and laboratory studies of CRP and ESR to aid in differentiating infections.

Healing The stage of healing may be assessed by MRI. This study is not appropriate for screening but may be useful in assessing progress in chronic cases.

Management

Management of stress injuries is simple—rest. In most situations, rest is relative. The frequency and magnitude of training are reduced, and other less stressful activities are substituted. The challenge is in preventing recurrence. This requires an understanding of the cause.

Rest If activity modification is insufficient, cast or splint immobilization may be necessary.

Modify factors contributing to stress injuries These are commonly categorized as *extrinsic* or *intrinsic* [C]. Identify and modify these factors, provide pain control, and rehabilitate before returning the patient to activity.

Return to sports should be carefully supervised and gradual.

Prognosis Most stress injuries and fractures heal with rest and cause no long-term disability. Stress injuries are rarely serious.

Displaced stress fractures are rare but may occur if the activity continues, even when pain occurs. The most serious fractures include the femoral neck and tibia.

Spondylolisthesis is common in gymnasts. Displacement progresses to the severity that fusion becomes necessary.

Growth plate injuries, such as the distal radius in gymnasts and proximal tibia in runners, may lead to growth arrest and bone shortening.

Osteochondritis dissecans commonly causes permanent joint damage with premature degenerative arthritis and long-term disability.

Bony overgrowth, such as a permanent prominence of the tibial tubercle or radial head, may cause mild long-term disability.

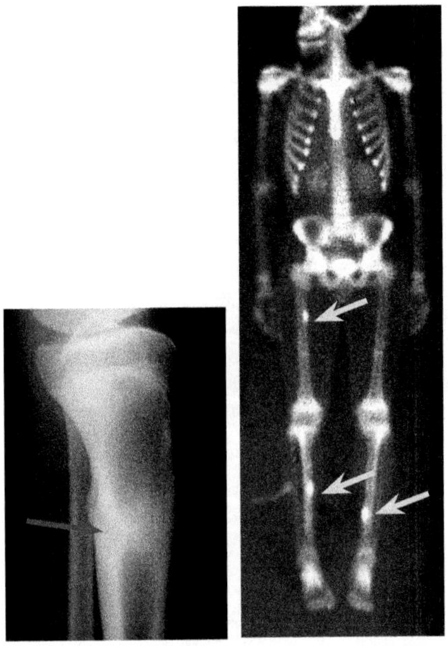

A Imaging stress fractures Often the location and radiographic appearance of stress fractures is diagnostic on plain radiographs, such as this proximal tibia (red arrow). Stress fractures may be multiple, as shown by a bone scan (yellow arrows).

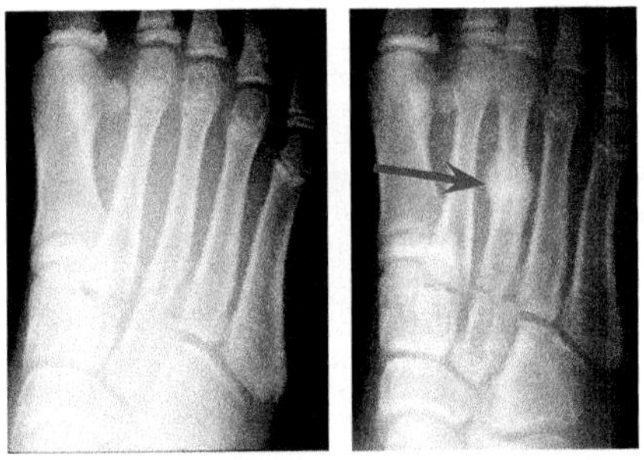

B Metatarsal stress fracture This 14-year-old runner complained of foot pain and demonstrated localized tenderness over the third metatarsal. Initial radiographs (left) were negative. Radiographs three weeks later show the fracture and callus (arrow).

Factors contributing to overuse injuries

Extrinsic factors that contribute include:

- Adult or peer pressure
- Incorrect sport technique
- Hard or rough surfaces
- Excessively rapid progression of training
- Too little rest
- Inappropriate equipment

Intrinsic factors

- Core weakness, poor hip stability
- Anatomic malalignment
- Psychological factors
- Inadequate conditioning
- Prior injury
- Growth
- Limited Range of Motion

C Factors contributing to overuse injuries in children Modified from DiFioni (1999).

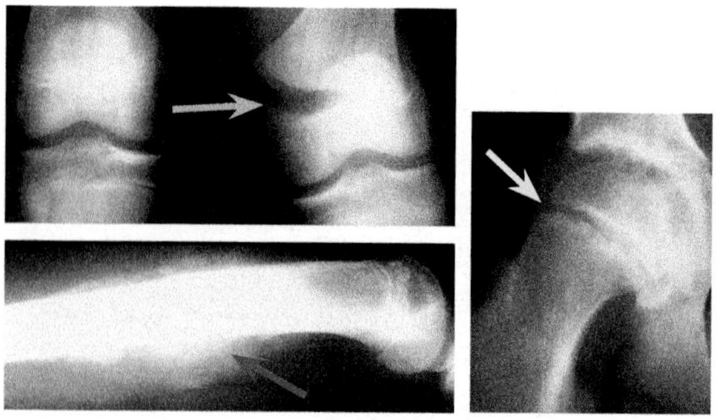

A Pitfalls in diagnosis Epiphyseal fractures (orange arrow) can be confused with ligament injury. Malignant tumors (red arrow) may be confused with intrinsic knee problems. Slipped capital femoral epiphysis (yellow arrow) may be confused with anterior knee pain.

More Significant	Less Significant
Night pain	Long duration
Unilateral	Bilateral
Onset with significant trauma	Poorly localized
History of feeling a "pop"	No localized tenderness
Inability to walk or run	Pain lasting only seconds
Local signs of swelling	Stable joint
Short duration	
Localized tenderness	
Instability	
Joint effusion	

B Features and significance Features that suggest the problem is more serious (left) versus less serious (right).

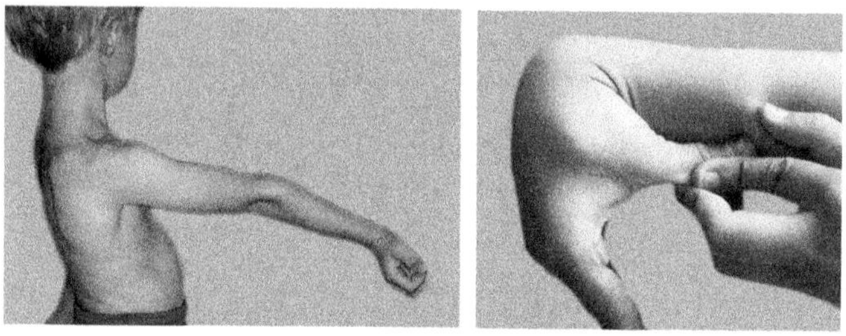

C Joint laxity Individuals with excessive joint laxity show exceptional wrist flexion, finger extension, and hyperextension of the elbows and knees.

Evaluation

Be prepared for difficulty in evaluating the injured athlete. Some players, fearful of being pulled from the game or letting down teammates, may understate the significance of their injury. The parents may have their own agenda and overstate or understate the problem. The coach may push for the player to return to the game.

History

Keep in mind the pitfalls in management [A]. A common mistake is to attribute the problem to trauma based on a history of an injury. Injuries are a normal part of a child's daily activity. Many serious tumors and infections have been missed because the problem was erroneously attributed to an injury. Some features of the history are more significant than others [B]. A report of feeling or hearing a "pop" is significant. Be suspicious of a history of night pain (for a tumor).

Physical Examination

Assess joint laxity to help establish what is normal for the child [C]. Joint laxity is more common in the younger child and in girls. Excessive laxity occurs in about 5% of adolescents and predisposes them to sprains and joint dislocations. Examine the uninjured side and consider the child's joint laxity when assessing possible ligamentous injury.

Localize tenderness and pain to help in pinpointing the site of injury. *Knee pain* should prompt a check of the hips. Perform the hip rotation test to rule out the hip as the source of the pain.

Assess active motion during screening. Unguarded full movement usually means the part is not injured.

Determine instability by applying the appropriate test.

Ankle stability is assessed by stressing the ligaments between the leg and foot. Stabilize the leg and attempt to move the foot forward [D]. Note any instability.

Lachman test is performed with the knee flexed to 20°. One hand stabilizes the thigh while the other applies anterior and posterior forces to the upper leg [E]. Instability of the anterior cruciate ligament is determined.

Collateral ligament stability should be assessed with the knee flexed to 30° with varus and valgus stress applied [F]. Consider the patient's joint laxity evaluation in assessing the significance of laxity of the knee. Grade the findings to include the quality of the endpoint.

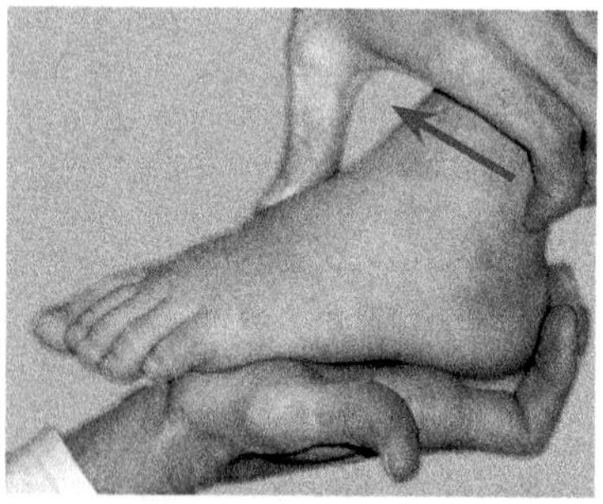

D Ankle stability assessment Stabilize the foot against a flat surface or by hand. Attempt to displace the ankle (talus) forward (arrow) to demonstrate ankle instability.

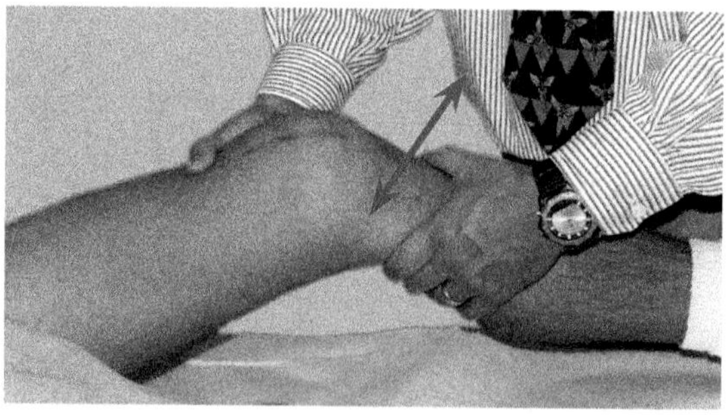

E Lachman test Flex the knee to an angle of about 20° and apply anterior and posterior forces (arrow). Note any instability.

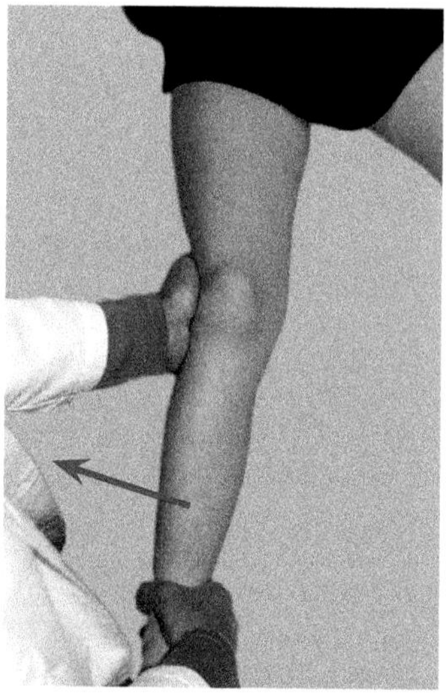

F Medial collateral ligament stability testing Flex the knee 20°–30° and apply valgus stresses to the knee (arrow). Note any instability.

Assess flexibility by manipulating the joint or checking mobility. Stiffness is often a sign of an injury, whereas limited motion is often indicative of disease [A]. The loss of mobility may be either a cause or an effect of the disease. Order imaging studies thoughtfully.

Imaging

Request plain radiographs first. Radiographs are most readily available, least likely to be misread, and least expensive. Comparison views are sometimes helpful. Each study has special indications [B]. Stress views to differentiate physeal fractures and ligament injuries are neither necessary nor appropriate. They may add further injury to an already traumatized physis.

Arthroscopy

Few arthroscopic studies are necessary in children as compared to adults. Arthroscopy is useful for the knee, ankle, elbow, shoulder, and hip [C], but it is most commonly used for evaluating knee problems. Because hip arthroscopy requires distracting the joint, it is less commonly used.

Arthroscopy is useful when noninvasive methods do not provide a diagnosis or when treatment can be part of the arthroscopic procedure. Knee arthroscopy is appropriate for the traumatic hemarthrosis associated with instability. Arthroscopy is helpful in evaluating osteochondritis dissecans of the ankle, knee, hip, and elbow. Arthroscopy is useful for removal of loose bodies in joints, meniscal repairs, reconstruction of cruciate tears or avulsions, and replacement and fixation of osteochondral fractures and osteochondral lesions from osteochondritis dissecans.

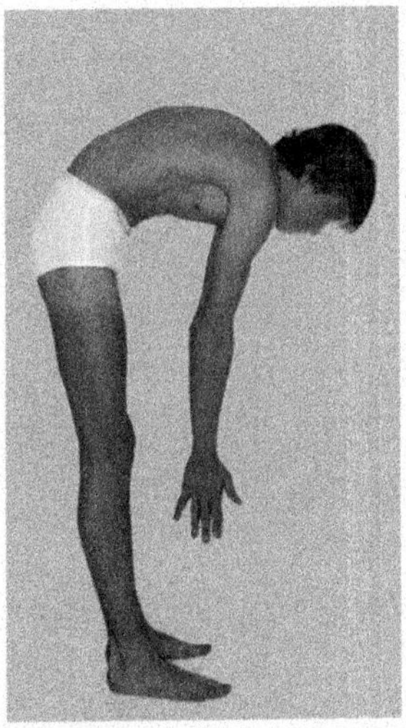

Limited motion	Problem
Forward bending	Spine problem
Backward bending	Spondylolysis (olisthesis)
Straight leg raising	Spondylolysis (olisthesis)
Hamstring-quad	Osgood-Schlatter disease
Quadriceps	Patellofemoral disorders
Medial hip rotation	Hip injuries and inflammation
Subtalar motion	Tarsal coalition
Elbow motion	Little league elbow

A Significance of limited motion Limited motion is often associated with specific disorders. A child should be able to reach to mid-tibial level on forward bending.

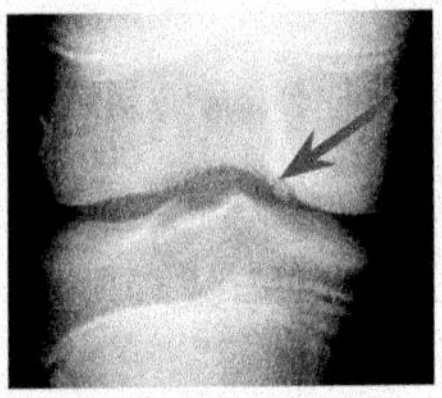

Conventional radiographs

Order before any other imaging study
Osteochondritis dissecans (arrow)

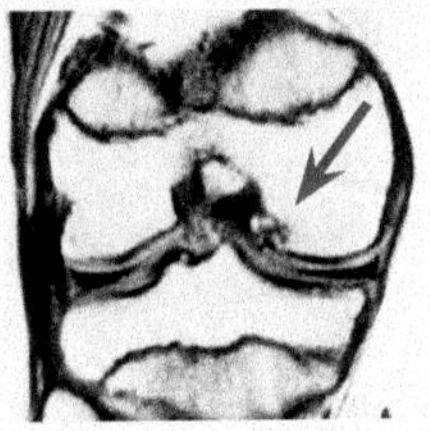

Magnetic resonance imaging

Meniscal injuries
Herniated intervertebral disc
Ring apophyseal fracture
Early stress injuries
Physeal bridges
Loose bodies in joints
Osteochondritis dissecans (arrow)

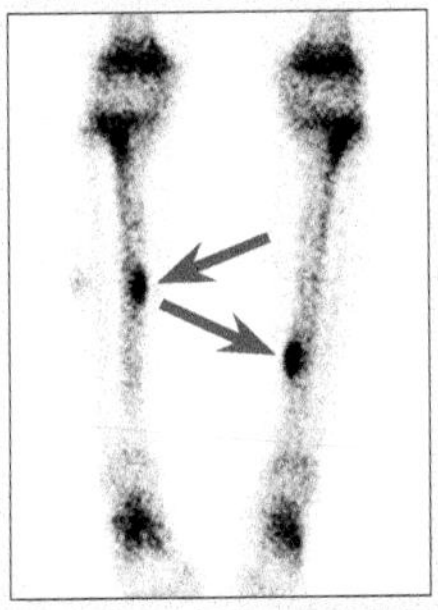

Bone scans

Stress injuries (arrows)
Occult fractures
Spondylolysis
Osteomyelitis

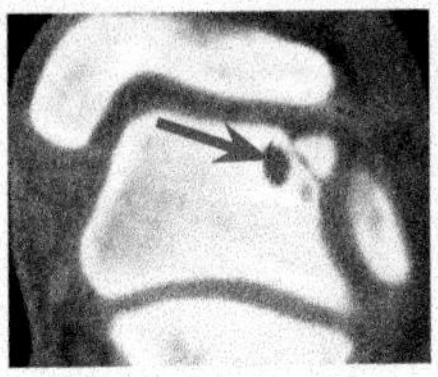

Computer tomography

Complex fractures
Bony lesions
Osteochondritis dissecans (arrow)

B Imaging choices This table shows the studies most likely to establish a diagnosis.

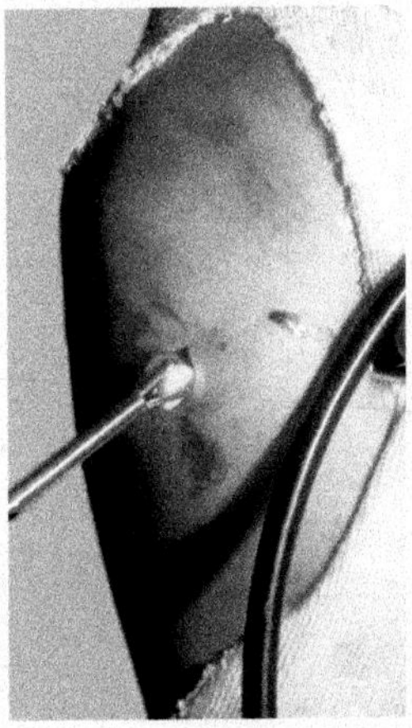

Diagnosis

Acute instability
Loose bodies
Osteochondritis dissecans
Meniscal injuries
Impingement problems

Treatment

Removal of loose bodies
ACL reconstruction
Repair of meniscus
Repair of OCD lesions

C Indications for arthroscopy Some of the diagnostic and therapeutic indications are listed.

Management Principles

Management of sports injuries is unique because these injuries are sometimes predictable and often preventable. Management is complicated by pressures to return the child to sports before healing is complete. Being the child's advocate and protector is important and sometimes difficult.

Acute Injury

Manage the acute injury by using the RICE sequence [A]. Ice in a plastic bag or plastic cup works well. The ice minimizes pain. Advise the family to discontinue the cold if the skin becomes numb. This initial management is designed to minimize swelling and is continued for the first 24 hours, then tapered.

Nonsteroidal antiinflammatory drugs (NSAIDs) are useful in reducing pain and inflammation. Tolmetin, naproxen, and ibuprofen are acceptable drugs for children and adolescents. Ibuprofen is widely used because it is inexpensive and available without a prescription.

Establish a Diagnosis

Be certain the diagnosis is accurate. Make radiographs of sites of tenderness over bones or joints. Follow with additional imaging studies or seek consultation. Be very careful in managing injuries around joints such as the elbow and knee.

Preparing Family and Coach

Patients, family, and coaches need to be advised in advance about the predicted healing time.

Establish a Management Plan

Develop a plan to manage the acute problem and the rehabilitation [B]. The child should not return until the acute effects of the trauma and the secondary effects on muscle strength, endurance, and joint stiffness have resolved.

Identify causative factors that may have contributed to the current problem.

Training regimens are the most common cause of overuse syndrome. These regimens should not add more than about 10% per week of additional load [C]. Avoid overhead lifting and full squats. Discourage excessive pressure from the trainer or family.

Anatomic features may predispose the child to injury. Such problems include rotational malalignment (femoral and tibial torsion), ligamentous joint laxity, tarsal coalitions, and tight heel cords.

Environmental problems contributing to the injury should be identified. These factors include surfaces, equipment size, and condition.

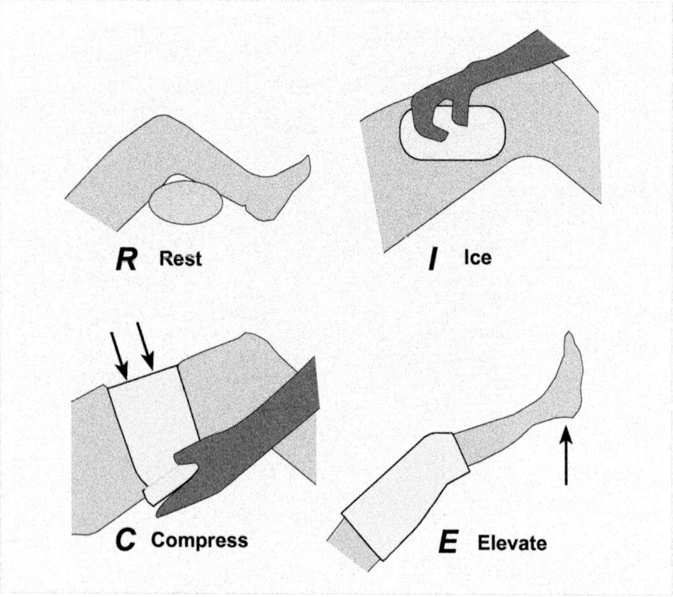

A RICE management for acute injuries R for rest, I for ice, C for compression, and E for elevation.

Management Plan

1. Acute management: RICE
2. Identify causative factors:
   Training factors
   Anatomic factors
   Environmental factors
3. Establish plan to modify these factors before child returns to activity
4. Provide adequate period of rest to heal injury
5. Maintain strength, endurance, and flexibility during healing period
6. Reintroduce activity in progressive fashion.

B Management plan Include each step in the overall plan. Discuss plan with coaches, trainers, and parents.

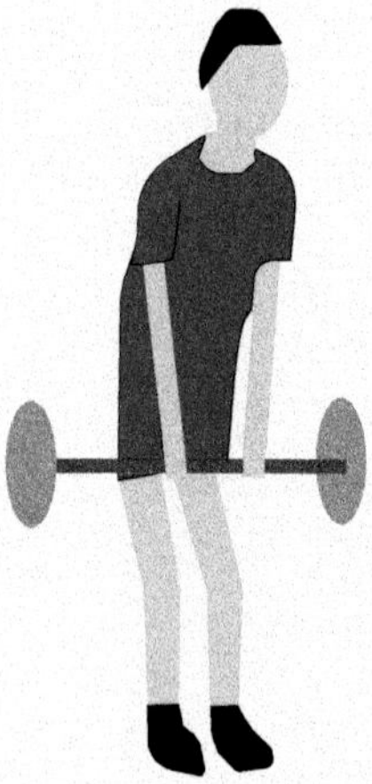

Sample exercise list for strength training in adolescents

Beginner: 1 set of 10 repetitions
Intermediate: 2 sets of 10 repetitions
Advanced: 3 sets of 10 repetitions

1. Biceps curls
2. Triceps extensions
3. Abdominal flexion
4. Back extensions
5. Knee extensions
6. Knee flexion
7. Bench press
8. Leg press

Increase load no more than 10% per week.

C Strength training program This program is the type often prescribed for adolescents. Weekly increases should be limited to 10%.

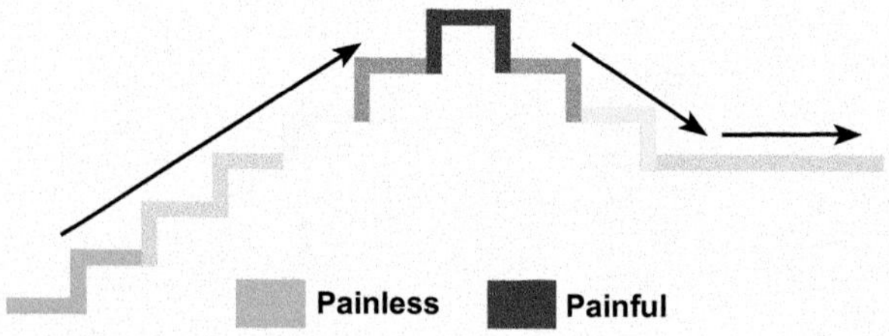

D Activity staircase Activities are gradually increased (left, green), and if overuse symptoms develop (red), the activity is reduced to the maximum level at which the child remains entirely pain free (right, green).

Modify causative factors while the child is recovering to prevent recurrence of the problem. Emphasize proper sports techniques.

Provide adequate time for healing of the bone, collagen, or muscle tissue because time, not treatment, is the principal factor in healing. The secondary effect of muscle atrophy and joint stiffness can be prevented by an exercise program. Do not underestimate the seriousness of soft tissue injuries, as they also require considerable time for recovery.

Prevent muscle atrophy during convalescence. Rest the injured part but plan an exercise program to maintain strength in nonaffected muscle groups. Isometric exercises may be used around an injured part. Avoid exercises that cause pain.

Prescribing "relative rest" involves reducing the training regiment, but allowing participation at a lower level.

Reintroduce activities progressively after healing is complete. Healing requires a minimum of 6 weeks (and sometimes longer) for bone, cartilage, ligaments, and tendons. Reintroduce activities by using the step model [D, previous page]. Break down sports into components and add progressively to the repetitions. If the new level of activity is performed without pain, then progress to the next level. If pain recurs, then move to the next lower level of activity.

Return to sports participation gradually Add sport-specific tasks with progressively increasing speeds prior to returning the patient to sports. Then start with practice sessions.

Return to competition Allow only after healing and rehabilitation are complete. Make certain the initial causative factors are corrected to avoid repeating this cycle.

Strength Training

Exercise programs for children and adolescents can increase strength and should be undertaken to overcome muscle weakness that may contribute to further injuries. Make the programs fun and varied. Children become bored quickly. Avoid many repetitions. Strictly adhere to the 10% rule and decrease the load promptly if symptoms develop [D, previous page]. Tailor strength to fit the specific condition and site. The options for exercises fall into several types:

Closed chain exercises are performed with the hand or foot stabilized.

Open chain exercises are performed with the hand or foot free.

Range of motion exercises fall into three types: passive, active, and active assistive.

Isotonic allows free motion.

Isometric restricts motion.

Isokinetic controls speed of contraction utilizing exercise machines.

Usually 20 to 30 repetitions are prescribed, which may be closed or open chain. Isokinetic exercises are most effective but require special equipment.

Exercises for Rehabilitation

Prescribe exercises with an understanding of the terminology [A]. Exercises should be tailored to the child [B]. Exercises help in maintaining or restoring strength following injury and in preparing the individual for the demands of certain sports.

Braces and Splints

Providing immobilization and protection is useful following sprains and fractures. A splint is often used in place of a cast when only protection is required. Commercial splints [C] can be more expensive than casts but less expensive than custom braces from an orthotist.

Female Sports Triad

This triad includes delayed menarche, eating disorders, and early osteopenia. This problem is commonly seen in sports that emphasize a low percentage of body fat such as gymnastics, ballet, and endurance running.

Term	Definition
Strength training	The use of resistance methods
Core strengthening	Focus on strengthening trunk stabilizers
Set	Group of repetitions separated by rest
Reps	An abbreviation for repetitions
One-rep	Jumping sports, mainly basketball
Concentric contractions	Muscle shortens during contractions
Eccentric contractions	Muscle lengthens during contraction
Isometric contraction	Muscle length unchanged during contraction
Isokinetic contraction	Speed of muscle contraction fixed during range of motion
Progressive resistive exercises	Regiment with progressive increases in amount of weight lifted and/or number of reps
Plyometric exercises	Repeated concentric and eccentric muscle contractions
Weight lifting	Competitive sport of maximum lifting
Power lifting	Max lifting ability and dead lift, squat, and bench press
Bodybuilding	Competition judging muscle size, symmetric, and definition

A Definitions This table provides definitions from the AAP. PEDIATRICS 2008 vol. 121:835-840.

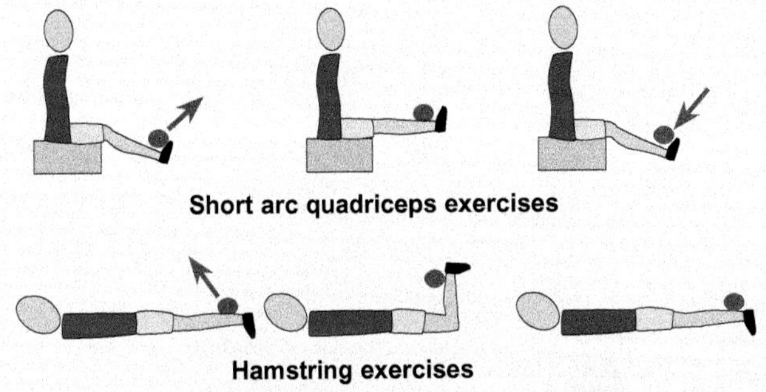

B Exercises Tailor the exercise program to the needs of the child or adolescent. These are some commonly prescribed exercises.

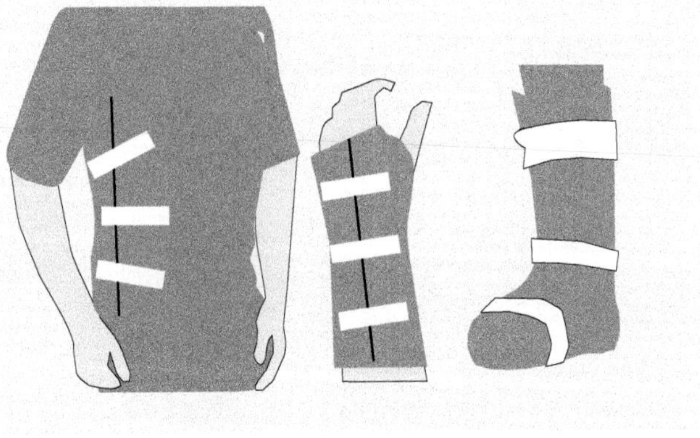

C Brace types Prefabricated splints and braces are often adequate. Their advantages are lower cost and immediate availability.

Injury	Description
Boxer fracture	Fracture of the fifth distal metacarpal
Breast-stroker knee	Medial collateral ligament or patellar tendon inflammation
Burners	Transient stretch injury to brachial plexus
Little league shoulder	Injury to proximal humeral growth pla
Dancer ankle	Inflammation of the os trigonum
Jogger ankle	Overuse injury of heel-cord insertion
Jumper knee	Patellar tendonitis
Little league elbow	Medial epicondyle, capitellum, or radial head injury
Pointers	Contusion over iliac crest
Skier thumb	Injury to ulnar collateral ligament
Stingers	Transient stretch injury to brachial plexus
Tennis elbow	Lateral epicondylitis

A Terms describing sports injuries These common terms are used to describe injuries common to various sports.

Contact	Noncontact
American Football	Tennis
Soccer	Track
Boxing	Volleyball
Ice Hockey	Cycling
Wrestling	Gymnastics
Basketball	Skateboard
	Skiing
	Skating

B Classification This is a list of sports considered as contact and noncontact types.

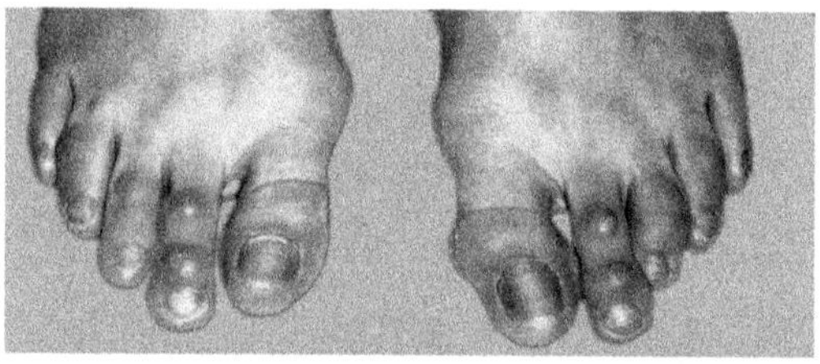

C Dancer toes These are the toes of a ballerina. Note the callosities over the second toe.

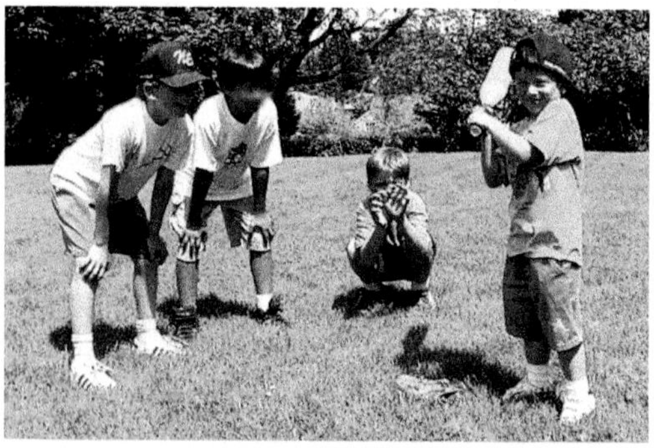

D Baseball in young children Baseball's low-velocity injuries are seldom serious. Being struck with the bat is the most serious risk.

Sport-Specific Problems

Knowledge of a sport's demands, lore, and jargon aids in understanding the athlete's problems [A]. Sports are often classified as contact or noncontact. Contact sports [B] are consider to be most likely to result in injury.

American Football

High risk. Most injuries are due to collisions in this most risky sport. Catastrophic head and neck injuries can be reduced by using a well-fitting helmet and by avoiding spearing (initial head contact in blocking and tackling). A quarter of American football players are obese. Injury rates increase with maturation. Long-term osteoarthritis of the knee and hip are possible sequela from major injuries of these joints. Most problems result from acute injury and are due to joint and neurological damage. Try to control pushy coaches and educate parents.

Ballet Dancing

Moderate risk. Reports of specific injuries, which include stress fractures of the pars, distal fibula, and base of the second metatarsal; Achilles tendonitis; cuboid subluxation; os trigonum impingement syndrome; and trigger toes. Toes are severely stressed [C]. Delay in puberty and emphasis on slenderness is a problem for girls and can lead to eating disorders. Be aware that the dancer's self-image is one of an artist, not an athlete, despite the high level of athletic demands.

Baseball and Softball

Moderate risk, depending upon the child's age [D]. Most acute injuries are associated with sliding, collisions, and ball or bat strikes. Most deaths occur from ball strikes to the head, neck, or chest. Overuse injuries, such as little league elbow, are preventable but potentially serious problems. Unusual injuries include apophysitis of the acromion, distal humeral epiphyseal separation, persistence of the olecranon physis, and avulsion of the iliac crest apophysis while swinging a bat.

Basketball

Moderate risk. Injuries as compared with other sports occur more often but usually are mild. Injuries in children under age 12 involve mainly contusions, sprains, lacerations, and rarely a fracture. Seldom are there serious injuries. Adolescent injuries are more common and more likely to be serious, such as contusions, sprains, and sometimes fractures. Ankles and knees are affected most. Most serious are ACL injuries. Ankle injuries require rehabilitation to prevent recurrence.

Cycling

High risk [B, next page]. Most serious accidents are due to collisions with motor vehicles. Prevention is essential through education of children, use of helmets, and avoidance of congested roadways. Potential long-term disability from head injury is significant.

Diving

High-risk [D, next page]. There is a risk of head and cervical spine injury with quadriplegia. Attention to diving height, water depth, and technique are essential in prevention.

Gymnastics

Moderate risk. Overuse injuries commonly produce spondylolysis [A] and wrist problems. Wrist pain occurs in about 75% of gymnasts, and radiographic changes of the distal radial physis were found in 25%. Long-term problems may result from growth arrest of distal radial epiphysis and spondylolisthesis. The great focus on slimness may cause eating disorders and menstrual and growth problems in girls. Stress injuries of the elbow in 19 adolescent elite gymnasts have been reported.

Elbow changes include avascular necrosis of the capitellar epiphysis, distortion of the articular surface, and osteochondritis of the radial head. Olecranon changes are common with fragmentation of the epiphysis to chronic Salter Type I stress fractures of the growth plate.

Specifically, rapid periods of growth and advanced levels of training and competition have appeared to be related to injury proneness.

Ice Hockey

Moderate to high risk. Shoulder injuries are common from collision and puck and stick strikes. Protective gear is essential and has resulted in fewer facial lacerations. Head injuries and joint damage may lead to long-term problems.

Horseback Riding

Moderate to high risk. Injuries are due to horse handling and falls. Serious falls with head and neck injuries and fractures are common. Protective helmets and special training for handling horses can reduce risks. Horseback riding is proposed as therapeutic for children with cerebral palsy, scoliosis, and other conditions, but proof of effectiveness is lacking.

Playground

The playground can be a dangerous place for children [F]. Soft surfaces and reduced height of playground equipment are important design features.

Running

Low to moderate risk. Overuse injury rates are high [E], but serious injuries are uncommon. Most injuries are preventable by appropriate training, shoes, and selection of proper running surface. Long-term sequelae are unlikely.

Skateboarding

High risk. Children 10 to 14 years old were injured with greatest frequency. Nontrivial injuries were more common among children younger than 5 years of age, reflecting a larger proportion of head and neck injuries. Boys sustained more frequent and more severe skateboard-related injuries. Observed injury patterns include head and neck injuries in younger children, and extremity injuries as well as more severe head and neck injuries in older children. Acute injury is common and is related to boards being difficult to control and being used on hard surfaces, unsupervised, with potential for collision [A, next page]. Skateboarders should use protective gear and avoid obstacles and high speed. Long-term sequelae risk is moderate and primarily results from head injury.

Skating (Inline)

Low to moderate risk. Collisions and falls cause forearm fractures and contusions. Skaters should use protective gear. Long-term sequelae are unlikely.

Skiing

Moderate to high risk. Jumping and racing injuries [C] pose the greatest risks. Tibial fractures, medial collateral ligament injuries, and thumb and shoulder injuries are common. Collision injuries are the most serious, as head, spine, and extremity injuries may have long-term sequelae [B, next page]. The most common injuries were contusions of the knee in children and sprains of the ulnar collateral ligament of the thumb in adolescents. With increasing age, lower extremity injuries decrease but upper extremity injuries increase.

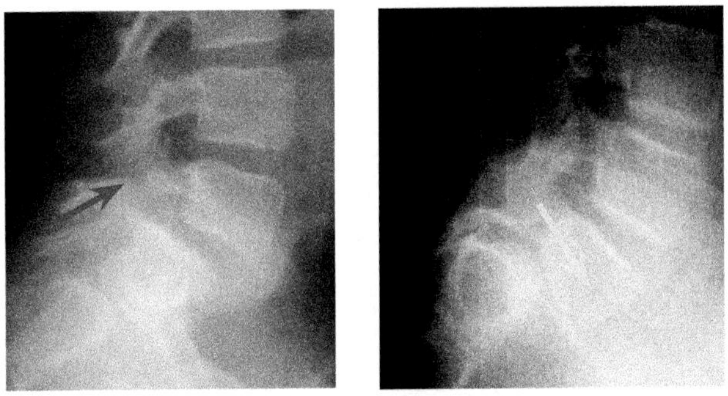

A Spondylolisthesis Grade 1 (red arrow) and grade 3 (yellow arrow) displacements are shown.

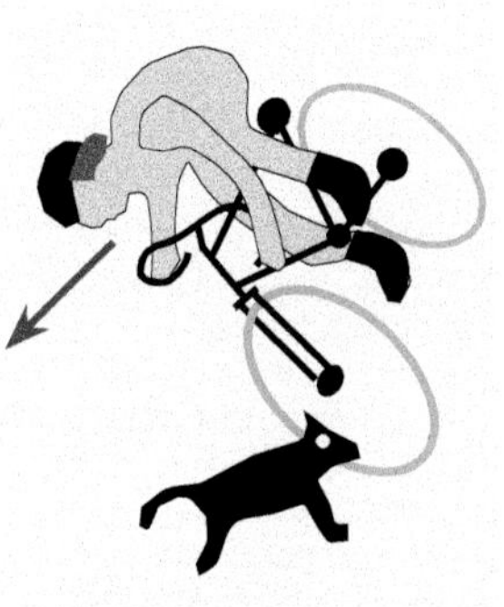

B Cycling Striking objects or collisions with cars pose serious risks.

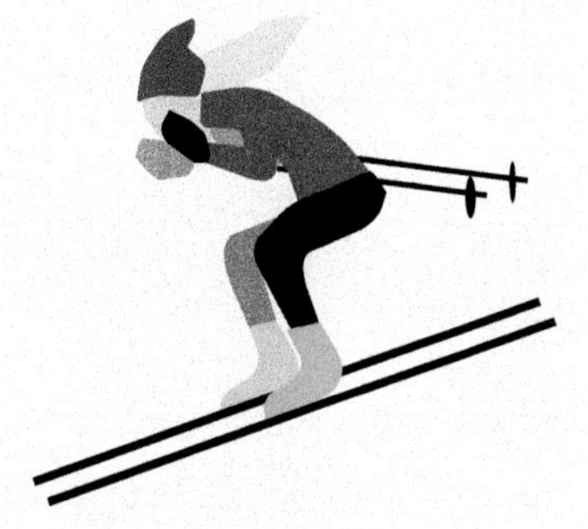

C Ski Racing These activities increase the risk of serious injury.

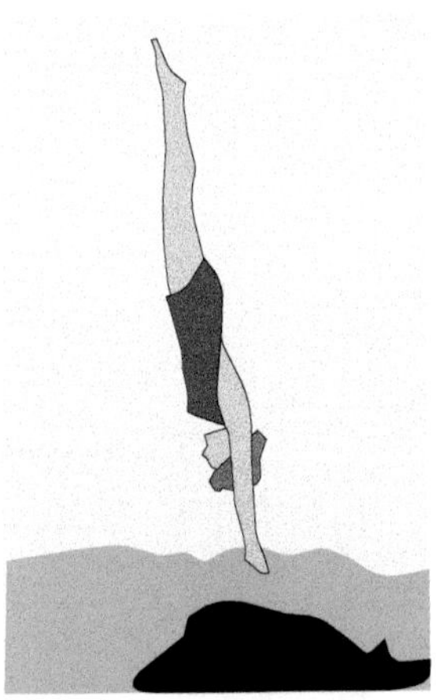

D Diving The greatest risk is striking an underwater object.

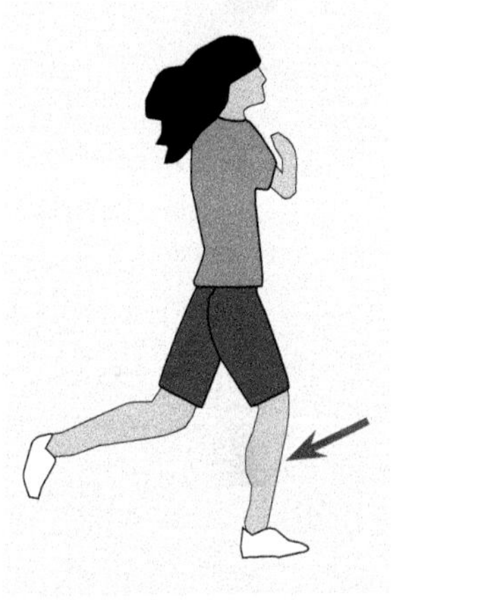

E Running injuries Most are overuse problems, with the tibia being vulnerable.

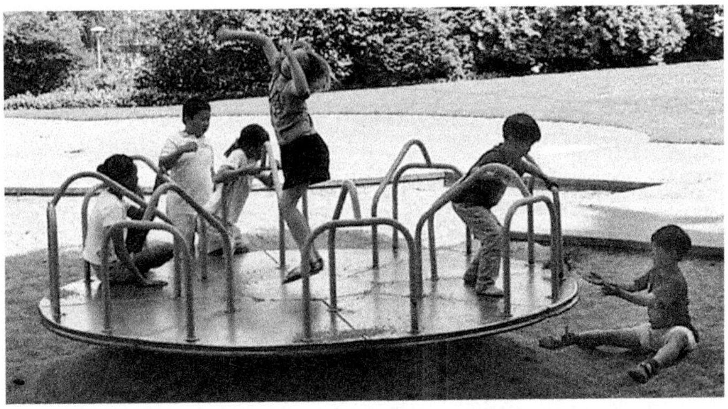

F Playground equipment Reduce risk by providing soft surfaces (sand) and playground equipment of limited height to reduce fall distance.

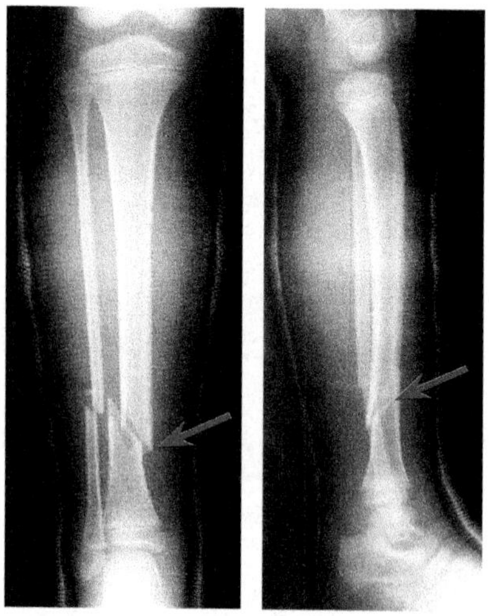

A Skateboarding Fractures such as this tibial fracture are common.

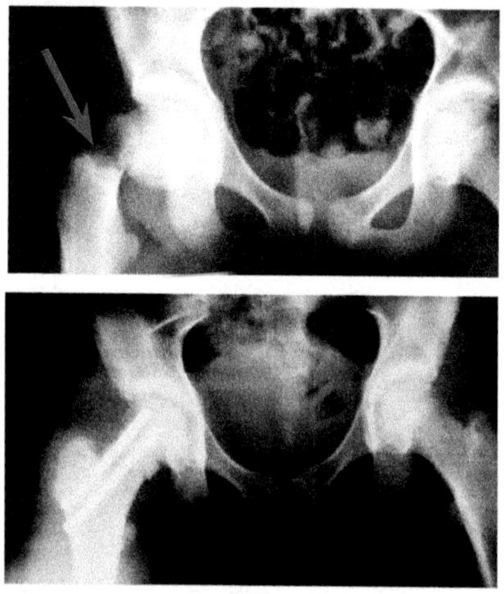

B Skiing collision fracture This 12-year-old girl was struck by an airborne adolescent skier. She sustained this displaced femoral neck fracture. The fracture was reduced, fixed with two screws, and healed. Avascular necrosis of the femoral head occurs in a third of femoral neck fractures.

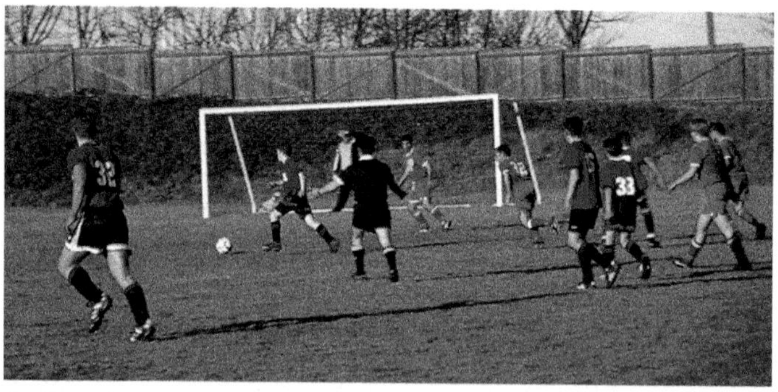

C Soccer These high school soccer players have a greater risk of injury than those of younger age.

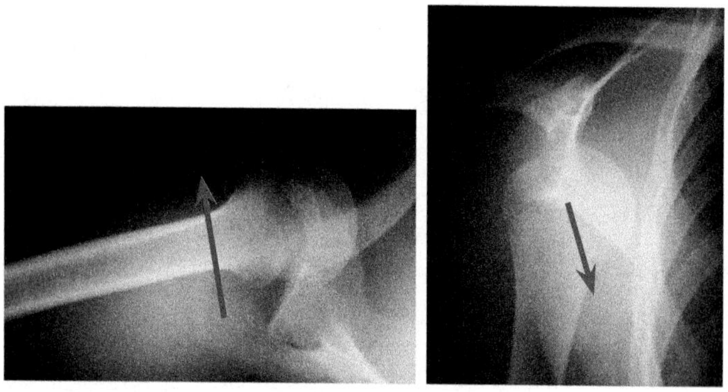

D Anterior shoulder dislocation Shoulder dislocations are common injuries in wrestling.

Snowboarding

Moderate to high risk. Injuries are due to impact. More ankle and upper extremity injuries occur in this sport than in skiing, but there are fewer torsional, knee, and thumb injuries. Snowboarders were younger, predominantly male, and were more often beginners than were skiers. They most commonly sustained ligament strains, dislocations, and fractures, with the hand, forearm, and shoulder most affected.

Soccer

Moderate risk [C]. Overuse and injuries involving the ankle and knee are common. ACL injuries are 2–3 times greater in girls. Long-term disability risk is low to moderate. The incidence increases with age, and injuries are more common in girls. Seventy percent of the injuries are located in the lower extremities, particularly the knee (26%) and ankle (23%). Back pain occurs in 14% of players. Fractures, which account for 4% of injuries, are more often in the upper extremities. Indoor soccer is the most risky.

Swimming

Low risk. Overuse injuries of the shoulder, back, and knee are common, but long-term disability risk is low. Good training and modification of swimming strokes are important in preventing and managing these problems. Shoulder pain is due to impingement or instability. Preparedness for swimming is optimal between ages 5 and 6 years.

Tennis

Low risk. Acute injuries involving the lower limbs with sprains are the most common injuries. Upper extremity injuries, often due to overuse, are preventable with appropriate training, stroke technique, and equipment. Long-term disability risk is low.

Trampoline

Very high risk. Most injuries occur from falls on hard surfaces to the side of the device. Head and cervical spine injuries are relatively common, and the potential for long-term disability is great. Discourage families from allowing children to play on trampolines.

Strength Training

Low to moderate risk. With proper supervision and low weights, this sport is relatively safe. Overuse is the most common cause of injury. Fractures of the distal radius and ulna and avulsion of the iliac apophysis occur. Long-term sequelae are low. It appears that a training frequency of twice per week is sufficient to induce strength gains in children.

Wrestling

High risk. More injuries occur in large adolescents and more during competition than in practice. The upper limb and knee are the most common sites of injury, and dislocations are more common than fractures [D]. Most injuries are acute sprains. Medial epicondyle fractures, olecranon epiphyseal stress fractures, scapular avulsion fractures, and unusual injury patterns are common. The long-term disability risk is low to moderate.

Foot and Ankle Problems

Foot and ankle problems are common in nearly all sports [A and B]. Most problems are generic and occur during play or athletic participation. Sports add intensity to normal activity and may bring out problems that might otherwise remain unnoticed. For example, a congenital tarsal coalition may remain silent only to become painful during adolescence. Some problems cause pain in adolescence and then subside in early adult life once activity is reduced. A girl may have anterior knee pain playing sports during her teens, but this resolves once she starts college and physical activity diminishes. Tight heel-cords may cause added stress on the tendon-bone interfaces around the calcaneus and cause pain in the 10-year-old soccer player. The two most common problems are detailed here.

Heel Pain

Heel pain is common during late childhood and adolescence and may occur at one of several levels [C]. Pain may occur at the insertion of the Achilles tendon into the calcaneus or at the origin of the plantar fascia as it attaches to the calcaneus. Irregular ossification of the calcaneal apophysis is often seen in asymptomatic children and is not a cause of pain. A stress fracture of the calcaneus is a rare cause of heel pain. If the condition is at all unusual or unilateral, make a radiograph of the calcaneus to rule out other problems.

Manage most heel problems by elevating and padding the heel and modifying activities. Do the least that controls the pain. Unlike some other overuse problems, resolution occurs with time, and no disability follows. Start with modifying the activity if the family concurs. Next, recommend shoes with a slightly elevated heel and a cushioned sole. If necessary, add a foam wedge of compressed felt, 3/4 inch in maximum thickness, in the heel of a high-top shoe. Flexibility exercises of the triceps are useful in preventing recurrence and reducing symptoms. Most soccer shoes have little cushioning, which contributes to recurrence.

Ankle Sprains

Ankle sprains are the most common injury in sports. They occur in classic locations. Most involve the lateral collateral ligament complex [E]. Sprains are common in children and often involve avulsion of fragments of bone or cartilage. Sprains may become chronic and pose disability in adulthood. Sprains are usually classified into three grades [D].

Evaluation Mild sprains damage only the anterior leaf of the lateral collateral ligament. Moderate sprains involve the middle (calcaneofibular ligament), and severe sprains damage the whole complex. Except for mild sprains with classic findings, order AP and lateral radiographs of the ankle to rule out other problems. Be aware that SH-1 epiphyseal injuries of the distal fibular (tenderness over mid-distal fibula), tears of the peroneal retinaculum (localized tenderness just behind the distal fibula), and tenderness inferior to the tip of the malleolus (os subfibulare, [B]), may suggest a different diagnosis. Less common locations for sprains include the medial collateral ligaments (much stronger than laterals) and the calcaneocuboid ligaments.

Management Ankle sprains are the most undertreated sports injury and have the highest rate of recurrence. In young children, undisplaced SH-1 fibular physeal fractures should be considered. These sprains are usually managed as mild sprains because they produce no late instability.

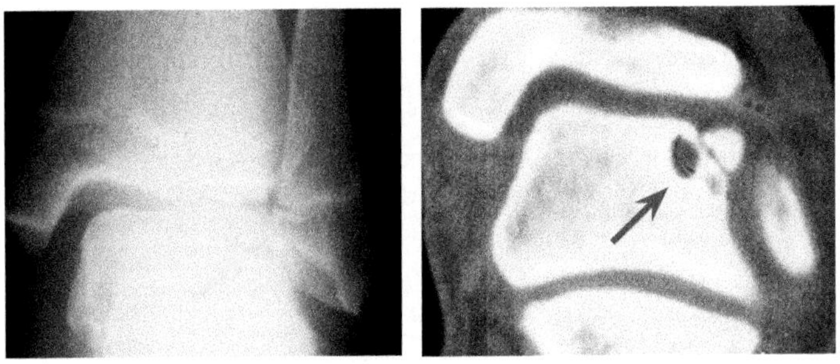

A Osteochondritis dissecans of the talus This 15-year-old runner complained of ankle pain. Radiographs showed an indistinct lesion of the lateral talus (yellow arrow). A CT scan shows the lesion well (red arrow).

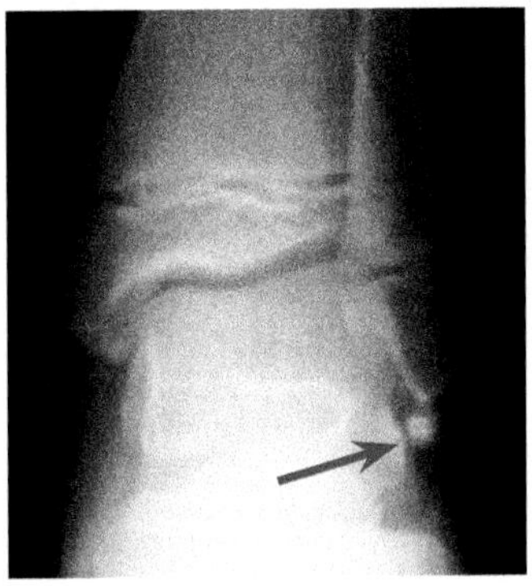

B Os subfibulare This ossicle lies just below the tip of the fibula (red arrow). Once the synchondrosis has fractured, it becomes painful.

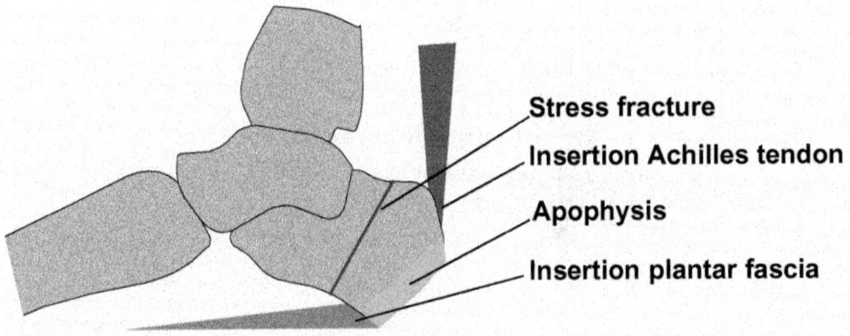

C Sites of heel pain The common sites of heel pain include the point of insertion of the heel-cord, the apophysis of the calcaneus, and insertion of the plantar fascia. Stress fractures may occur through the calcaneus.

Grading of ankle sprains

1. Attenuation	Mild swelling and tenderness
2. Partial tears	Moderate swelling, unable to bear weight
3. Complete tears	Marked swelling, bleeding, instability, and disability

D Classic grading of ankle sprains

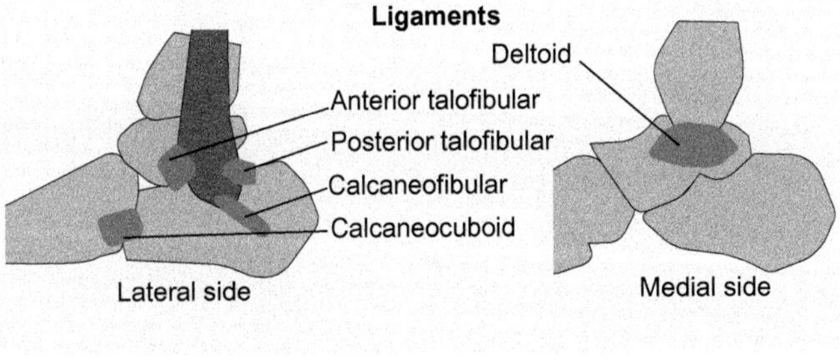

E Ankle ligaments These ligaments may be sprained: anterior talofibular, calcaneofibular, posterior talofibular, calcaneocuboid, and deltoid.

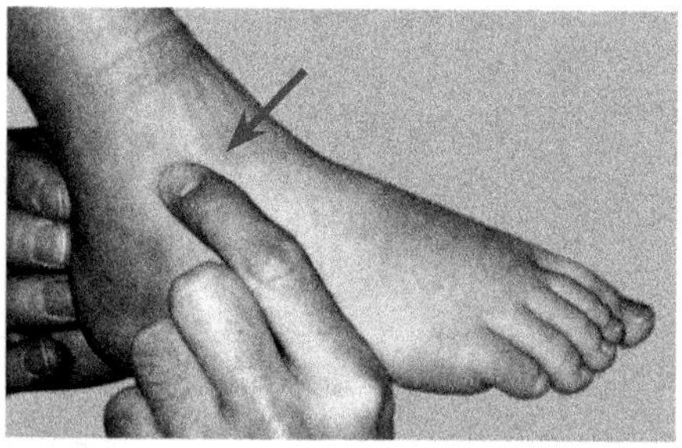

A Classic grade 1 ankle sprain This 15-year-old basketball player twisted his ankle during play. He had mild swelling and well-localized tenderness just anterior to the distal fibular, the site of the anterior talofibular ligament.

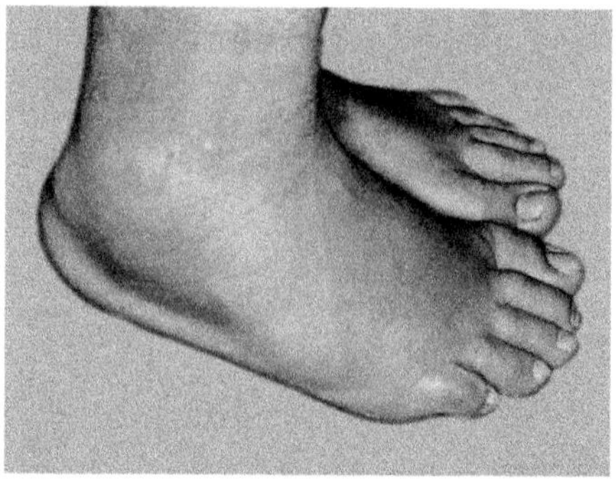

B Severe sprains Severe swelling, ankle discoloration, and broad areas of tenderness are often associated with osteochondral injuries and are best managed by immobilization.

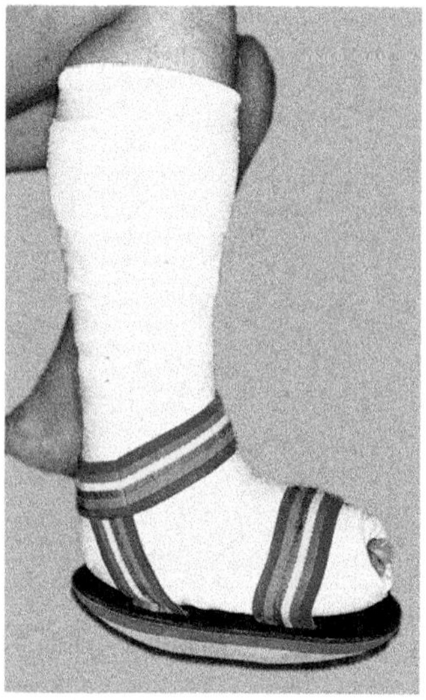

C Immobilization of sprains This may be accomplished by a short-leg walking cast.

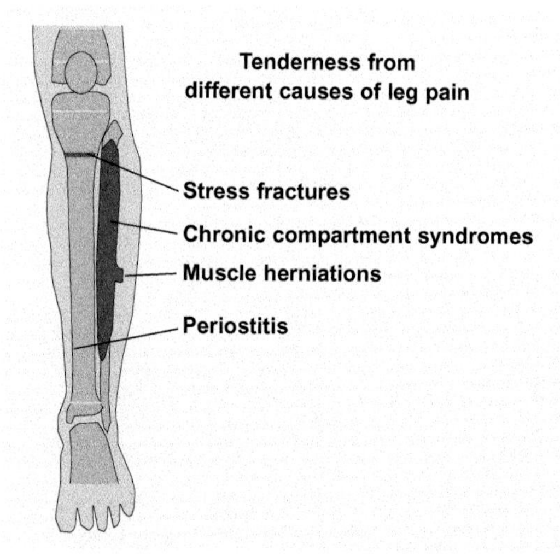

D Tenderness in types of leg pain Localizing tenderness is helpful in separating the different types of midleg pain.

Manage sprains with RICE overnight and exercises to maintain muscle strength about the foot and ankle during convalescence.

Mild sprains are those with minimal swelling and tenderness. The classic example is the anterior talofibular ligament with localized tenderness just anterior to the distal fibula [A]. Manage by rehabilitation to prevent recurrence. Sometimes an air-stirrup splint improves comfort.

Moderate sprains have more swelling and a wider area of tenderness with little or no instability. Manage by resting the ankle with a plastic splint or a cast for 2–3 weeks allowing weight bearing as tolerated. Allow return to activities once muscle strength is regained, tenderness resolved, and range of motion restored.

Severe sprains produce severe swelling, and instability may be demonstrated [B]. Management of ankle instability for sprains is controversial but repairs of chronic instability may be necessary. Most may be managed by cast immobilization [C] for not more than three weeks. Return to sports with a laceup ankle brace for about three months.

Return to sports Teach proprioceptive exercise to reduce the risk of recurrent injury. Delay return until the child is able to walk normally, run a straight line and change direction at full speed without discomfort.

Tibia Problems

The common problems include fractures (covered in Chapter 4), stress fractures, and shin splints. Because leg pain and shin splints are common and sometimes perplexing, the subject is detailed here.

Leg Pain

Leg pain is caused by a variety of disorders that include periostitis, compartment syndromes, stress fractures, and muscle herniation. The most common cause is a periostitis at the origin of the soleus muscle on the posteromedial aspect of the lower leg.

Evaluate by localizing the tenderness [D], palpate for swelling and muscle hernia, and image with AP and lateral radiographs of the tibia. Consider other possibilities, such as tumors or infection.

Periostitis (shin splints) are common. It occurs in the older adolescent and is often bilateral. Tenderness covers a broader area than a stress fracture. The tenderness is localized to the posteromedial aspect of the distal tibia, and radiographs are negative.

Stress fractures cause localized tenderness over bone [E].

Chronic compartment syndromes are less common and are characterized by a history of pain with activity, relief with rest, and, rarely, tenderness and swelling over the involved compartment.

Muscle herniation is identified by palpating a protruding muscle, usually over the distal lateral leg.

Manage by applying the standard management principles of RICE, gradual conditioning, appropriate shoes, and NSAIDs.

Determine the underlying cause(s) of the initial pain and make modifications before returning the adolescent back to full activity, to prevent recurrence.

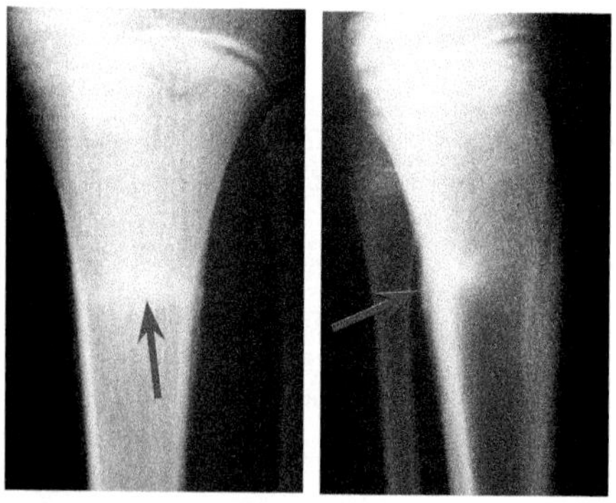

E Tibial stress fractures The classic location for tibial stress fractures is in the proximal posterior tibia (red arrows). When stress fractures occur over the tibial shaft, they are more likely to be included in the differential diagnosis of shin splints. This boy had multiple stress fractures involving the right femur and both tibiae.

Knee Problems

Knee problems are common. Knee problems are covered in Chapter 10. Because most anterior cruciate ligament injuries occur with sports, this injury and management are presented here.

Anterior Cruciate Ligament Insufficiency

Anterior cruciate ligament tears are becoming more common in adolescents, especially among girls playing basketball or soccer. Nonoperative management is typically unsatisfactory. Without repair, return to competitive sports is unsatisfactory, as many have repeated injuries, including meniscal damage.

Rehabilitation Start with exercises, activity modification, and possibly bracing. Bracing clearly communicates that the problem is legitimate but hinders performance and doubtfully protects the knee.

Indications for repair Several situations make repair appropriate.

Persisting disability Once rehabilitation is complete, activity modification has gone to the acceptable limit, and if disability is unacceptable, surgical reconstruction is appropriate.

Associated meniscal injury Reconstruct the ligament and repair the meniscus during the same procedure.

Noncompliance Return to sports without repair puts the patient at risk for meniscal injury.

ACL repair Assess bone age and Tanner staging to determine level of maturation. Repair any meniscal tears with ACL reconstruction. Avoid placing any bone or hardware across a clearly open physis to avoid arrest.

Extraarticular repairs Because these repairs are not anatomic, stretching occurs and the dissection may damage the physis.

Intraarticular repairs may be physeal sparing, partial transphyseal through the central tibia, or completely transphyseal through the femur and tibia [A]. Preferably use autogenous hamstring. If performed in a growing patient, follow limb lengths and knee angles frequently to diagnose any growth disturbance promptly.

Hip and Thigh Problems

Varied sports-related problems occur about the hip and thigh. The usual injuries, such as avulsion fractures, dislocations, and acute slipping of the proximal femoral epiphysis, are common in sports.

The thigh is heavily muscled and more protected than the tibia. It is also more difficult to examine because localization of tenderness is less exact. A variety of problems may occur, including fractures, stress fractures, and contusions. Contusions of the quadriceps may cause myositis ossificans.

Myositis Ossificans

Blunt trauma to the front of the thigh may cause the accumulation of a hematoma, which may lead to myositis ossificans. Treat the acute injury by applying RICE. Some recommend immobilization in flexion. Immobilize for 5–7 days, then encourage active knee flexion. Ossification in the damaged muscle progresses in a sequence of changes [B] that are sometimes difficult to distinguish from that of osteogenic sarcoma. The lesions of myositis ossificans tend to be better localized, are often mid-anterior thigh in location, and arise in the muscle rather than the bone. Consider excision in the rare case when the mass is troublesome.

Overuse Injuries

Overuse injury of muscle attachments can occur in the same location as avulsion injuries [C].

Bursitis

Bursitis may involve the greater trochanteric bursa and the iliopectineal bursa located anterior to the hip joint [C]. Manage bursitis with NSAIDs and rest.

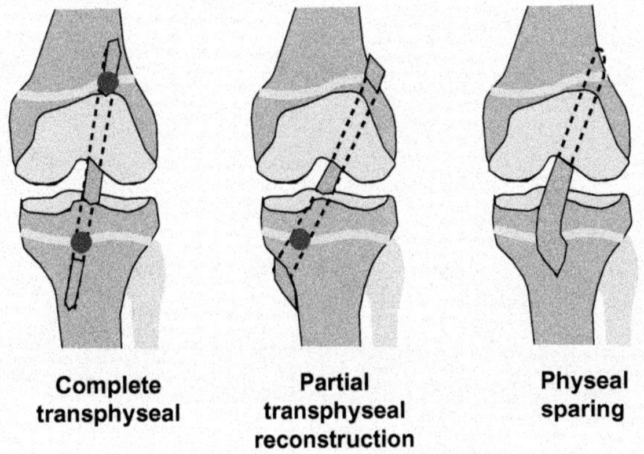

A Options for ACL repair before skeletal maturity Repair may extended across both or one physes (red circles), or spare both physes. Based on Stanitski (1995).

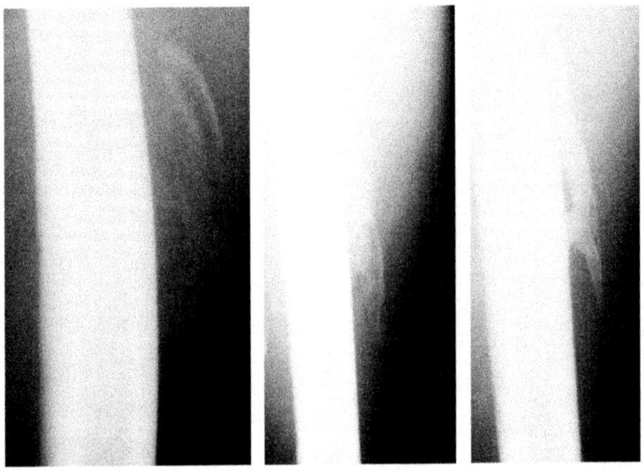

B Myositis ossificans Serial radiographs show the evolution of the lesion at 3 weeks, 6 weeks, and 6 months following injury.

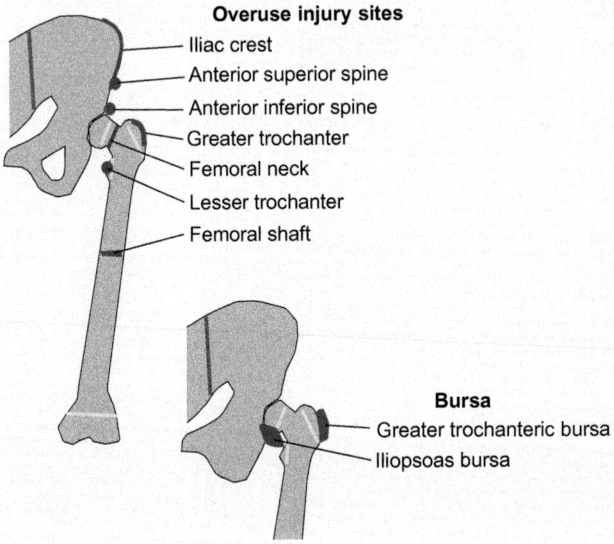

C Overuse problems about the hip These problems include fractures, apophysitis, or bursitis.

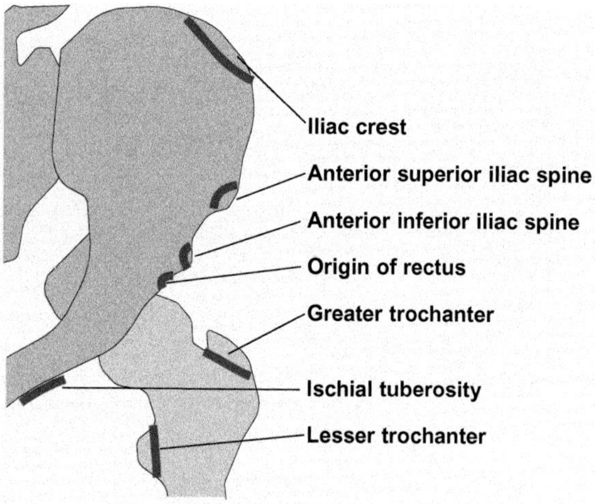

A Sites of avulsion injuries about the hip.

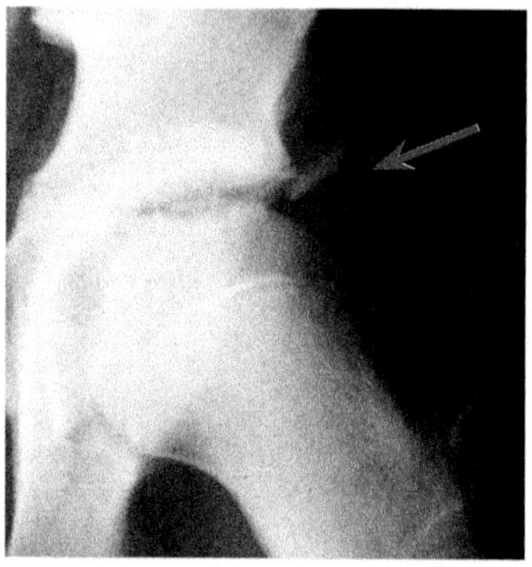

B Avulsion of the origin of rectus The fleck of bone is attached to the straight head of the rectus femoris. Tenderness was present over the avulsion. The fragment healed with time, and no residual disability was present.

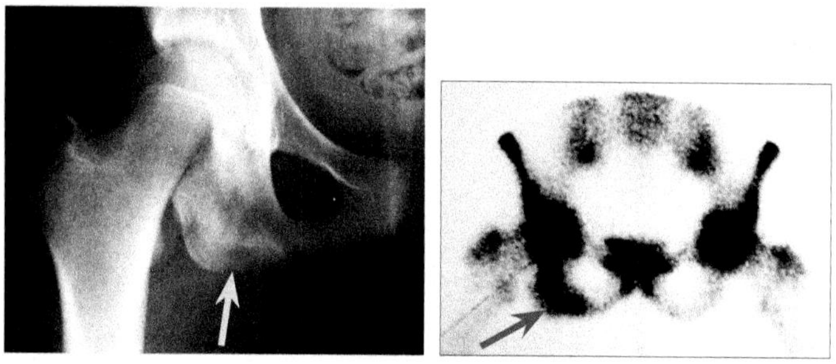

C Ischael avulsion This 16-year-old runner sustained an avulsion of the hamstring origin on the ischium. Note the prominence (yellow arrow) and increased uptake (red arrow) on the bone scan. The bone scan was unnecessary.

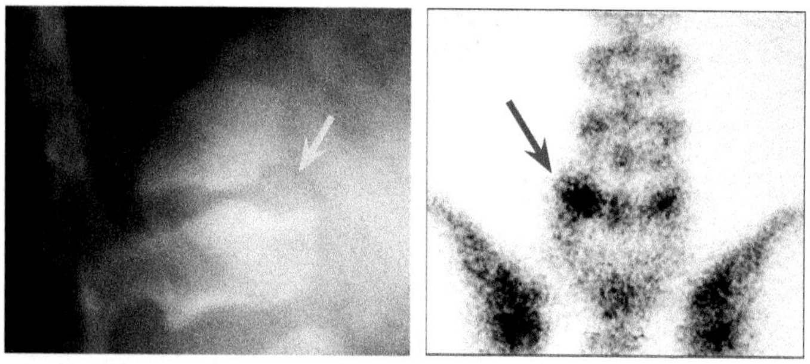

D Back pain in the athlete Herniation of the nucleus pulposus into the vertebral body causes narrowing of the disc space (yellow arrow). The lesions may be painful. The radiographic defect is sometimes called a lumbar *Schmorl node*. Bone scans in spondylolysis show increased uptake. The condition may be unilateral (red arrow).

Pelvis Problems

Avulsion Injuries

Avulsion injuries occur in a variety of locations about the hip and pelvis [A–C]. Most of these injuries are managed by rest because healing of the fracture occurs spontaneously. Some surgeons recommend replacing displaced large avulsion fractures of the ischium, but this is controversial.

Hip Pointers

A hip pointer is a contusion over the iliac rim or gluteal muscular seen in American football and other contact sports. These injuries are usually managed by RICE and NSAIDs, but may be slow to recover.

Sports Hernia (Athletic Pubalgia)

A sports hernia is a strain or tear of soft tissue in the lower abdomen or groin area. It may be difficult to diagnose. It is usually treated by rest, physical therapy, and NSAIDs. Operative repair is rarely necessary. Always differentiate from a slipped capital femoral epiphysis that requires immediate diagnosis and treatment.

Stress Injuries

Osteitis pubis is an overuse syndrome that occurs in the adolescent. Tenderness is localized over the symphysis. Lower extremity malalignment may contribute to the problem. Manage by rest and NSAIDs.

Pubic ramus stress fractures may occur. The diagnosis is suspected by the location of the tenderness and confirmed by a positive bone scan.

Spine Problems

Spine injuries and back pain [D] are common sports injuries that are discussed in Chapter 12.

Neck Problems

Some of the most catastrophic injuries in sports involve the cervical spine. Fortunately, such injuries are rare. They have reduced in frequency since the ban of "spearing" (deliberate use of the head for primary contact in American football) and with improved football helmet design. Most cervical spine injuries occur in diving, trampoline use, and American football. Quadriplegia and death are potential consequences of such injuries.

Stingers and Burners

These are injuries resulting in burning pain in the arm that may be transient (stingers) or persist for several hours (burners). These injuries result from nerve root traction from sport-induced trauma. They are most common in American football and in individuals who have congenital narrowing of the cervical canal. These injuries resolve, but they should be recognized as a warning to be careful.

Sports in Children with Down Syndrome

Physicians are frequently asked to assess the child with trisomy-21 who wish to participate in sports. These children are at risk due to instability of C1– C2 caused by stretching of the apical ligament and possibly dens hypoplasia. Down syndrome children have extreme joint laxity, and C1–C2 instability is one of the more serious outcomes of this underlying defect. Evaluation and management are controversial.

Evaluation About 15% of Down children have atlantoaxial hypermobility. About 1–2% have neurological manifestations that include easy fatiguability, an abnormal gait, neck pain, limited neck mobility, torticollis, uncoordination and clumsiness, sensory deficits, spasticity, and hyperreflexia. Make lateral flexion and extension views of the neck. Measure the atlanto-dens interval (ADI).

Management Depends upon the clinical and radiographic evaluation.

Asymptomatic and stable Allow full participation; additional radiographs are probably not necessary.

Hypermobile and asymptomatic Be concerned if the ADI measure is >5 mm and discourage participation in contact sports.

Symptomatic If patients are symptomatic, consider surgical stabilization.

Upper Limb Problems

Shoulder

A variety of lesions occur about the shoulder. Swimmers commonly develop impingement syndrome, American football players often injure the medial or lateral aspects of the clavicle [A], and wrestlers dislocate their shoulders. Overuse injuries of the upper humeral epiphysis occur in pitchers (little league shoulder).

Elbow

Elbow injuries are common in sports. The elbow is vulnerable because of its anatomic complexity and its position in the upper limb, where it is subjected to excessive loads.

Little League Elbow

The elbow is easily overloaded during the act of overhand throwing or during serves in racket sports. This is aggravated by poor throwing mechanics when pitching is done with more enthusiasm than skill. This causes excessive valgus loading of the joint. This overloading causes traction on the medial side and compression on the lateral side of the elbow joint [B]. The most common injury is the traction injury to the medial epicondyle, the common origin of the forearm flexors and pronators. Less common but more serious are the compression injuries on the capitellum and radial head. Compression injuries usually occur in the adolescent.

Ulnar collateral ligament injuries occur in the older child or adolescent. They may result from overuse or rupture. Manage by rest and graded return to activity.

Medial epicondylar injuries may result in an inflammation or frank separation from the humerus. Because the medial epicondyle is extraarticular, this injury is less serious. Persisting instability may require operative stabilization.

Capitellar osteochondritis is more serious because it can lead to damage to the joint. Compressive loading causes osteochondritic lesions that may separate and create loose bodies in the joint. This condition is different from *Panner disease*, which occurs in younger children, is often asymptomatic, and resolves spontaneously.

Radial head osteochondritis more commonly leads to overgrowth and joint incongruity.

Diagnosis is usually not difficult. The child is often a baseball pitcher, tenderness is localized over the site of the problem, and radiographs often show changes. Range of motion of the elbow is usually reduced.

Manage the acute problem with the usual RICE and NSAIDs. Insist that any throwing be avoided for 4–6 weeks. Encourage the child to bike or run as a diversion. Evaluate and correct poor throwing mechanics. Reintroduce throwing gradually. Initially limit throwing to 20–30 feet. Use the 10% rule. To prevent recurrence, limit pitching to a specific number of throws or innings per game [C]. The number depends upon the physiologic age and condition of the child. Imposing limits on throws is very difficult to enforce. If the joint is damaged, the adolescent should switch to another sport.

Forearm, Wrist, and Hand

The forearm is frequently fractured in falls (see Chapter 4). The wrist may be injured by overuse in gymnastics. Gymnastic injuries may damage the distal radial physis and cause impingement from hyperextension and fractures. For hand problems, see Chapter 13.

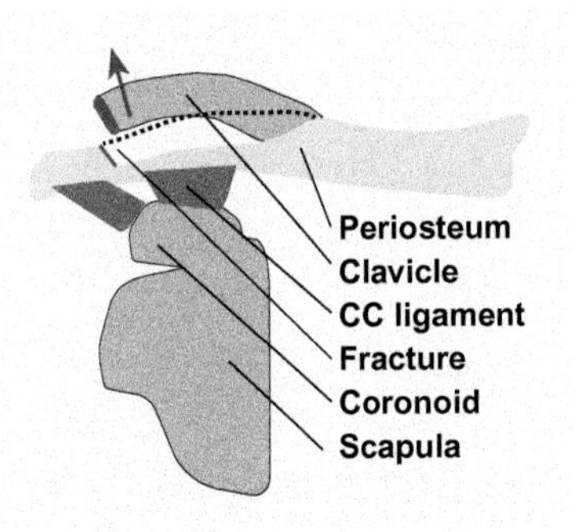

A Fracture of distal clavicle This type of fracture through the growth plate of the distal clavicle may be confused with an AC separation. The clavicle is often displaced upward through a tear in the periosteum. The coracoclavicular (CC) ligament remains intact. Reduction is not necessary, as remodeling rapidly corrects the deformity.

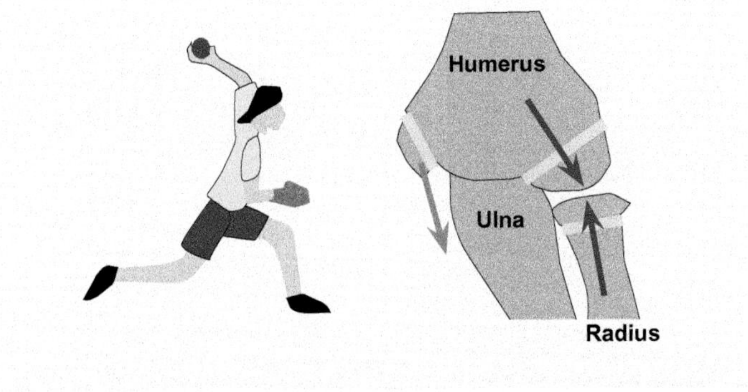

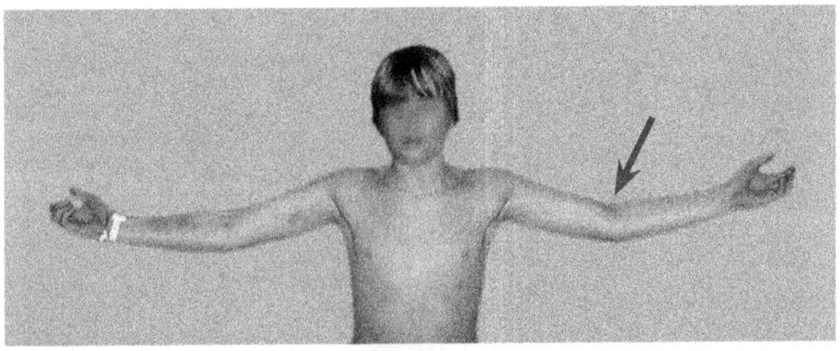

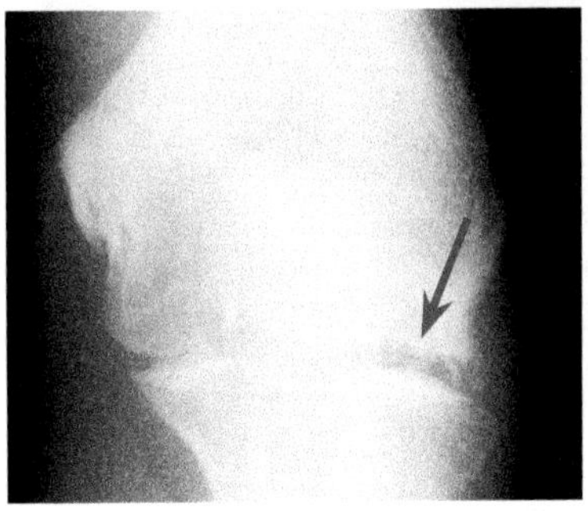

B Little league elbow The adolescent above has osteochondritis of the capitellum (red arrows), which causes limited extension of the left elbow. The act of throwing causes medial traction (blue arrow, upper drawing), which tends to avulse the medial epicondyle. Throwing also causes lateral compression of the capitellum and radial head (red arrows, upper drawing).

Pitching Guidelines

Age
- Before 8 yrs - throwing only
- After 8 yrs - allow pitching
- After 14 yrs - allow curve balls

Games per week -
- About 2

Pitches per game
- Progress from about
  - Age 8 - 50 pitches
  - Age 17- 100 pitches

C Pitching guidelines This is a rough guide. Tailor to fit the child. Based on Whiteside (1999).

GENERAL

Cawley J. The economics of childhood obesity. Health Affairs, 29(3):364-371, 2010.

Faigenbaum AD, Myer GD. Resistance training among young athletes: safety, efficacy and injury prevention effects. Br. J. Sports. Med. 44(1):56-63, 2010.

Halstead ME, Kevin D, Walter KD, Council on Sports Medicine and Fitness. Clinical report: sport-related concussion in children and adolescents. Pediatrics 126(3):597-615, 2010.

König F. Veber freie korper in der gehenken. Dtsch. Z. Chir. 27:90–109, 1888.

Lippi G, Longo UG, Maffulli N. Genetics and sports. Br. Med. Bull. 93(1):27-47, 2010.

Norton C, Nixon J, Sibert J. Playground injuries to children. Arch Dis Child. 89(2):103–108, 2004.

Wilt F, Yessis M. Soviet Theory, Technique and Training for Running and Hurdling. Vol 1. Championship Books, 1984.

ANKLE

Berndt AL, Harty M. Transchondral fractures (osteochondritis dissecans) of the talus. J. Bone Joint Surg. 41-A:988–1020, 1959.

Flick AB, Gould N. Osteochondritis dissecans of the talus (transchondral fractures of the talus): review of the literature and a new surgical approach for medial dome lesions. Foot Ankle 5:165–185, 1985.

Tol JL, Struijs PAA, Bossuyt PMM, Verhagen RAW, van Dijk CN. Treatment strategies in osteochondral defects of the talar dome: a systematic review. Foot Ankle Int 21:119–126, 2000.

ACL

Frosch, K. H., et al. (2010). "Outcomes and risks of operative treatment of rupture of the anterior cruciate ligament in children and adolescents." Arthroscopy 26(11): 1539-1550.

Lawrence, J. T., et al. (2011). "Degeneration of the knee joint in skeletally immature patients with a diagnosis of an anterior cruciate ligament tear: is there harm in delay of treatment?" Am J Sports Med 39(12): 2582-2587..

Spindler, K. P., et al. (2011). "The prognosis and predictors of sports function and activity at minimum 6 years after anterior cruciate ligament reconstruction: a population cohort study." Am J Sports Med 39(2): 348-359.

van Eck, C. F., et al. (2012). "Prospective analysis of failure rate and predictors of failure after anatomic anterior cruciate ligament reconstruction with allograft." Am J Sports Med 40(4): 800-807.

Wright, R. W., et al. (2011). "Ipsilateral graft and contralateral ACL rupture at five years or more following ACL reconstruction: a systematic review." J Bone Joint Surg Am 93(12): 1159-1165.

Xu, Y., et al. (2013). "Prospective randomized comparison of anatomic single- and double-bundle anterior cruciate ligament reconstruction." Knee Surg Sports

KNEE

Hefti F, Beguiristain J, Krauspe R. Osteochondritis dissecans: a multicenter study of the European Pediatric Orthopedic Society. J. Pediatr. Orthop. 8(4)-B: 231-245, 1999.

Hui C, Roe J, Ferguson D, Waller A, Salmon L, Pinczewski L. Outcome of anatomic transphyseal anterior cruciate ligament reconstruction in Tanner stage 1 and 2 patients with open physes. Am. J. Sports Med. 40(5):1093-2008, 2012.

Joo SY, Park KB, Kim BR, Park HW, Kim HW. The 'fourin-one' procedure for habitual dislocation of the patella in children: early results in patients with severe generalised ligamentous laxity and aplasis of the trochlear groove. J. Bone Joint Surg. 89(12)-B:1645-1649, 2007.

Kennedy A, Coughlin DG, Metzger MF, Tang R, Pearle AD, Lotz JC, Feeley BT. Biomechanical evaluation of pediatric anterior cruciate ligament reconstruction techniques. Am J. Sports Med. 39(5):964-971, 2011.

Kocher MS, DiCanzio J, Zurakowski D, Micheli LJ. Diagnostic performance of clinical examination and selective magnetic resonance imaging in the evaluation of intraarticular knee disorders in children and adolescents. Am. J. Sports Med. 29:292-296, 2001.

Lawrence JT, Argawal N, Ganley TJ. Degeneration of the knee joint in skeletally immature patients with a diagnosis of an anterior cruciate ligament tear: is there harm in delay of treatment? Am J. Sports Med. 39(12):2582-2587, 2011.

MacIntosh DL, Darby TA. Lateral substitution reconstruction. J. Bone Joint Surg. 58-B:142-146, 1976.

MacNab I. Recurrent dislocation of the patella. J. Bone Joint Surg. 34(4)-A:957-967, 1952.

Nelitz M, Dornacher D, Dreyhaupt J, Reichel H, Lippacher S. The relation of the distal femoral physis and the medial patellofemoral ligament. Knee Surg. Sports Traumatol. Arthrosc. 19(12):2067-2071, 2011.

Rohren E, Kosarek FJ, helms CA. Discoid lateral meniscus and the frequency of meniscal tears. Skeletal Radiol. 30:316-320, 2001.

Stanitski CL, Harvell JC, Fu F. Observations on acute knee hemarthrosis in children and adolescents. J. Pediatr. Orthop. 13(4):506-510, 1993.

Vavken P, Murray MM. Treating anterior cruciate ligament tears in skeletally immature patients. Arthroscopy 27(5):704-716, 2011.

Wilson JN. A diagnostic sign in osteochondritis dissecans of the knee. J. Bone Joint Surg. 49(3)-A: 477-480, 1967.

Young R. The external semilunar cartilage as a complete disc. In Cleland J, Mackey JY, Young RB eds, Memoirs and Memoranda in Anatomy, Williams and Norgate, London, 179-187, 1987.

SHOULDER

Bottoni CR, Smith EL, Berkowitz MJ, Towle RB, Moore JH. Arthroscopic versus open shoulder stabilization for recurrent anterior instability. A prospective randomized clinical trial. Am. J. Sports Med. 34(11):1730-1737, 2006.

Dotter WE. Little leaguer's shoulder - fracture of the proximal humeral epiphyseal cartilage due to baseball pitching. Guthrie Clin. Bull. 23:68-72, 1953.

Hovelius L, Augustini BG, Fredin H, Johansson O, Norlin R, Thorling J. Primary Anterior Dislocation of the Shoulder in Young Patients. A Ten-Year Prospective Study. J. Bone Joint Surg. 78(11)-A:1677-1684, 1996.

Pasque CB, McGinnis DW, Griffin LY. Shoulder. In Sullivan JA, Anderson ST (eds), Care of the Young Athlete. Rosemont, IL: American Academy of Orthopaedic Surgeons, and Elk Grove Village, IL: American Academy of Pediatrics, 2000.

ELBOW

Bennett GE. Elbow and shoulder lesions of baseball players. Am. J. Surg. 98:484–492, 1959.

Diab M, Poston JM, Huber P, Tencer AF. The biomechanical effect of radial shortening on the radiocapitellar articulation. J. Bone Joint Surg. 87(6)-B:879-883, 2005.

Takahara M, Mura N, Sasaki J, Harada M, Ogino T. Classification, treatment, and outcome of osteochondritis dissecans of the humeral capitellum. J. Bone Joint Surg. 89(6)-A:1205-1214, 2007.

OTHER

Goldschneider KR. Complex regional pain syndrome in children: asking the right questions. Pain Res Manag. 17(6):386-390, 2012.

Johnson DP, Eastwood DM, Witherow PJ. Symptomatic synovial plicae of the knee. J. Bone Joint Surg. 75(10)-A:1485-1496, 1993.

Mavor GE. The anterior tibial syndrome. J. Bone Joint Surg. 38(2)-B:513-517, 1956.

Mitchell SW, Morehouse GR, Kean WW. Gunshot Wounds and Other Injuries of Nerves. New York: Lippincott, 1864.

Nallamothu N, Pancholy SB, Lee KR, Heo J, Iskandrian AS. Impact on exercise single-photon emission computed tomographic thallium imaging on patient management and outcome. J. Nucl. Cardiol. 2(4):334-338, 1995.

Pedowitz RA, Hargens AR, Mubarak SJ, Gershuni DH. Modified criteria for the objective diagnosis of chronic compartment syndrome of the leg. Am. J. Sports Med. 18:35–40, 1990.

CHAPTER 6

INFECTION

Infections involving the musculoskeletal system are common [A] and can cause severe disability. With optimum management, practically all infections may be cured, and deformity and disability may be prevented.

The prevalence of osteomyelitis is declining and changing character. Long-bone infections caused by *Staphylococcus aureus* and septic arthritis caused by *Haemophilus influenza* have declined most. Osteomyelitis has changed forms, with more complex and unusual patterns [B]. The incidence of infection with resistant strains is increasing.

Infections are still important and often challenging, but improved management makes poor outcomes less common and less acceptable.

Pathogenesis

An understanding of the pathogenesis of musculoskeletal infections facilitates management.

Portals of Entry

Most infections are hematogenous, with the primary site of entry in the ear; oropharynx; or respiratory, gastrointestinal (GI), or genitourinary (GU) tracts [C] . Skin infections such as occur after chicken pox, penetrating injuries such as nails in the sole of the foot, or infections from surgical procedures are less common [D]. Extension of contiguous infections are least common, although adjacent joint infections are relatively common when associated with adjacent osteomyelitis [B].

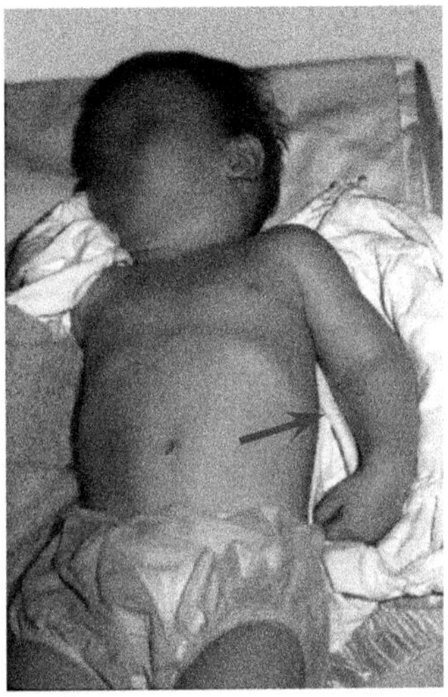

A Infection causes systemic illness This infant has septic arthritis of the elbow and is systemically ill.

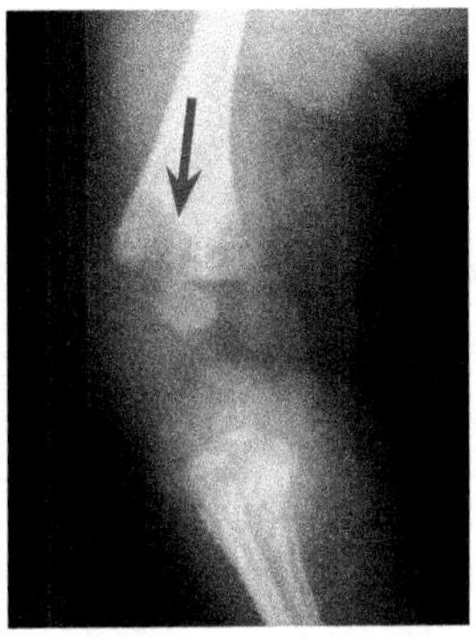

B Local spread Infection from metaphyseal osteomyelitis may spread into adjacent joints in the infant.

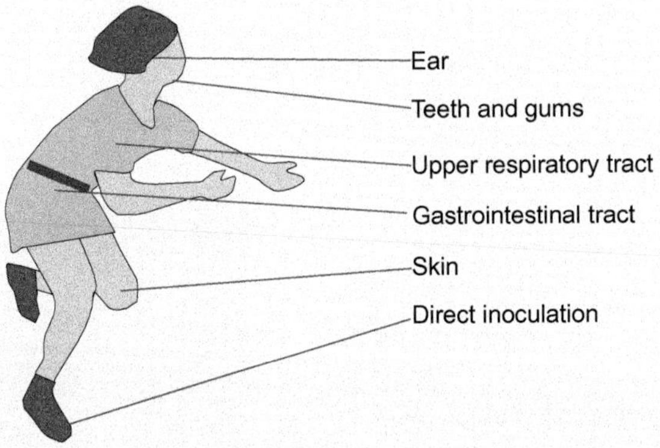

C Portals of bacterial entry

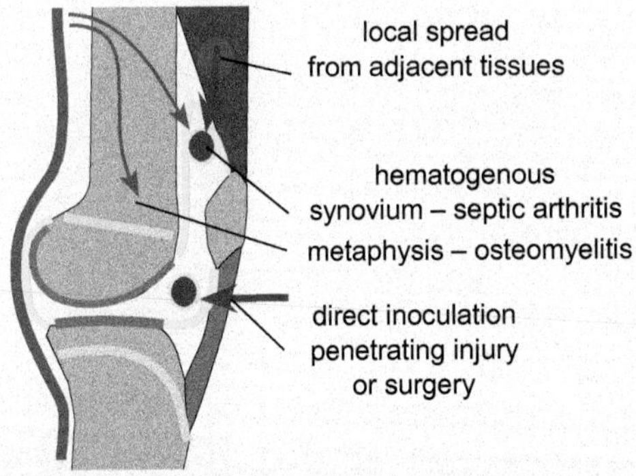

D Spread to bone and joints Infection is commonly hematogenous but may occur by local spread or from direct inoculation.

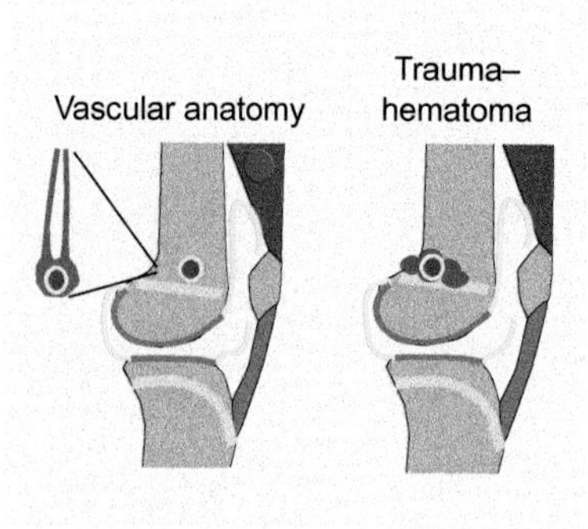

A Vascular anatomy of the metaphysis Bacteria may accumulate in vascular loops in the metaphysis. Traumas with hematoma formation provide good environments for bacterial proliferation.

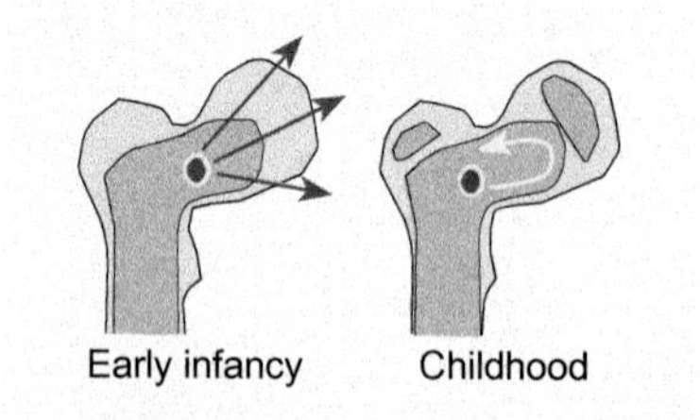

B Transphyseal spread Transepiphyseal vessels allow spread of infection from the metaphysis into the joint (red arrows). The presence of a physis blocks this spread (yellow arrow).

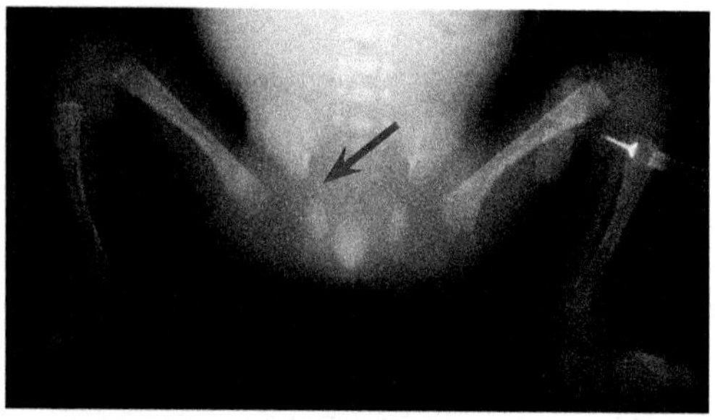

C Neonatal septic arthritis of the hip Note the widening of the joint space. This is a late finding.

Initial Deposition

Bacteremia is a common event but rarely results in tissue infections. When infections occur, bone and joints are vulnerable. The reason for this vulnerability is unknown.

Bone is usually infected in the metaphysis. Bacteria are deposited in capillary loops adjacent to the physeal plate. Nearly always, these bacteria are quickly destroyed by phagocytosis. Trauma is a factor that reduces resistance by causing the formation of a hematoma [A]. Bacterial proliferation is enhanced by the elaboration of a *biofilm,* which enhances bacterial adhesion to bone and provides protection from phagocytosis or antibiotics.

Joints may be infected by hematogenous spread via the synovium, by a penetrating injury of a joint, by direct spread from a contiguous infection, or by bacterial transport by way of transphyseal vessels. Transphyseal vessels are present in early infancy before the formation of the growth plate [B]. This may account for the frequency of septic arthritis of the hip in the neonate [C]. In children, about a third of long-bone osteomyelitis is associated with septic arthritis of the adjacent joint.

Natural History of Infection

It is probable that the vast majority of bacterial colonies are destroyed by systemic and local mechanisms. The likelihood of progression is based on the balance between organism virulence and host resistance [D].

Spontaneous resolution is common. Host resistance exceeds the virulence of the organism.

Subacute osteomyelitis is less common. Host resistance and virulence are about equal. A bone abscess forms reactive sclerotic bone walls off the abscess. No equivalent of this subacute form exists for septic arthritis.

Classic acute osteomyelitis, or septic arthritis, results from a virulent organism and a normal host. The patient becomes systemically ill, and if untreated may develop septicemia and die, or extensive local bone necrosis may occur, and chronic osteomyelitis follows.

Impaired host may allow development of a bone or joint infection from organisms of relatively low virulence, as seen in such conditions as sickle cell disease [E].

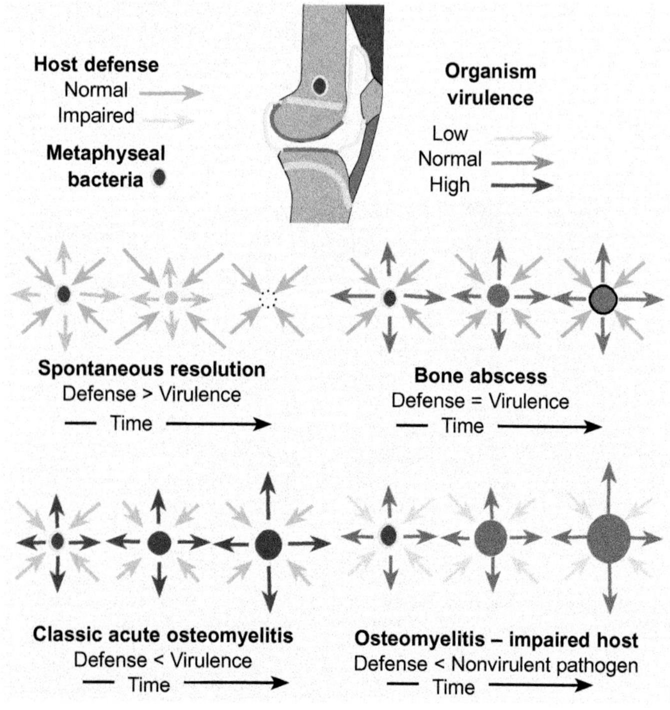

D Natural history of osteomyelitis This is often determined by host resistance and organism virulence.

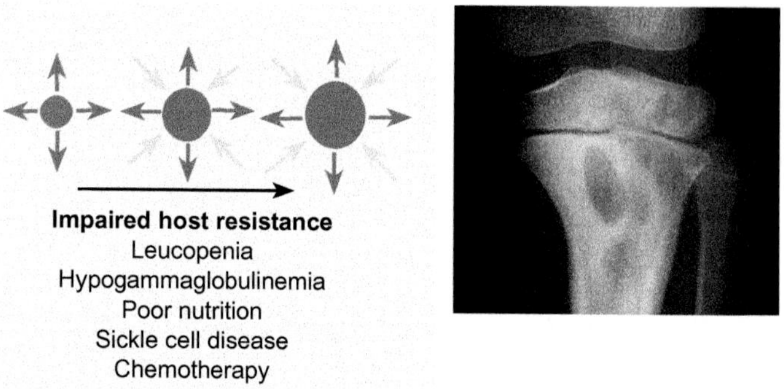

E Impaired host resistance. Organisms of low virulence may cause infections when host resistance is impaired.

Organisms

The organisms that infect the musculoskeletal system are numerous, varied, continually changing, and have predilection for the site, tissue, and age of the host [A].

Staphylococci

Gram-positive organisms are the most common causes of infections. The incidence is declining, however. *Staphylococcus aureus* includes a variety of pathogenic strains. New strains may be methicillin or vancomycin resistant. *Staphylococcus epidermidis* may cause infection in impaired hosts.

Streptococci

Streptococcal infections cause soft tissue and bony infections. Common pathogens are b-hemolytic streptococci. *Streptococcus pneumonia* may cause septic arthritis. *Streptococcus agalactiae* is a common cause of neonatal osteomyelitis. *Streptococcus pyogenes* is a less common pathogen.

Neisseria meningitidis

Meningococcal septicemia causes acute and chronic orthopedic problems. The disseminated intravascular coagulation and focal infections acutely cause necrotizing fasciitis and damage physeal circulation, causing physeal arrest and limb deformities [B].

Pseudomonas aeroginosa

This gram-negative rod is chondrophilic, and a common cause of joint infections of the foot from penetrating injuries.

Escherichia coli

This gram-negative rod is a rare cause of musculoskeletal infections.

Salmonella

This gram-negative rod is most likely to be encountered in sickle cell osteomyelitis.

Mycobacteria tuberculosis

This acid-fast organism has a resurgence of worrisome drug-resistant strains. It causes bone and joint infections in children. Tuberculous spondylitis with kyphosis is a common and serious deformity [C].

Kingella kingae

This gram-negative coccobacillus is common in the respiratory system, slow growing, aerobic, and fastidious. It is difficult to culture. Only recently has it been found to cause musculoskeletal infections. It remains susceptible to most antibiotics.

Haemophilus influenza

This was previously a common cause of septic arthritis in infants. Now it is rare due to immunization programs.

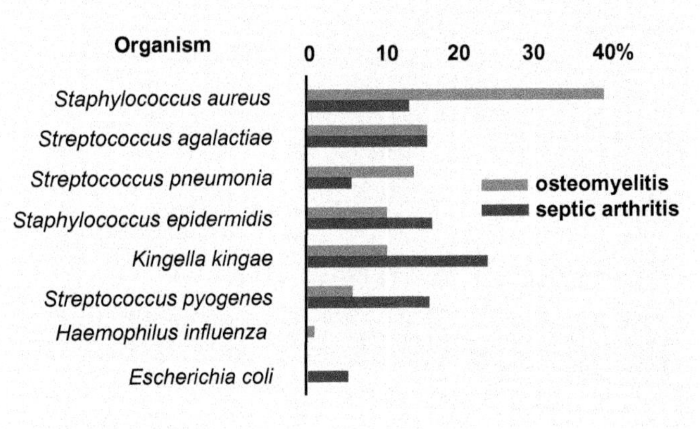

A Infecting organism in bone and joint infections in children under 36 months of age The percentage of 30 cases of osteomyelitis (blue bars) and 30 cases of septic arthritis (red bars) caused by different organisms. From data of Lundy and Kehl (1998).

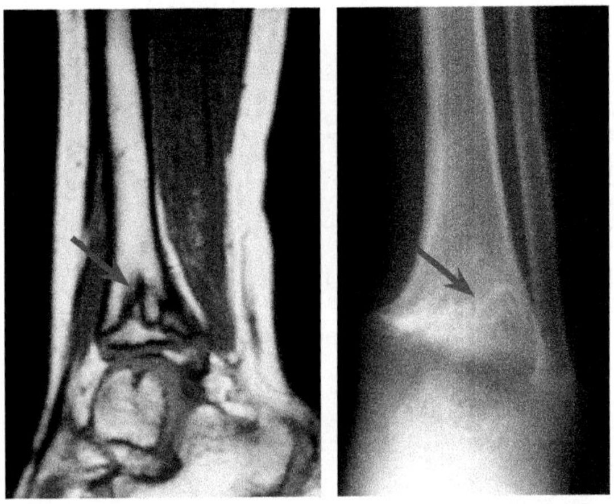

B Septic physeal fusion This child with meningococcemia developed a fusion of the distal tibial growth plate (arrows).

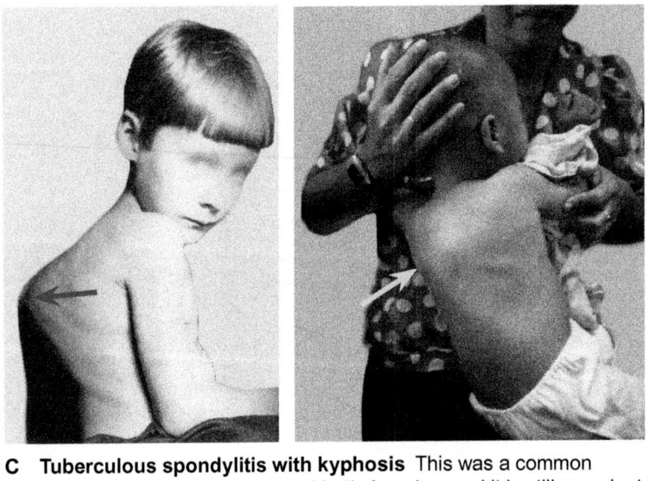

C Tuberculous spondylitis with kyphosis This was a common condition in the past (red arrow) in North America, and it is still prevalent in developing countries (yellow arrow).

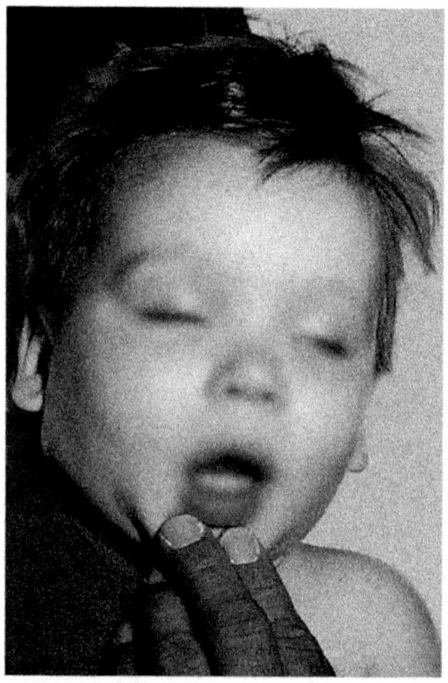

A Ill Child This child is systemically ill from septic arthritis. Note the lethargy and dehydration.

Evaluation

The child's medical history is important in the assessment of any previous injury or medical problem in the course of the current illness. The duration of symptoms in septic arthritis is of prognostic significance. Infections that are present for more than three days may cause residual joint damage, especially in the newborn. It is important to inquire about previous antibiotic treatment.

Physical Examination

Perform a screening examination first. Does the child appear ill [A]? The presence of systemic signs distinguishes septic arthritis from toxic synovitis. Is spontaneous movement present? The most reliable sign of septic arthritis of the hip in the newborn is a reduction of spontaneous movement of the limb. The reduction of movement from infection is described as *pseudoparalysis*. Swelling, erythema, and increased temperature are signs of inflammation, often due to infection. Note the position of the limb. Most infected limbs are positioned with the joints in slight flexion to reduce the intraarticular pressure. The hip is usually positioned in slight flexion, lateral rotation, and abduction [B].

Note the extent of soft tissue swelling and joint effusions. Try to localize the area of tenderness about the knee, ankle, wrist, or elbow to determine whether the primary problem is in the joint or the adjacent metaphysis. This is helpful in differentiating septic arthritis from osteomyelitis.

Move the joint through a gentle range of motion to assess guarding or limitation of the arc of motion. Medial rotation is limited by inflammation about the hip.

Imaging

Conventional radiographs may show soft tissue swelling [C] and obliteration of the soft tissue planes, but little else during the early course of an infection. A reduction of bone density of about 30% is necessary before radiographic changes are present. This usually requires 10–14 days [D].

Bone scans are useful in evaluating infection in the early stages of the illness. Technetium scans in septic arthritis are usually "warm." Scans in osteomyelitis are usually warm or hot but may be cold early in the disease. In the early phase of the disease, uptake may be reduced and a cold segment of bone may indicate the presence of a severe infection. In early osteomyelitis, the phasic scan may be useful. The early phase includes vascular perfusion that parallels the physical findings of swelling and inflammation. In the second or osseous phase, uptake is greater over the site of involvement. Bone scans are not necessary if radiographic changes are already present. Often the bone scan is helpful in localizing the site of involvement [E]. Order a high-resolution scan for increased resolution. The bone scan is unaffected by bone or joint aspiration.

SPECT scans Single-photon emission computed tomography (SPECT) scans are tomographic bone scans to identify focal inflammatory lesions of bone.

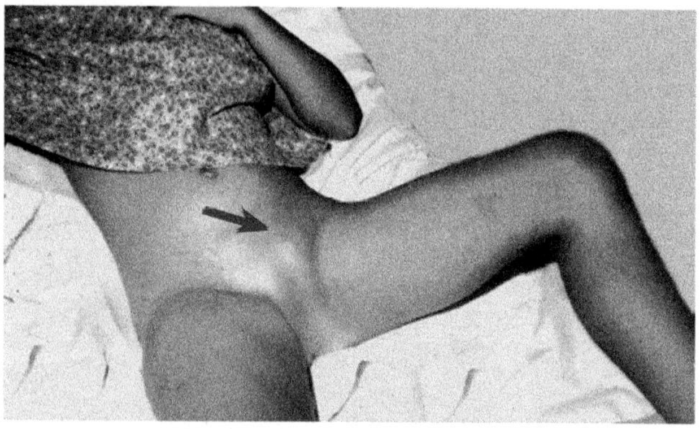

B Cellulitis involving the hip This child has cellulitis about the left hip (arrow). The limb is held in a position of flexion and abduction that reduces soft tissue pressure and minimizes discomfort.

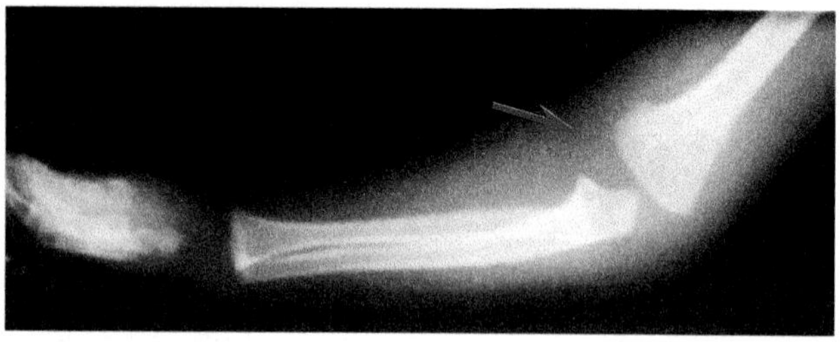

C Soft tissue swelling Soft tissue swelling is present in this infant with septic arthritis of the elbow.

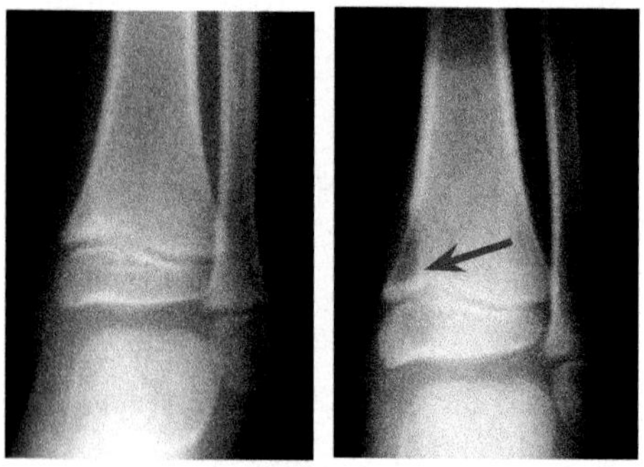

D Delay in radiographic appearance of osteomyelitis. This original film at the onset of the disease was normal (left). At 2 weeks (right), the lytic lesion is seen in the metaphysis (red arrow).

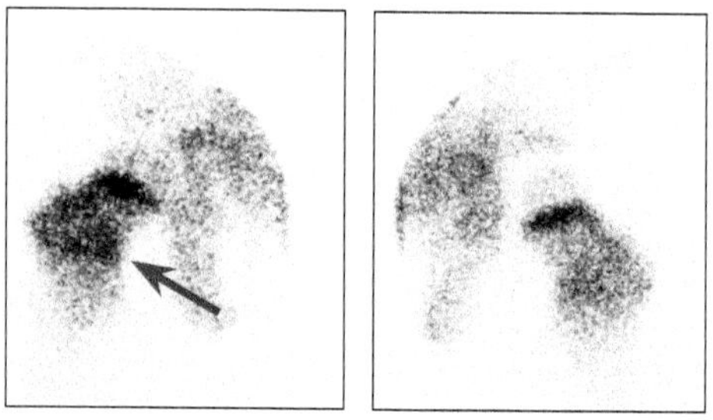

E Osteomyelitis of proximal femur Bone scans aid in localizing the site of infection. The metaphysis of the proximal femur on the right hip (arrow) shows more uptake than the opposite femur. The bone scan may be useful in determining the site for surgical drainage.

Ultrasound evaluation for hip joint effusions [A] may be helpful if the ultrasonologist is experienced. A negative study should not delay a diagnostic aspiration if the clinical signs suggest the possibility of an infected joint. Ultrasound is also useful in localizing abscess formations around long bones, and its use is underutilized.

MRI studies of infection may be useful in localizing an abscess [B]. MRI studies of discitis may be alarming and can lead to overtreatment. Use newer imaging techniques only as adjuncts to conventional well-understood techniques.

CT studies are sometimes useful in evaluating deep infections, such as those about the pelvis. CT and MRI studies may be helpful in localizing abscess and planning the surgical approach for drainage.

Laboratory Studies

The erythrocyte sedimentation rate (ESR), C-reactive protein (CRP), and cultures are the most valuable laboratory tests. Serial measures are useful in following the course of infection. Often the white blood count (WBC) is normal.

ESR is still valuable. Following the onset of infection, the ESR slowly rises to peak at 3–5 days and remains elevated for about 3 weeks if treatment is successful [C].

CRP peaks in 2 days and follows most closely the clinical course of the infection. If treatment is successful, the values return to normal in about a week.

Cultures are essential and usually include blood, joint fluid, wound, and biopsy samples. Blood cultures are positive in 30–50% of patients. Be aware that negative cultures are common in both osteomyelitis and septic arthritis.

PCR Molecular methods are being applied to the microbiology of bone and joint infections. Amplification techniques using polymerase chain reaction (PCR) have been shown to be very sensitive and specific when DNA probes are used for such specific infections as tuberculosis and Lyme disease. In settings of polymicrobial infections and infections where the likely organism is unknown, the ability of molecular techniques to identify the organism is as yet not superior to standard cultures. Further evolution of these techniques will likely increase their use in clinical medicine in the future.

Differentiation from Neoplasm

The differentiation of infection from neoplasm is sometimes difficult. Infections are more common, especially in younger subjects, and often show signs of inflammation. Subacute osteomyelitis may be confused with osteoid osteoma, osteosarcoma, chondroblastoma, Ewing sarcoma, fibrosarcoma, or eosinophilic granuloma. If necessary, establish the diagnosis with biopsy, curettage, and cultures. If the lesion is well demarcated, making a malignant tumor less likely, consider prescribing a course of oral antibiotics. If the lesion is due to an infection, the treatment is both diagnostic and therapeutic.

Eosinophilic granuloma may show inflammatory features.

Ewing sarcoma differentiation may pose a major problem. MRI and bone scans may be helpful [D]. Sometimes biopsy and cultures are necessary.

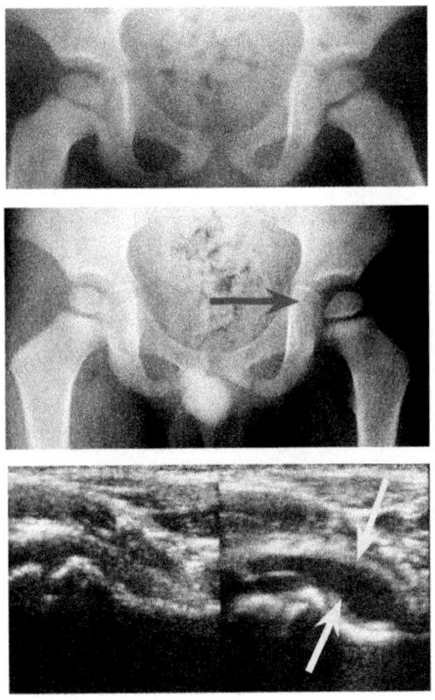

A Imaging in septic arthritis This child developed hip pain and guarding. The initial radiograph (top) was negative. The family refused aspiration. When seen the next day, the radiograph showed widening of the joint space (red arrow), and the ultrasound showed a joint effusion (yellow arrow).

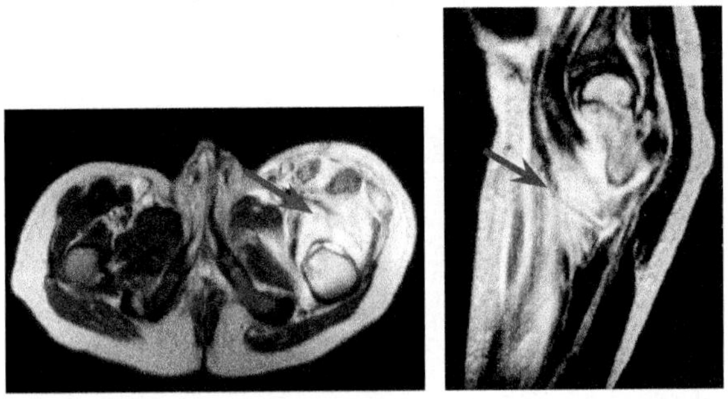

B MRI showing a thigh abscess This study shows the massive upper thigh abscess (arrows) secondary to femoral osteomyelitis.

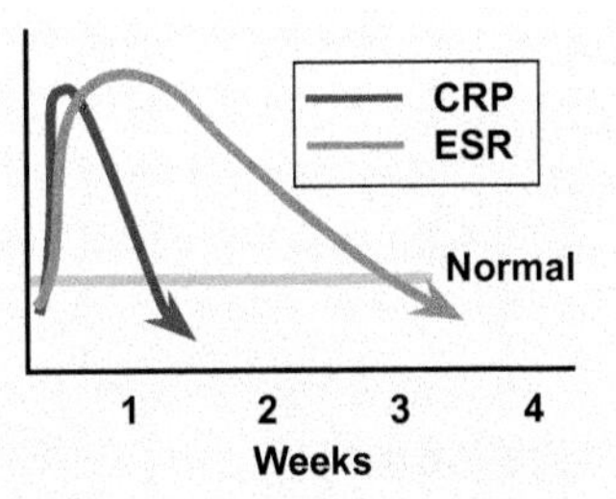

C CRP and ESR changes with time Following a musculoskeletal infection, the CRP declines more rapidly than the ESR. Based on Unkila-Kallio (1993).

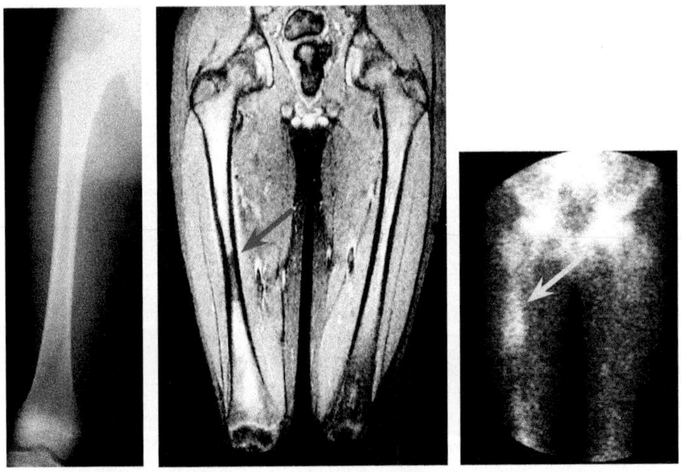

D Differentiating diaphyseal osteomyelitis from Ewing sarcoma In this child with osteomyelitis, note that the conventional radiograph was negative (left). This differentiation was aided by the MRI study, which showed little soft tissue involvement (arrow). The bone scan (yellow arrow) showed that only the femur was involved.

Management Principles

Management of infections in children is guided by a number of principles that often differ from those that apply to adults.

Greater Healing Potential

The potential for healing infection is remarkable in children. For example, discitis usually resolves with time with or without treatment. Bone damaged by osteomyelitis heals. Infection of bone may be contained and localized to only a residual abscess or it may resolve completely without treatment. Chronic osteomyelitis can nearly always be cured in children. Operative wound infections are uncommon in children.

Antibiotics

The selection of an antibiotic agent is complex. Consider the disease, organism, and special features of the child. These features include the age, concurrent illness, and the family situation. The route of administration and duration of treatment are other factors to consider. Initial therapy should be intravenous or, if access is difficult, intramuscular. Certain antibiotics are most commonly used for musculoskeletal infections [A and D].

Oral antibiotic therapy is justified if the infection is minor, the agent is well absorbed, and the family is reliable. In most serious infections, treatment may begin with parenteral antibiotics and switch to oral agents when the disease is under control. Before switching to the oral route of administration, be certain that adequate blood levels are documented following oral administration and that the family is reliable.

Methicillin-resistant organisms Consider the incidence of methicillin-resistant *Staphylococcus aureus* (MRSA) in the community. If the child appears ill, the empiric choice is vancomycin, with modifications made after the culture and sensitivities are determined.

Duration of antibiotic treatment is controversial. Several factors should be considered in determining the duration. Consider the severity and potential for disability that the infection poses, the rapidity of response to treatment [B], serial determinations of the ESR and CRP, the results of published studies, and the age of the child. Treat older children slightly longer. There are, however, some generalizations that can be made [C]. These can be modified according to the situation. Joint suppuration in septic arthritis reduces the effectiveness of the antibiotic treatment. For duration and dose of antibiotic selection, use the AAP Red Book [E].

Agent	Dose
Oxacillin	150-200 mg/kg/day
Nafcillin	150-200 mg/kg/day
Dicloxacillin	75-100 mg/kg/day
Cephealexin	100-150 mg/kg/day
Cefazolin	100-150 mg/kg/day
Cefotaxime	100-150 mg/kg/day
Cefuroxime	150-200 mg/kg/day
Gentamicin	5-7.5 mg/kg/day
Clindamycin	30-40 mg/kg/day

A Daily dosage of antibiotic treatment These are some broad generalizations for infants over 1 month of age and for children.

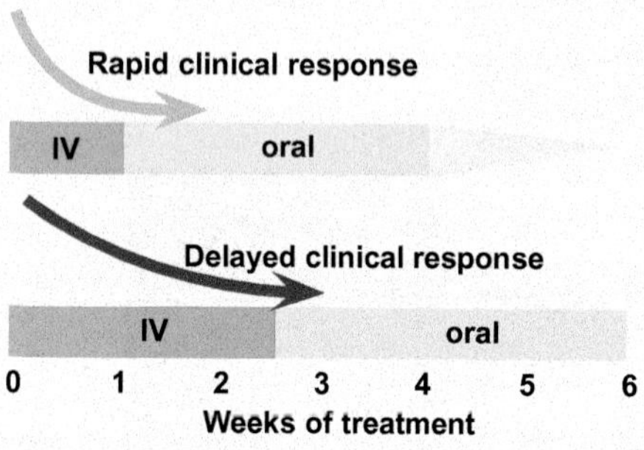

B Duration of IV antibiotic treatment Base duration of parenteral antibiotics on clinical response.

Disease	Comment
Septic arthritis	7 days IV, 3-4 weeks total
Osteomyelitis	7 days IV, 4-6 weeks total or until ESR normal
Cellulitis	10-14 days
Surgical prophylaxis	Single dose prior to incision

C Duration of antibiotic treatment These broad generalizations serve as an average duration of treatment.

Condition	Organism	Agent
Sepsis		
Neonate	Group A and B strep, coliforms	Oxacillin + gentamicin
Infant	*H. flu*, pneumococcus, meningococcus	Ceftriaxone or cefotaxime
Septic Arthritis		
Neonate	Group A and B strep, coliforms	Oxacillin + gentamicin
Infant	*H. flu*, staph A, group A and B strep	Cefotaxime
Child	*Staph. aureus*	Nafcillin
Osteomyelitis		
Neonate	Group A and B strep, coliforms	Nafcillin + gentamicin
Infant/Child	Staph A	Nafcillin
Nail Puncture		
Through Shoes	Pseudomonas	Ceftazidime or ticarcillin
Barefoot	*S. aureus*	Nafcillin
Discitis	*S. aureus*	Nafcillin
Open Fractures	*S. aureus*	Nafcillin
Operative prophylaxis	*S. aureus*	Nafcillin

D Commonly used antibiotics for musculoskeletal infections

RED BOOK ONLINE
The Report of the Committee on Infectious Diseases

E See: http://aapredbook.aappublications.org

Indication	Comment
Abscess	Open drainage
Hip Joint	Open drainage
Other Joints	Drain by aspiration
Osteomyelitis	Drain abscess open
Brodie Abscess	Drain open if necessary
Sequestrum	Excise

F Methods of drainage These are the common methods of drainage.

Operative Drainage

Drainage may be accomplished by needle aspiration, arthroscopic decompression, or open procedures [F, previous page].

Indications Drainage is necessary whenever antibiotic penetration into the infected site is impaired. This penetration is most often due to the presence of an abscess or an accumulation of pus within a joint [A]. Impaired penetration may also be due to a loss of vascularity, as occurs in chronic osteomyelitis with sequestration or in soft tissue with poor vascularization due to thrombosis of vessels and acute inflammation. The presence of an abscess may be demonstrated by clinical examination, imaging such as ultrasound or MRI, needle aspiration, or suggested by a failure of clinical response to antibiotic treatment. This failure of response to antibiotics [B] is the failure of reduction in fever, pain, local inflammatory signs, and CRP during the first 48–72 hours after instituting antibiotic treatment. Keep in mind that this failed response may also be due to an ineffective antibiotic agent or to an immunocompromised child.

Technique may be simply needle aspiration [C], as is feasible for most joints, arthroscopic, or open drainage. Open drainage of abscess due to acute infections requires simply draining the abscess through a small window in the cortex. If the abscess is near a growth plate, take care to avoid injuring the physis [D and F]. Monitor the position of the curette with fluoroscopy.

The techniques for drainage of septic arthritis and osteomyelitis are presented on the next two pages.

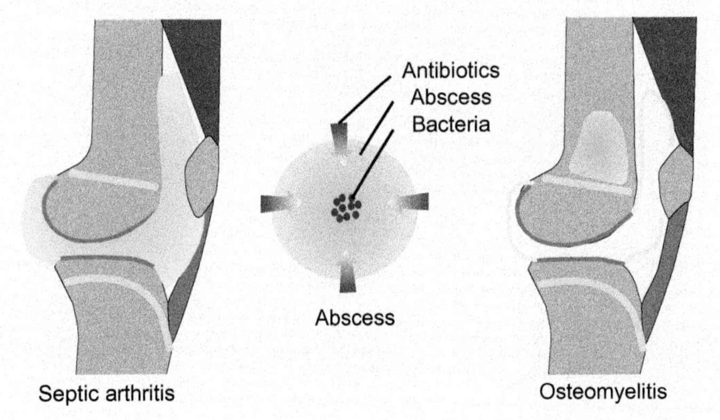

A Abscess protects bacteria from antibiotics The abscess prevents antibiotic penetration, protecting bacteria.

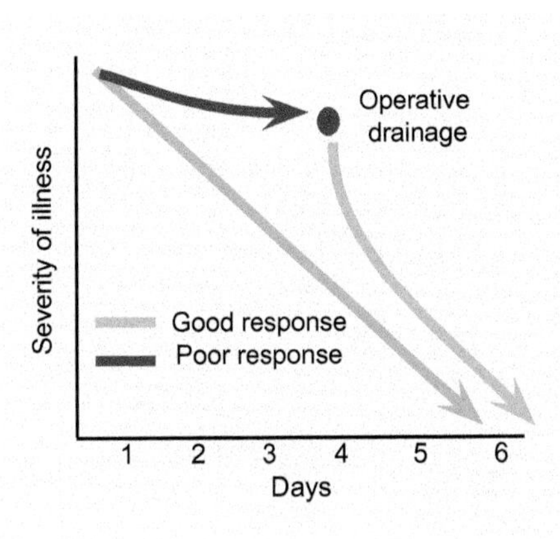

B Indication for operative drainage The failure of response to antibiotic treatment is often an indication for drainage.

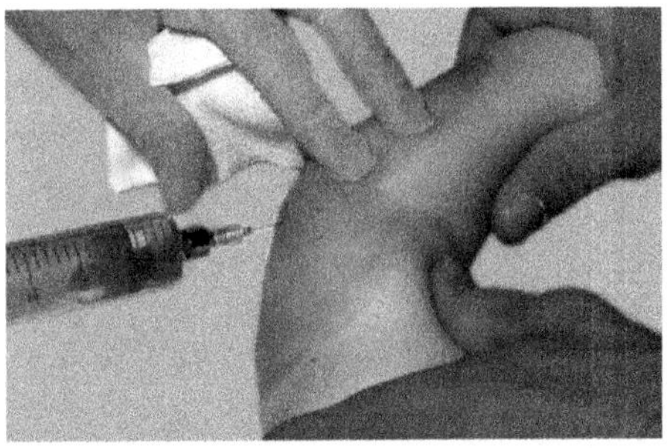

C Needle aspiration This drainage is usually adequate for most joints with septic arthritis.

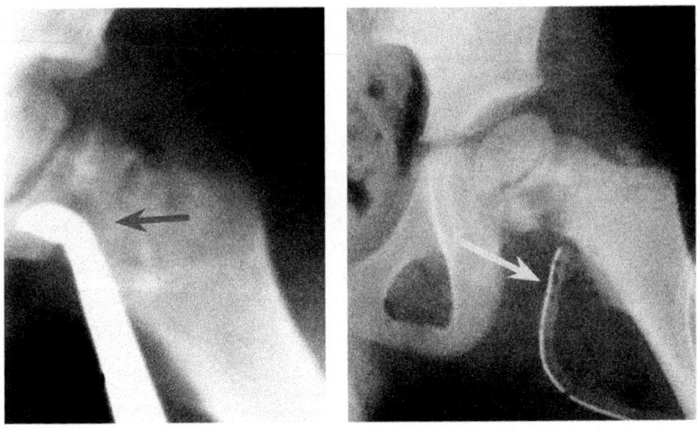

D Drainage in difficult locations Monitor position of curette with fluoroscopy and avoid the physis (red arrow). Usually, a drain is placed (yellow arrow).

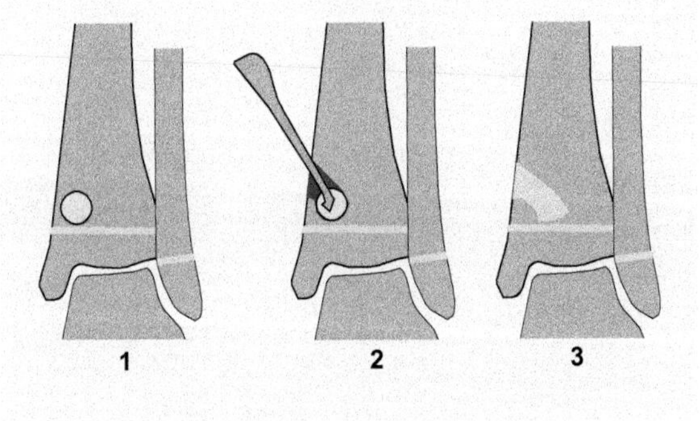

E Surgical drainage of acute or subacute osteomyelitis The infection is drained locally, with care taken to avoid injury to the growth plate. With time, bone fills in the defect.

Osteomyelitis

Osteomyelitis is an infection of the bone [A]. The infection may be acute, subacute, or chronic, and may involve any bone [B]. Osteomyelitis in the preantibiotic era often caused death or severe disability. Currently, osteomyelitis remains a relatively common problem but with a much better prognosis.

Natural History

The natural history of osteomyelitis depends upon the virulence of the organism, the resistance of the host, and the age of onset [C]. Virulent organisms may cause the death of a child due to overwhelming sepsis or, if localized, osteomyelitis progresses to chronic osteomyelitis. Chronic osteomyelitis develops through stages, which include bone and soft tissue abscesses causing sequestrum formation [D], intermittent drainage, and a lifelong disability. Chronic drainage may lead to development of squamous cell carcinoma of the sinus tracts during adult life.

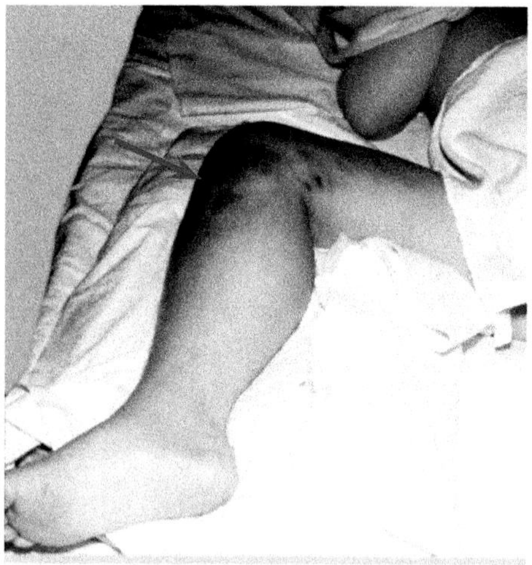

A Osteomyelitis This boy has osteomyelitis of the upper tibia with an associated soft tissue abscess (arrow).

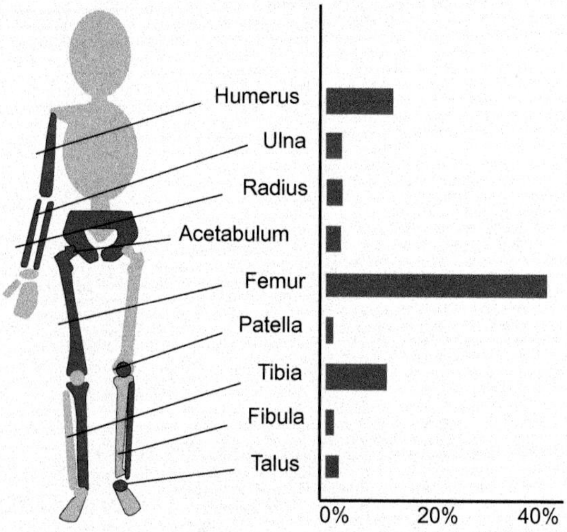

B Distribution of osteomyelitis From a series of 66 patients reported by Perlman (2000).

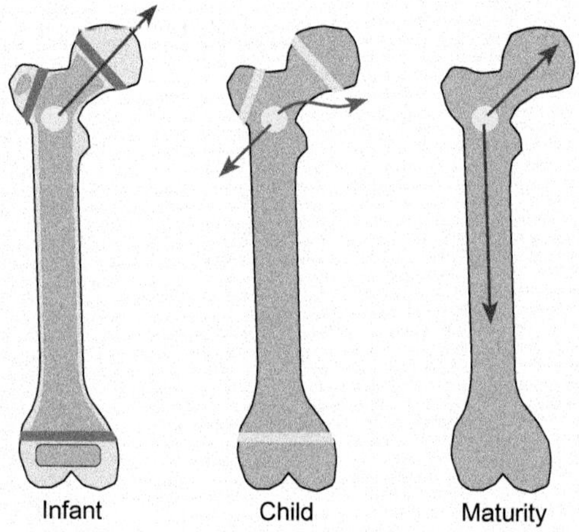

C Spread of osteomyelitis by age Bone structure affects the spread of osteomyelitis (red arrows). In the infant, the absence of an epiphyseal plate may allow spread into a joint. In the child, the path of least resistance is through the adjacent cortex to an extramedullary abscess. In the mature adolescent, the thick cortex and absence of growth plates allow extension throughout the medullary cavity.

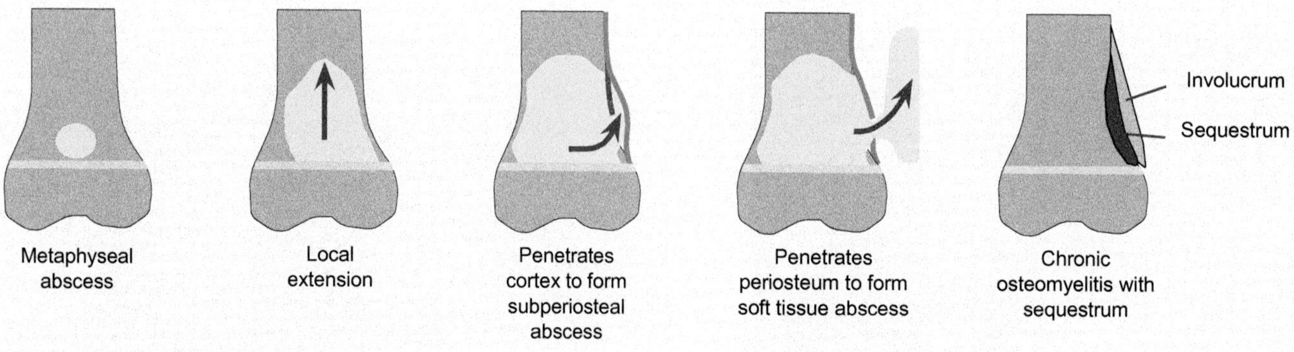

D Natural history of osteomyelitis The infection starts in the metaphysis. Contained by the growth plate, the infection spreads through the metaphysis, and then penetrates the cortex, creating a subperiosteal abscess. This may penetrate the periosteum to produce a soft tissue abscess. During healing, new bone (involucrum) forms around the devitalized cortical bone. This dead bone is called a "sequestrum."

Acute Osteomyelitis

Acute osteomyelitis produces local pain, swelling, warmth, erythema, tenderness, and systemic manifestations of fever and malaise. Laboratory findings usually include a leukocytosis and elevated CRP and ESR. The CRP and ESR elevations are the most consistent laboratory findings.

Image with conventional radiographs to provide a baseline, and assess for soft tissue swelling. A bone scan may be useful in localizing the site of involvement. Ultrasound and MRI studies may be helpful in localizing any abscess. To isolate the organism, culture the blood and consider aspirating the site of infection. Aspiration is most successful if a subperiosteal abscess is present.

Management When planning management, estimate the stage of the disease [D, previous page]. Antibiotic treatment is usually successful without the need for drainage if the osteomyelitis is discovered early before suppuration has occurred. Start antibiotic treatment while awaiting the results of the cultures. Agent selection is done empirically, taking into consideration the age of the patient and the presence of any special features. Antibiotics are first given parenterally to ensure effective blood levels. The clinical course is monitored. If the antibiotic is effective against the organism and no suppuration is present, clinical improvement will occur with reduction in local signs of inflammation and systemic manifestations. If such improvement fails to occur over a period of 24–48 hours, the most likely cause is the formation of an abscess. An abscess requires operative drainage [A].

Subacute Osteomyelitis

Subacute osteomyelitis is an infection with a duration longer than 2–3 weeks. Often this type of osteomyelitis is the residual of acute osteomyelitis that has been contained but not eradicated [B]. The child may show no or little systemic response but experience local swelling, warmth, and tenderness. Sometimes the complaint concerns a limp.

Evaluation Radiographs will show the lesion. The appearance will be variable [D] and may be confused with a primary bone tumor, especially when diaphyseal and showing periosteal elevation. The differentiation between infection and Ewing sarcoma or leukemia is usually not difficult.

Management Manage classic metaphyseal lesions by antibiotic treatment without drainage. Drain and culture if lesions are atypical, if concern exists about a neoplastic etiology, if the child is immunologically impaired, or if the lesion or symptoms persist following antibiotic treatment [C].

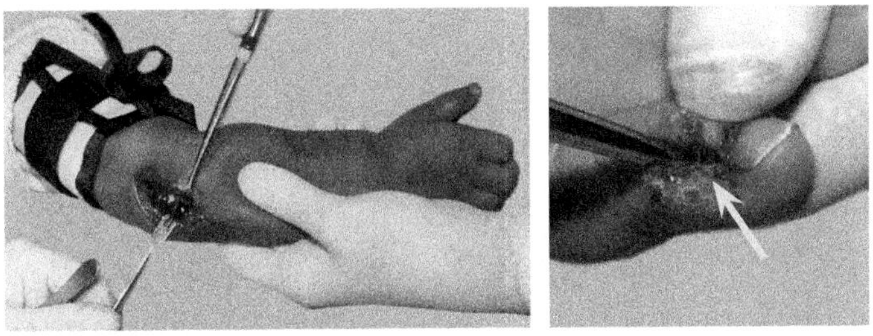

A Drainage of osteomyelitis Drain by windowing the cortex and exploring adjacent bone with a curette (yellow arrow).

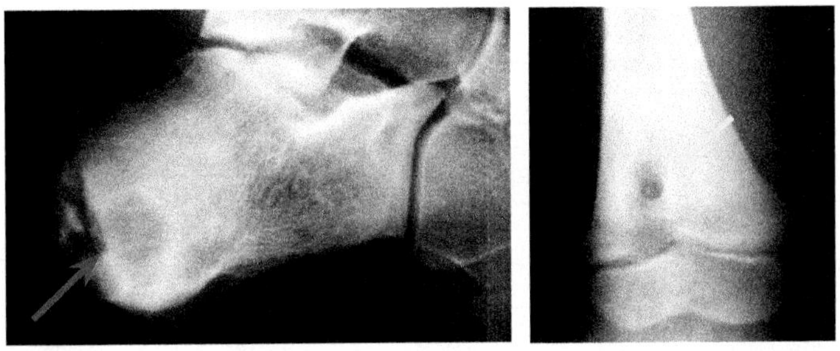

B Subacute osteomyelitis Osteomyelitis is contained in a bone abscess (arrows).

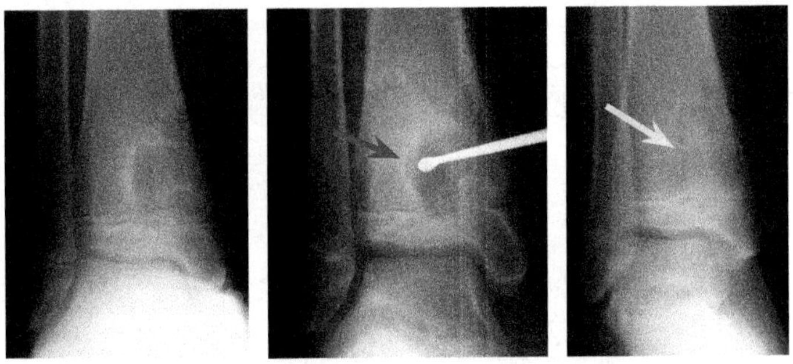

C Drainage of persistent subacute distal tibial osteomyelitis Tenderness and inflammation and radiographic changes were indications for operative drainage. Avoid placing the curette across the physis (red arrow). Defect is healing four weeks later (yellow arrow).

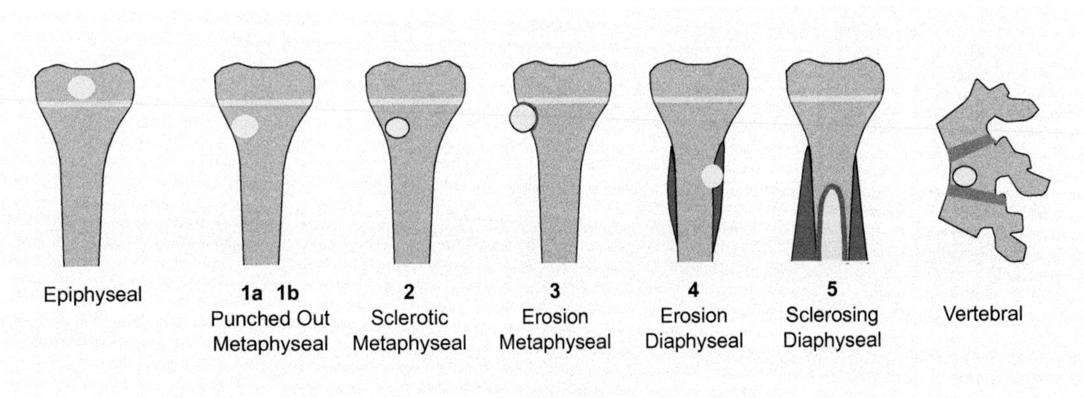

D Types of subacute osteomyelitis Redrawn from Roberts (1982).

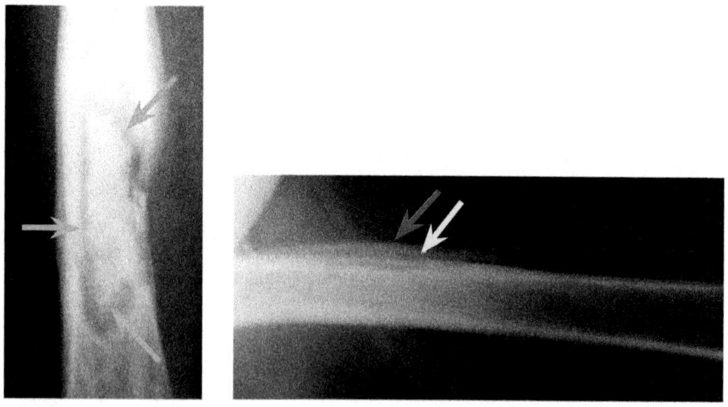

A Diaphyseal osteomyelitis Note the classic appearance of a well-established sequestrum in the tibia (orange arrows). This uncommon pattern of osteomyelitis of the femoral diaphysis is present in an 8-year-old girl. New bone formation (red arrow) surrounds a linear sequestrum (yellow arrow). This sequestrum was removed surgically.

Chronic Osteomyelitis

Untreated acute osteomyelitis usually becomes chronic, with the disease localized to a segment of bone. Long bones are most likely to develop chronic osteomyelitis, as a segment of cortex may be devascularized to form a sequestrum [A]. Flat bones, such as those of the pelvis, are primarily cancellous, with better blood supply, and less likely to develop chronic disease. The patterns of chronic osteomyelitis are numerous [B and C].

Management requires operative sequestrectomy and resection of infected tissue by saucerization to allow filling of the dead space with viable tissue [D]. In very long-standing infections, complex sinus tracts may develop. Assess the condition preoperatively with MRI, CT scans, and possibly by contrast injection of the sinus tract to determine its location, path, and the depth of the sinus. Before resection, consider injecting dye into the sinus to stain the infected tissue [E]. Plan the operative approach that will allow excision of all infected tissue. Provide antibiotic coverage based on preoperative sinus cultures. If the periosteum is viable, new bone will fill in the surgically created bony defect.

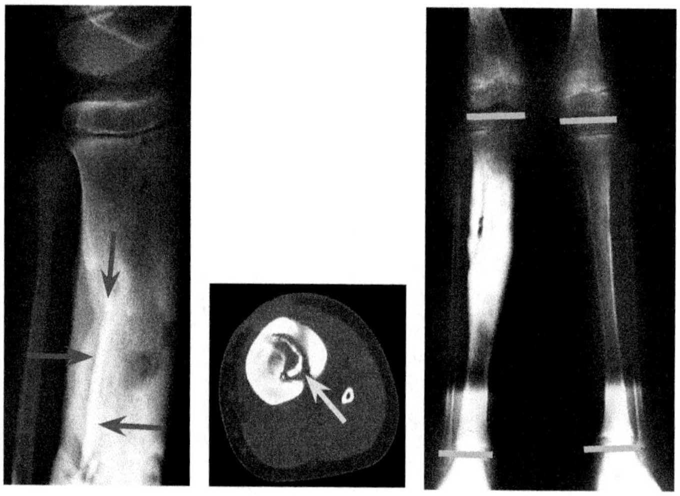

B Chronic osteomyelitis in a 12-year-old boy The sequestrum is clearly shown on the lateral radiograph (red arrows) and CT scan (yellow arrow). Note the overgrowth and valgus deformity of the boy's right tibia (green lines).

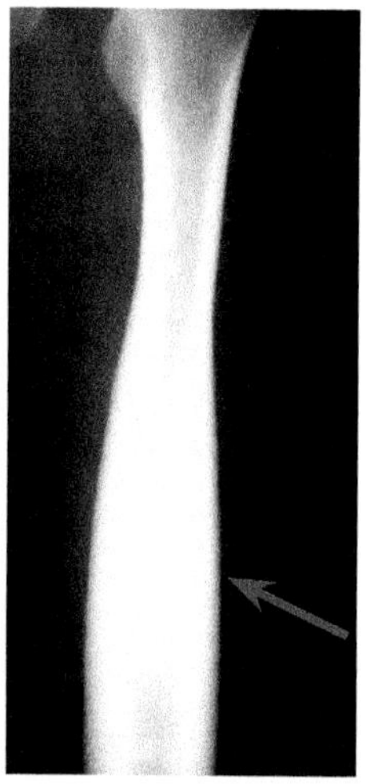

C Sclerosing osteomyelitis The entire shaft of the femur was converted into an abscess cavity in this adolescent boy.

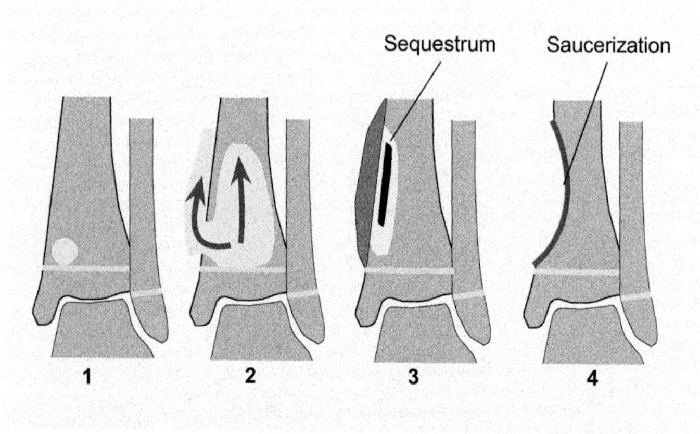

D Saucerization of chronic osteomyelitis If the infection spreads and devascularizes a segment of bone, this dead bone becomes a sequestrum (black) under the involucrum (dark brown). Manage by *saucerization* to remove the sequestrum and infected tissue. The healthy overlying soft tissue fills in the saucer.

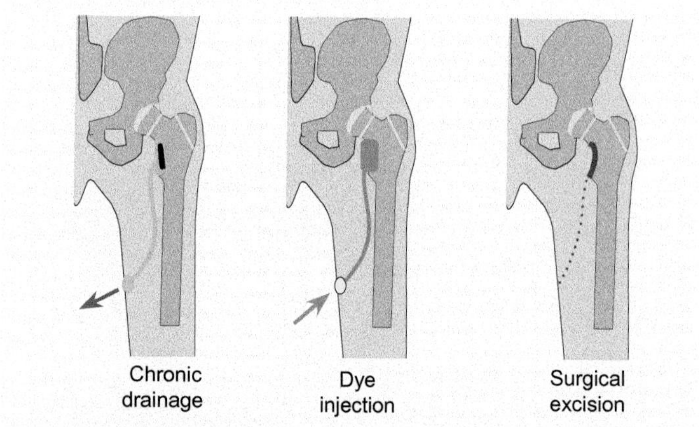

E Operative debridement The site of drainage of chronic osteomyelitis (proximal medial thigh—red arrow) may be distant from the sequestrum. Define the sinus tract and infected tissue with a sinogram with methylene blue dye. Excise the sequestrum and all infected tissue (red).

Complications of Osteomyelitis

Systemic complications Untreated osteomyelitis may lead to systemic infections such as bronchopneumonia and septic pericarditis with life-threatening consequences.

Local complications are uncommon with current treatment. Complications due to deformity of bone can usually be reconstructed with a satisfactory outcome. This is in contrast to the complications of septic arthritis, which often damage joints with no satisfactory reconstruction usually possible.

Pathological fracture is a serious complication of osteomyelitis [A]. Often the extent of the deossification is not appreciated, and the child is discharged with the affected limb unprotected. Pathological fractures are slow to heal and may heal in a deformed position. The deossification resulting from osteomyelitis lags the activity of the infection by 2–3 weeks. The risk of pathological fracture should be anticipated, and a protective cast should be applied before the deossification occurs.

Sequestrum formation is usually due to delay in diagnosis. Sequestrectomy is usually effective and curative for chronic disease.

Growth disturbance may be due to initial damage from the infection or operative drainage. Infections that destroy the growth plate or epiphysis may cause significant deformity [B and C].

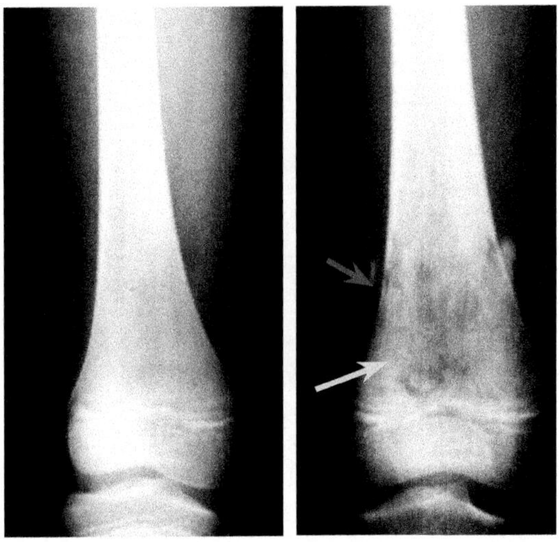

A Pathological fracture complicating osteomyelitis This girl was treated only with antibiotics for a metaphyseal osteomyelitis. Her discharge radiographs showed no deossification. She returned three weeks later with a pathological fracture (red arrow) through the deossified metaphysis (yellow arrow).

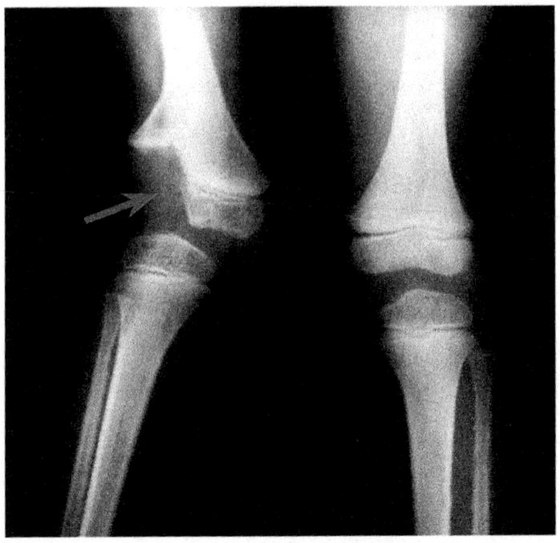

B Severe genu valgum due to infection This child lost the lateral half of the distal femoral growth plate due to osteomyelitis in early infancy. The deformity is progressive and difficult to correct.

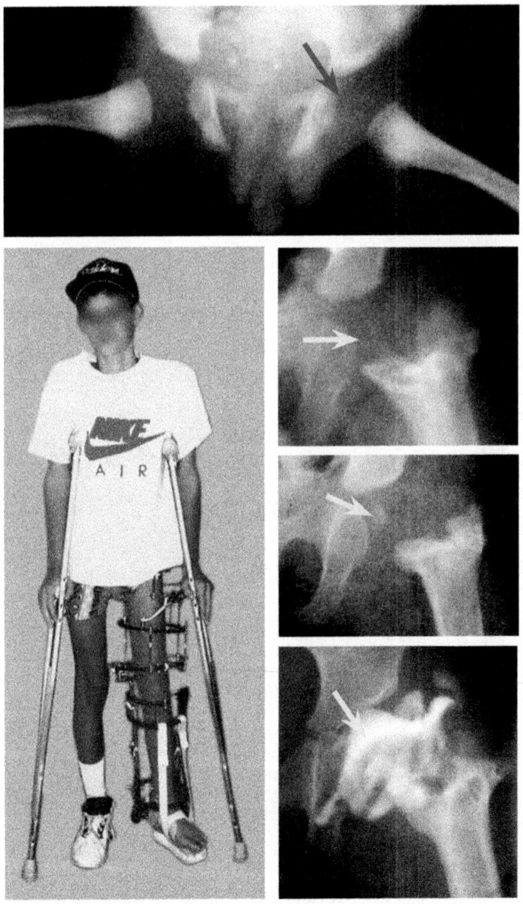

C Limb lengthening for residual of osteomyelitis This boy developed osteomyelitis of the left upper femur in the neonatal period (red arrow). The growth plate was damaged, resulting in deformity of the femoral head (yellow arrows) and limb shortening of 8 cm. The shortening was corrected by an Ilizarov leg lengthening technique. The bone is divided and gradually distracted while being stabilized with the external fixator.

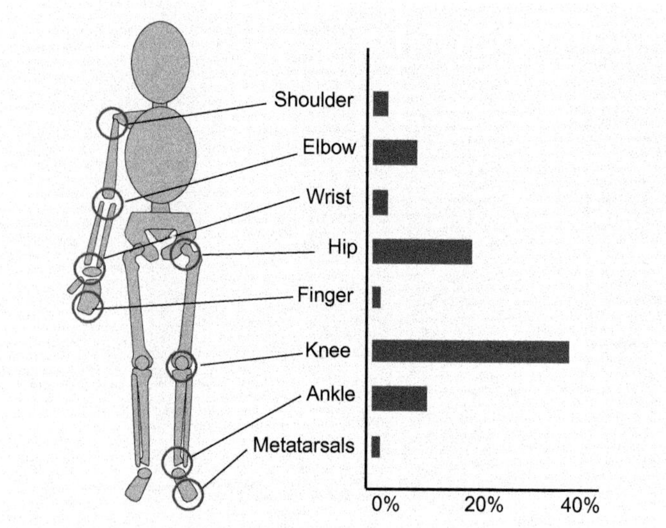

A Distribution of septic arthritis From data of Jackson and Nelson (1982).

Organism	Comment
Staphylococcus	Most common
Hemophilus	Becoming rare
Streptococcus	
Meningococcus	Primary or secondary
Pneumococcus	Infant
E. coli	Infant
Gonococcus	Adolescent
Lyme Disease	
Tuberculosis	Increasing frequency
Fungal Infections	Certain areas endemic
Viral Infections	Rare

B Organisms in septic arthritis These organisms are listed according to relative frequency.

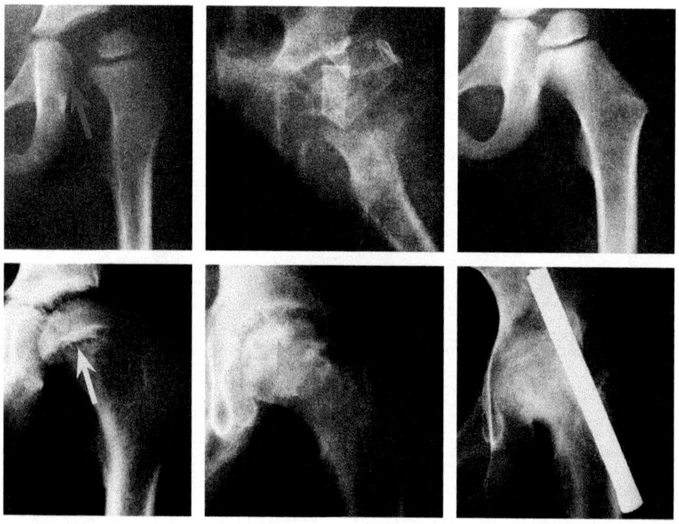

D Sequence of late-treated septic arthritis Treatment was delayed. Note the widening of the joint (red arrow). Open drainage was performed, but avascular necrosis (yellow arrow) and joint destruction (orange arrow) followed. The hip was eventually fused.

Septic Arthritis

Septic arthritis is a joint inflammation due to an infection usually involving synovial joints [A]. Many agents may cause septic arthritis [B], but the vast majority are due to various strains of *Staphylococcus* and *Streptococcus* and *Kingella kingae*. Septic arthritis can cause severe deformity and disability, especially when involving the hip during the neonatal period. The joint is damaged by enzymes produced by the bacteria and leukocytes, causing proteoglycan loss and collagen degradation. Inflammation may cause secondary vascular damage from thrombosis or direct compression of vessels.

Natural History

Unlike osteomyelitis, which may resolve without treatment, septic arthritis causes joint damage [C and D]. This makes septic arthritis a more serious disease than osteomyelitis.

Diagnosis

Clinical features are age related.

Neonate with septic arthritis may show few clinical signs. The most consistent finding is a loss of spontaneous movement of the extremity and posturing of the joint at rest. The hip is positioned in flexion, abduction, and some lateral rotation. Fever is often absent, and the neonate may not appear ill.

Infant and child septic arthritis produces local and systemic signs of inflammation. The joint is swollen and tender, and the child resists movement. Hip infections result in severe limitation of rotation, a useful sign in separating septic arthritis from osteomyelitis. Radiographs early in the disease may be deceptive [E]. A negative study is not significant. Widening of the joint is significant. Ultrasound studies may show joint effusions. Bone scans show slight to moderate increased uptake over the joint.

The most useful laboratory studies are the sedimentation rate and CRP. The ESR is usually elevated above 25 mm/hour. This test is not reliable for diagnosis in the neonate.

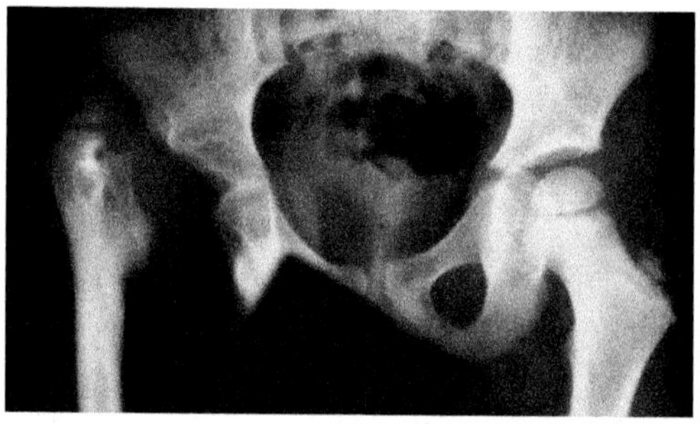

C Residual deformity of septic arthritis of the hip Note the severe deformity or Choi type 4 (see E, next page).

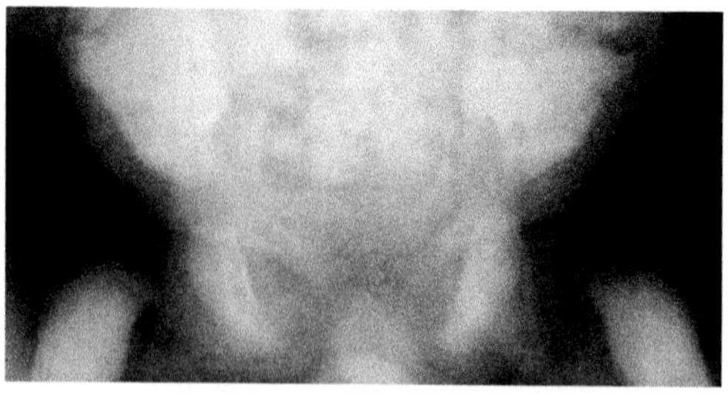

E False negative radiograph The radiograph was read as negative, no treatment was given, and the hip was destroyed by the septic arthritis.

The diagnosis of septic arthritis is established by joint aspiration [A]. This evaluation should be performed early and not delayed to obtain a bone scan or other imaging studies. Joint fluid in septic arthritis is cloudy, with leukocyte counts above 50,000 and PMNs predominating. Perform a Gram stain and culture. Cultures will be negative in 20–30% of cases of septic arthritis and thus a negative study does not rule out a joint infection. Culture the blood before starting antibiotic treatment.

Differential diagnosis includes poststreptococcal reactive arthritis, rheumatoid arthritis, and toxic synovitis. Differentiate toxic synovitis by considering four signs [B]. If three or four of these signs are present, the diagnosis is >90% likely to be septic arthritis rather than toxic synovitis.

Management

Manage with antibiotics and drainage.

Antibiotic treatment Start with an agent, that is, statistically most likely to be effective [C]. Later, the antibiotics may be changed based on the culture reports. Parenteral treatment is continued for several days and the clinical course monitored. Failure to improve suggests that the antibiotic is ineffective or that the drainage is incomplete. The duration of parenteral antibiotics should be based on the rapidity of clinical response in reduction of fever, local inflammation, and CRP response. Arbitrary rigid regimens prolong hospitalization and increase costs and patient discomfort without improving results. Most septic arthritis may be managed with parenteral antibiotics for 3 to 21 days followed by oral antibiotics for a total of about four weeks.

Joint drainage is necessary for all cases and should be done promptly.

Serial needle aspiration is a traditional method of drainage. Aspirate initially and as necessary to keep the joint free of pus. Most joints should be drained several times. If response to needle aspiration is slow, consider open or arthroscopic drainage.

Open drainage is mandatory for the hip. Consider open drainage for other joints if the diagnosis is delayed or if the situation is complicated.

Arthroscopic drainage is an option for large joints in children [D]. Place a drain.

Immobilization in septic arthritis is unnecessary. Avoid placing the child in traction, as the child will naturally hold the limb in the position of greatest comfort, which is the position in which intraarticular pressure is least.

Residual Deformity

Knee Residual deformity is most likely if the infection occurs in infancy and treatment is delayed. Usually a valgus or varus deformity develops due to displacement or loss of the physis. The deformity is usually permanent and often progressive.

Hip Ischemic changes in the hip are common and varied, including absence of or delayed ossification, loss and then return of ossification, or most severe complete loss or collapse. In this most severe form, increasing deformity may be present. Deformity varies, depending upon the extent of articular and physeal cartilaginous damage [E].

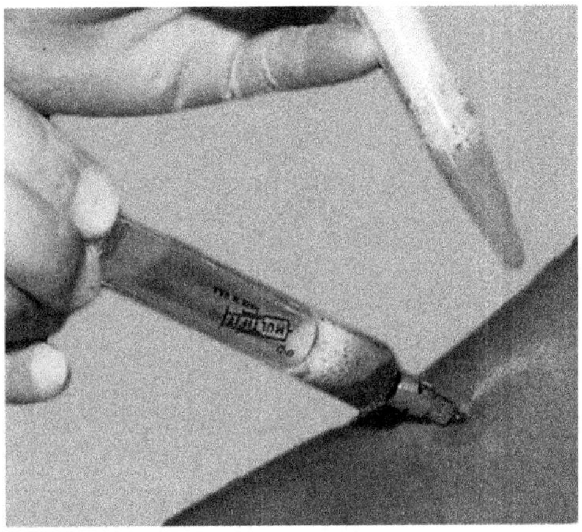

A Hip aspiration for diagnosis Open drainage is required for septic arthritis of the hip.

Features of Septic Arthritis

- Fever
- Unwilling to bear weight on the leg
- CRP > 0.8 mg/dl
- ESR > 40 mm/hr
- Leukocytosis >12,000

B Signs differentiating septic arthritis from toxic synovitis of the hip If three or four of these signs are present, the diagnosis is 90% likely to be septic arthritis. From Kocher (1999).

Age	Organism	Antibiotic	Dose
Neonate	Group B streptococcus *S. aureus* *E. coli*	Cefotaxime	150 mg/kg/day
Infant	*S. aureus* Group A streptococcus Pneumococcus	Nafcillin	150-200 mg/kg/day
Child	*S. aureus*	Nafcillin	150-200 mg/kg/day

C Antibiotic management of septic arthritis by age group The usual infecting organism and appropriate antibiotic are categorized by age group.

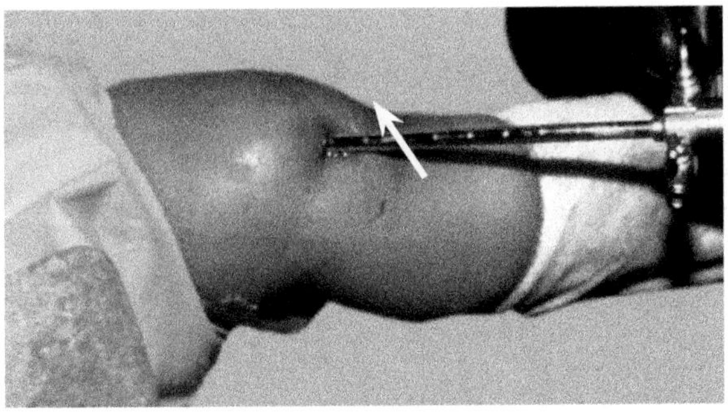

D Arthroscopic drainage of septic arthritis of the knee This is an acceptable method of drainage.

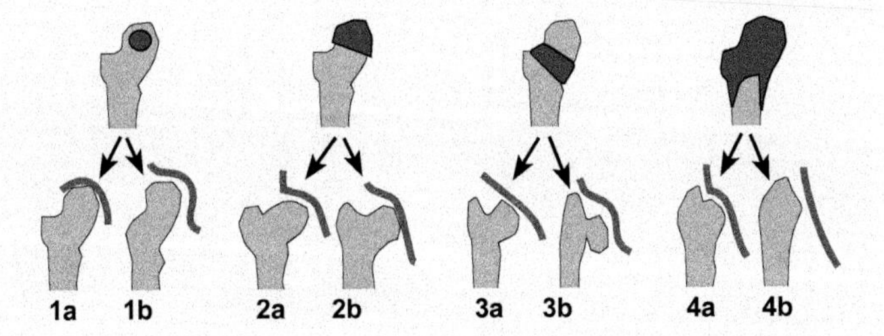

E Classification of sequelae from septic arthritis of the hip This classification demonstrates that the initial necrosis (red) determines the severity of the final deformity. From Choi (1990).

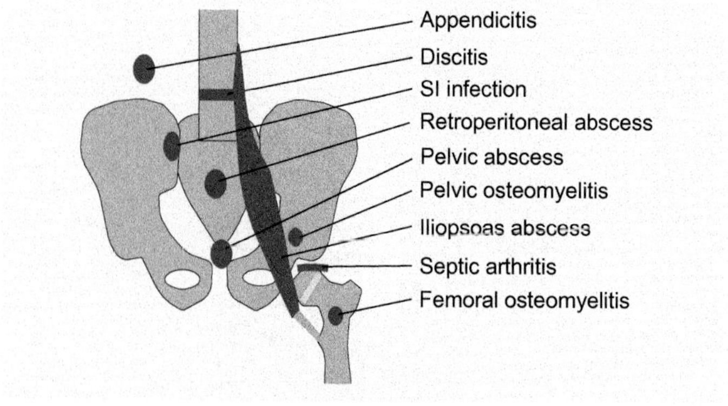

A Sites of infections about the pelvis Consider these possibilities in the differential diagnosis.

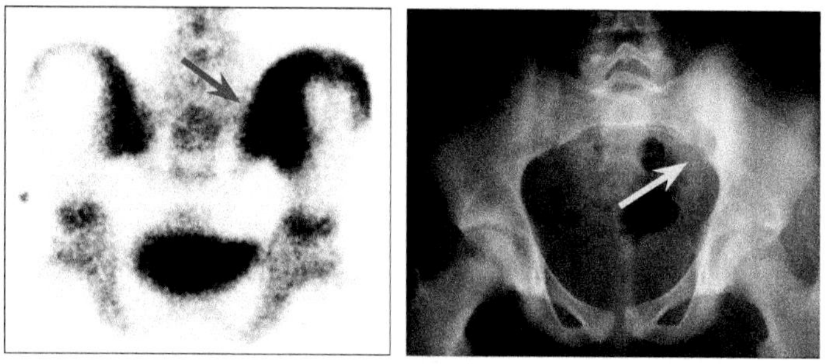

B Sacroiliac joint infection Initial radiographs were negative, but a bone scan demonstrated involvement of the SI joint (red arrow). Radiographs one month later demonstrated a bone abscess (yellow arrow).

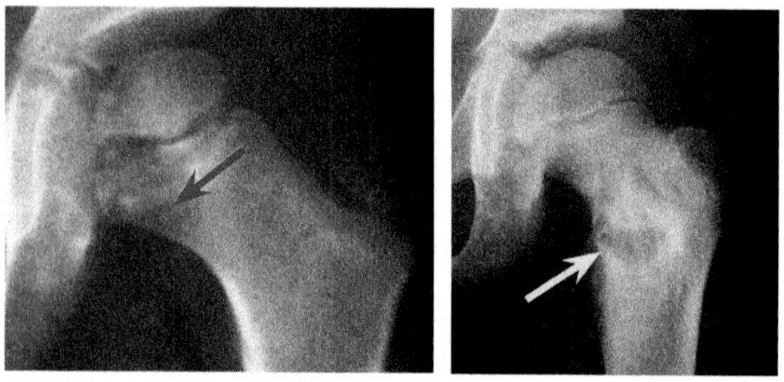

C Osteomyelitis proximal femur These lesions may be lytic (red arrow) or, when chronic, become more sclerotic (yellow arrow).

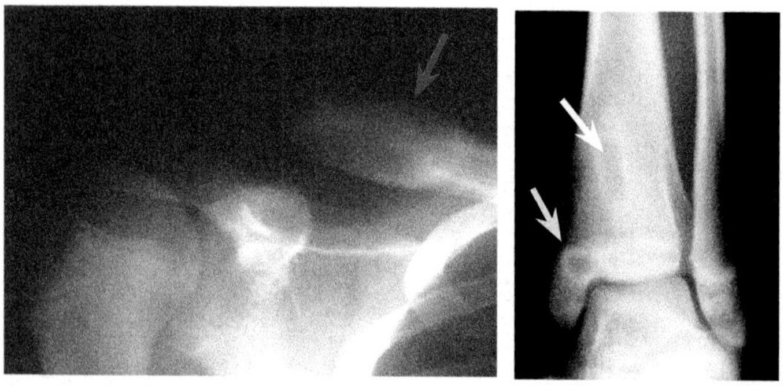

D Unusual forms of osteomyelitis Chronic osteomyelitis of the clavicle produces bony overgrowth with a cystic appearance, often confused with a neoplasm (red arrow). Rarely, lesions occur in the epiphysis (yellow arrow). A metaphyseal lesion was also present (white arrow).

Pelvic Infections

The combination of hip or flank pain, limp, and fever suggests an infection about the pelvis [A]. Because these infections are deep in location, localization by physical examination is more difficult than for infections of the extremities. Each infection has some unique characteristics that aid in diagnosis.

Evaluation

Physical examination may localize the infection. Tenderness and pain in the back or abdomen suggest discitis or an abdominal problem. Limitation of hip rotation suggests septic arthritis of the hip. Tenderness over the SI joints or proximal femur may help localize the process to those sites. Performing a rectal examination may help localize the problem.

Imaging is usually necessary. A bone scan is most helpful in localizing the infection [B, left]. CT scans may show soft tissue swelling. Ultrasound evaluation may demonstrate inflammatory changes in muscles.

Laboratory Growth of *Staphylococcus aureus* from a pelvic abscess indicates that the process is musculoskeletal in origin. Growth of fecal flora suggests an intraabdominal cause that warrants further study.

Differential Diagnosis

Septic arthritis of the hip requires most urgent management. Pain on passive rotation of the leg suggests this diagnosis. Confirm by aspiration. Urgent open drainage is necessary.

Iliopsoas abscess causes pain and positioning of the hip in flexion. Extension is painful. Iliopsoas abscess can be readily diagnosed by ultrasonography or computed tomography and treated by percutaneous retroperitoneal drainage.

SI infection of the joint or adjacent bone are best demonstrated by bone scan [B]. Manage with antibiotic treatment. Drainage is usually not necessary.

Pelvic osteomyelitis may occur in varied sites. Localize with bone scan, demonstrate any abscess by ultrasound or CT scans. Treat with antibiotics. If unresponsive, consider aspiration with image guidance.

Femoral osteomyelitis is very serious, with the potential for joint or growth damage [C]. Open drainage is often necessary.

Unusual Forms of Osteomyelitis

Osteomyelitis of the Clavicle

The clavicle responds to osteomyelitis with thickening and cystic changes that give the appearance of a neoplasm [D, left]. CT scans may demonstrate a bone abscess, which may be drained. Cultures may be negative. Consider chronic recurrent multifocal osteomyelitis in the differential. Treat bacterial infections with drainage and antistaphylococcal antibiotics.

Epiphyseal Osteomyelitis

Primary hematogenous osteomyelitis rarely affects the epiphysis primarily [D, right]. The infection may spread through the growth plate from a metaphyseal origin. The physeal erosion allowing this transphyseal spread usually heals without the formation of a physeal bridge. The exception is in meningococcemia and severe infections with delayed treatment.

Salmonella Osteomyelitis

Salmonella and staphylococcal aureus osteomyelitis occur in children with sickle cell disease [A, next page]. The infection is characterized by polyostotic distribution, extensive diaphyseal involvement, massive involucrum, and frequent complications due to compromised immune status and poor circulation of blood in bone. Manage by decompression and parenteral antibiotics.

Soft Tissue Infections

Chicken Pox (Varicella)

Group A streptococcal infections may cause cellulitis, abscesses, septic arthritis, or extensive necrotizing fasciitis.

Toxic Shock Syndrome

Toxic shock syndrome (TSS) is due to a toxin elaborated by different types of *S. aureus* and streptococcus. TSS has been reported about two weeks following orthopedic procedures and under casts in children. About half are nonmenstrual. The characteristic features include high fever, vomiting, diarrhea, rash, hypotension, pharyngitis, headache, and myalgia. Management is directed toward controlling the effects of the toxemia.

Pyomyositis

Muscle abscesses are infrequent, as skeletal muscle is resistant to bacterial infections. A bacteremia seeds muscle abscess [B]. In some cases, some underlying condition reduces resistance. Untreated, the generalized inflammation becomes focal with abscess formation in 2–3 weeks. The child becomes progressively more ill, with the potential of death. *Tropical pyomyositis* often occurs in anemic and malnourished children.

Initial stage The child presents with poorly localized aching pain and fever. The most common sites are the hip and thigh. Clinical and laboratory signs of infection are present. Radiographs show soft tissue swelling, the bone scan shows increased uptake [C], and the MRI is most specific and diagnostic. Treat with parenteral antistaphylococcal antibiotics.

Suppurative stage The child shows more systemic signs and focal tenderness. The MRI demonstrates a muscle abscess. Confirm the diagnosis and determine the organism by aspiration of the abscess. In some, this is adequate, but most require operative drainage.

Lyme Disease

Lyme arthritis in children may mimic other pediatric arthritides. The natural history of untreated Lyme disease in children may include acute infection followed by attacks of arthritis and then by keratitis, subtle joint pain, or chronic encephalopathy. Treat with amoxicillin, doxycycline, and ceftriaxone. With treatment complete, resolution is expected within 2–12 weeks and prognosis is excellent.

Puncture Wounds

Foot infections are often due to puncture wounds. The classic example is the nail puncture wound of the foot. When these occur through shoes, the infecting organism is *Pseudomonas*. Puncture wounds in other situations are usually due to *Staphylococcus*. Retention of foreign material such as wood may be best imaged by ultrasound [D]. Removal of foreign bodies is often more difficult than expected.

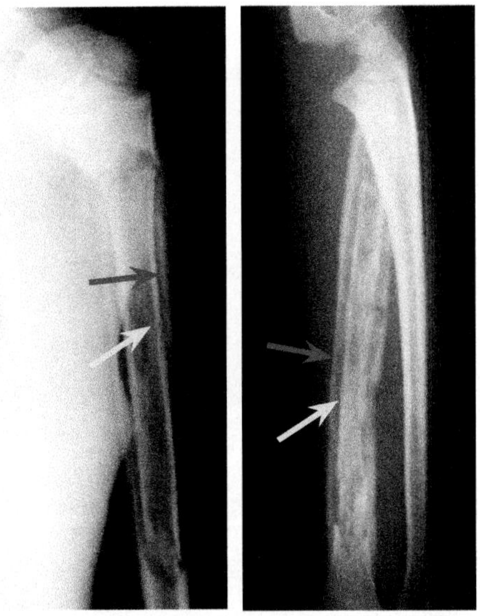

A Salmonella osteomyelitis in sickle cell disease This osteomyelitis elicits an extensive subperiosteal new bone formation (red arrows) that completely surrounds the original diaphysis (yellow arrows).

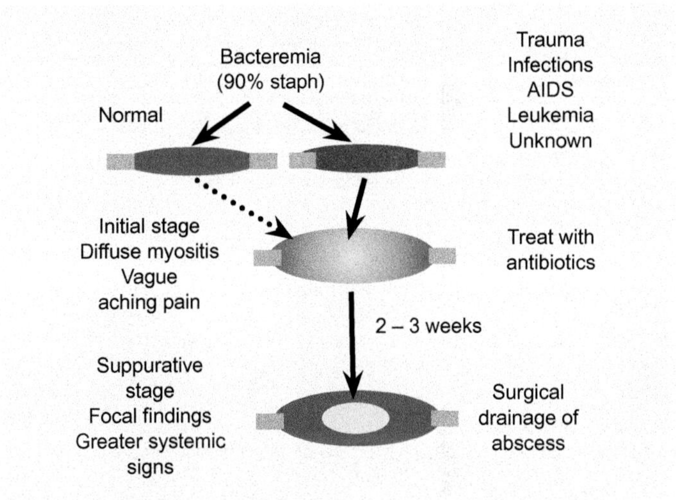

B Natural history of polymyositis The natural history of this infection includes cellulitic and suppurative stages.

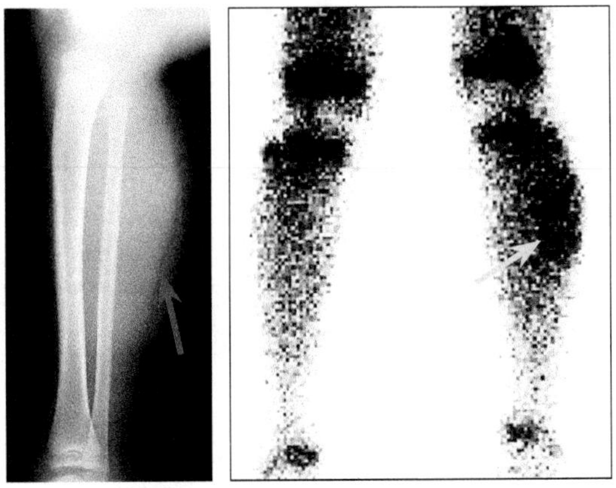

C Polymyositis Note the soft tissue swelling (red arrow) and increased muscle uptake (yellow arrow) on bone scan.

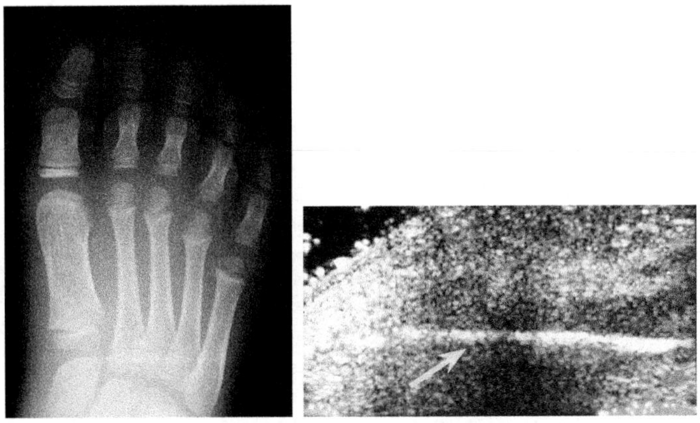

D Foreign body infections The foot is swollen but without bony change. The ultrasound shows the wood fragment (yellow arrow).

Tuberculosis

More new cases of tuberculosis are being seen throughout the world. This is due to an increasing number of people with suppressed immune systems, drug resistant strains of *Mycobacterium*, an aging population, and more exposed health care workers. Musculoskeletal tuberculosis most often involves the spine [A].

Spinal Tuberculosis

In children, the infection usually involves only bone [B], leaving the disc and cartilaginous end plates intact. This improves prognosis and allows spontaneous correction of the kyphosis with growth. Medical management is the primary treatment. Treat all patients with at least three drugs for a prolonged period.

Operative management is controversial. Undisputed indications include a significant neurological deficit, a neurological deficit or kyphosis progressing despite adequate medical management, or compromised pulmonary function from the abscess.

Tuberculous Osteomyelitis

In young children, this may be associated with BCG vaccination. The children are usually afebrile and show local swelling and discomfort, which may alter function. Mild leukocytosis and increased ESR are common. The CRP is usually normal. Radiographs show metaphyseal lesions with soft tissue swelling. Manage with operative drainage and immediate wound closure. Avoid leaving wounds open to prevent fistula formation. Provide antituberculosis chemotherapy for about one year.

Tuberculous Arthritis

In contrast to pyogenic arthritis, tuberculosis causes a slow, progressive joint disintegration that involves both sides of the joint [C]. Management usually requires medical management, joint debridement, and closure of the skin over drains. Later joint stabilization by arthrodesis may be necessary.

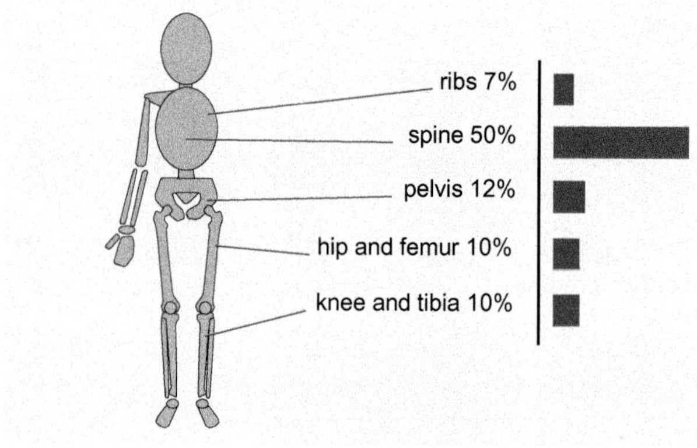

A Distribution of musculoskeletal tuberculosis

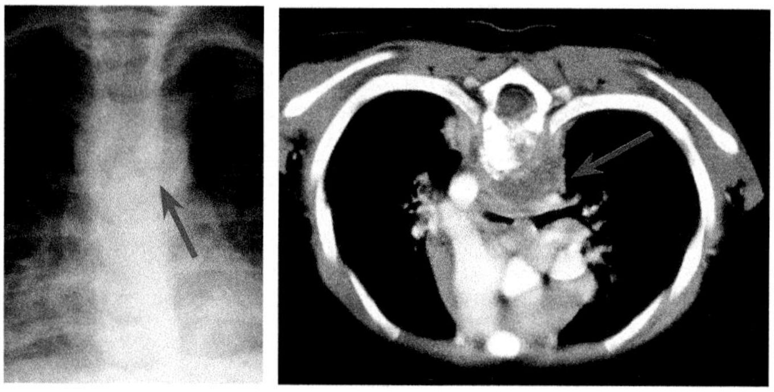

B Tuberculous paravertebral abscess The abscess can be seen both on the chest radiograph and the CT scan (red arrows).

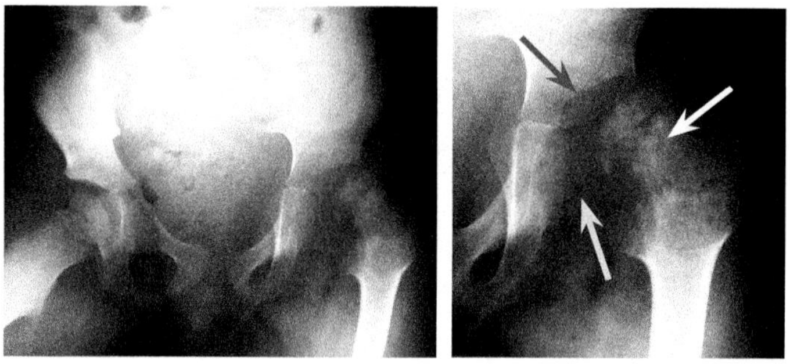

C Tuberculous hip infection Note that the infection involves the proximal femur (white arrow), joint (yellow arrow), and acetabulum (red arrow).

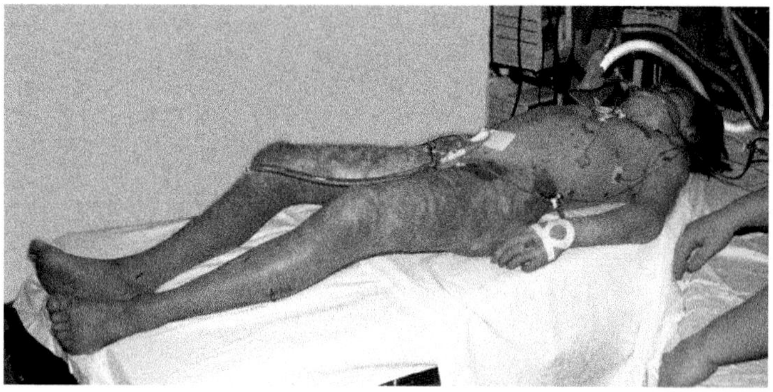

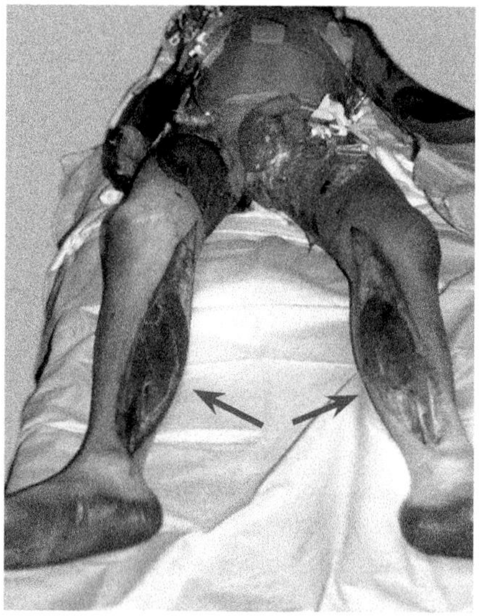

D Necrotizing fasciitis This 12-year-old boy developed meningococcemia and four-extremity involvement. Despite fasciotomies (arrows), the limbs became gangrenous. The disease was fatal.

Meningococcal Infections

The current practice of immunization for meningococcal infections may reduce the prevalence of all such infections.

Purpura Fulminans

The clinical course includes a premonitory illness, rapid development of fever, shock, and disseminated intravascular coagulation. This results in extensive soft tissue damage with compartment syndromes and skin necrosis most evident in the extremities [D, previous page]. Management requires aggressive debridement and fasciotomy and the management of multiple organ failure. Multiple amputations of gangrenous limbs may be required.

Meningococcal Multifocal Osteomyelitis

This infection is unique because it often affects the growth plate, causing physeal fusions and severe deformities [A and B].

Chronic Nonbacterial Osteomyelitis

Chronic nonbacterial osteomyelitis (CNO) is a sterile inflammatory bone disorder possibly of autoimmune or autoinflammatory etiology [C and D]. This is not an infection but included in this chapter as the condition is often confused with bacterial osteomyelitis.

Diagnosis

The onset is usually mid-childhood, about 2/3 are girls, about half have a comorbidity autoimmune disease (common in their families), and showed more bone lesions. The bone lesions are most often located at the metaphyseal region of tubular bones and the clavicle, but can occur also at the spine, ischiopubic bone, and the sacroiliac joint. Progressive sclerosis and hyperostosis occurs mostly in the clavicle and occasionally in the tibia, femur, metatarsal, and ischiopubic bone, similar to those sclerosing bacterial osteomyelitis. Less common is unilateral involvement [C].

Management

Antibiotic treatment is ineffective. Traditionally, NSAIDs were the first line of treatment. More recently, immunosuppressive treatment with methotrexate, corticosteroids, and TNF (tumor necrosis factor) inhibitors have been reported to be more effective. Using this treatment at two years, about half of the children will experience remission. Others advocate bisphosphonate therapy.

Prognosis

The long-term prognosis is good. Pathological fractures may complicate management. Bone overgrowth and deformity are rare.

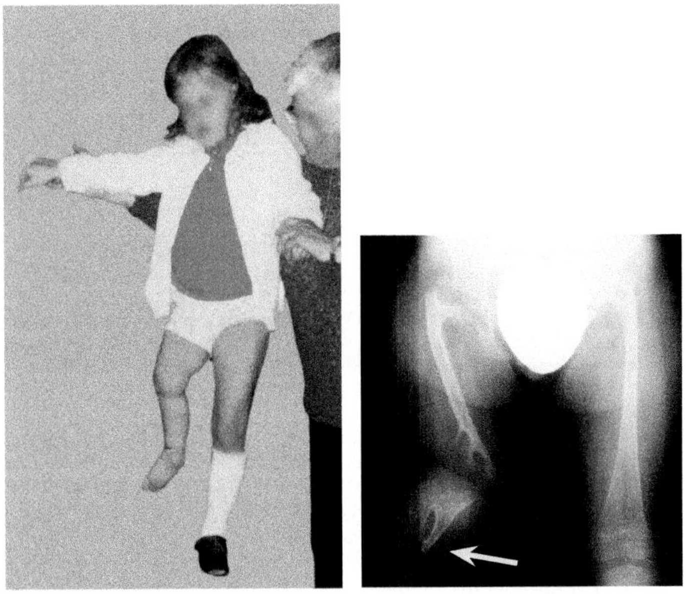

A Meningococcemia with growth plate injury This child developed meningitis and meningococcemia. Meningococcal osteomyelitis damaged the growth plate, causing severe residual shortening of the right leg. A below-the-knee amputation was performed to make prosthetic fitting possible (yellow arrow).

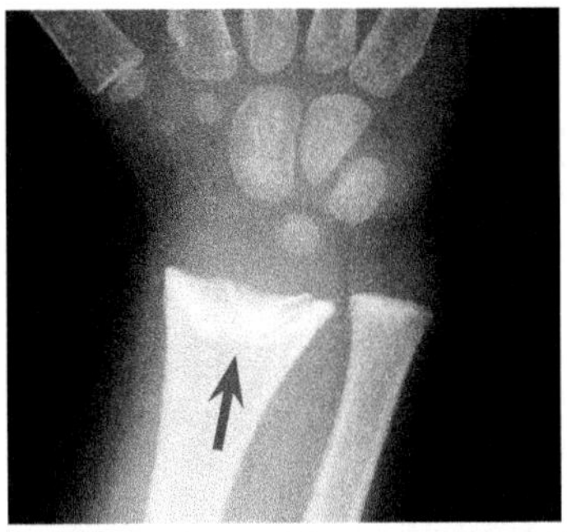

B Physeal arrest from meningococcemia Note the sclerosis and shortening of the radius.

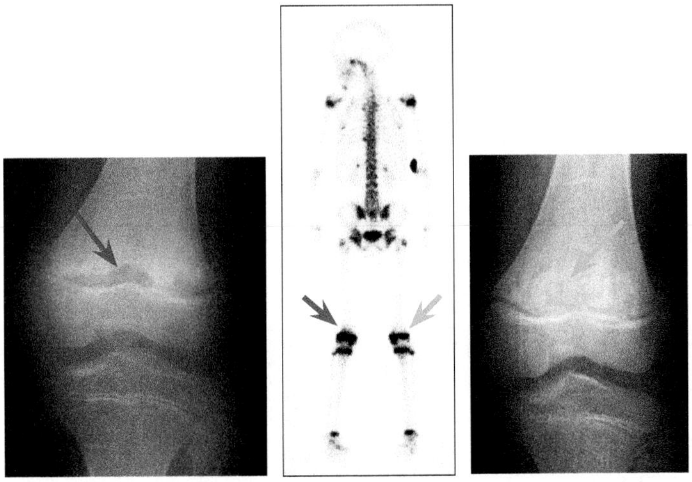

C Unilateral chronic nonbacterial osteomyelitis Note the unilateral right distal femoral metaphysis involvement (red arrows). The left femur (green arrows) is not affected.

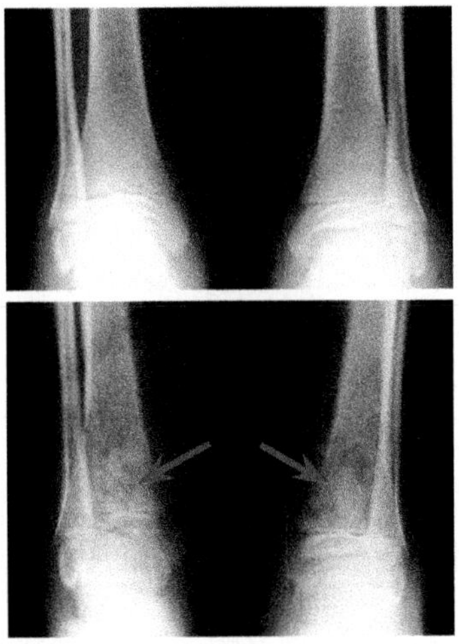

D Bilateral chronic nonbacterial osteomyelitis This atypical form of osteomyelitis produces symmetrical bone lesions in early disease before radiographic findings (top) and two months later when extensive metaphyseal changes are seen (bottom, red arrows).

Abernethy LJ, Lee YC, Cole WG. Ultrasound localization of subperiosteal abscesses in children with late-acute osteomyelitis. J Pediatr Orthop 1993:13:766.

Appel M, Pauleto AC, Cunha LA. Osteochondral sequelae of meningococcemia: radiographic aspects. J Pediatr Orthop 2002 Jul-Aug;22(4): p511-6.

Aroojis AJ, Johari AN. Epiphyseal separations after neonatal osteomyelitis and septic arthritis. J Pediatr Orthop 2000 Jul-Aug;20(4): p544-9.

Bickels J, Ben-Sira L, Kessler A, et al. Primary pyomyositis. J Bone Joint Surg Am 2002;84-A:2277–86.

Bos CF, et al. Late sequelae of neonatal septic arthritis of the shoulder. J Bone Joint Surg 1998:80B:645.

Brodie BC. An account of some cases of chronic abscess of the tibia. Med Chir Trans. 1832;17:239-49

Brook I. Microbiology and management of infectious gangrene in children. J Pediatr Orthop 2004 Sep-Oct;24(5): p587-92.

Cavalier R, Herman MJ, Pizzutillo PD, Geller E. Ultrasound-guided aspiration of the hip in children: a new technique. Clin Orthop 2003 Oct;(415): p244-7.

Chambers JB, Forsythe DA, Bertrand SL, Iwinski HJ, Steflik DE. Retrospective review of osteoarticular infections in a pediatric sickle cell age group. J Pediatr Orthop 2000 Sep-Oct;20(5): p682-5.

Choi IH, et al. Sequelae and reconstruction after septic arthritis of the hip in infants. J Bone Joint Surg 1990:72A:1150.

Dhillon MS, Nagi ON. Tuberculosis of the foot and ankle. Clin Orthop 2002 May;(398): p107-13.

Duffy CM, Lam PY, Ditchfield M, Allen R, Graham HK. Chronic recurrent multifocal osteomyelitis: review of orthopaedic complications at maturity. J Pediatr Orthop 2002 Jul-Aug;22(4): p501-5.

Ezra E, Cohen N, Segev E, Hayek S, Lokiec F, Keret D, Wientroub S. Primary subacute epiphyseal osteomyelitis: role of conservative treatment. J Pediatr Orthop 2002 May-Jun;22(3): p333-7.

Garron E, Viehweger E, Launay F, Guillaume JM, Jouve JL, Bollini G. Nontuberculous spondylodiscitis in children. J Pediatr Orthop 2002 May-Jun;22(3): p321-8.

Giedion, A., Holthusen, W., Masel, L. F., Vischer, D. Subacute and chronic 'symmetrical' osteomyelitis. Ann. Radiol. 15: 329-342, 1972.

Girschick HJ, Zimmer C, Klaus G, Darge K, Dick A, Morbach H. Chronic recurrent multifocal osteomyelitis: what is it and how should it be treated? Nature Clinical Practice Rheumatology 3:733-738, 2007.

Gram, HC. "Über die isolierte Färbung der Schizomyceten in Schnitt- und Trockenpräparaten". Fortschritte der Medizin (in German) 1884, 2: 185–189.

Grimes J, Carpenter C, Reinker K. Toxic shock syndrome as a complication of orthopedic surgery. J Pediatr Orthop 1995:15:666.

Gristina AG, Shibata Y, Giridhar G, Kreger A, Myrvik QN. The glycocalyx, biofilm, microbes, and resistant infection. Semin Arthroplasty. 1994 Oct;5(4):160-70.

Grogan DP, et al. Chondro-osseous growth abnormalities after meningococcemia. A clinical and histopathological study. J Bone Joint Surg 1989:71A:920.

Hammond PJ, Macnicol MF. Osteomyelitis of the pelvis and proximal femur: diagnostic difficulties. J Pediatr Orthop B 2001 Apr;10(2): p113.-9.

Harrington P, Scott B, Chetcuti P. Multifocal streptococcal pyomyositis complicated by acute compartment syndrome: case report. J Pediatr Orthop B 2001 Apr;10(2): p120-2.

Harris NH, Kirkaldy-Willis WH. Primary subacute pyogenic osteomyelitis. J Bone Joint Surg Br. Aug 1965;47:526-32.

Hodgson AR, Stock FE, Fang HS, Ong GB. Anterior spinal fusion. The operative approach and pathological findings in 412 patients with Pott's disease of the spine. Br J Surg 48:172-178, 1960.

Jaberi FM, Shahcheraghi GH, Ahadzadeh M. Short-term intravenous antibiotic treatment of acute hematogenous bone and joint infection in children: a prospective randomized trial. J Pediatr Orthop 2002 May-Jun;22(3): p317-20.

Jung ST, Rowe SM, Moon ES, Song EK, Yoon TR, Seo HY. Significance of laboratory and radiologic findings for differentiating between septic arthritis and transient synovitis of the hip. J Pediatr Orthop 2003 May-Jun;23(3): p368-72.

Khachatourians AG, Patzakis MJ, Roidis N, Holtom PD. Laboratory monitoring in pediatric acute osteomyelitis and septic arthritis. Clin Orthop 2003 Apr;(409): p186-94.

Kim HK, Alman B, Cole WG. A shortened course of parenteral antibiotic therapy in the management of acute septic arthritis of the hip. J Pediatr Orthop 2000 Jan-Feb;20(1): p44-7.

Kocher MS, Mandiga R, Zurakowski D, Barnewolt C, Kasser JR. Validation of a clinical prediction rule for the differentiation between septic arthritis and transient synovitis of the hip in children. J Bone Joint Surg Am 2004 Aug;86-A(8): p1629-35.

Konyves A, Deo SD, Murray JR, Mandalia VI, Von Arx OA, Troughton AH. Septic arthritis of the elbow after chickenpox. J Pediatr Orthop B 2004 Mar;13(2): p114-7.

Kucukkaya M, Kabukcuoglu Y, Tezer M, Kuzgun U. Management of childhood chronic tibial osteomyelitis with the Ilizarov method. J Pediatr Orthop 2002 Sep-Oct;22(5): p632-7.

Lowden CM, Walsh SJ. Acute staphylococcal osteomyelitis of the clavicle. J Pediatr Orthop 1997:17:467.

Luhmann SJ, Jones A, Schootman M, Gordon JE, Schoenecker PL, Luhmann JD. Differentiation between septic arthritis and transient synovitis of the hip in children with clinical prediction algorithms. J Bone Joint Surg Am 2004 May;86-A(5): p956-62.

Lundy DW, Kehl DK. Increasing prevalence of Kingella kingae in osteoarticular infections in young children. J Pediatr Othrop 1998:18:262

Maraqa NF, Gomez MM, Rathore MH. Outpatient parenteral antimicrobial therapy in osteoarticular infections in children. J Pediatr Orthop 2002 Jul-Aug;22(4): p506-10.

Odio CM, Ramirez T, Arias G, AbdelNour A, Hidalgo I, Herrera ML, Bolan W, Alpizar J, Alvarez P. Double blind, randomized, placebo-controlled study of dexamethasone therapy for hematogenous septic arthritis in children. Pediatr Infect Dis J. 22(10):883–8, 2003.

Orlicek SL, Abramson JS, Woods CR, Givner LB. Obturator internus muscle abscess in children. J Pediatr Orthop 2001 Nov-Dec;21(6): p744-8.

Peltola H, Unkila-Kallio L, Kallio MJ. Simplified treatment of acute staphylococcal osteomyelitis of childhood. The Finnish Study Group. Pediatrics 1997; 99(6): 846-50.

Perlman MH, Patzakis MJ, Kumar PJ, Holtom P. The incidence of joint involvement with adjacent osteomyelitis in pediatric patients. J Pediatr Orthop 2000 Jan-Feb;20(1): p40-3.

Piehl FC, Davis RJ, Prugh SI. Osteomyelitis in sickle cell disease. J Pediatr Orthop 1993:13:225.

Pott P. The chirurgical works of Percivall Pott, F.R.S., surgeon to St. Bartholomew's Hospital, a new edition, with his last corrections. 1808. Clin Orthop Relat Res. May 2002;4-10.

Rasool MN. Hematogenous osteomyelitis of the calcaneus in children. J Pediatr Orthop 2001 Nov-Dec;21(6): p738-43.

Rasool MN. Osseous manifestations of tuberculosis in children. J Pediatr Orthop 2001 Nov-Dec;21(6): p749-55.
Roderick MR, Ramanan AV. Chronic recurrent multifocal osteomyelitis. Adv Exp Med Biol. 2013;764:99-107 Rose CD, et al. Pediatric Lyme arthritis: clinical spectrum and outcome. J Pediatr Orthop 1994:14:238.

Scott RJ, et al. Acute osteomyelitis in children: a review of 116 cases. J Pediatr Orthop 1990:5:649.

Segev E, Hayek S, Lokiec F, Ezra E, Issakov J, Wientroub S. Primary chronic sclerosing (Garre's) osteomyelitis in children. J Pediatr Orthop B 2001 Oct;10(4): p360-4.
Skaggs DL, Kim SK, Greene NW, Harris D, Miller JH. Differentiation between bone infarction and acute osteomyelitis in children with sickle-cell disease with use
Lower Limb / Topic Heading X8X9
of sequential radionuclide bone-marrow and bone scans. J Bone Joint Surg Am 2001 Dec;83-A(12): p1810-3.

Song J, Letts M, Monson R. Differentiation of psoas muscle abscess from septic arthritis of the hip in children. Clin Orthop 2001 Oct;(391): p258-65.

Spiegel DA, et al. Pyomyositis in children and adolescents: report of 12 cases and review of the literature. J Pediatr Orthop 1999:19:143.

Tong CW, et al. The conservative management of acute pyogenic iliopsoas abscess in children. J Bone Joint Surg 1998:80B:83.

Tudisco C, et al. Influence of chronic osteomyelitis on skeletal growth: analysis at maturity of 26 cases affected during childhood. J Pediatr Orthop 1991:11:358.

Tuson CE, Hoffman EB, Mann MD. Isotope bone scanning for acute osteomyelitis and septic arthritis in children. J Bone Joint Surg 1994:76B:306.

Unkila-Kallio L, Kallio MJ, Peltola H. The usefulness of C-reactive protein levels in the identification of concurrent septic arthritis in children who have acute hematogenous osteomyelitis. A comparison with the usefulness of the erythrocyte sedimentation rate and the white blood-cell count. J Bone Joint Surg 1994:76A:848.

Walsh S, Phillips F. Deep vein thrombosis associated with pediatric musculoskeletal sepsis. J Pediatr Orthop 2002 May-Jun;22(3): p329-32.

Wang MNH, et al. Tuberculous osteomyelitis in young children. J Pediatr Orthop 1999:19:151.

Willis AA, Widmann RF, Flynn JM, Green DW, Onel KB. Lyme arthritis presenting as acute septic arthritis in children. J Pediatr Orthop 2003 Jan-Feb;23(1): p114-8.

Wilson B. "Necrotising Fasciitis". Am Surg 18 (4): 416–31, 1952.

Yokoe DS, Mermel LA, Anderson DJ, et al. A compendium of strategies to prevent healthcare-associated infections in acute care hospital. Infect Control Hosp Epidemiol 2008:29:S12-S21.

CHAPTER 7

Tumors

About 2,000 to 3,000 new cases of malignancies of the musculoskeletal system are diagnosed each year in the United States. The number of benign neoplasms is estimated to be about ten times this number. A timely diagnosis of malignant tumors reduces the likelihood of metastasis and dramatically increases survival rates.

Evaluation

Evaluate tumors by taking the patient's history, performing a careful physical examination, and obtaining necessary laboratory and imaging studies. The diagnosis of a tumor usually is made by the presence of pain, a mass, or a pathologic fracture. It may be an incidental finding [A].

History

Tumors usually present as a soft tissue mass, produce pain, or cause disability. How long a mass has been present is often difficult to determine from a history. Frequently, a large lesion, such as a slow-growing osteochondroma, is not noticed until shortly before the consultation. The family may incorrectly conclude that the tumor had grown quickly.

Pain is a more reliable indicator of the time of onset of a tumor. Inquire about the onset, progression, severity, and character of the pain. Night pain is common for both malignant tumors and some benign lesions, such as osteoid osteoma. Malignant lesions produce pain that increases over a period of weeks or months. Night pain in the adolescent is especially worrisome and should be evaluated first with a conventional radiograph. An abrupt onset of pain is usually due to a pathologic fracture. Such fractures most commonly occur through bone cysts typically found in the humerus and femur.

Age of the patient is helpful. A bone lesion in a child under age 5 years is likely to be due to an infection or eosinophilic granuloma. Giant cell tumors and osteoblastomas occur in the late teen period.

Race is notable, as blacks seldom develop Ewing sarcoma.

Examination

The initial examination is usually performed for a mass or pain. Some lesions, such as osteochondromas, are usually multiple. Look for asymmetry, deformity, or swelling. Palpate for masses. If a mass is present, measure its size, assess for tenderness, and note any associated inflammation. Malignant tumors are typically firm, are nontender, and may produce signs of inflammation.

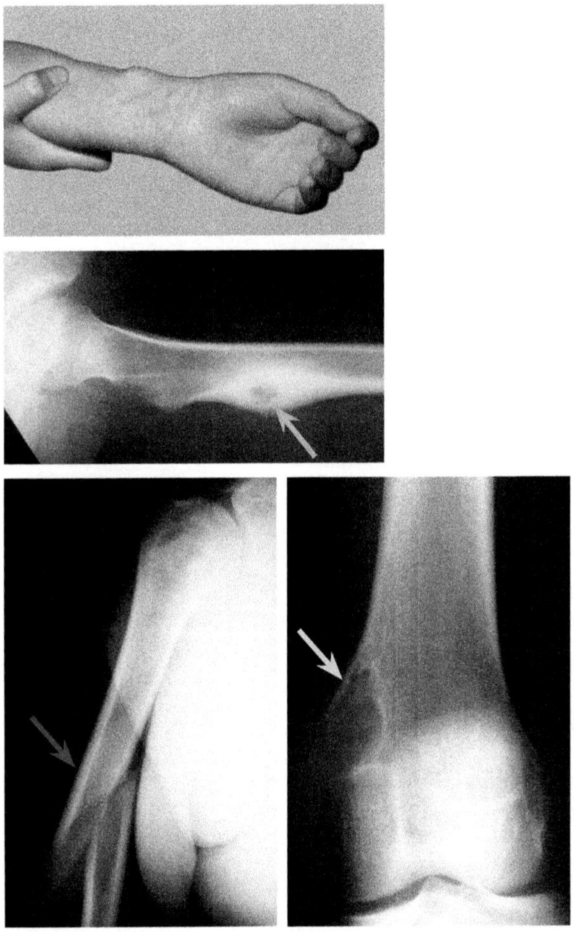

A Presentations of tumors in children The common modes of presentation are with a mass, as in osteochondroma (green arrow); with pain, as in osteoid osteoma (orange arrow); with a pathologic fracture, as in osteosarcoma (red arrow); or as an incidental finding, such as this small nonossifying fibroma (yellow arrow).

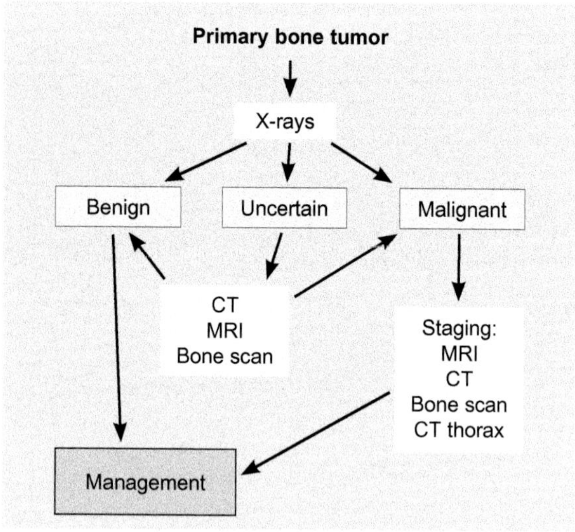

A Flowchart for imaging primary bone tumors

Imaging

Order imaging studies with a plan in mind [A]. Start with good-quality radiographs. Conventional radiographs remain the basic tool for diagnosis. Consider several features in assessment.

Location Lesions tend to occur in typical locations both with respect to the bone involved [B] and the position in the bone [A, next page].

Effect of lesion Note the lesion's effect on the surrounding tissue [C, next page].

Effect of lesion on bone Sharply punched out lesions are typical of eosinophilic granuloma. Osteolytic lesions are typical of most tumors; few are osteogenic on radiographs.

Effect on normal adjacent bone is useful in determining the invasiveness of the lesion. An irregular, moth-eaten appearance suggests a malignant lesion or an infection. A lesion that expands the adjacent cortex is usually benign and typical for aneurysmal bone cysts.

Diagnostic features suggest the aggressiveness of the lesion. Sclerotic margination suggests that the lesion is long-standing and benign. Periosteal reaction suggests a malignant, traumatic, or infectious etiology.

Special imaging Consider special types of conventional radiographs, such as for soft tissue or bone detail [B, next page].

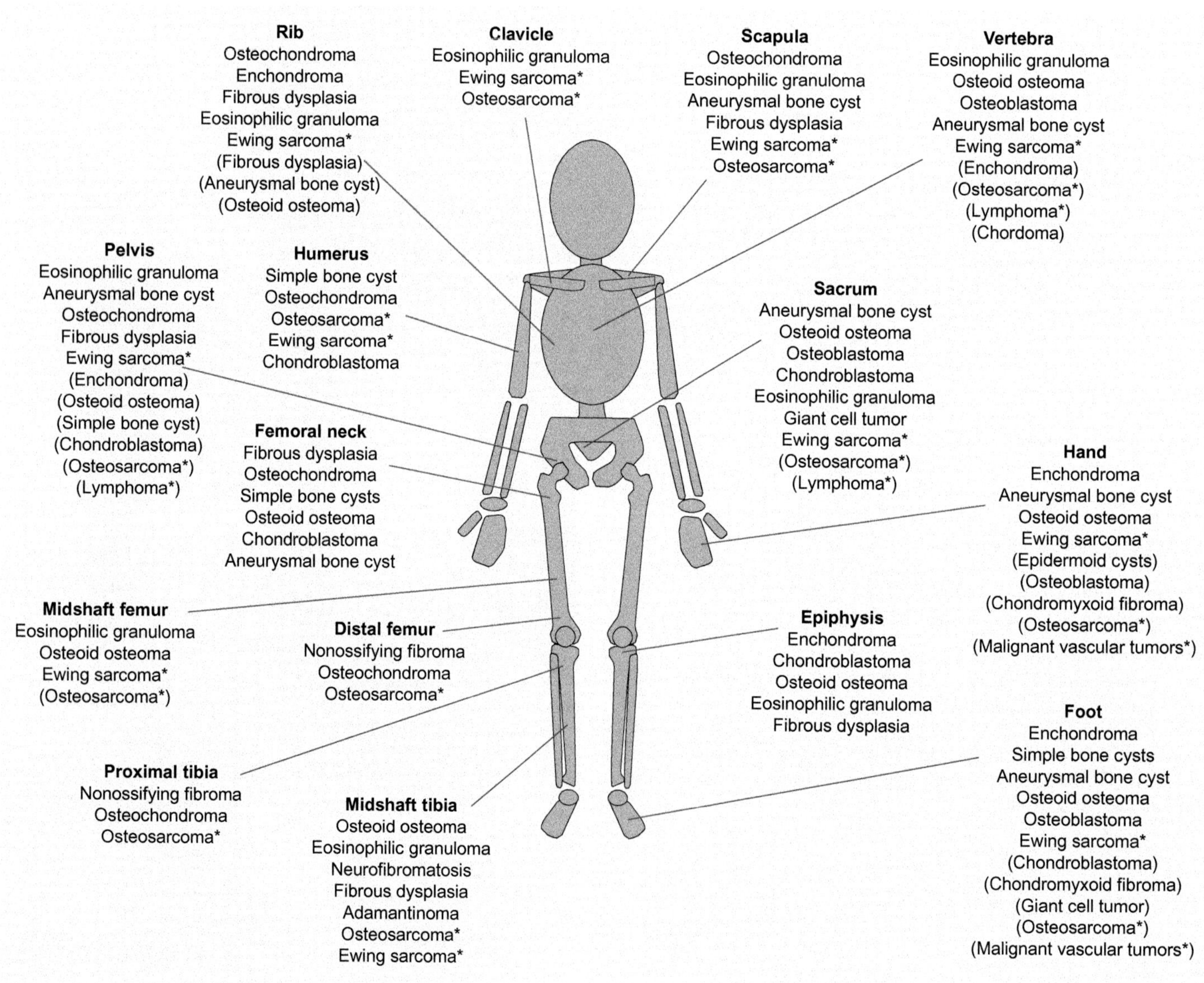

B Tumor types per site Less common tumors at each site are in parentheses. Asterisks (*) indicate malignant tumors. Based on Adler and Kozlowski (1993).

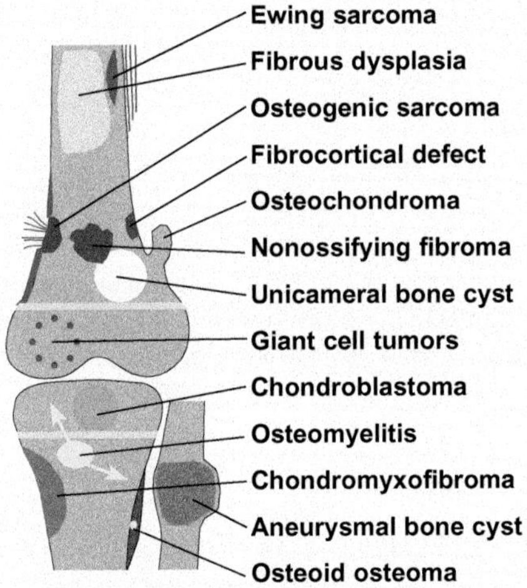

A Typical locations for various tumors Note the location in the epiphysis, metaphysis, or diaphysis.

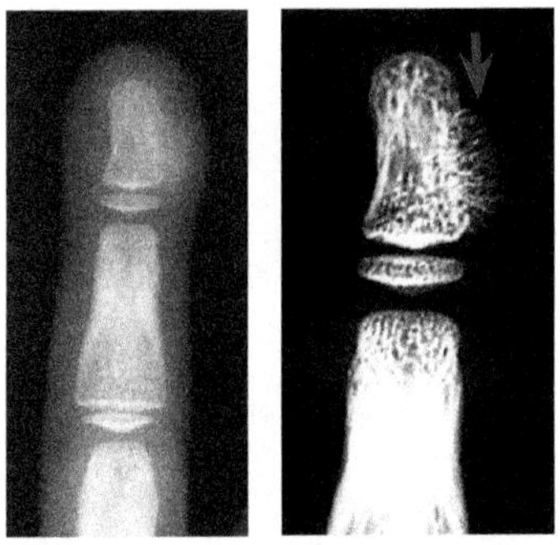

B High-resolution radiographs Compared to conventional radiography (left), note the increased bony detail shown by the high-resolution radiograph (red arrow).

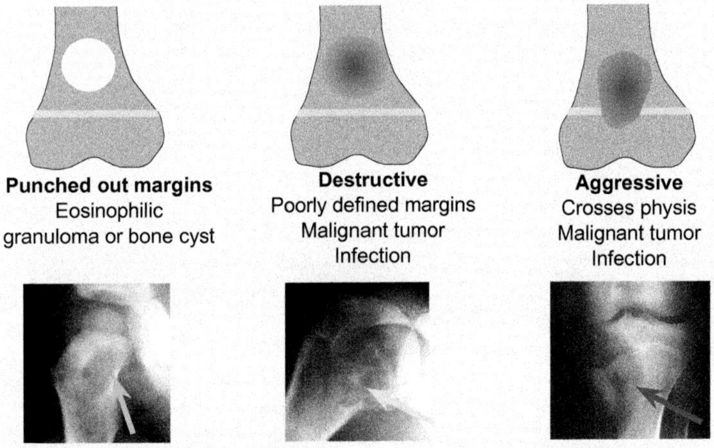

Effect of lesion on bone Bone destruction from eosinophilic granuloma in an infant (green arrow), destructive lesion in osteogenic sarcoma (yellow arrow), and aggressive osteogenic sarcoma that readily crosses the physis (red arrow).

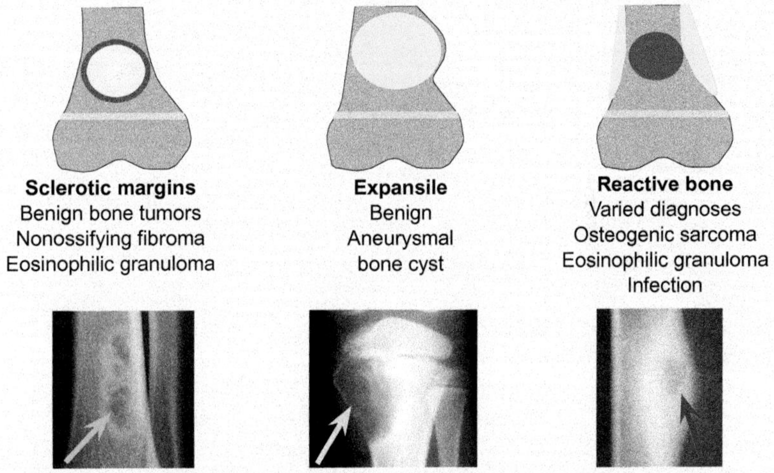

Effect of lesion on normal adjacent tissue Note the sclerotic margins in the nonossifying fibroma (green arrow), expanded cortex in an aneurysmal bone cyst (yellow arrow), and marked periosteal reaction in an eosinophilic granuloma (red arrow).

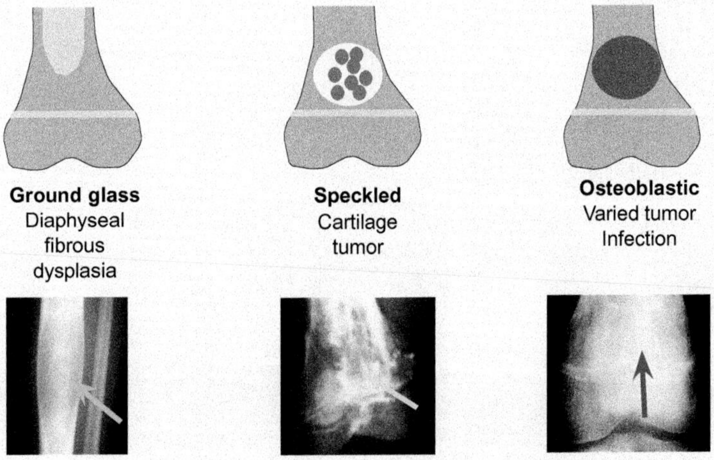

Special diagnostic features of lesion Note the ground glass appearance of fibrous dysplasia (green arrow), speckled calcification in a cartilage tumor (yellow arrow), and osteoblastic features of an osteoblastic osteogenic sarcoma (red arrow).

C Diagnostic features by conventional radiography Note the effect of the lesions on bone (top), the effect on normal adjacent tissues (middle), and special diagnostic features (bottom).

Special studies may be essential to establish the diagnosis [A].

CT scans are useful in assessing lesions of the spine or pelvis. Whole lung CT studies are highly sensitive for pulmonary metastases.

MRI is the most expensive diagnostic tool and is limited in young children due to the need for sedation or anesthesia. However, it is the most sensitive in making an early diagnosis and excellent for tissue characterization and staging of tumors, so it should be made of all malignant soft tissue and bone tumors.

Bone scans are the next most useful diagnostic tools. These scans are helpful in determining whether a lesion is solitary or other lesions are present. The uptake of the lesion is important to note. A cool or cold scan suggests that the lesion is inactive, and only observation may be necessary. Warm scans are common in benign lesions. Hot scans suggest that the lesion is very active and that it may be either a malignant or benign lesion, such as an osteoid osteoma. Biopsy or excision is required.

Positive emission tomography PET scans are expensive but useful in evaluating malignant soft tissue and bone tumors, and especially in assessing the response to chemotherapy.

Laboratory

Complete blood count (CBC) is useful as a general screening battery and helpful in the diagnosis of leukemia.

C-reactive protein (CRP) is elevated in inflammatory conditions.

Erythrocyte sedimentation rate (ESR) is often elevated in Ewing sarcoma, leukemia, lymphomas, eosinophilic granuloma, and infection. ESR values rise more slowly and elevations persist for longer durations than CRP values.

Alkaline phosphatase (AP) values may be elevated in osteosarcoma, Ewing sarcoma, lymphoma, and metastatic bone tumors. The value of the study is limited because of the natural elevation of this value during growth, especially in the adolescent.

Biopsy

A biopsy is a critical step in management and should be performed thoughtfully by an experienced surgeon. In most cases, an open biopsy is appropriate. Needle biopsy is indicated for lesions located at inaccessible sites and for special circumstances. The biopsy should provide an adequate sample of involved tissue, and the tissue should be cultured unless the lesion is clearly neoplastic. The biopsy procedure should not compromise subsequent reconstructive procedures.

Biopsies can be incisional, excisional, or compartmental in type. Excisional biopsy is appropriate for benign lesions such as osteoid osteoma or for other lesions when the diagnosis is known before the procedure and the lesion can be totally resected.

Staging

Staging of malignant tumors provides a means of establishing a prognosis. Prognosis depends on the grade of the lesion (potential for metastases), the extent and size of the lesion, and the response to chemotherapy. The extent of the lesion is categorized by whether the lesion is extracompartmental or intracompartmental [B] and whether any distant metastases are present. A knowledge of the response to chemotherapy helps the surgeon to determine the appropriateness of limb salvage procedures and how wide the surgical margins must be to avoid local recurrence following resection.

Differential Diagnosis

Differentiating myositis ossificans Differentiating bone tumors from myositis ossificans (MO) is sometimes difficult. MO lesions have reactive bone that is most active on the margins. MRI studies are rarely necessary, but will show an inflammatory lesion with a tumor core.

Differentiating neoplasms, infection, and trauma Sometimes a child presents with pain and tenderness over a long bone (usually the tibia or femur). The radiographs may be negative or show only slight periosteal elevation. The differential diagnosis often includes osteomyelitis, a stress fracture, or Ewing sarcoma. The evaluation usually requires a careful physical examination, radiographs, a bone scan, MRI, and a determination of the ESR and CRP.

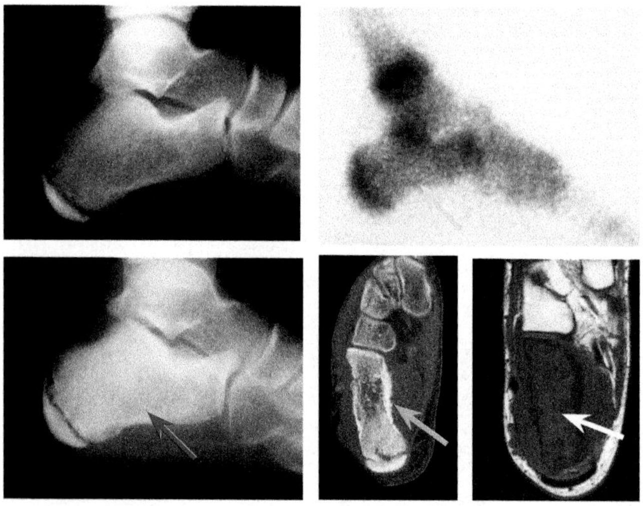

A Evaluation by imaging This child had foot pain and a negative radiograph (upper left). A month later, the patient was seen again because of increasing night pain. At that time, a bone scan showed increased uptake (yellow arrow), the radiograph showed increased density of the calcaneus (red arrow), a CT scan showed erosion of the calcaneus (orange arrow), and MRI showed extensive marrow involvement (white arrow). Ewing sarcoma was suspected by these findings.

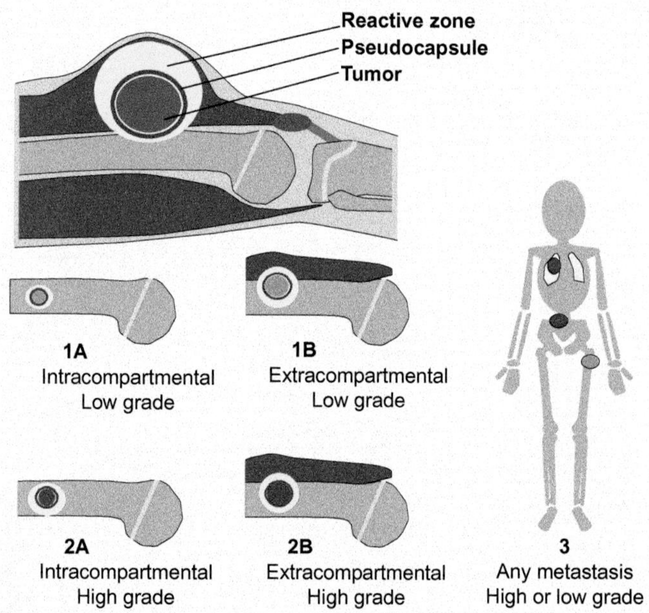

B Staging of musculoskeletal tumors Staging is determined by the grade and extent of the lesion. Intracompartmental lesions are those within a fascial compartment between deep fascia and bone; intraarticular lesions and those within bone. Based on Wolf and Enneking (1996).

Unicameral Bone Cysts

Simple, solitary, or unicameral bone cysts (UBCs) are common lesions of unknown cause that generally occur in the upper humerus or femur [A]. Theories of etiology include a defect in enchondral bone formation or altered hemodynamics with venous obstruction, causing increased interosseous pressure and cyst formation. The cysts are filled with yellow fluid and lined with a fibrous capsule [B].

Diagnosis

UBCs are most often first diagnosed when complicated by pain or a pathologic fracture [C]. Their radiographic appearance is usually characteristic. The lesions are usually metaphyseal, expand the bone, have well-defined margins, evoke little reaction, and appear cystic with irregular septa. Sometimes a fragment of cortical bone (called *fallen leaf sign*) can be seen in the bottom of the cavity.

Active cysts abut the growth plate and occur in children less than 10 to 12 years of age. They are more likely to recur after treatment and are associated with growth arrest that may follow a fracture.

Inactive cysts are separated from the plate by normal bone and usually occur in adolescents over 12 years of age.

Fractures are usually the presenting complaint. Sometimes the fracture line is difficult to separate.

Management Principles

Management is complicated by recurrence. The usual natural history of these cysts is to become asymptomatic following skeletal maturation. The objective of treatment is to minimize the disability when cysts are likely to fracture. These lesions are not precancerous.

Humeral cysts Place the child in a sling to allow the fracture to heal and to reestablish stability. Seldom does the effect of the trauma result in permanent healing of the cyst. Plan to manage the cyst by a series of injections [D] with steroid, bone marrow, or bone matrix. Some doctors recommend breaking up the adhesion by forceful injections or perforating the septa with a trochar. Recurrence can be managed by repeated injections or curettage and grafting with autogenous or bank bone. Opinions differ regarding how aggressively recurrence is managed.

Femoral cysts are much more difficult to manage because of the load carried by the femur. Plan to curette and graft the cyst and stabilize the fracture with flexible intramedullary fixation. Complications include malunion with coxa vara and avascular necrosis with displaced neck fractures. This fixation is permanent and may prevent additional fractures even if some recurrent cyst formation occurs. An alternative approach is injection followed by spica cast protection for 6 weeks.

Calcaneal cysts asymptomatic cysts may be managed by observation. Symptomatic or expanding cysts may do better by curettage and bone grafting. Small lesions may be treated by injection [E].

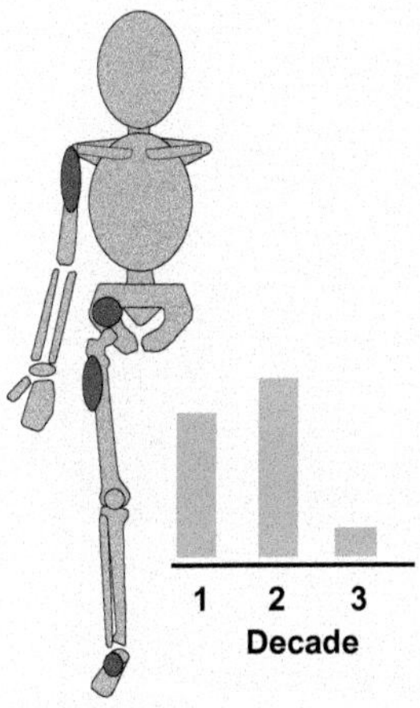

A Unicameral bone cysts Common locations (red) and age pattern of involvement (blue) are shown.

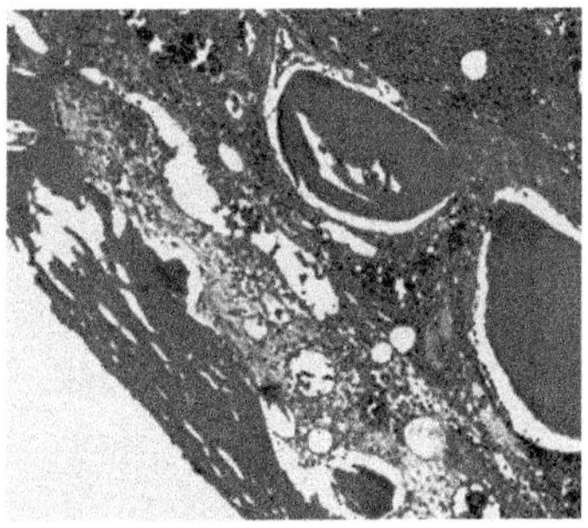

B Unicameral bone cyst lining This shows the synovial lining of a cyst wall.

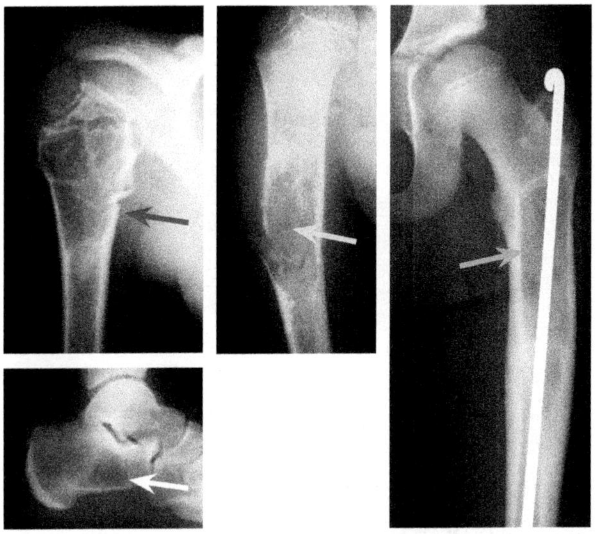

C Unicameral bone cysts in varied locations Note the typical active (red arrow) and inactive (yellow arrow) cysts with fractures. Flexible intramedullary rod fixation of an upper femoral cyst (orange arrow) is shown. A calcaneal cyst is an additional common site (white arrow).

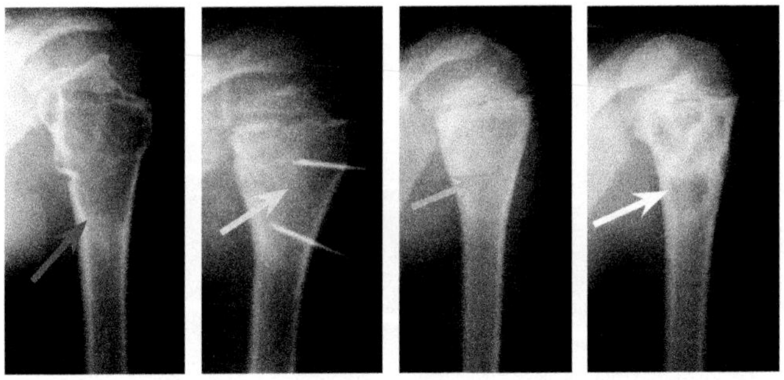

D Steroid injection treatment This is the classic location for a unicameral bone cyst. This 12-year-old boy developed pain in the right upper arm; a radiograph showed the typical cyst with a pathologic fracture (red arrow). The lesion was treated by steroid injection (yellow arrow) with satisfactory healing (orange arrow). A year later, the cyst recurred (white arrow), but not to a degree that required additional treatment.

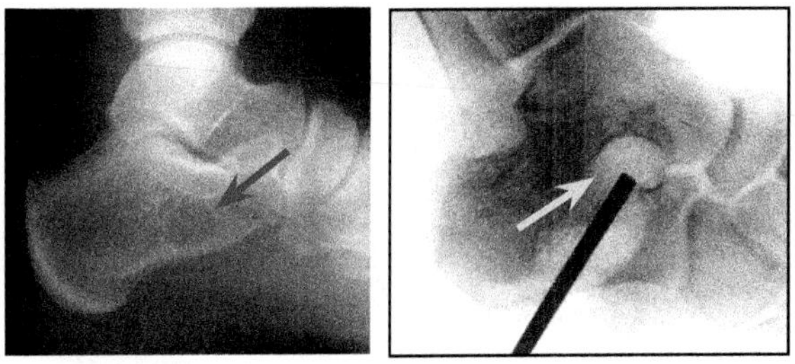

E Small calcaneal unicameral bone cyst This 14-year-old complained of pain and demonstrated a limp. X-rays demonstrated a small cystic lesion (red arrow). This was managed by perforating the cortex and septa with a trochar and injecting bone marrow (yellow arrow).

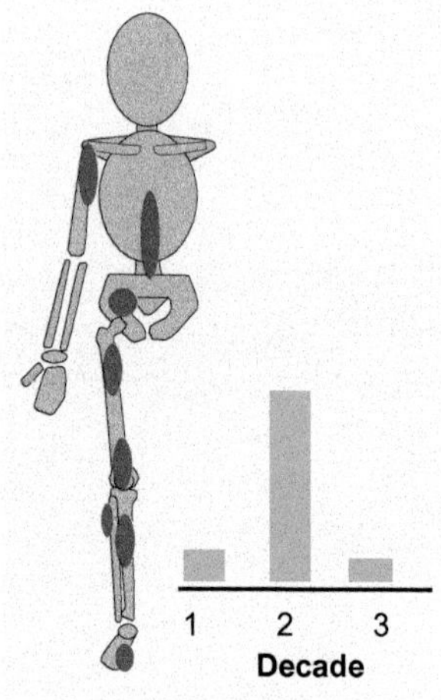

A Aneurysmal bone cysts Common locations (red) and age pattern of involvement (blue) are shown.

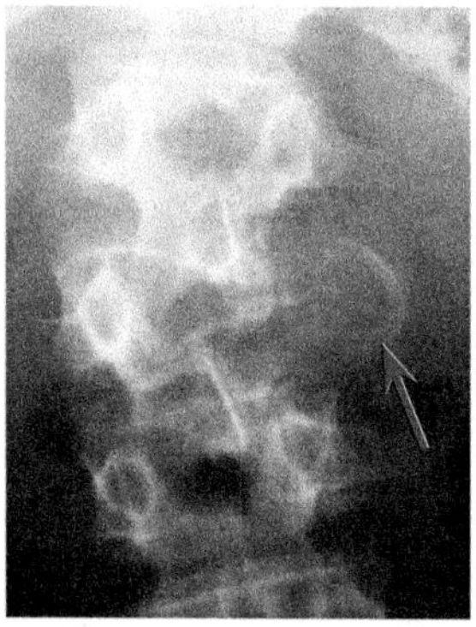

B Aneurysmal bone cyst of the vertebral column

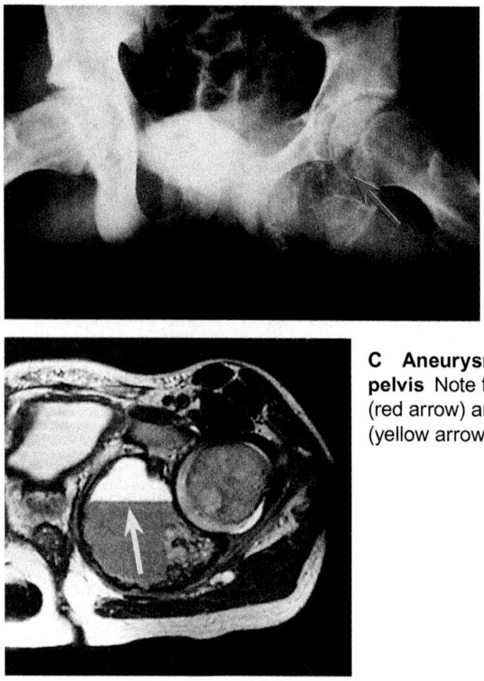

C Aneurysmal bone cyst of the pelvis Note the extensive lesion (red arrow) and the fluid level (yellow arrow) on the MRI.

Aneurysmal Bone Cysts

An aneurysmal bone cyst (ABC) is considered to be a pseudotumor possibly secondary to subperiosteal or interosseous hemorrhage or a transitional lesion secondary to some primary bone tumor.

Diagnosis

The diagnosis can usually be established by a combination of the location of the lesion, the age of the patient [A], and the appearance on conventional radiographs [B]. ABCs are eccentric, expansile, cystic lesions with a high recurrence rate. Lesions present in a variety of patterns and are sometimes difficult to differentiate from simple bone cysts [D].

Activity of the lesion The activity level can also be assessed by the appearance of the lesion's margins.

Inactive cysts have intact, well-defined margins.

Active cysts have incomplete margins but the lesion is well defined.

Aggressive cysts show little reactive bone formation and poorly defined margins.

Other imaging is often necessary, especially in aggressive cysts. Fluid levels are common and can be seen on CT scans and MRI studies [C].

Management

Manage ABCs on the basis of the patient's age, as well as the site and size of the lesion.

Spine About 10–30% of ABC lesions are in the spine. They most commonly occur in the cervical and thoracic levels. Lesions arise in the posterior elements but may extend to involve the body. Study posterior elements with CT and MRI preoperatively. The possible need for a combined approach, complete excision, and stabilization, as well as the risk of recurrence, complicates management.

Long bones Options include complete excision or saucerization, leaving a cortical segment intact, or curettage with cryotherapy or with a mechanical burr.

Pelvis Manage most lesions by curettage and bone grafting. Some recommend selective embolization. Be prepared for extensive blood loss.

Complications Bleeding can pose a significant problem.

Recurrence may require more aggressive management that might include more extensive excision. Expect a recurrence rate of 20–30% following curettage. Recurrence is 10-60% higher in children under 10 years of age.

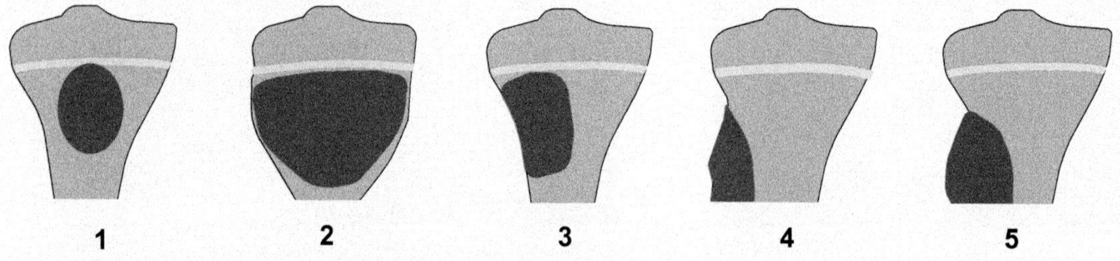

D Classification of aneurysmal bone cysts. Types 1–5 are various common patterns of lesions of long bones. Based on Capanna et al. (1985).

Fibrous Tumors

Fibrocortical Defects

Fibrocortical defects (or *fibrous metaphyseal defects*), fibrous lesions that are the most common bone tumor, occur in normal children, produce no symptoms, resolve spontaneously, and are found incidentally. They occur at the insertion of a tendon or ligament near the epiphyseal growth plate, which may be related to the etiology. They have a characteristic appearance that is eccentric and metaphyseal, with scalloped sclerotic margins. These lesions often cause concern that sometimes leads to inappropriate treatment. Fortunately, the lesions have a characteristic radiographic appearance that is usually diagnostic. They are small, cortical in location, and well-delineated by sclerotic margins. They usually resolve spontaneously over a period of 1 to 2 years.

Nonossifying Fibroma

A larger version of the fibrocortical defect is called a *nonossifying fibroma*. These lesions are present in classic locations and are usually diagnosed during adolescence [A]. They are metaphyseal, eccentric with scalloped sclerotic margins [B and C], and may fracture when large or if present in certain locations. Manage most by cast immobilization. Resolution of the lesion occurs with time. Rarely, curettage and bone grafting are indicated if the lesion is unusually large or if a fracture through the lesion occurs with minimal trauma.

Fibrous Dysplasia

Fibrous dysplasia includes a spectrum of disorders characterized by a common bony lesion. The neoplastic fibrosis replaces and weakens bone, causing fractures and often a progressive deformity. Ribs and the proximal femur are common sites, and the lesions are most common in adolescents [D].

Fibrous dysplasia can be monostotic or polystotic. The polystotic form is more severe and is more likely to cause deformity. This deformity is often most pronounced in the femur, where a "shepherd's crook" deformity is sometimes seen [E], and may show extensive involvement of the femoral diaphysis. Rarely, fibrous dysplasia is associated with café-au-lait skin lesions and precocious puberty, as described with Albright syndrome.

Medical management using drugs that inhibit osteoclastic activity have not been widely used in children but offer an alternative to surgical management.

Surgical management of fibrous dysplasia involves strengthening weakened bone using flexible intramedullary rods. Leave these rods in place indefinitely to prevent fractures and progressive deformity [E].

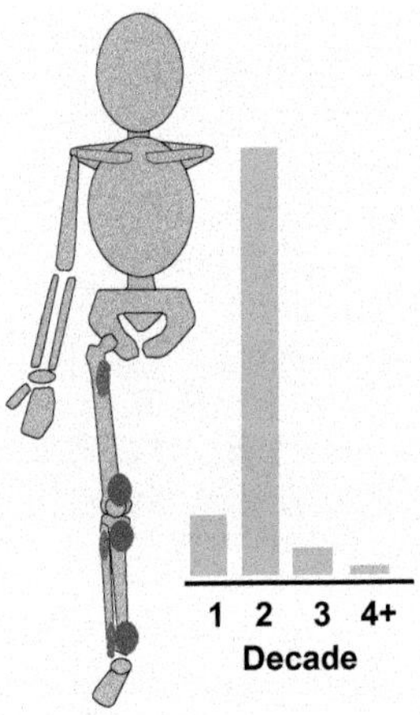

A Nonossifying fibroma Common (red) and less common (gray) locations are shown. Age pattern of involvement is shown in blue.

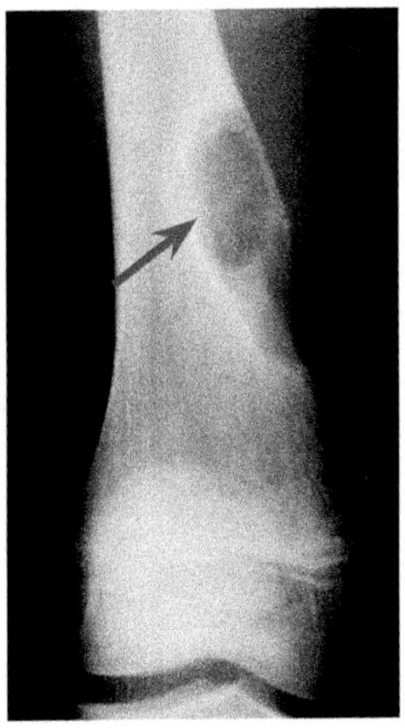

B Nonossifying fibroma of the distal femur

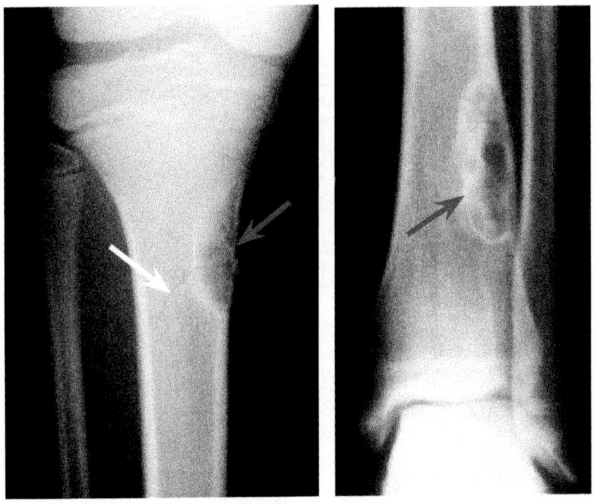

C Typical nonossifying fibroma These are typical features and locations (red arrows). Note the fracture line (white arrow) through the proximal tibia, with its origin in the fibroma.

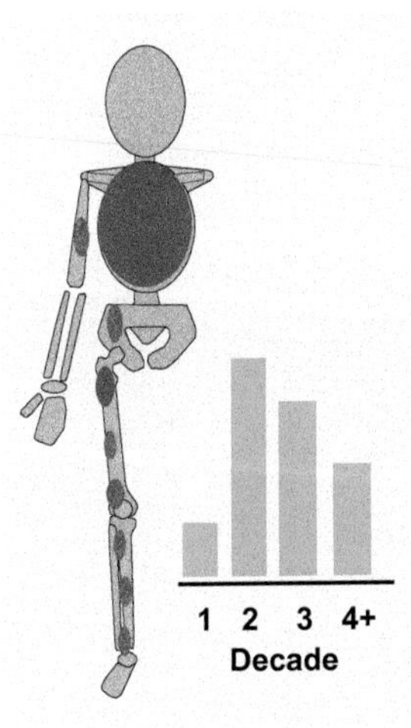

D Fibrous dysplasia Common (red) and less common (gray) locations are shown. Age pattern of involvement is shown in blue.

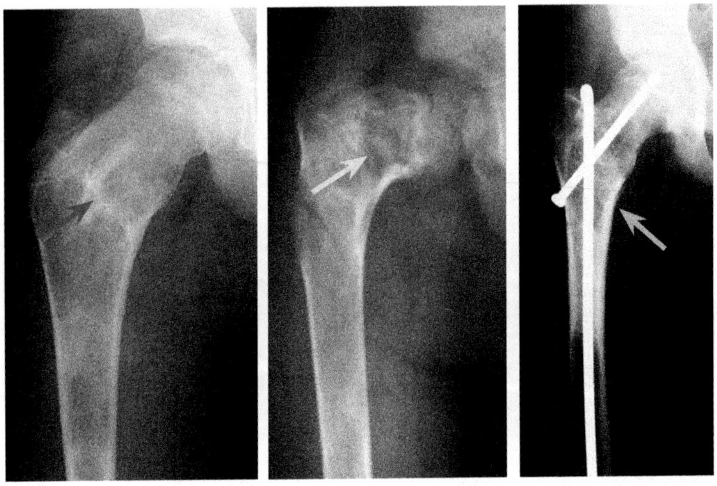

E Fibrous dysplasia of proximal femur These patients show a femur at risk for deformity (red arrow), varus deformity (yellow arrow), and intramedullary fixation to prevent deformity (orange arrow).

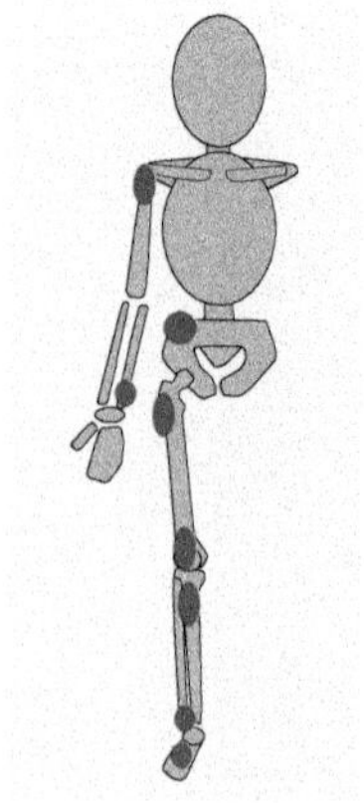

A Common locations of solitary osteochondromas

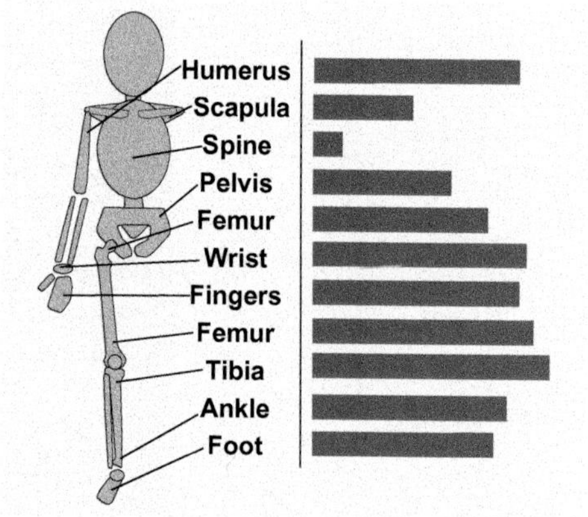

B Multiple familial osteochondromas Note the widespread involvement. Based on data by Jesus-Garcia (1996).

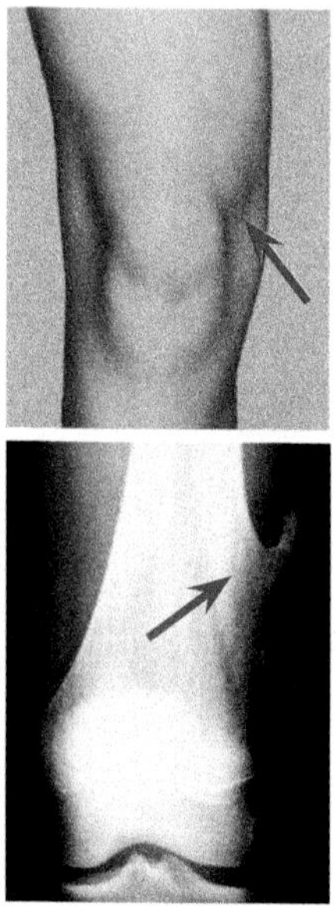

C Typical location for symptomatic lesions Lesions about the knee are frequently irritated and painful (red arrows).

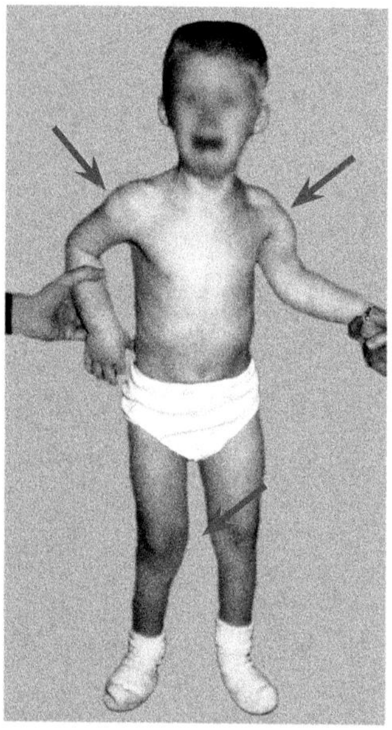

D Multiple osteochondromas This child has multiple lesions (arrows).

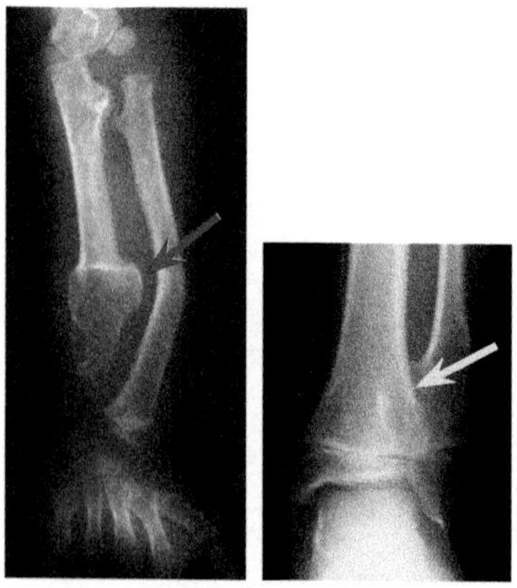

E Common deformities that cause disturbed growth These are common about the wrist (red arrow) and ankle (yellow arrow).

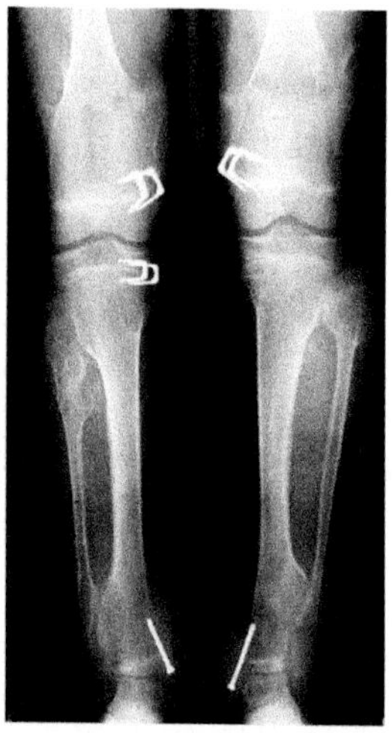

F Deformity correction Correction of knee and ankle valgus by placement of staples and medial malleolus screws.

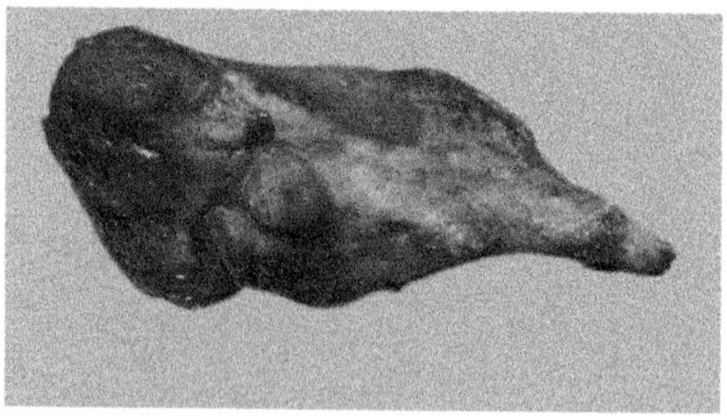

G Removed osteochondroma This resected lesion is large and irregular.

Benign Cartilagenous Tumors

Osteochondroma

Osteochondromas (osteocartilagenous exostoses) include solitary [A] and multiple [B] lesions. The multiple form is inherited but thought to be due to a loss or mutation of two tumor suppressor EXT 1 and 2 genes. Lesions sometimes develop after chemotherapy and radiation therapy. Most tumors develop by enchondral ossification under a cartilage cap.

Diagnosis Osteochondromas are usually first noted as masses that are painful when injured during play [C]. These lesions are usually pedunculated but may be sessile. They may grow to a large size. Osteochondromas are so characteristic in appearance that the diagnosis is made by conventional radiographs.

Solitary osteochondromas These lesions are most common in the metaphyses of long bones. They occur sporadically and present as a mass, often about the knee. Presentations in the spine may be associated with neurologic dysfunction.

Multiple osteochondromas The common multiple form [D] is inherited in an autosomal dominant pattern and is more common in boys. Multiple lesions about the wrist and ankle often cause progressive deformity [E]. Others may cause valgus deformities about the knee.

Management depends on the location and size of the tumor.

Pain is the most common indication for removal [G]. Often several lesions are removed in one operative setting. Complications of excision include peroneal neuropraxia, arterial lacerations, compartment syndromes, and pathologic fracture.

Valgus knee can be managed by medial femoral or tibial hemistapling [F] in late childhood.

Limb length inequality may require correction by an epiphysiodesis.

Wrist deformities result from growth retardation and bowing of the distal ulna. Management of these deformities is complex and controversial. Studies in adults show surprisingly little pain and functional disability, considering the magnitude of the deformity and the unsightly appearance.

Ankle deformities result from growth retardation of the distal fibula, producing ankle valgus. Studies in adults show significant disability and suggest that prevention or correction of tibiotalar valgus should be undertaken in late childhood or adolescence. Consider resecting the osteochondroma and performing an opening wedge osteotomy of the distal tibia to correct the valgus. When identified in childhood, consider placing a medial malleolar screw [F] to prevent excessive deformity. Deformities are often complex, and operative correction must be individualized.

Prognosis Very rarely, malignant transformation to chondrosarcoma occurs during adult life. This transformation is most common in solitary lesions, usually from lesions involving flat bones, and occurs about two decades earlier than primary chondrosarcomas. Most tumors are low grade. Because the transformation is very rare, prophylactic removal of exostoses is not appropriate.

Enchondroma

These cartilage tumors are located within bone. They are common in the phalanges and long bones and increase in frequency during childhood [A]. They produce the classic characteristic of cartilage tumors of speckled calcification within the lesion [B].

Types There are several different types of enchondromas.

Solitary lesions occur most commonly in the hands [C] and feet. Removal and grafting is indicated if the lesions cause disability.

Ollier disease is a generalized disorder with cartilaginous enchondromas as one feature. Children with Ollier disease often have limb shortening and varus deformities [B] involving one side of the skeleton. About one-fourth develop chondrosarcoma in adult life.

Maffucci syndrome is a rare disorder with subcutaneous hemangiomatas and multiple enchondromas. Malignant transformation is not uncommon in adult life.

Chondromyxoid Fibroma

This is a rare primary bone tumor that occurs mostly about the knee during the second decade. The radiographic appearance is often characteristic [D] with an eccentric position, a sclerotic rim with lobulated margins, and prominent septa. Manage with local resection and grafting.

Chondroblastoma

These uncommon tumors occur in the epiphysis of long bones often during adolescence [E]. They occur most commonly in the upper humerus, femur, and tibia. They can be confused with infection or arthritis. They are aggressive and prone to recur. Treat by thorough curettage and possibly cryotherapy or phenolization and bone grafting. Operative injury to the growth plate or articular cartilage is due to the juxtaarticular location. Anticipate local recurrence in about 20% of lesions.

Dysplasia Epiphysialis Hemimelica

Dysplasia epiphysialis hemimelica (Trevor disease) is a rare cartilaginous tumor that arises from the growth plate or articular cartilage [F]. The most common sites of involvement are the distal tibia and the distal femur. Lesions often involve one side of the epiphysis and may show multilevel involvement in the same limb. The diagnosis is often difficult early on, as the lesion is primarily cartilaginous and poorly imaged with conventional radiographs. MRI is helpful in showing the extent of the tumor and separating the lesion from the normal epiphysis or joint cartilage. Excise extraarticular lesions. Remove intraarticular lesions and correct secondary deformity with an osteotomy as necessary. Recurrence of the tumor is common, due to its periarticular location and extensive involvement of adjacent bone. Multiple resections throughout childhood are often necessary.

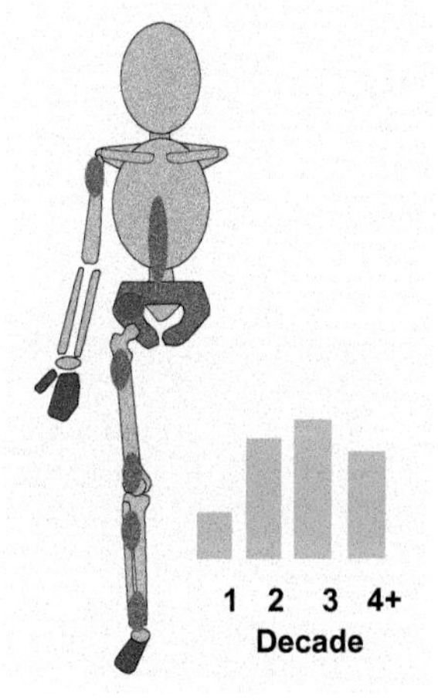

A Enchondromas Common (red) and less common (gray) locations are shown. Age pattern of involvement is shown in blue.

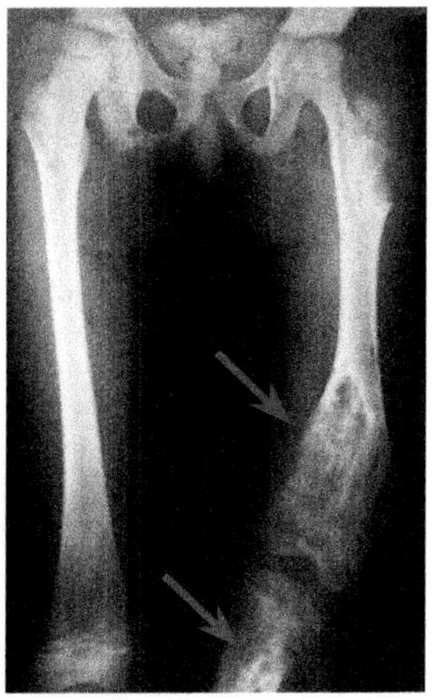

B Ollier disease Note the extensive lesions of the distal femur and tibia (red arrows) with shortening and varus deformity.

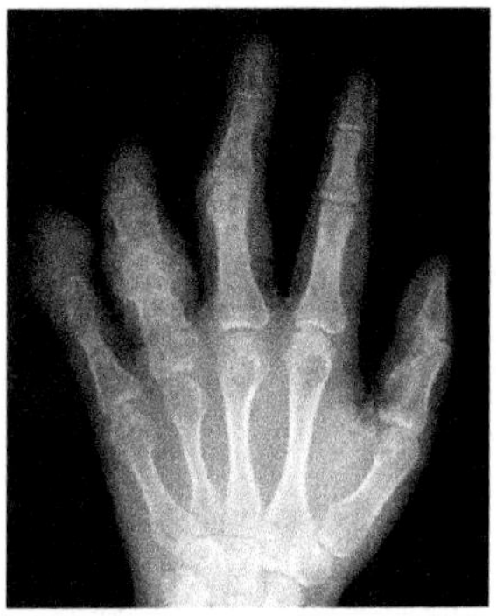

C Multiple enchondromas Note the extensive involvement of several fingers.

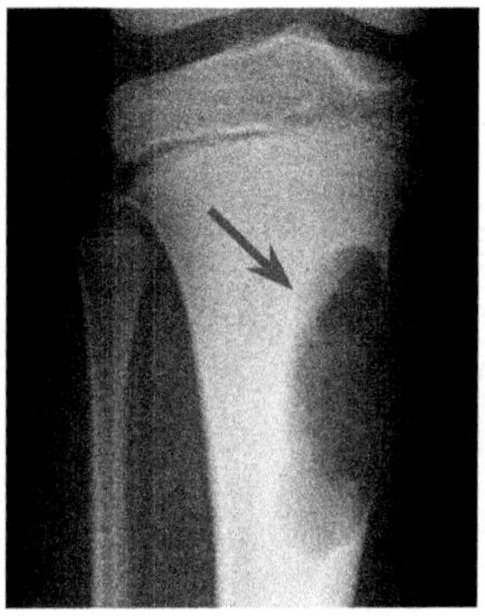

D Chondromyxoid fibroma Note the characteristic features.

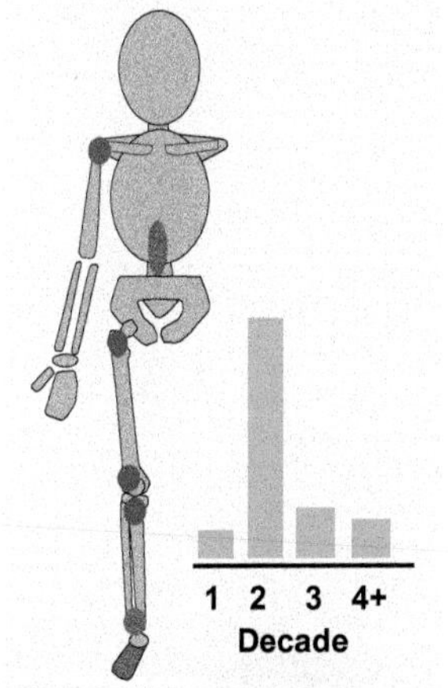

E Chondroblastoma Common (red) and less common (gray) locations are shown in the drawing. Age pattern of involvement is shown in blue. Based on Schuppers (1998). Radiographs (below) show typical locations in the epiphysis of the greater trochanter (red arrow) and proximal tibia (white arrow). Note that the proximal tibial lesion is aggressive, as it crossed the physis (yellow arrow).

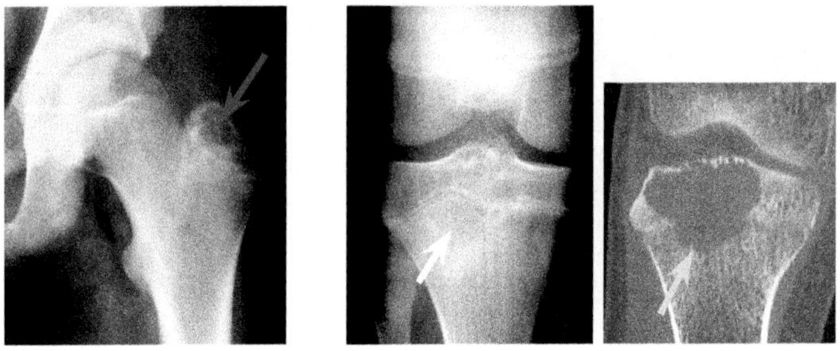

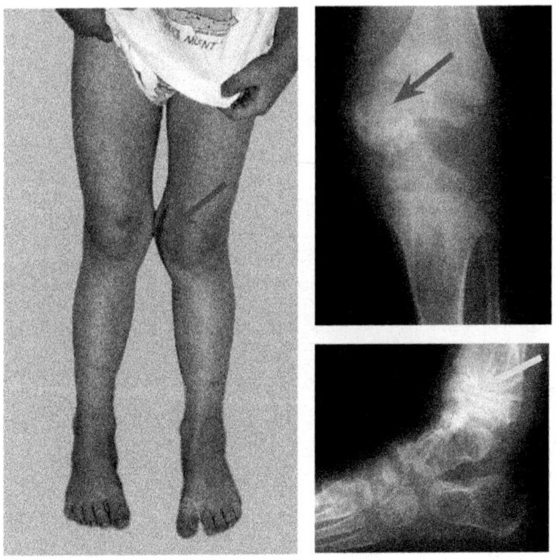

F Dysplasia epiphysialis hemimelica Note the swelling of the knee (red arrows) and ankle involvement (yellow arrow).

Osseous Tumors

Osteoid Osteoma

This benign, bone-producing, highly vascular tumor induces an intense bony reaction and a characteristic pain pattern. These tumors occur most commonly in long bones during the second decade [A].

Diagnosis The pain typically occurs at night, is well localized, and is often relieved by aspirin. Spine lesions occur in the posterior elements of the spine and may cause secondary scoliosis. Lesions are tender and, if close to a joint, cause joint inflammation that may be confused with primary arthritis. Lesions may cause hemideossification due to chronic pain and a limp [B]. The radiographic appearance is often characteristic for well-established lesions. A radiolucent nidus is surrounded by reactive bone [C]. The bone scan is diagnostic, with intense localized uptake at the nidus. Image with MRI and CT scans to fully evaluate the lesion.

Management New options for management supplement the traditional approach of open excision.

Antiinflammatory Lesions eventually resolve over many years. This option is rarely acceptable to families.

Percutaneous ablation using CT for localization and radio frequency ablation is preferred in most cases [D].

Open excision is a reasonable option but carries a significant risk of an incomplete resection and local recurrence.

Osteoblastoma

This benign bone-producing tumor is similar to the osteoid osteoma but larger and shows clear differences. Pain is less intense and not relieved by aspirin. Lesions are not surrounded by reactive bone. These lesions occur in the spine and long bones most frequently during the second decade [E]. One-third of these lesions occur in the spine [F], causing back pain and often scoliosis and sometimes localized tenderness. Laboratory studies are normal. CT and bone scans are useful. They are sometimes difficult to differentiate from osteosarcoma. Spinal lesions are most difficult to manage because of the adjacent vertebral artery in a cervical spine lesion. Manage by complete resection. Expect a recurrence rate of about 20–30%.

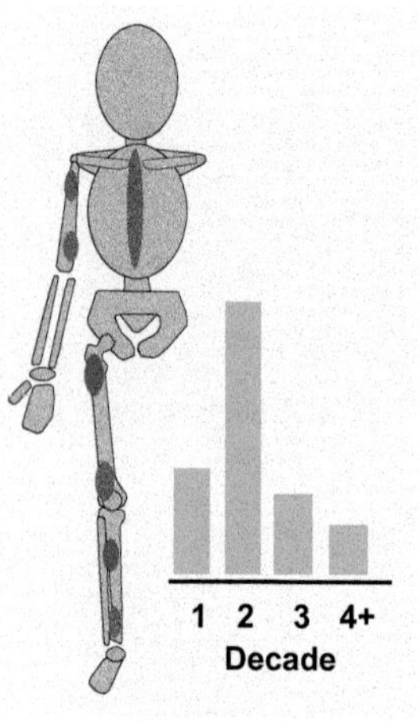

A Osteoid osteoma Common (red) and less common (gray) locations are shown. Age pattern of involvement is shown in blue.

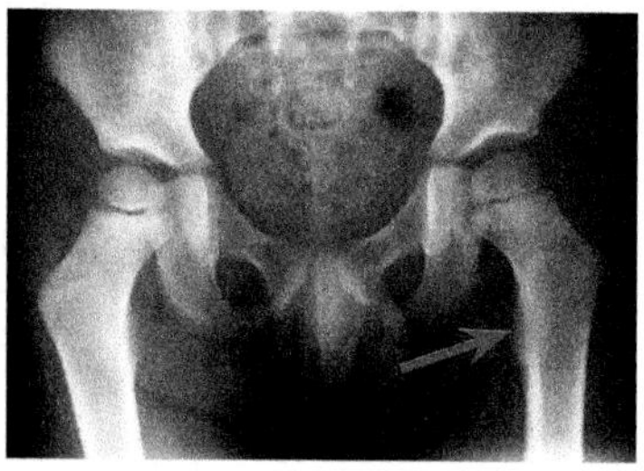

B Osteoid osteoma Note the hemideossification of the left pelvis and femur. This is due to pain and limp over a period of months from a proximal femoral lesion.

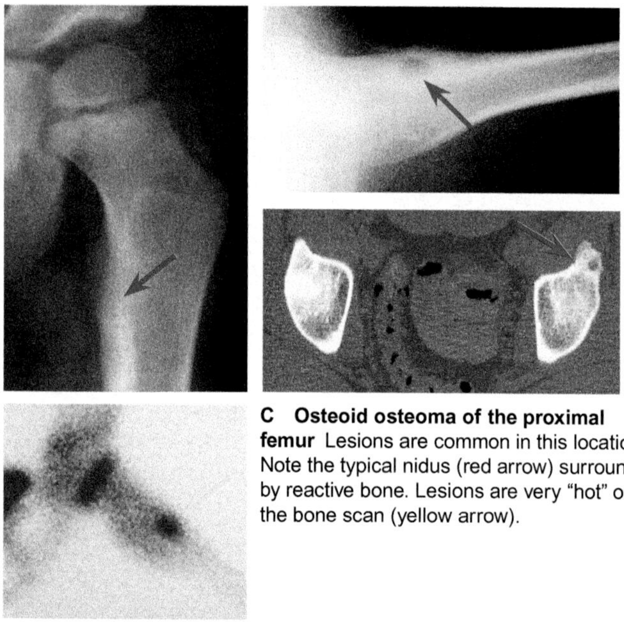

C Osteoid osteoma of the proximal femur Lesions are common in this location. Note the typical nidus (red arrow) surrounded by reactive bone. Lesions are very "hot" on the bone scan (yellow arrow).

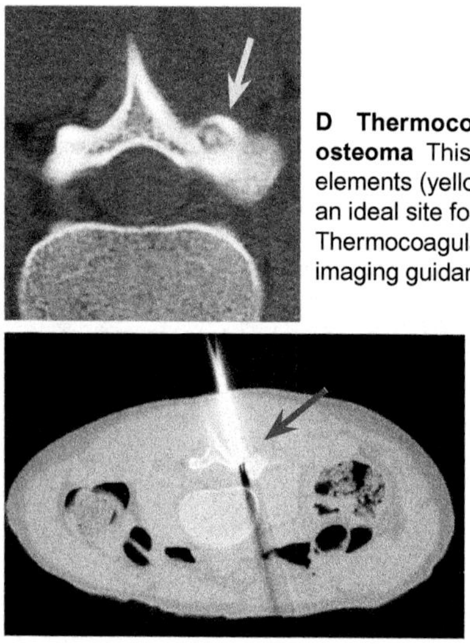

D Thermocoagulation of osteoid osteoma This lesion of the posterior elements (yellow arrow) is located in an ideal site for percutaneous ablation. Thermocoagulation was performed under CT imaging guidance (red arrow).

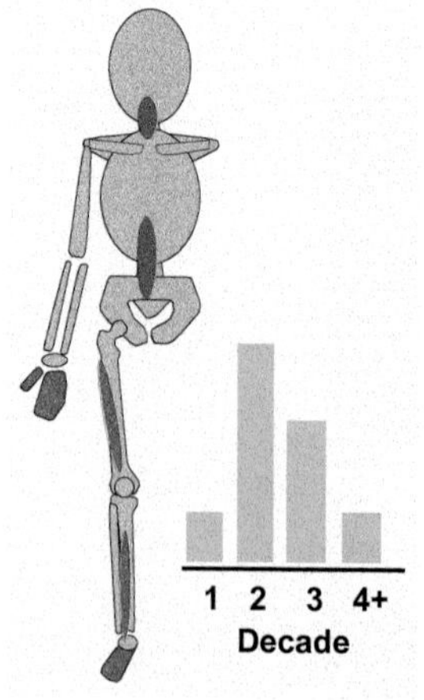

E Osteoblastomas Common (red) and less common (gray) locations are shown. Age pattern of involvement is shown in blue.

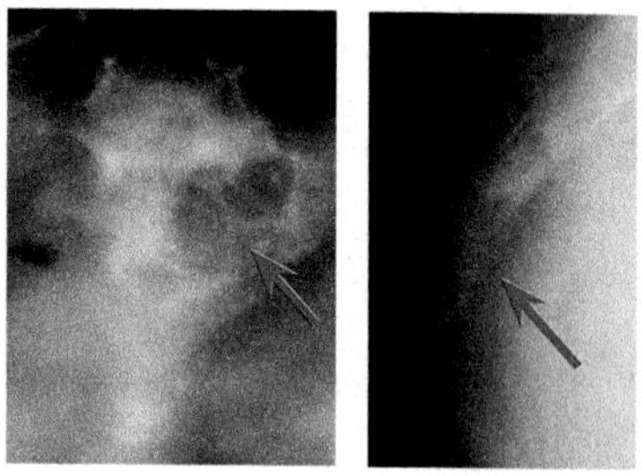

F Osteoblastoma of the sacrum

Miscellaneous Bone Tumors

Eosinophilic Granuloma

Eosinophilic granuloma is the localized form of Langerhans' cell histiocytosis or histiocytosis X.

Diagnosis The peak age of onset is between 1 and 3 years of age [A]. This tumor has been described as the "great imitator" of bone tumors. Lesions are painful and are most often confused with osteomyelitis or sometimes Ewing sarcoma. Lesions often appear "punched out" on conventional radiographs [B and C], but sometimes elicit periosteal reactions, suggesting a sarcoma. The child may have a low-grade fever and elevated ESR and CRP, making the differentiation from an infection difficult. Consider ordering skull films because the skull is the most common site of bony involvement. Sometimes the diagnosis must be established by biopsy.

Management The natural history is of spontaneous resolution over a period of many months. Management options include simple observation, immobilization to improve comfort and reduce the risk of pathologic fracture, injection with steroid, limited curettage, or radiation treatment.

Spine lesions cause collapse (vertebra plana) and sometimes neurologic involvement. Manage by observation or brace immobilization. Rarely, curettage is necessary to hasten resolution.

Lower limb long-bone lesions, if large enough, may pose a risk of pathologic fracture. Curettage and cast protection may be appropriate.

Giant Cell Tumors

Giant cell tumors (GCT) are aggressive tumors that occasionally occur in adolescents. Lesions are usually metaphyseal or epiphyseal, eccentric, expansive, and show little sclerosis or periosteal reaction [D]. These tumors are locally invasive and often recur. Manage by curettage, thermoablation, and grafting. Provide careful follow-up because recurrence develops in about a quarter of cases.

Neurofibroma

Neurofibromatosis causes widespread pathology [E], including scoliosis, pseudoarthrosis of long bones, thoracic lordoscoliosis, protrusio acetabuli, and abnormal bone growth (see details in Chapter 12).

Osseous Hemangioma

This is often present in the vertebrae or skull but may appear in the extremities [F]. Lesions are diffuse and suggest a malignant tumor [G]. Wide resection is necessary, and recurrence is common.

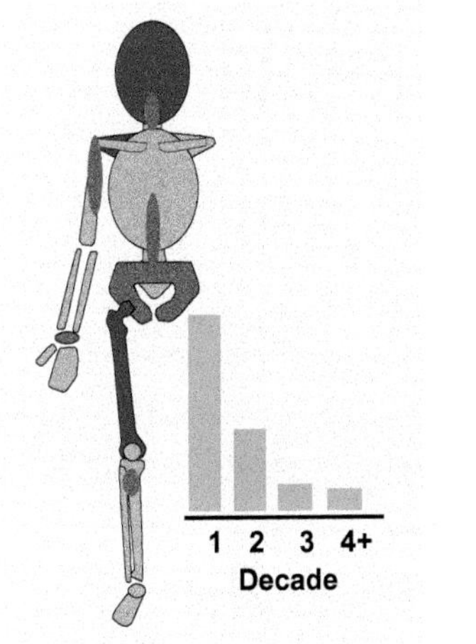

A Eosinophilic granuloma Common (red) and less common (gray) locations are shown. Age pattern of involvement is shown in blue.

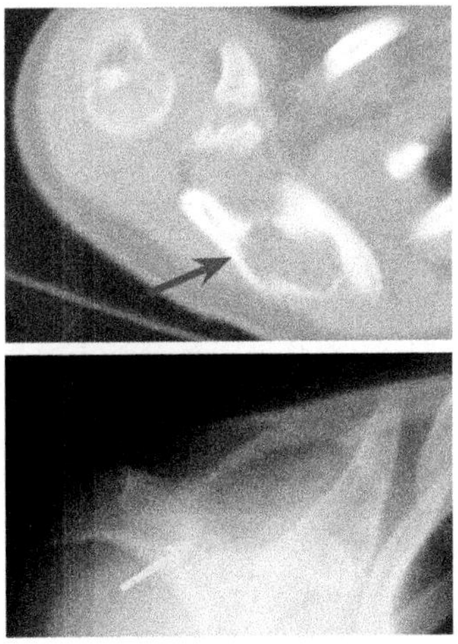

B Eosinophilic granuloma of the scapula This lesion is shown by CT scan (red arrow) and conventional radiograph (yellow arrow).

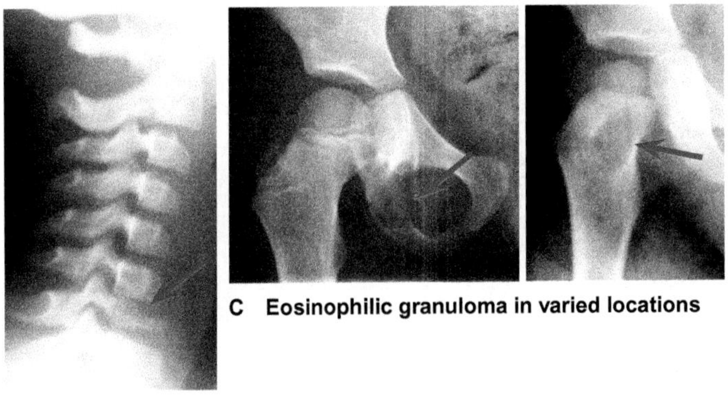

C Eosinophilic granuloma in varied locations

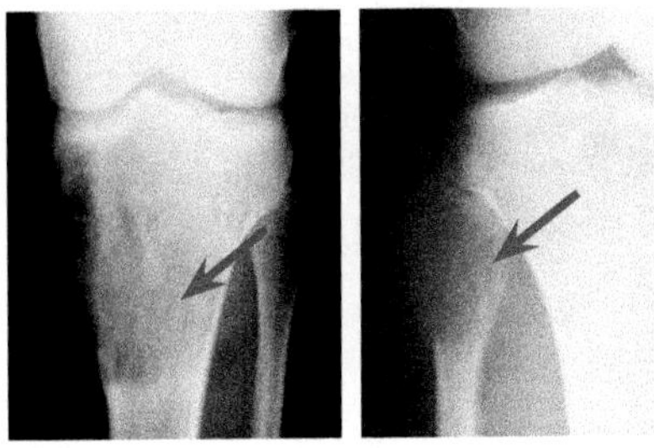

D Giant cell tumor of bone These lesions (arrows) occurred shortly after the end of growth. Note the lack of periosteal reaction.

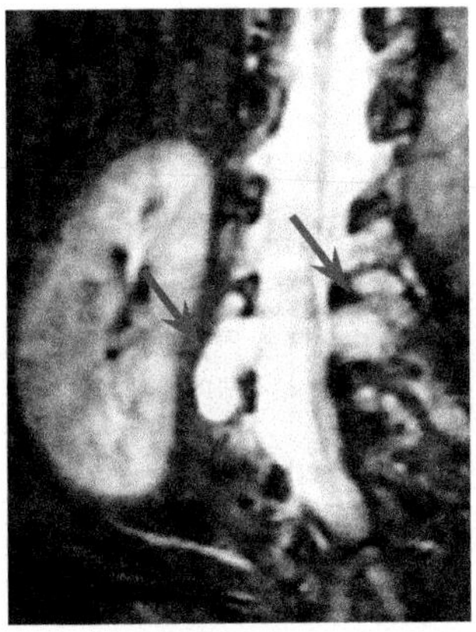

E Neurofibromatosis Note the dural ectasia (red arrows).

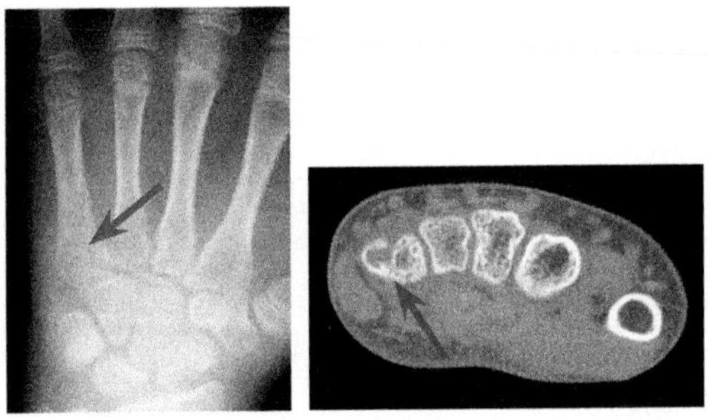

F Hemangioma of bone This hemangioma involved the fifth metacarpal, which was painful clinically and destructive in its radiographic appearance (red arrows).

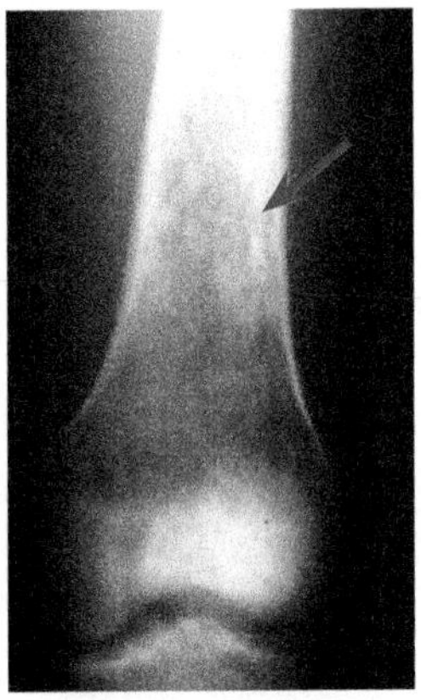

G Hemangioma of bone These lesions (arrow) are often difficult to differentiate from malignant lesions.

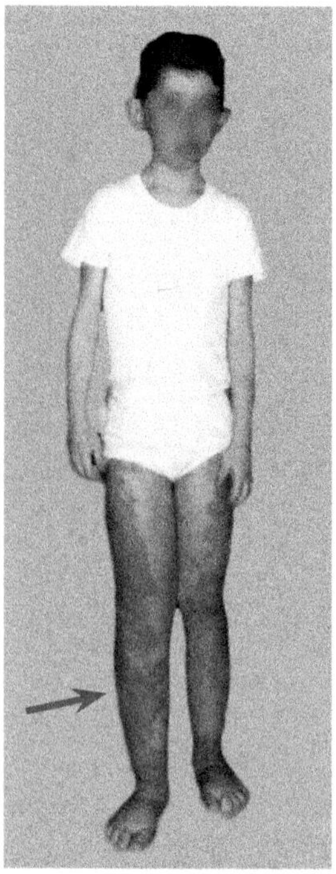

A Hemangioma This boy has Klippel-Weber-Trenaunay syndrome with extensive hemangioma and limb hypertrophy (red arrow).

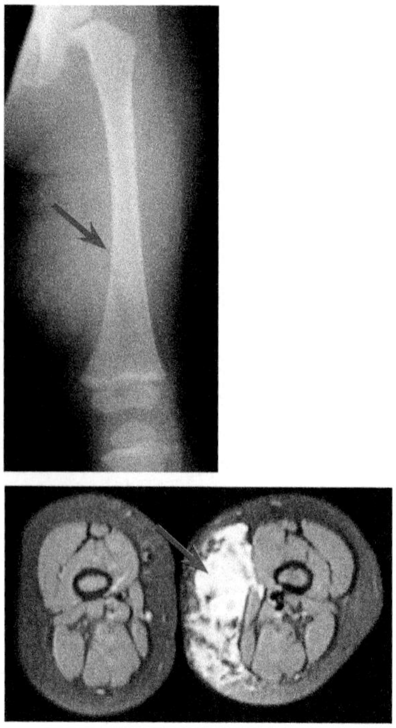

B Extensive thigh hemangioma This large lesion involves much of the medial thigh muscles (red arrows).

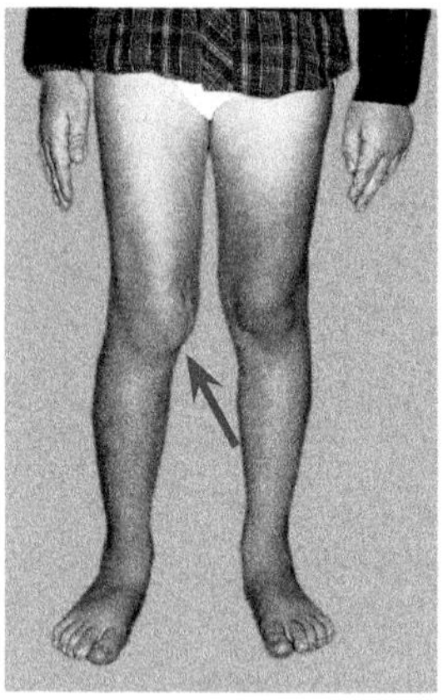

C Synovial hemangioma This child had a swollen knee with frequent bloody effusions. Repeated resections over a period of many years were required.

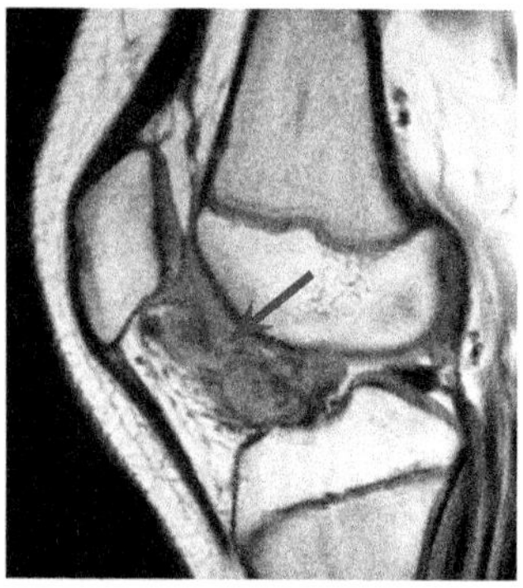

D Pigmented villonodular synovitis This lesion presented with a pain and joint swelling.

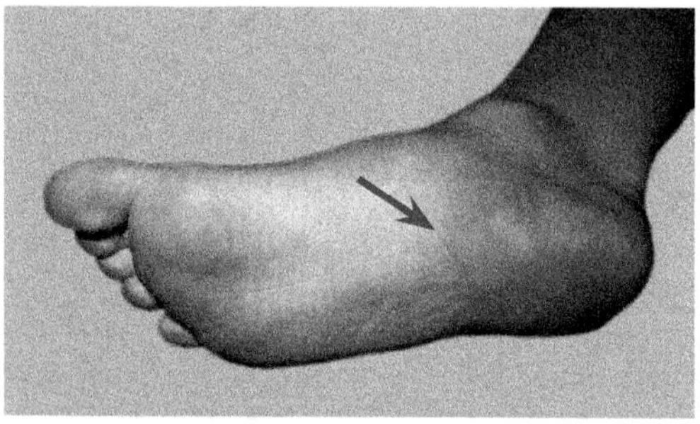

E Plantar fibromatosis Note the plantar thickening with overlying thickening of the skin.

Benign Soft Tissue Tumors

Hemangioma

Hemangiomas are common during childhood. They may be part of a systemic condition [A] or an isolated lesion [B].

Diagnosis The clinical features depend on the location and size of the lesions. Subcutaneous lesions are usually locally tender. Intramuscular lesions cause pain and fullness, and very large or multiple lesions may cause overgrowth or bony deformity.

Imaging Punctate calcification in the lesion is diagnostic. CT and MRI are most useful for diagnosis and preoperative planning.

Management Many patients are diagnosed clinically and treated symptomatically. Large and very painful lesions may require resection. Resection is often difficult, as the lesions are poorly defined and may be extensive. Recurrence is common.

Synovial Hemangioma

Hemangioma of the knee is a cause of pain and recurrent hemarthroses in the pediatric age group [C]. The diagnosis may be delayed and the condition misdiagnosed as an internal derangement of the knee. Historically, long delays in diagnosis have occurred. Conventional radiographs show soft tissue swelling. MRI is usually diagnostic. Diffuse lesions are difficult to excise arthroscopically, and open wide excision is often required. Recurrence is common.

Pigmented Villonodular Synovitis

These lesions are rare in children. They should be considered in the differential diagnosis of a hemarthrosis of joints. They occur in varied sites, may involve joints [D] and tendon sheaths, can be multifocal, and may present as popliteal cysts. Manage by total synovectomy. Recurrence is common.

Plantar Fibroma

Fibromas may occur in infants with a lump on the anteromedial portion of the heel pad. Most remain small and asymptomatic, some disappear, but most persist, and if painful require excision.

In the child, plantar fibroma usually occurs as nodular thickening of the plantar fascia [E]. Observe to determine the potential for enlargement. Resect enlarging lesions. Be aware that mitotic figures are common in the specimen. Recurrence is frequent, and overtreatment is common. Differentiating fibrosarcoma from desmoid tumors is difficult.

Other Tumors

A variety of other tumors occur in childhood, including lipomas [F], lymphangiomas, and benign fibrous tumors.

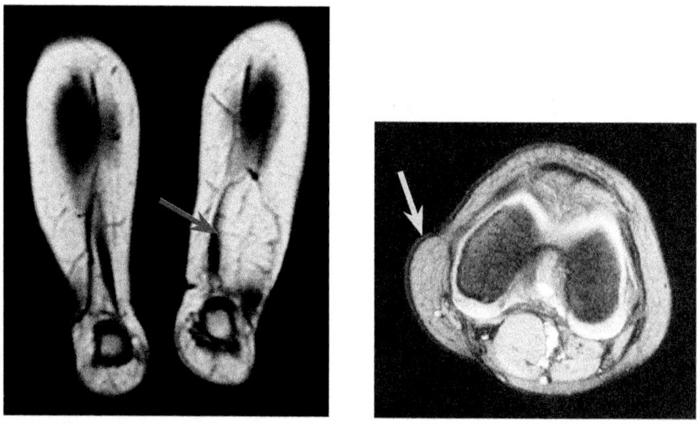

F Lipoma Note the large lipoma (red arrow) of the distal leg in a 16-month-old infant, and the smaller, more typical lesion in a subcutaneous location (yellow arrow) in a child.

Malignant Soft Tissue Tumors

These tumors account for about 7% of malignant tumors of childhood. About half are rhabdomyosarcomas. These soft tissue malignancies are divided into five general categories [A]. Features that suggest a soft tissue lesion to be malignant include being firm, deep, nontender, and greater than 5 cm in diameter.

Rhabdomyosarcoma

This is a sarcoma of the skeletal muscle. It is the most common pediatric soft tissue sarcoma [B]. Extremity tumors account for 20% and carry a poorer prognosis.

Lesions are firm, nontender, and within the muscle compartment [C]. Tumors occur in childhood, and metastasize to lymph nodes and later to bone. Manage by total excision and chemotherapy. Expect the 5-year survival to be in the 65–75% range.

Malignant Fibrous Tumors

Desmoid tumors or fibromatosis are sometimes considered to be benign. However, because of their high rate of recurrence, they are sometimes considered as low-grade fibrosarcomas. Most occur in the extremities, creating a soft tissue mass and sometimes erosion or deformity of the adjacent bone [D]. The natural history of fibromatoses is variable; lesions often recur and undergo spontaneous remission. Fibromatoses seldom metastasize or cause death.

Manage by total resection when possible. If surgical margins cannot be achieved without sacrificing the limb or its function, excisional resection is an acceptable alternative. The role of adjuvant chemotherapy is controversial. Radiation therapy is effective but often complicated by growth arrest when the radiation field includes centers of bone growth.

Synovial Sarcoma

These tumors occur most commonly in adolescents [E] and adults. Most occur in the lower extremities. The tumor may be confused with a synovial cyst. Primary metastases are usually to regional lymph nodes or the lungs. Manage by chemotherapy, nonmutilating resection, and radiation. Expect 70–80% survival.

Round Blue Cell Tumors

These tumors include primitive neuroectodermal tumors, soft tissue Ewing sarcomas, and Askin tumors. Askin tumors are round-cell tumors involving the central axis and chest wall.

Miscellaneous Sarcomas

Peripheral nerve sheath sarcomas Malignant degeneration occurs in 5–10% of patients with neurofibromatosis (NF1). Enlarging lesions in these patients should be documented by MRI and excised or biopsied.

Other sarcomas These include a variety of tumors [F]: leiomyosarcoma, liposarcoma, angiosarcoma, and many others.

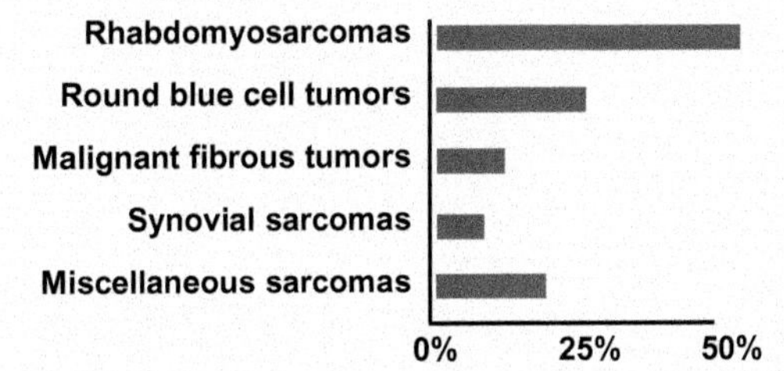

A Soft tissue sarcomas From data of Conrad et al. (1996).

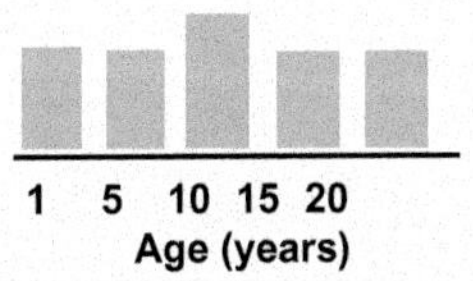

B Rhabdomyosarcoma age distribution These tumors are common in infancy and early childhood.

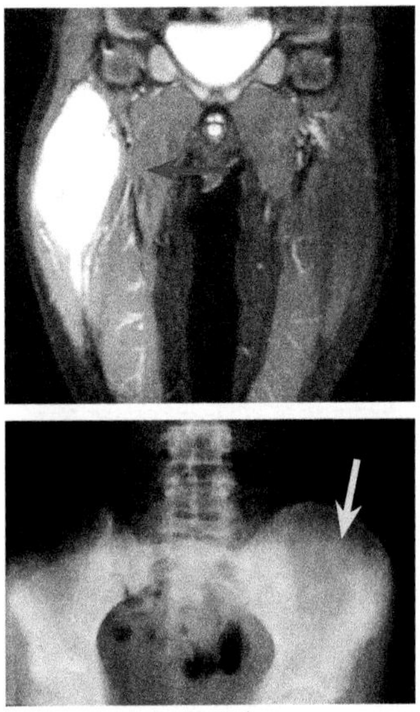

C Rhabdomyosarcomas These tumors develop within muscle compartments (red arrow). Rarely, they spread to bone (yellow arrow).

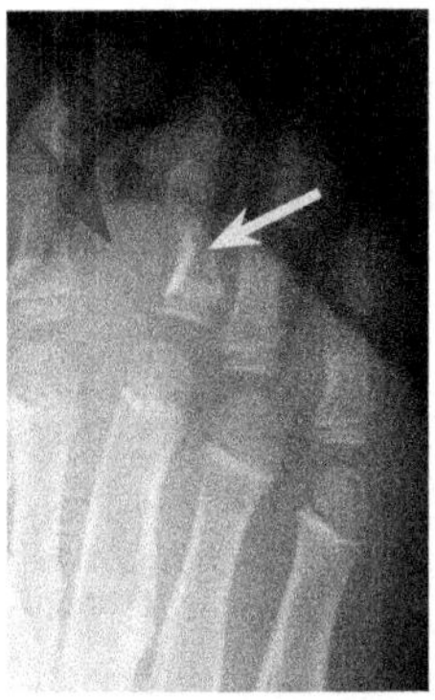

D Desmoid tumors Note the large soft tissue mass (red arrow) and deformation of the second proximal phalanx (yellow arrow).

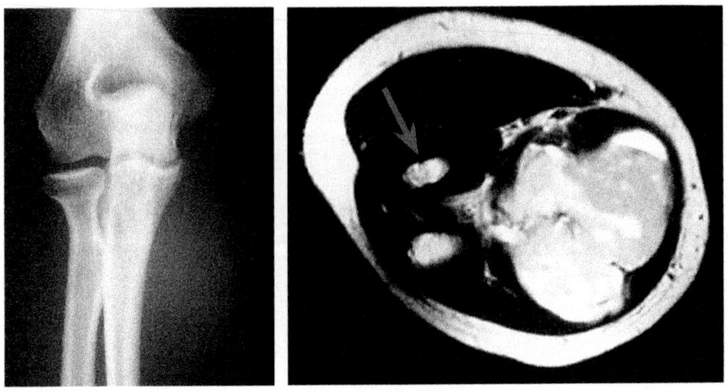

E Synovial sarcoma This lesion in a 16-year-old boy involving the elbow joint is poorly seen on conventional radiographs but readily imaged by MRI (red arrow).

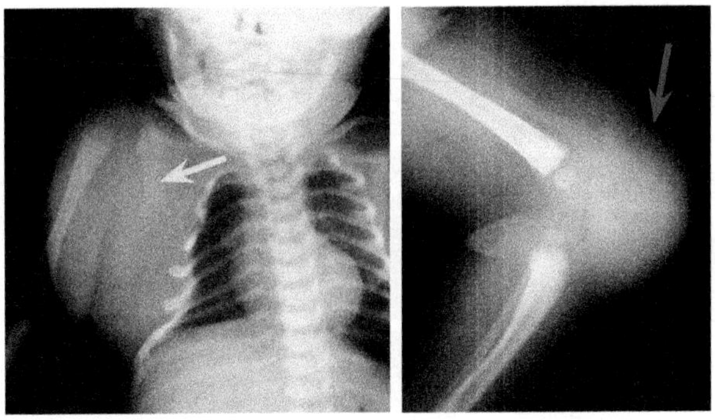

F Soft tissue malignancies in infants This liposarcoma (red arrow) and fibrosarcoma (yellow arrow) have become massive lesions.

Feature	Osteosarcoma	Ewing sarcoma
Activity pain	85%	64%
Night pain	21%	19%
History minor trauma	47%	26%
Palpable mass	39%	34%
Diagnosis: tendonitis	31%	21%
Delayed diagnosis	9 weeks	19 weeks

A Presenting features of childhood bone tumors Differences in presentation of the two common childhood bone tumors are shown. Based on Widhe B and Widhe T. JBJS 82A:667, 2000.

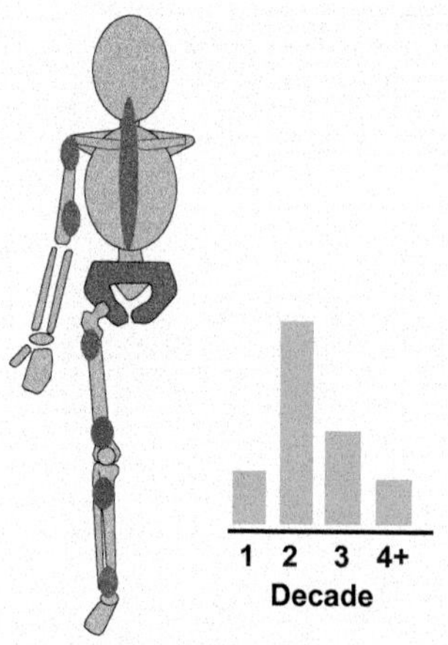

B Osteosarcoma Common (red) and less common (gray) locations are shown. The age of onset is shown in blue.

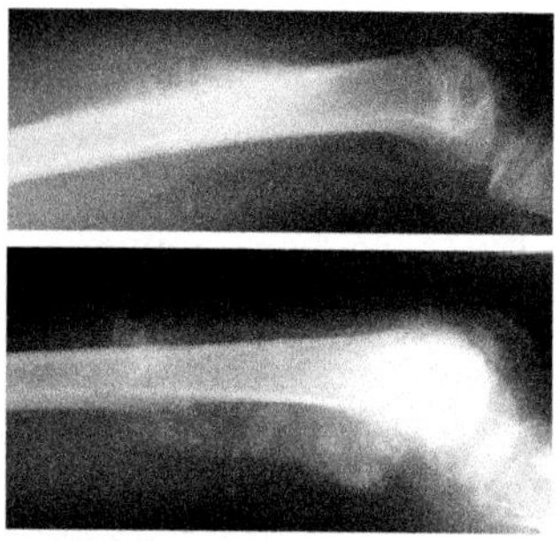

C Classic radiographic appearance of osteosarcoma These studies show the classic osteogenic features of the lesion in the most common location.

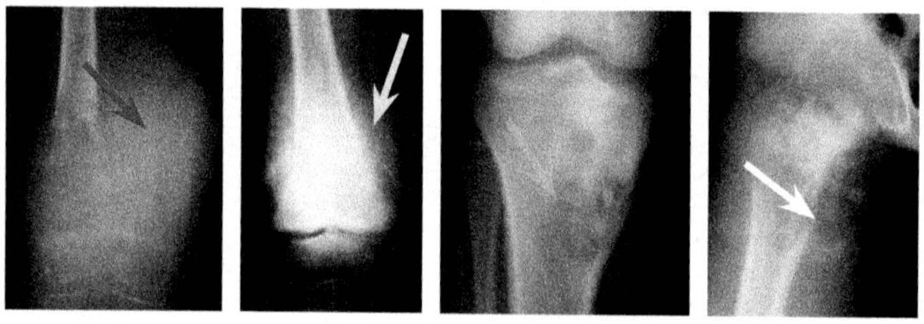

D Varied radiographic appearance of osteosarcoma Lesions may be destructive (red arrow), osteogenic (yellow arrow), cause a moth-eaten appearance (orange arrow), or show combined osteoblastic and lytic features (white arrow).

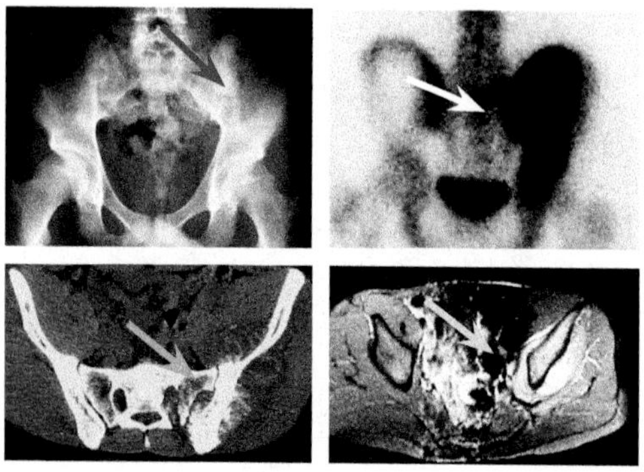

E Osteogenic sarcoma of the pelvis Note that the lesion is not readily identified on conventional radiographs (red arrow), but it is well imaged by bone scan (white arrow), CT (orange arrow), and MRI (yellow arrow).

Malignant Bone Tumors

The early diagnosis of malignant bone tumors is an important factor in improving survival. The features of osteosarcoma and Ewing sarcoma at presentation should be kept in mind [A]. A careful history and physical examination are important. Be aware that the history of pain is often intermittent, especially for Ewing sarcoma, and a misleading history of minor trauma is common. About a third of the patients present with a palpable mass.

Osteosarcoma

Osteogenic sarcoma is the most common malignant tumor of bone. Primary osteosarcoma occurs in children and adolescents, with a peak incidence at age 14 years.

Diagnosis Osteosarcoma commonly occurs during the second decade of life and often occurs about the knee [B]. Pain with activities and a palpable mass are often early findings. Sometimes the patient presents with a pathologic fracture.

For pain lasting more than 6 weeks, consider evaluating by an x-ray and/or ESR and CRP studies. Radiographs may show the classic features of an osteogenic lesion [C]. Lesions may be either an osteolytic or osteogenic lesion of metaphyseal bone [D]. Bone scans are helpful in identifying other affected sites. CT and MRI are helpful in assessing the osseous and soft tissue components of the lesion and in staging the tumor [E]. The histology [F] shows tumor cells with primitive bone matrix formation.

Variants Osteosarcoma has several types with prognostic significance.

Parosteal osteosarcoma These well-differentiated lesions develop on the surface of the bone, such as the posterior femoral metaphysis, with little or no medullary involvement. Manage by wide local resection.

Periosteal osteosarcoma develops on long tubular bones, especially the tibia and femur. In contrast to parosteal osteosarcoma, periosteal osteosarcoma is less differentiated, resulting in a poorer prognosis.

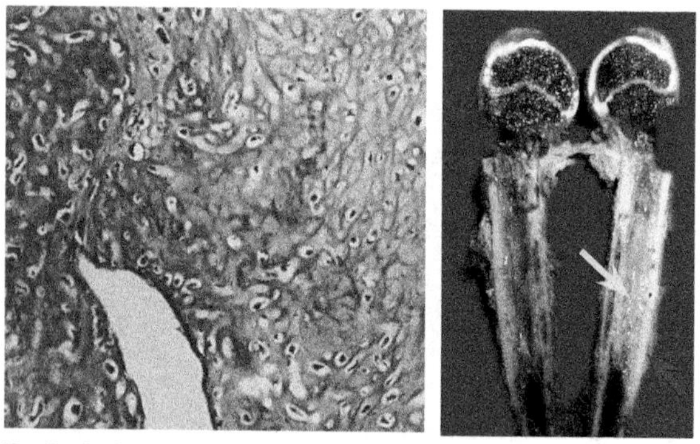

F Pathology of osteosarcoma This photomicrograph (left) shows tumor cell and primitive bone matrix formation. The gross specimen of the proximal humerus from an adolescent (right) shows the intramedullary tumor (yellow arrow) and periosteal new bone formation (red arrow).

Ewing Sarcoma

Ewing sarcoma is the second most common childhood malignant bone tumor.

Diagnosis The tumor is most common in the second decade [A] and occurs most commonly in the pelvis, femur, and tibia [B]. These tumors cause pain and sometimes present with a soft tissue mass. The lesion is usually diaphyseal [C] and osteolytic or permeative in character. Bone scans and MRI are useful. Because the tumor may cause fever, leukocytosis, anemia, and an elevated sedimentation rate, it can be confused with osteomyelitis. Confirm the diagnosis by biopsy. This is a very malignant round cell tumor [D].

Management Management principles are similar for both osteosarcoma and Ewing sarcoma [E]. In general, Ewing sarcoma is primarily managed by chemotherapy and resection and often adjunctive radiation therapy.

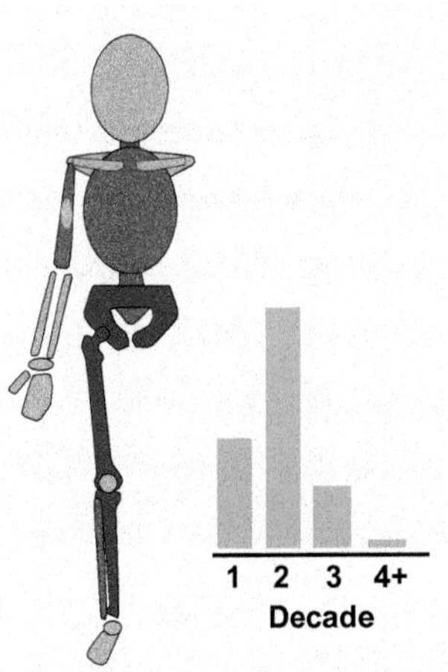

A Ewing sarcoma Common (red) and less common (gray) locations are shown. The age of onset is shown in blue.

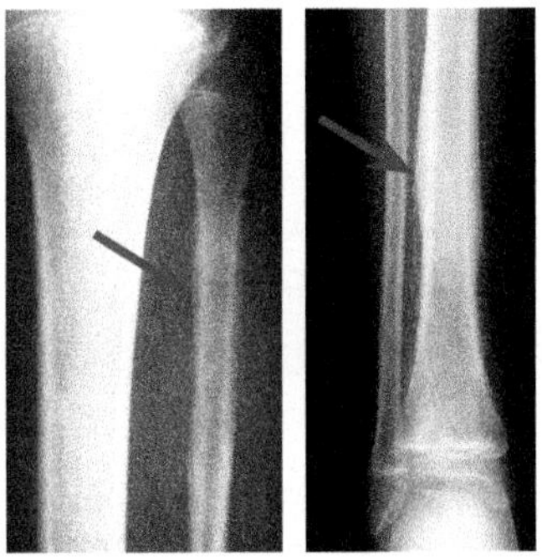

B Typical radiographic features of Ewing sarcoma Note the diaphyseal location with periosteal reaction.

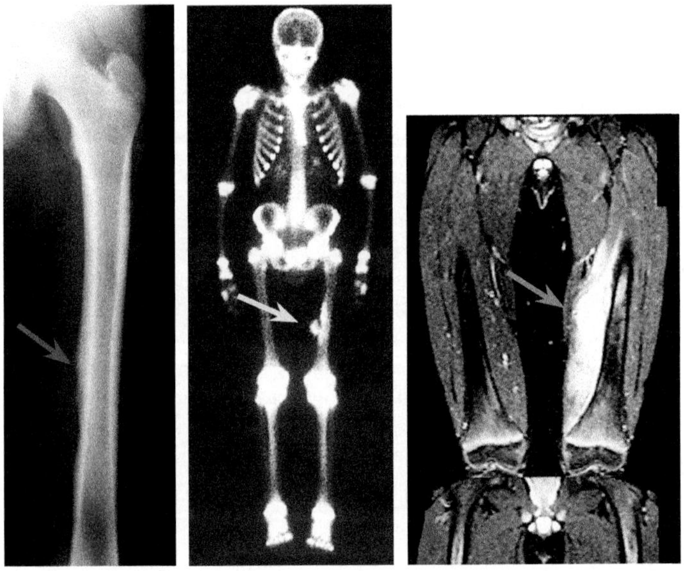

C Appearance of Ewing sarcoma Note the diaphyseal location (red arrow), the positive bone scan (yellow arrow), and extensive soft tissue involvement (blue arrow).

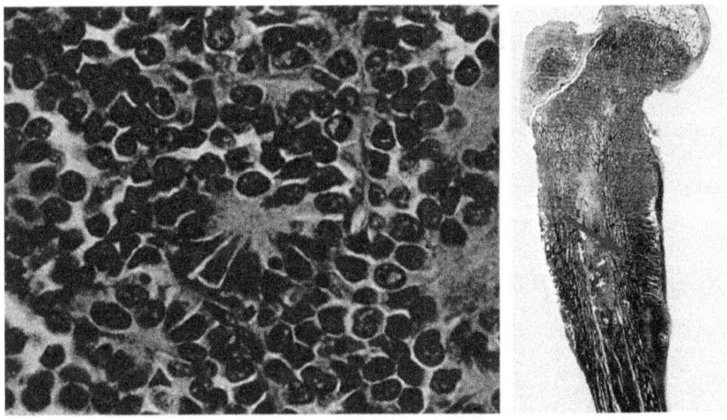

D Pathology of Ewing sarcoma This photomicrograph (left) shows small round cell tumor cells. Note the cortical destruction and extracortical extension in the proximal femur (right, arrow).

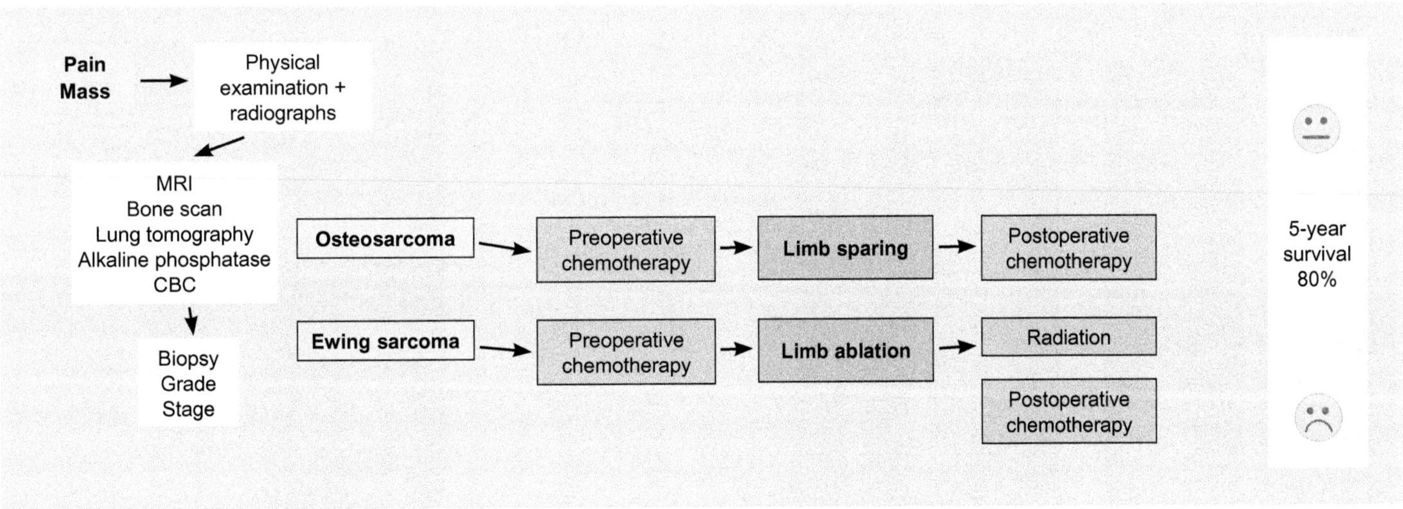

E Management scheme Management of typical cases of osteosarcoma and Ewing sarcoma are shown.

Agent	Common name	Comment
Doxorubicin	Adriamycin	Cytotoxic antibiotic
Methotrexate		Antimetabolite
Cisplatin		Heavy metal
Cycloprosphamide	Adriamycin	Like nitrogen mustard
Ifosfamide		Synthetic cytoxan
Vincristine		Alkaloid
Bleomycin		Cytotoxic glycopeptide
Actinomycin D	Dactinomycin	Antibiotic

A Chemotherapeutic agents These agents are used together in various regimens for treating malignant tumors in children.

Contraindications to limb-sparing procedures
Estimated leg-length discrepancy >8 cm in immature child
Inappropriately performed biopsy or biopsy-site complications
Poor response to preoperative chemotherapy
Major infection in the operative field
Extensive soft tissue or muscle involvement by the tumor
Pathologic fracture with hematoma extending beyond compartment boundary
Major neurovascular structures penetrated by tumor and vascular bypass not feasible

B Relative contraindications for limb salvage Consider management by limb ablation when these features are present. Based on DiCaprio MR and Friedlaender GE, JAAOS 11:25, 2003.

Outcome	Amputation	Limb sparing
Local recurrence	5–10%	5%
Survival	70%	70%
Function	Fair	Good
Initial cost	Low	High
Long-term cost	More	Less if uncomplicated

C Comparison of outcomes of amputation and limb-sparing procedures Note that the outcomes are similar.

Management of Malignant Bone Tumors

Some general principles apply to most lesions.

Chemotherapy Chemotherapeutic agents [A] are commonly used in regimens of 3 to 5 agents given over a period of about 9 to 12 months. Typically, a third is administered preoperatively for a period of 4 to 6 weeks and the rest following resection for an additional 6 to 9 months.

Operative options Make the choice based on a discussion with the patient and family. Outcomes for various procedures are often comparable, and the choice is often best made based on the features of the tumor. Limb-sparing procedures [A, next page] have the greatest appeal to the child and family and have become the standard of care for most patients.

Amputation versus limb-sparing procedures Each method has its indications and contraindications [B]. Functional outcomes are about the same. Patients managed by amputation have slightly lower functional scores but experience fewer complications from the surgery [C].

Endoprosthesis Modular prosthetic management is gaining favor with time. Modern prostheses are strong, lightweight, and nonreactive [D]. Rehabilitation can commence immediately, and acceptance is good. Infection and loosening are major problems. Problems with tendon and ligament attachments can occur. Replacements about the knee, especially the proximal tibia, are most problematic and demonstrate the highest failure rates. Between 30% and 40% require revisions within the first decade following replacement. Most infections and loosening problems can be resolved by revisions.

Expandable endoprosthesis For children, provide an option to maintain equal limb lengths. Design allows 6-9 cm with 1.5–2 cm expansion by minimally invasive procedures. Design improvements allow greater excursion and stable design.

Allografts Allografts may be intercalary, osteoarticular, or composites, combined with an endoprosthesis. Nonunion is the most common problem [E]. The allografts never completely incorporate, but they stabilize with time. This provides improved long-term function, making this a good choice for young people with long-bone diaphyseal tumors. In addition, attachments of tendons and ligaments are more satisfactory than with endoprostheses. Although intercalary allografts have the best results, osteoarticular reconstructions may be considered, especially about the knee. Because of tendon-ligament attachment capability, use around the knee has advantages over endoprostheses. Allograft outcomes may be improved by tissue typing in the future.

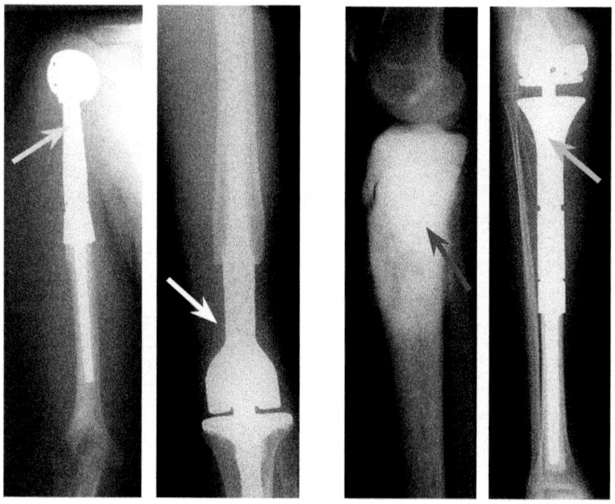

D Endoprostheses Shown are replacements for the proximal humerus (yellow arrow) and distal femur (white arrow). The proximal tibial osteosarcoma (red arrow) resection was managed by a proximal tibial endoprosthesis (green arrow).

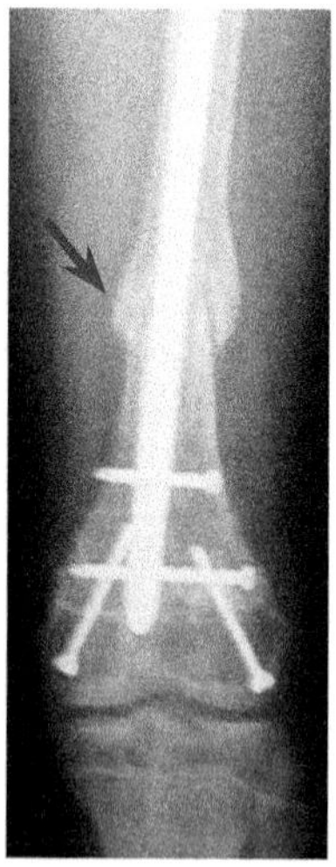

E Allograft This intercalary allograft shows a nonunion (arrow) at its proximal junction.

Rotationplasty This option provides the most energy-efficient outcome, best suited for children under 10 years of age with extensive tumors. Complications are few, and outcome allows a prosthetic fitting that is durable and functional. Most children function in sports. The major drawback is the complexity of the reconstruction and the appearance of the reconstructed limb. Preoperative meetings with other patients who have had the procedure are recommended. Although not in vogue, some suggest the procedure is better suited for boys than girls.

Other alternatives These include vascularized grafts, bone transport for lengthening, and arthrodesis. These options are less commonly considered, but may have a role for specific needs.

Management of malignant tumors is difficult, as the disease is potentially lethal. The options are numerous, making it necessary to integrate management and tailor management to the unique features of each child.

Leukemia

About 20% of children with leukemia present with bone pain and may first be seen by an orthopedist or rheumatologist. Common findings include bone pain, joint pain and swelling, antalgic gait, mild lymphadenopathy and hepatosplenomegaly, and a moderate fever. Radiographic findings include diffuse osteopenia, metaphyseal bands, periosteal new bone formation [B], sclerosis, and a combination of sclerosis and lytic features. Usual laboratory findings include an elevated ESR or CRP, thrombocytopenia, anemia, decreased neutrophils, increased lymphocytes, and blast cells on the peripheral blood smear. Confirm the diagnosis with a bone marrow biopsy.

Metastatic Bone Tumors

The most common primary tumors are neuroblastoma followed by rhabdomyosarcoma [C]. Metastatic tumors to bone are most likely to involve the axial skeleton [D]. Vertebrae metastases are most common in the lumbar spine, whereas thoracic and cervical involvements are less common. The primary site of tumors with spinal involvement are neuroblastoma and astrocytoma, depending on the patient's age. Complications of spinal metastasis include paralysis, pathologic fractures, and kyphoscoliosis. Assess children with neuroblastoma and Ewing sarcoma for bony metastatic disease by CT, MRI, scintigraphy, or bone marrow biopsy. Extensive bony involvement is a relatively late finding [E].

Limb-sparing options
Modular endoprosthesis
Allograft
Osteoarticular allograft
Allograft-prosthetic composites
Expandable prostheses
Rotationplasty
Bone transport (lengthening)
Vascularized grafts
Arthrodesis

A Limb-sparing options Consider these options for limb salvage.

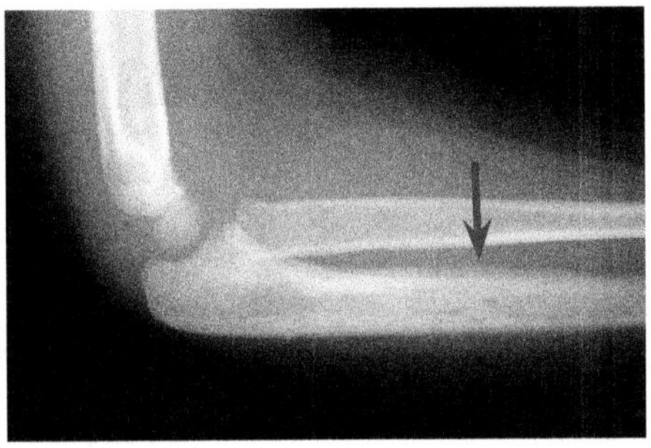

B Leukemia Note the periosteal bone of the proximal ulna (arrow).

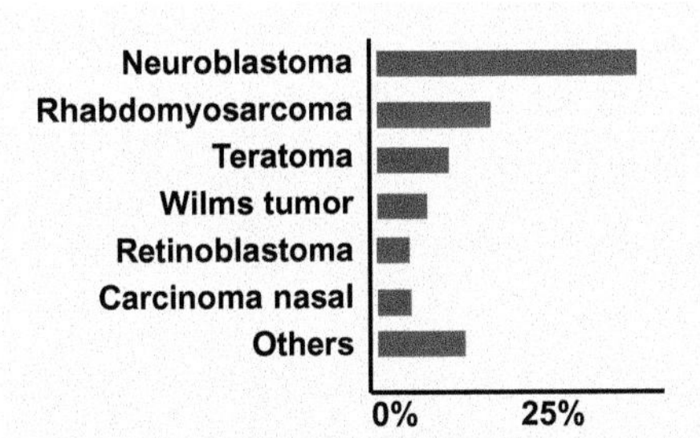

C Tumors producing skeletal metastasis From data of Leeson et al. (1985).

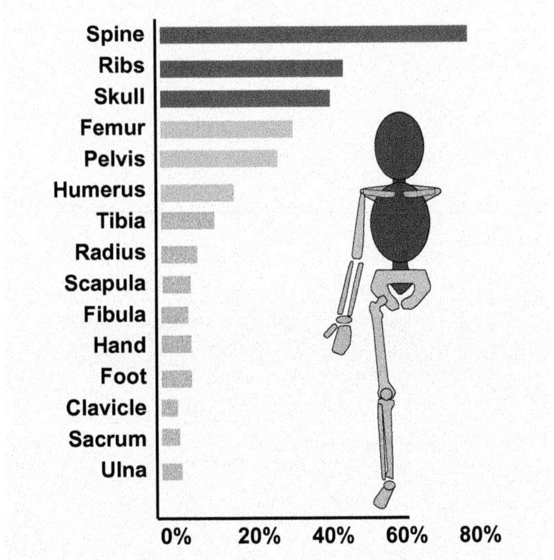

D Site and frequency of skeletal metastasis From data of Leeson et al. (1985).

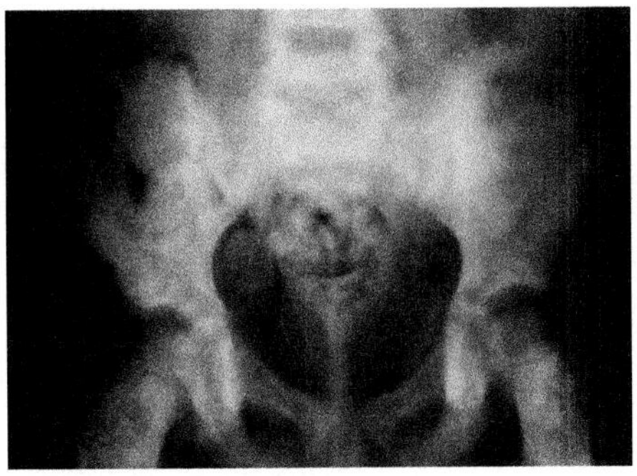

E Metastatic neuroblastoma Note the extensive metastases in the pelvis and proximal femora.

BENIGN BONE TUMORS

Bell SN, Campbell PE, Cole WG, Menelaus MB. Tibia vara caused by focal fibrocartilaginous dysplasia: Three case reports. J. Bone Joint Surg. 67-B:780-784, 1985.

Bergstrand H. Uber eine eigenartige, warscheinlich bisher nicht beschriebene osteoblastische Krankheit in den langen Knochen in der Hand und des Fusses. Acta Radiol. 11:596-613, 1930.

Bianco, P., Riminucci, M., Majolagbe, A., Kuznetsov, S. A., Collins, M. T., Mankani, M. H., Corsi, A., Bone, H. G., Wientroub, S., Spiegel, A. M., Fisher, L. W., Robey, P. G. Mutations of the GNAS1 gene, stromal cell dysfunction, and osteomalacic changes in non-McCune-Albright fibrous dysplasia of bone. J. Bone Miner. Res. 15:120-128, 2000.

Campanacci M, Ruggieri P, Gasbarrini A, Ferraro A, Campanacci L. Osteoid osteoma. Direct visual identification and intralesional excision of the nidus with minimal removal of bone. J. Bone Joint Surg. 81-B:814-819, 1999.

Canavese F, Soo BC, Chia SK, Krajbich JI. Surgical outcome in patients treated for hemangioma during infancy, childhood, and adolescence: a retrospective review of 44 consecutive patients. J. Pediatr. Orthop. 28(3):381- 386, 2008.

Couture, J., Mitri, A., Lagace, R., Smits, R., Berk, T., Bouchard, H.-L., Fodde, R., Alman, B., Bapat, B. A germline mutation at the extreme 3-prime end of the APC gene results in a severe desmoid phenotype and is associated with overexpression of beta-catenin in the desmoid tumor. Clin. Genet. 57:205-212, 2000.

Garg S, Mehta S, Dormans JP. Langerhans cell histiocytosis of the spine in children: long-term follow-up. J. Bone Joint Surg. 86-A(8):1740-1750, 2004.

Godette GA, O'Sullivan M, Menelaus MB. Plantar fibromatosis of the heel in children: a report of 14 cases. J. Pediatr. Orthop. 17(1):16-17, 1997.

Geschickter CF, Keasbey LE. Tumors of blood vessels. Am. J. Cancer 23:568-591, 1935.

Green JA, Bellemore MC, Marsden FW. Embolization in the treatment of aneurysmal bone cysts. J. Pediatr. Orthop. 17(4):440-443, 1997.

Guille JT, Kumar SJ, MacEwen GD. Fibrous dysplasia of the proximal part of the femur. Long-term results of curettage and bone-grafting and mechanical realignment. J. Bone Joint Surg. 80-A:648-652, 1998.

Jaffe H., Liechtenstein L. Non-osteogenic fibroma of the bone. Am. J. Pathol. 18:205-221, 1942.

Jaffe HL, Lichtenstein L. Solitary unicameral bone cyst with emphasis on the roentgen picture, the pathologic appearance and the pathogenesis. Arch. Surg. 44:1004-1025, 1942.

Kolodny A. Bone sarcoma: the primary malignant tumors of bone and the giant cell tumor. Surg. Gynec. Obstet. 44(1):214-241, 1927.

Mammano S, Candiotto S, Balsano M. Cast and brace treatment of eosinophilic granuloma of the spine: long- term follow-up. J. Pediatr. Orthop. 17(6):821-827, 1997.

Möller E, Mandahl N, Mertens F, Panagopoulos I. Molecular identification of COL6A3-CSF1 fusion transcripts in tenosynovial giant cell tumors. Genes Chromosomes Cancer 47(1):21-5, 2008.

Ramirez AR, Stanton RP. Aneurysmal bone cyst in 29 children. J. Pediatr. Orthop. 22(4):533-9, 2002.

Scaglietti O, Marchetti PG, Bartolozzi P. The effects of methylprednisolone acetate in the treatment of bone cysts. Results of three years follow-up. J. Bone Joint Surg. 61-B(2):200-204, 1979.

Stanton RP, Abdel-Mota'al MM. Growth arrest result- ing from unicameral bone cyst. J. Pediatr. Orthop. 18(2):198-201, 1998.

BENIGN CARTILAGE TUMORS

Chew DK, Menelaus MB, Richardson MD. Ollier's disease: varus angulation at the lower femur and its management. J. Pediatr. Orthop. 18:202-208, 1998.

Codman EA. Epiphyseal chondromatous giant cell tumors of the upper end of the humerus. Surg. Gynecol. Obstet. 52:543, 1931.

Dadfarnia T, Velagaleti GV, Carmichael KD, Eyzaguirre E, Eltorky MA, Qiu S. A t(1;9)(q10;q10) translocation with additional 6q23 and 9q22 rearrangements in a case of chondromyxoid fibroma. Cancer Genet. 204(12):666-670, 2011.

Jaffe HL, Lichtenstein L. Chondromyxoid fibroma of bone: a distinctive benign tumor likely to be mistaken especially for chondrosarcoma. Arch. Path. 19:541-551, 1943.

Konishi E, Nakashima Y, Iwasa Y, Nakao R, Yanagisawa A. Immunohistochemical analysis for Sox9 reveals the cartilaginous character of chondroblastoma and chondromyxoid fibroma of the bone. Hum. Pathol. 41(2):208-213, 2010.

Purandare NC, Rangarajan V, Agarwal M, Sharma AR, Shah S, Arora A, Paradar DS. Integrated PET/CT in evaluating sarcomatous transformation in osteochondro- mas. Clin. Nucl. Med. 34(6):350-354, 2009.

Yasuda T, Nishio J, Sumegi J, Kapels KM, Althof PA, Sawyer JR, Reith JD, Bridge JA. Aberrations of 6q13 mapped to the COL12A1 locus in chondromyxoid fibroma. Mod. Pathol. 22(11):1499 1506, 2009.

MALIGNANT SOFT TISSUE TUMORS

Barr FG, Galili N, Holick J, Biegel JA, Rovera G, Emanuel BS. Rearrangement of the PAX3 paired box gene in the paediatric solid tumour alveolar rhabdomyosarcoma. Nat. Genet. 3:113-117, 1993.

Deshmukh R, Mankin H.J, Singer S. Synovial sarcoma: The importance of size and location for survival. Clin. Orthop. 419:155-161, 2004.

Galili N, Davis RJ, Fredericks WJ, Mukhopadhyayl S, Rauscher FJ III, Emanuel BS, Rovera G, Barr FG. Fusion of a fork head domain gene to PAX3 in the solid tumour alveolar rhabdomyosarcoma. Nat. Genet. 5:230-235, 1993.

Kawai A, Woodruff J, Healey JH. Brennan MF, Antonescu CR, Ladanyi M. SYT-SSX gene fusion as a determinant of morphology and prognosis in synovial sarcoma. N. Engl. J. Med. 338(3):153-160, 1998.

Shapiro DN, Sublett JE, Li B, Downing JR, Naeve CW. Fusion of PAX3 to a member of the forkhead family of transcription factors in human alveolar rhabdomyosarcoma. Cancer Res. 53:5108-5112, 1993.

Sharp, R., Recio, J. A., Jhappan, C., Otsuka, T., Liu, S., Yu, Y., Liu, W., Anver, M., Navid, F., Helman, L. J., DePinho, R. A., Merlino, G. Synergism between INK4a/ARF inactivation and aberrant HGF/SF signaling in rhabdomyosarcomagenesis. Nature Med. 8:1276-1280, 2002.

Stout AP. Rhabdomyosarcoma of the skeletal muscles. Ann. Surg. 123:447-472, 1946.

MALIGNANT BONE TUMORS

Batson OV. The function of the vertebral veins and their role in the spread of metastasis. Ann. Surg. 112(1):138–149, 1940.

Delattre O, Zucman J, Melot T, Garau XS, Zucker J-M, Lenoir GM, Ambros PF, Sheer D, Turc-Carel C, Triche TJ, Aurias A, Thomas G. The Ewing family of tumors — a subgroup of small-round-cell tumors defined by specific chimeric transcripts. N. Engl. J. Med. 331:294-9, 1994. 1996.

Ottaviani G, Jaffe N. The etiology of osteosarcoma. Cancer Treat. Res. 152:15-32, 2009.

Pasic I, Shlien A, Durbin AD. Recurrent focal copy-number changes and loss of heterozygosity implicate two noncoding RNAs and one tumor suppressor gene at chromosome 3q13.31 in osteosarcoma. Cancer Res. 70(1):160-71, 2010.

Schimke RN, Lowman JT, Cowan AB. Retinoblastoma and osteogenic sarcoma in siblings. Cancer 134:2077- 2079, 1974.

OTHER TUMORS

Abe T, Tomatsu T, Tazaki K. Synovial hemangioma of the knee in young children. J. Pediatr. Orthop. 11-B(4):293-297, 2002.

Müller H, Horwitz A, Kuhl J. Acute lymphoblastic leukemia with severe skeletal involvement: a subset of childhood leukemia with a good prognosis. Pediatr. Hematol. Oncol. 15(2):121-133, 1998.

OTHER

Adler C-P, Kozlowski K. Primary Bone Tumors and Tumorous Conditions in Children: Pathologic and Radiologic Diagnosis. Springer-Verlag, Berlin, 1993.

Cheng EY, Thompson RC. New developments in the staging and imaging of soft-tissue sarcomas. J. Bone Joint Surg. 81-A(6):882-891, 1999.

Enneking WF, Spanier SS, Goodman MA. A system for the surgical staging of musculoskeletal sarcoma. Clin. Orthop. 153:106-120, 1980.

Lowry PA, Carstens MC. Occult trauma mimicking metastases on bone scans in pediatric oncology patients. Pediatr. Radiol. 27:114-118, 1997.

Malkin D, Li FP, Strong LC, Fraumeni JF, Nelson CE, Kim DH, Kassel J, Gryka MA, Bischoff FZ, Tainsky MA. Germ line p53 mutations in a familial syndrome of breast cancer, sarcomas, and other neoplasms. Science 250:1233-1238, 1990.

Mankin HG, Lange TA, Spanier SS. The hazards of biopsy in patients with malignant primary bone and soft-tissue tumors. J Bone Joint Surg. 64-A:1121-1127, 1982.

Mirels H. Metastatic disease in long bones. A proposed scoring system for diagnosing impending pathologic fractures. Clin. Orthop. 249:256-264, 1989.

Lower Limb

CHAPTER 8

This chapter covers problems of one or more lower limb segments and includes some of the most common problems seen in children's orthopedic clinics [A].

Lower Limb Development

Lower limb development shows a wide range of normal variability, both as variations of growth of children [A] and in the time of appearance of ossification [B and C]. The lower limb bud appears during the 4th embryonic week (see Chapter 1).

Ossification

Ossification appears first in primary centers [B] before birth. The secondary ossification centers appear in infancy and childhood [C].

Growth

Lower limb growth occurs earlier for girls than boys. In contrast with spine growth, the lower limbs show only a small secondary growth spurt [D]. Most growth of the foot occurs before the age of 10 years.

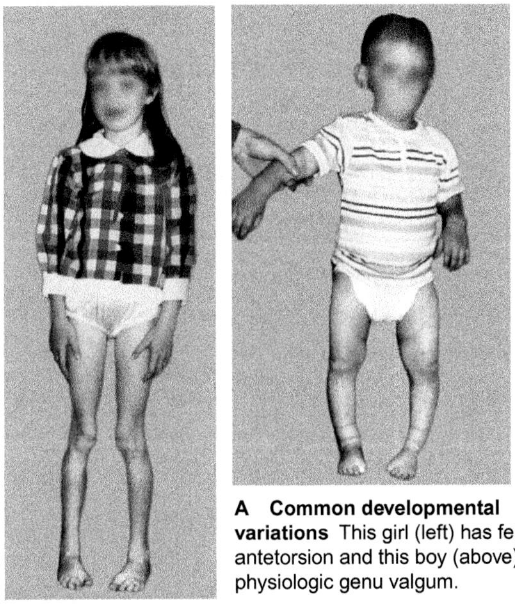

A Common developmental variations This girl (left) has femoral antetorsion and this boy (above) has physiologic genu valgum.

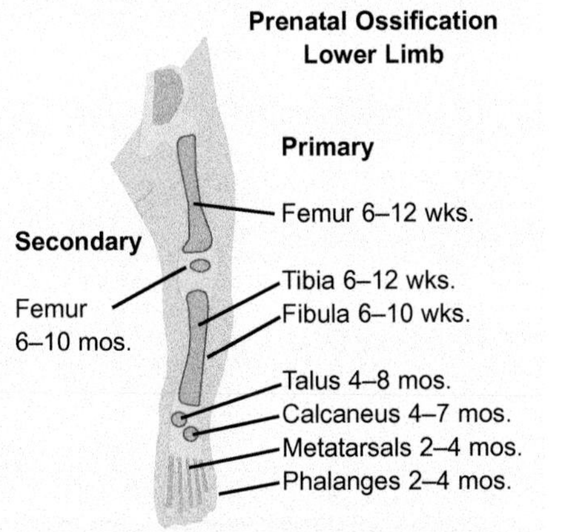

B Prenatal ossification Shown is the time schedule for the appearance of the primary and secondary ossification centers in the lower limb. Based on Caffey (1967).

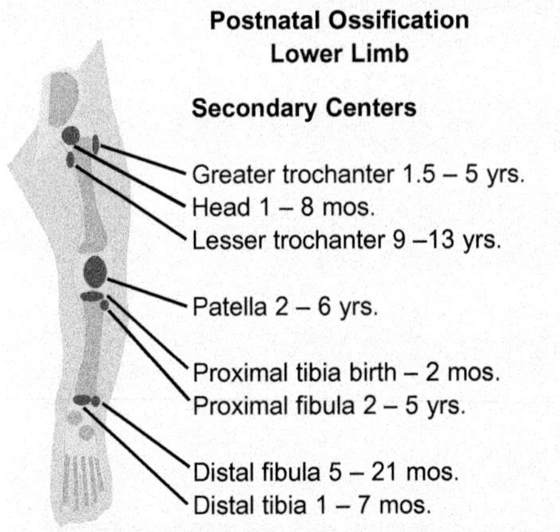

C Postnatal epiphyseal ossification The age range is shown for the appearance of epiphyseal ossification centers in the lower limb. In this range, ossification for girls occurs earlier than for boys. Based on Caffey (1967).

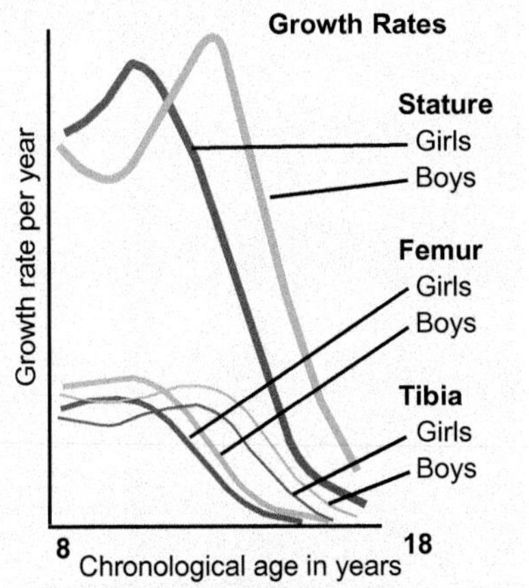

D Growth rates Shown are yearly growth rates for girls and boys for stature and femoral and tibial lengths. Based on Anderson (1963).

Limp

A limp is an abnormal gait that is commonly due to pain, weakness, or deformity. A limp is a significant finding and the cause should be established [A]. Be aware that a painless limp in a toddler maybe due to developmental hip dysplasia.

Evaluation

A presumptive diagnosis can usually be made by the history and physical examination. Age is an important factor to consider during evaluation.

History First, inquire about the onset [B]. When was the limp first noted? Was the onset associated with an injury or illness? Was it gradual or abrupt? If the limp has been present since infancy, inquire about developmental history because children with neuromuscular disorders have delayed motor development.

Observation The type of limp can usually be determined by observation. Remove outer clothing to allow the full view of the legs. Watch the child walk in the hallway of the clinic [C]. Observe in three phases: (1) Overview. Look for obvious abnormalities. Which side seems abnormal? Is the stance phase on each side equal in duration? Is lateral shoulder sway present? Is circumduction seen? (2) Study each leg *individually*. Look for more subtle changes. Is the normal heel-to-toe gait pattern present? Does the knee approach full extension during the stance phase? How is the hand carried? Elevation of the arm is seen in hemiplegia. (3) Make a presumptive diagnosis, and then make a final observation to be certain that this diagnosis is consistent with the characteristics of the limp.

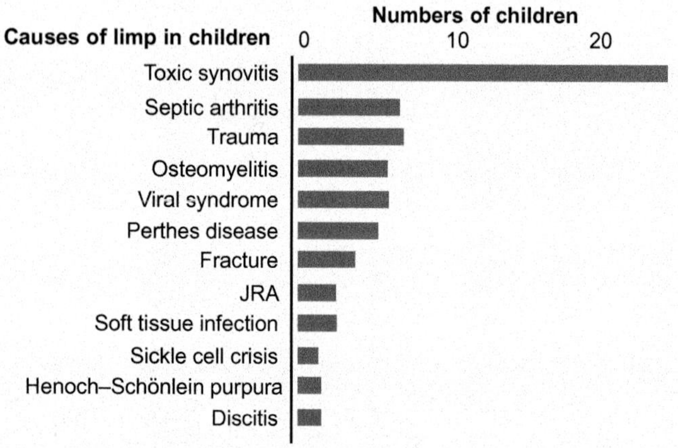

A Causes of limp in 60 young children Data from Choban and Killian (1990).

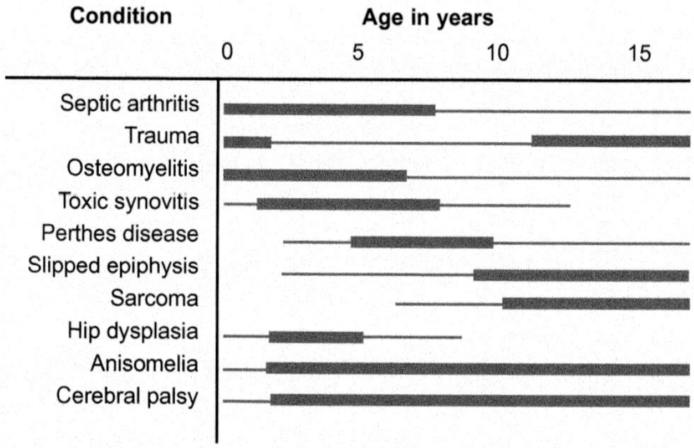

B Causes of limp by age The causes of limp are related to the age of the child. The fine red lines show the range and the heavy lines the most common age range of involvement.

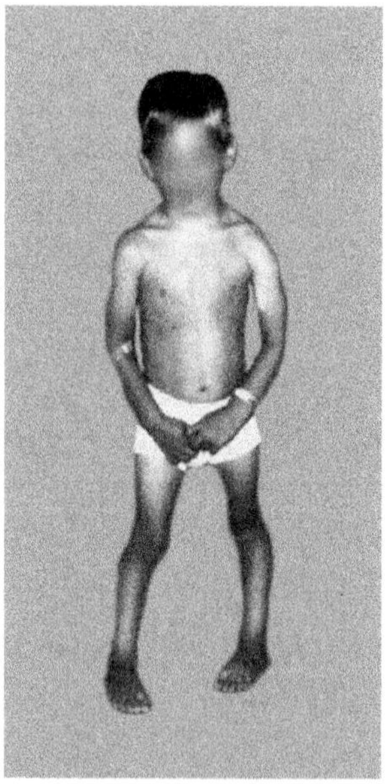

C Hallway observation
Evaluate the limp by studying the child's gait while the child walks in the clinic hallway.

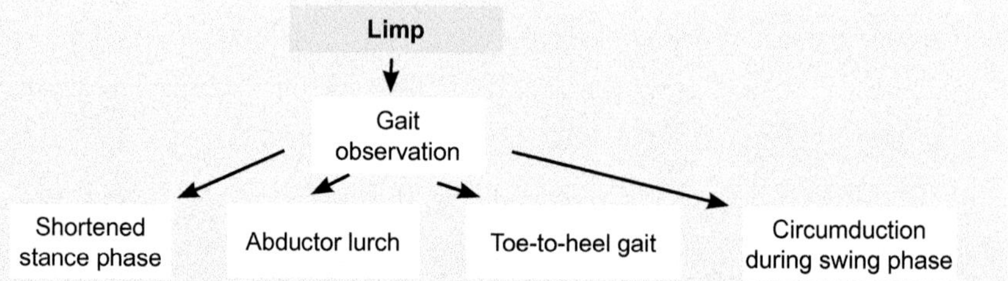

Gait type	Antalgic Gait	Abductor Lurch	Equinus Gait	Circumduction Gait
Physical examination	Tenderness Reduced range of motion	Trendelenburg sign	Heel-cord contracture Neurological exam needed	Assess limb lengths Neurological exam Check range of motion
Tests	Radiographs bone scan	Pelvis radiographs		Orthodiagrams
Common examples	Trauma Toddler's fracture Overuse syndrome Infection Inflammations	Hip dysplasia Cerebral palsy	Cerebral palsy Idiopathic toe walker Clubfoot	Painful foot Leg length inequality

D Algorithm for evaluation of limping The major causes of limping are shown. A general categorization is first possible by observation. The exact causes are established by physical examination and laboratory studies.

Types of Limps

The common types of limping may be classified into four groups [D, previous page].

Antalgic gait This is a painful limp. The most prominent feature is a shortened stance phase on the affected side. To minimize discomfort, the time of weight bearing on the affected side is shortened. The child is said to "favor" one side or the other. The term "favor" is ambiguous because it may be used to describe either the affected or unaffected side. Find the anatomic location of the problem by determining the site of tenderness, joint guarding, or limitation of motion. The hip is the most common site for the problem [A]. Follow-up with radiographs. Often a CBC and ESR or CRP are helpful. If the radiographs are negative, order a bone scan to localize the problem [B and C].

Abductor lurch results from weakness of the abductor muscles, usually due to hip dysplasia or a neuromuscular disorder. An abductor lurch is characterized by lateral shoulder sway toward the affected side or sides. In normal gait, the abductor muscles contract during the stance phase to maintain a level pelvis and a linear progression of the center of gravity of the body. If the abductors are weak, the pelvis tilts and falls on the unsupported side during stance. To maintain the center of gravity over the foot, the shoulder shifts toward the weak side. This shift is referred to as an *abductor lurch* or a *Trendelenburg gait*. Weakness of the abductors is demonstrated by the Trendelenburg test or sign. The test is positive if the pelvis drops on the unsupported side during single-leg standing. The cause of the abductor lurch is usually established by a standing radiograph of the pelvis and a neurological examination.

Equinus gait An equinus gait is due to a heel-cord contracture, which is usually due to cerebral palsy, residual clubfoot deformity, or idiopathic heel-cord tightness. Regardless of the etiology, the contracture causes a "toe-to-heel" sequence during the stance phase on the affected side. In the young child, equinus is often associated with a "back knee" or recurvatum deformity of the knee that occurs during the stance phase. Document the deformity by evaluating the range of dorsiflexion of the ankle with the knee extended. The ankle should dorsiflex more than 10°. If an equinus deformity is present, a thorough neurological examination is required. Be aware that this may be confused with a short leg gait due to developmental hip dysplasia.

Circumduction gait allows a functionally longer limb to progress forward during the swing phase. Circumduction is often due to a painful condition about the foot or ankle because circumduction requires less ankle movement, making walking more comfortable.

Management

The limp may be caused by something as simple as a stone in the shoe, or by something as serious as leukemia or osteogenic sarcoma. Thus, generalizations regarding management cannot be made. Sometimes the cause of the limp cannot be determined. Should the diagnosis be unclear, reevaluate the child weekly until the problem resolves or a diagnosis is established.

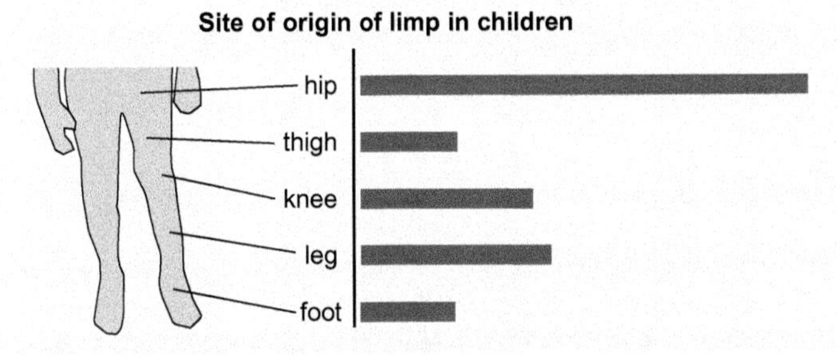

A Origin of limp in 60 young children Data from Choban and Killian (1990).

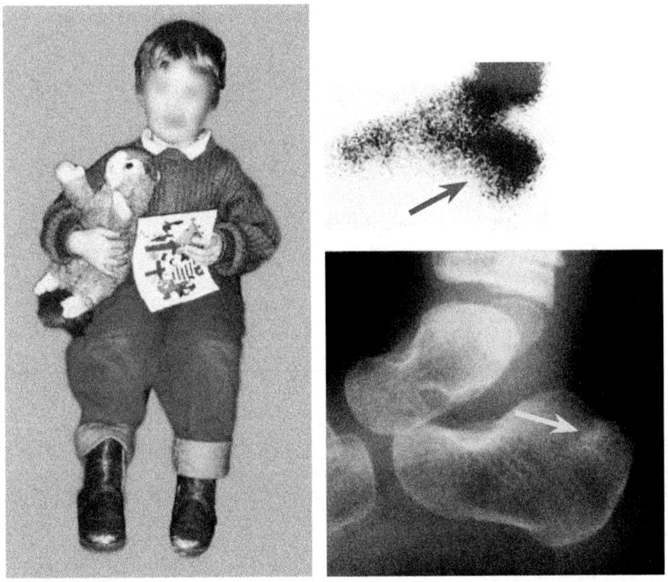

B Role of bone scan in limp evaluation This child had an antalgic limp with a negative physical examination, radiographs, and ESR. The bone scan showed increased uptake over the calcaneus (red arrow). This suggested a stress injury to the calcaneus. This was confirmed by a radiograph 2 weeks later, showing evidence of a stress fracture (yellow arrow). The child had been stressed by being taken on long walks in a shopping mall.

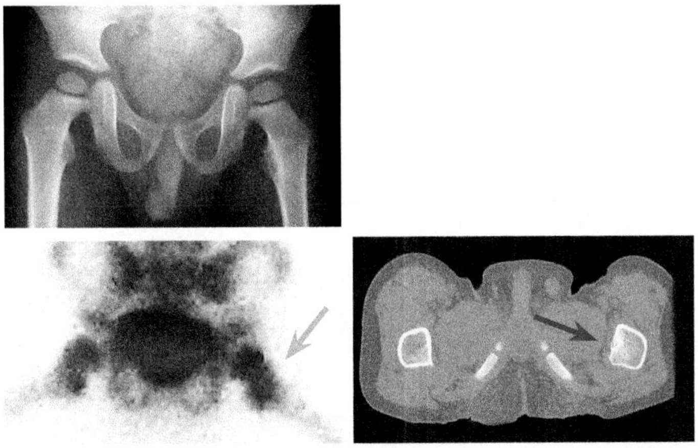

C Obscure limp from osteomyelitis This 2-year-old complained of night pain and showed a subtle limp during the day. Radiographs were negative, and the bone scan showed slight increased uptake in the upper femur (orange arrow). CT scan demonstrated an intracortical defect (red arrow). The differentiation from osteoid osteomy was made by a resolution with antibiotic treatment.

Feature	Growing Pain	Serious Problem
History		
Long duration	Often	Usually not
Pain localized	No	Often
Pain bilateral	Often	Unusual
Alters activity	No	Often
Causes limp	No	Sometimes
General health	Good	May be ill
Physical Examination		
Tenderness	No	May show
Guarding	No	May show
Reduced range of motion	No	May show
Laboratory		
CBC	Normal	± Abnormal
ESR	Normal	± Abnormal
CRP	Normal	± Abnormal

A Differentiating growing pains from more serious problems The features of growing pains are usually so characteristic that special studies are seldom required.

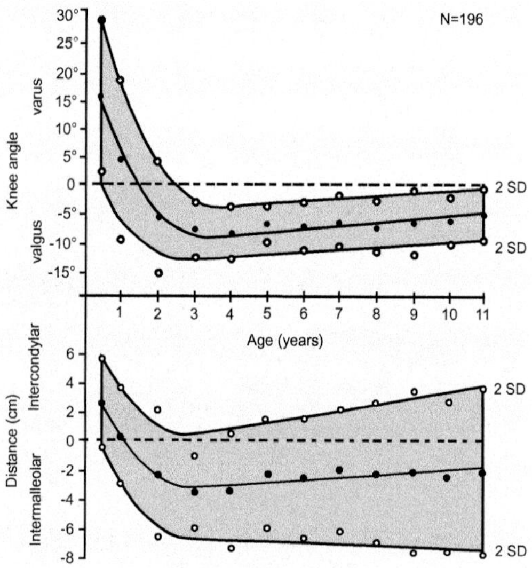

B Normal values for knee angle The normal values for the knee angle are shown in knee angle and intermalleolar or intercondylar distances. From Heath and Staheli (1993).

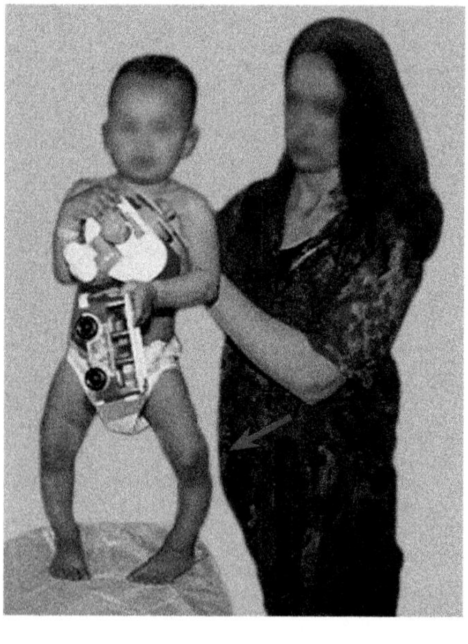

C Physiologic bowlegs This 18-month-old infant has moderate bowing.

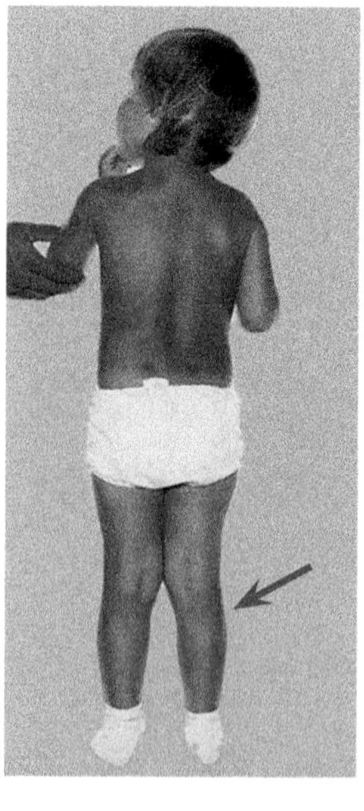

D Physiologic knock-knees This 3-year-old girl has mild physiologic knock-knees.

Leg Aches

Leg aches, or growing pains, are idiopathic, benign discomfort of extremities, which occur in 15–30% of children. The pains are most common in girls, usually occur at night, and primarily affect the lower limbs. The condition produces no functional disability or objective signs and resolves spontaneously without residua. The cause is unknown. Undocumented speculation on cause includes genetic, functional, or structural (hypermobility) etiology. Leg aches follow headaches and stomachaches as the most common sites of pain during childhood.

Clinical Features

The differential diagnosis of leg aches includes most of the painful conditions involving the musculoskeletal system in children. The diagnosis is made by exclusion [A].

History The pain from leg aches is typically vague, poorly localized, bilateral, nocturnal, and seldom alters activity. This condition does not affect gait or general health. A history of long duration is most consistent with the diagnosis of leg aches. This long duration is helpful in separating out more serious problems, which over a period of time will usually produce objective findings.

Screening examination Does the child appear systemically ill? Is deformity or stiffness present? Does the child limp?

Tenderness Systematically palpate the limbs and trunk for tenderness.

Joint motion Is joint motion guarded or restricted? Check for symmetry of medial rotation of hips.

Differential Diagnosis

Night pain may also be due to a tumor, such as osteoid osteoma, osteogenic, or Ewing sarcomas. Tumor pain is more localized, often associated with a soft tissue mass, progressive, and usually occurs later in childhood than growing pains.

Management

If the history is atypical for leg aches, or signs are found on examination, imaging and laboratory studies are required. If the findings are negative, a presumptive diagnosis of growing pains or leg aches is made. Provide symptomatic treatment with heat and an analgesic. Reassure the family about the benign, self-limited course of the condition, but advise them that if the clinical features change, the child should be reevaluated.

Genu Varus and Genu Valgus

Genu varum and genu valgum are frontal plane deformities of the knee angle that fall outside the normal range, ±2 SD of the mean. Knee angle variations that fall within the normal range are referred to as *bowlegs* or *knock-knees* or physiologic variations [A]. The range of normal for knee angle changes with age [B, previous page]. Lateral bowing of the tibia is common during the first year, bowlegs are common during the second year [C, previous page], and knock-knees are most prominent between ages 3 and 4 years [D, previous page]. Varus or valgus deformities are classified as either "focal," as seen in tibia vara, or "generalized," as occurs in rickets.

Evaluation

History Inquire about the onset. Was there an injury or illness? Is the deformity progressing? Are old photographs or radiographs available for review? Is the child's general health good? Does the family provide a normal diet? Are other family members affected?

Physical examination Start with a screening evaluation. Does the child have normal height and body proportions? Short stature is common in rickets and various syndromes. Are other deformities present? Is the deformity symmetrical [B]? Is the deformity localized or generalized? Are the limb lengths equal? Shortening and knee angle deformity may be due to epiphyseal injuries or some developmental problems such as fibular hemimelia. Measure the rotational profile. Frontal and transverse plane deformities often coexist; make a clear separation. Measure the deformity. With the patella directly forward, measure the knee angle with a goniometer. Measure the intermalleolar or intercondylar distance. Does the deformity increase when the child stands? If the collateral ligaments are lax, such as in achondroplasia, the varus deformity is worse in the upright position.

Laboratory If the child has a generalized deformity, order a metabolic screen, including calcium, phosphorus, alkaline phosphatase, and creatinine, plus a hematocrit.

Imaging If findings suggest the possibility of a pathological basis for the deformity, order a single AP radiograph of the lower limbs [C]. If knee ligaments are loose, make the radiograph with the infant or child standing. Position the child with the patella directly forward [C]. Use a film large enough to include the full length of femora and tibiae. A 36-inch film is often required. Study the radiograph for evidence of rickets, tibia vara, or other problems. Measure the metaphyseal-diaphyseal angle of the upper tibia (see D, pg. 142). Values above 11° are consistent with but not diagnostic of tibia vara. Measure the hip-knee-ankle angle. Complete the evaluation with other imaging studies if necessary. For knee deformities, a lateral radiograph is useful. CT or MRI studies may be useful in identifying and measuring a physeal bridge. Document the deformity by photography. A sequence of photographs provides a graphic record of the change with time.

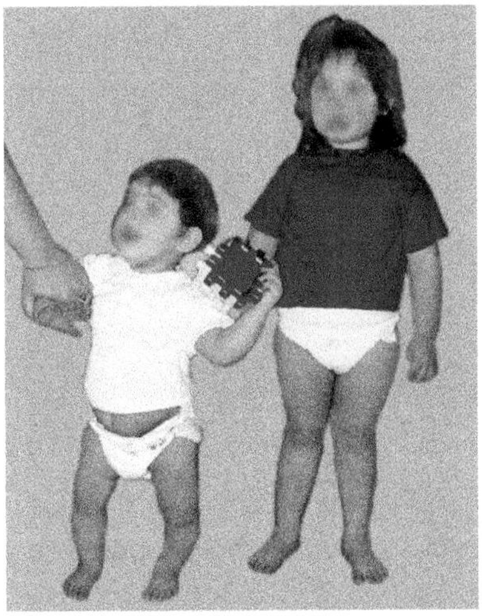

A Physiological bowlegs and knock-knees These siblings show the sequence, with the toddler having bowlegs and the older sister having mild knock-knees.

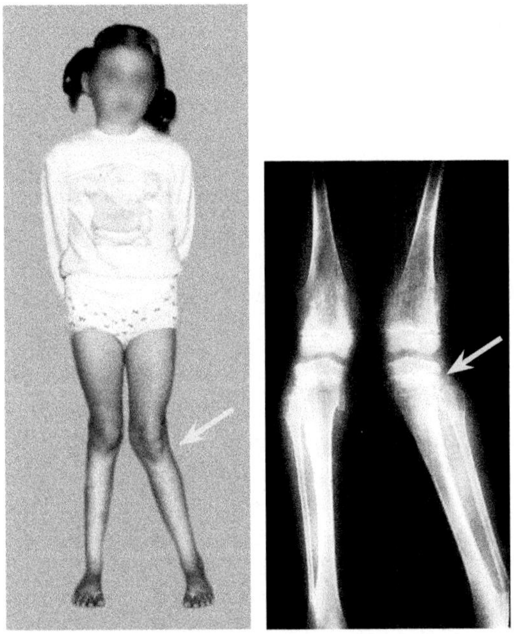

B Pathological genu valgum Deformity is asymmetrical and due to osteochondromatosis (yellow arrows).

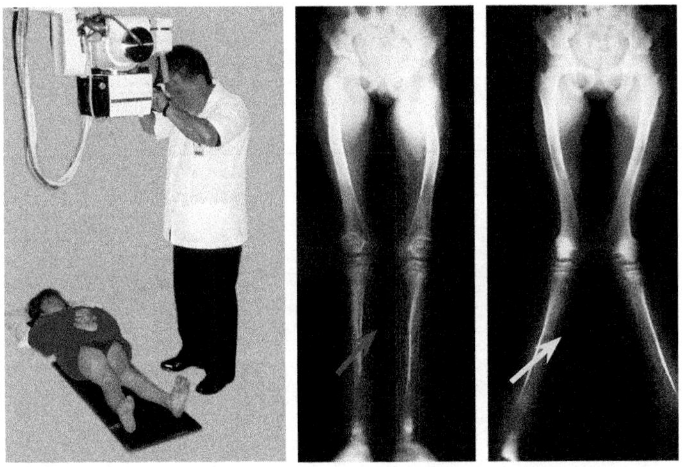

C Positioning for radiographs This girl is being carefully positioned to assure an accurate study. Positioning the patient to fit the legs on the radiograph (red arrow) results in misinformation. In the same patient, note the difference with a properly positioned study (yellow arrow).

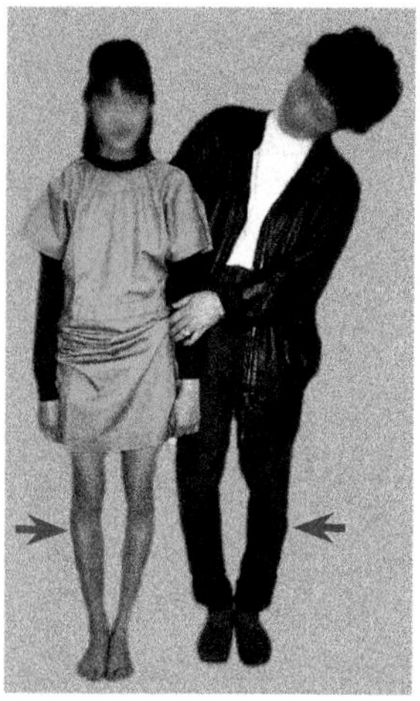

A Familial genu varum Asians tend to have more physiological bowing than other groups.

Diagnosis

Follow a plan [D and E]. First make the differentiation between physiologic and pathologic forms [A and B]. If a pathologic form is present, consider the different categories of causes [C]. Causes are varied, and usually the diagnosis is not difficult.

Evaluation

Mechanical axis Obtain a long, standing radiograph of the lower limbs. Be certain the child is positioned with the patella directly anterior when the exposure is made. Draw the axis of the femur and tibia connecting the center of the femoral head to the center of the distal femoral epiphysis [A, next page]. Construct a second line between the midpoint of the upper and lower tibial epiphyses. Mark the articular surfaces. Measure the degree of valgus or varus.

Zone system On a full-length radiograph, draw a line between the femoral head and ankle. Note the position of the knee relative to this axis [B, next page].

Feature	Physiologic	Pathologic
Frequency	Common	Rare
Family history	Usually negative	May occur in family
Diet	Normal	May be abnormal
Health	Good	Other MS abnormalities
Onset	Second year for bowing Third year knock-knees	Out of normal sequence Often progressive
Effect of growth	Follows normal pattern	Variable
Height	Normal	Less than 5th percentile
Symmetry	Symmetrical	Symmetrical or asym
Severity	Mild to moderate	Often beyond ±2 SD

B Differentiating physiologic and pathologic genu varum

Cause	Genu Valgum	Genu Varum
Congenital	Fibular hemimelia	Tibial hemimelia
Dysplasia	Osteochondrodysplasias	Osteochondro-dysplasias
Developmental	Knock-knee >2 SD	Bowing >2 SD Tibia vara
Trauma	Overgrowth Partial physeal arrest	Partial physeal arrest
Metabolic	Rickets	Rickets
Osteopenic	Osteogenesis imperfecta	
Infection	Growth plate injury	Growth plate injury
Arthritis	Rheumatoid arthritis knee	

C Classification of pathologic knee angle Causes of genu varum and genu valgum are listed.

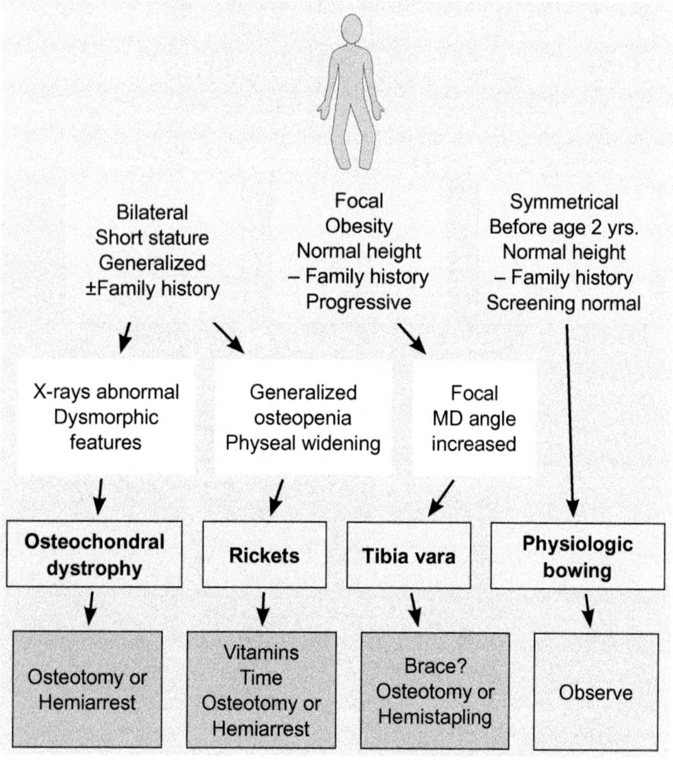

D Evaluation of genu varum or bowlegs This flowchart shows the differentiation of the common causes of change in knee angle.

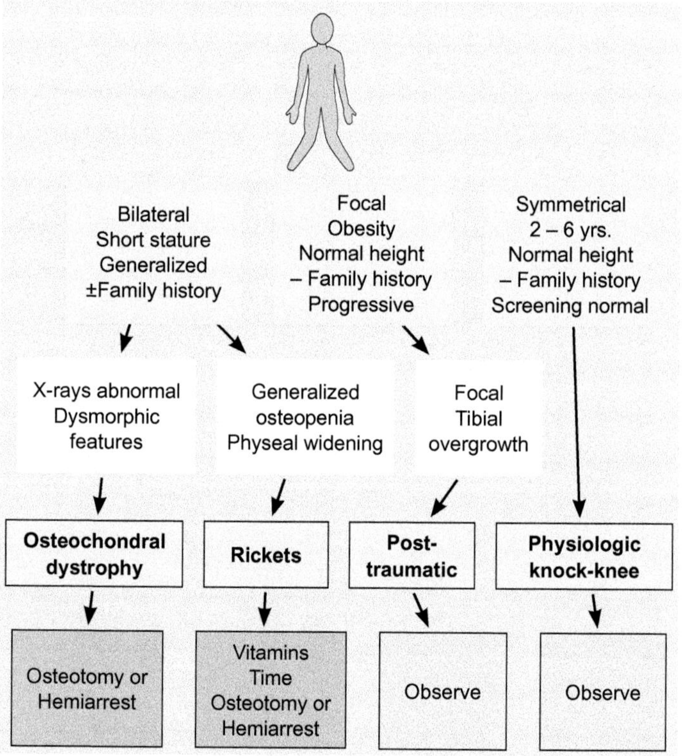

E Evaluation of genu valgum or knock-knees This flowchart shows the differentiation of the common causes of change in knee angle.

Management Principles

The vast majority of children have bowlegs or knock-knees that will resolve spontaneously. If the intracondylar and intramalleolar distances are >8 cm, consider a consultation.

Document these physiological variations with a photograph and see the child again in 3–6 months for follow-up. No radiographs are necessary. If the problem is pathological, establish the cause. Then consider treatment options.

Nonoperative treatment with shoe wedges is not effective and should be avoided. Long-leg bracing may be used for early tibia vara, but its effectiveness is uncertain. Avoid long-term bracing for conditions such as vitamin D–resistant rickets because the effectiveness of bracing is unclear and considerable disability results from brace treatment.

Operative correction options include osteotomy, or hemiarrest procedures either by hemiepiphysiodesis or unilateral physeal stapling. The objectives of operative treatment are to (1) correct knee angle, (2) place the articular surfaces of the knee and ankle in a horizontal position, (3) maintain limb length equality, and (4) correct any coexisting deformities. To achieve these objectives, preoperative planning is required.

Make corrective osteotomies as close to the site of deformity as practical.

Translation of the osteotomy may be necessary to position the joint within the mechanical axis.

Multilevel osteotomies are often necessary in generalized deformities from metabolic conditions and osteochondrodystrophies. Balance the number of osteotomies with risks.

Recurrent deformity is likely in certain conditions, so delay each correction as long as possible to reduce the number of procedures required during childhood.

Idiopathic Genu Valgum and Varum

Valgus deformity with an intermalleolar distance exceeding 8–10 cm is most common in obese girls. This deformity seldom causes functional disability; the problem is primarily cosmetic. If severe, with an intermalleolar distance of >15 cm, consider operative correction by hemiepiphysiodesis or stapling. Make a standing radiograph and construct the mechanical axis. Determine the site(s) of deformity. In most cases, the distal femur is most deformed near the appropriate site for correction.

Varus deformity is most common in Asians [A, previous page]. The varus deformity may be familial. Whether it increases the risk of degenerative arthritis of the knee is uncertain. This deformity seldom requires operative correction. Manage severe deformity by stapling or hemiepiphysiodesis.

Posttraumatic Genu Valgum

Posttraumatic genu valgum results from overgrowth following fracture of the proximal tibial metaphysis in early childhood [C]. Valgus may also be due to malunion or soft tissue interposition in the fracture.

Natural history The deformity develops during the first 12 to 18 months due to tibial overgrowth following the fracture. This is followed by a very gradual reduction of the valgus over a period of years. In the majority, this correction is adequate and no operative procedure is necessary.

Management Manage proximal tibial fractures by correcting any malalignment, and immobilize with a long-leg cast applied with gentle varus molding. Document reduction and position with a long film that includes the entire tibia. Advise the family of the potential of this fracture to cause a secondary deformity, which cannot be prevented. Avoid early osteotomy because recurrence is frequent and the deformity usually resolves spontaneously with time. Reassure the family that the knee will not be damaged by the deformity. Should the deformity persist, correct by osteotomy or by hemiepiphysiodesis or stapling near the end of growth.

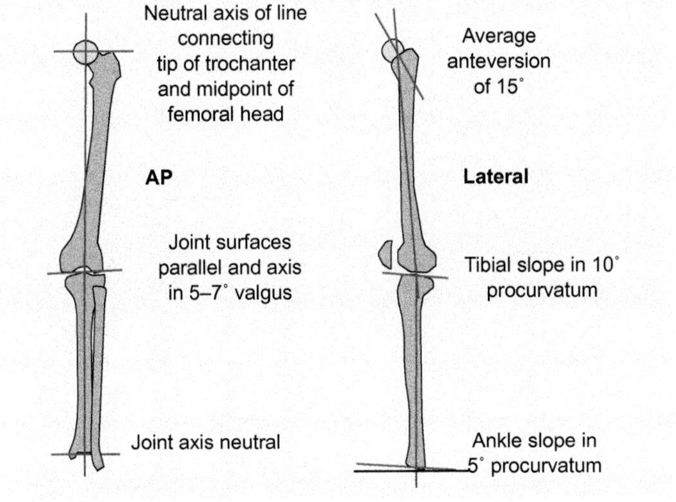

A Normal mechanical axis of lower limbs These are average values. Based on Paley and Tetsworth (1992).

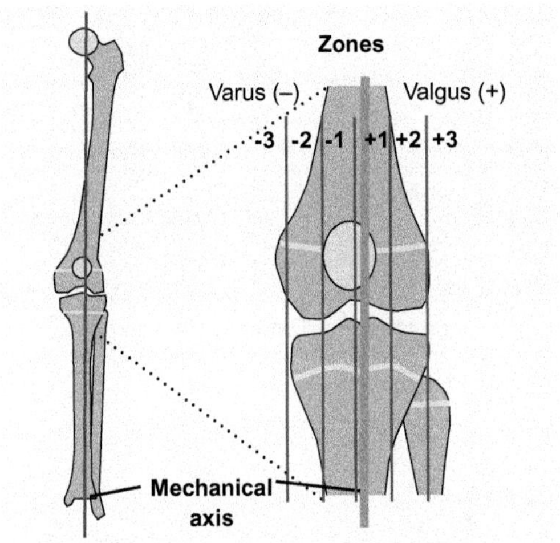

B Zone system for assessing mechanical axis The zone into which the mechanical axis falls is graded as a (–) for varus and a (+) for valgus, and into thirds with values ranging from 1 to 3. Based on Stevens et al (1999).

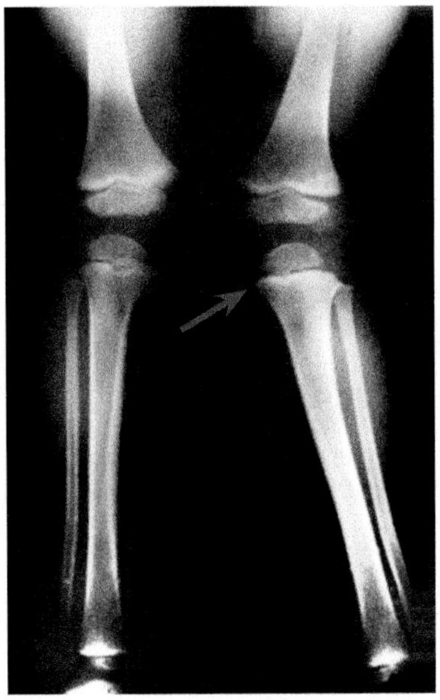

C Posttraumatic genu valgum This deformity is due to overgrowth of the tibia following proximal tibial metaphyseal fracture.

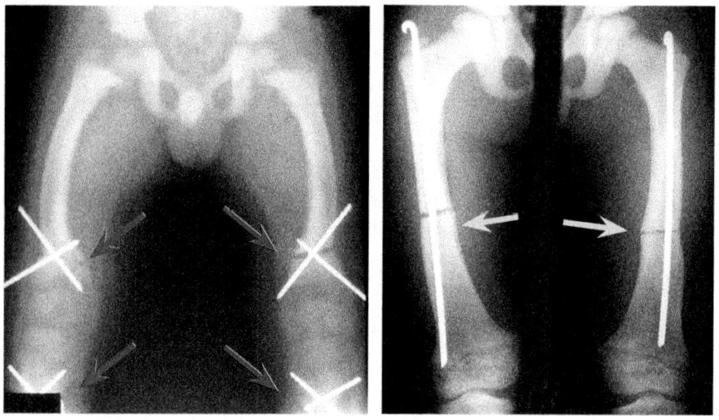

A Operative correction of rachitic deformity Multilevel correction is often necessary (red arrows). In some, intramedullary fixation can be used (yellow arrows).

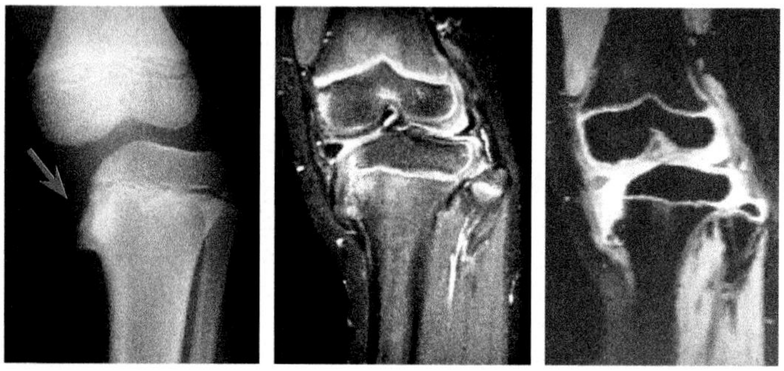

B Tibia vara These images are of a 6-year-old boy with moderate deformity. Note the deformity and medial subluxation of the femur on the tibia as it appears in standing and walking.

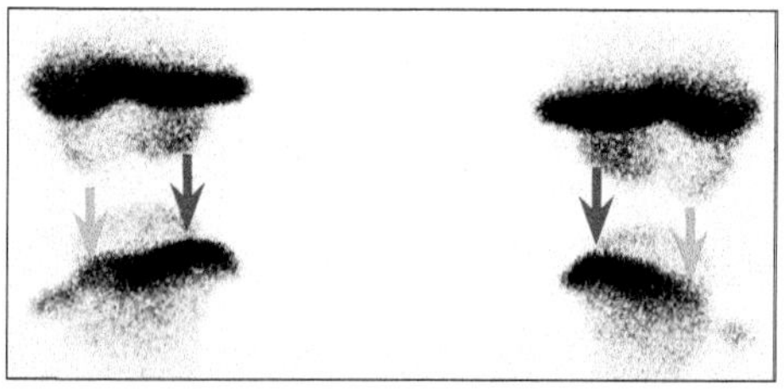

C Bone scan Bone scans early show increased uptake on the medial aspect of the proximal tibial epiphysis (red arrows) as compared with the lateral side (orange arrows). This may be helpful in differentiating early tibia from physiologic bowing.

Rickets

Suspect rickets in a child with increasing genu valgum, short stature, and a history of an atypical diet or similar deformities in other family members. Rickets produces a generalized genu valgum with bowing of the diaphysis and rarefaction of the epiphysis. Low calcium and phosphorus and a high alkaline phosphatase are confirming laboratory findings. Document severity with a 36-inch radiograph of the entire femur and tibia. Measure the hip-knee-ankle angle and mechanical axis zone.

Manage by first referring the child to an endocrinologist to optimize the medical management of the rickets. Despite optimal medical management, the deformities often persist in vitamin D–resistant forms of rickets.

Bracing The role of bracing is controversial, as long-term bracing imposes a major added burden on the child and the value of bracing has not been shown.

Surgery If possible, delay correction until late childhood for stapling or adolescence for osteotomy. Correction at the end of growth reduces the risk of recurrence. If deformity is severe, correction may be necessary in childhood [A]. Plan osteotomy as discussed earlier with long films and cutouts. Drape the entire limb free to visualize adequacy of correction. Correct at one or more levels on each bony segment following the preoperative plan. Immobilize for about 10 weeks, as healing may be slightly slower than normal.

If operative correction is performed before the end of growth, recurrence is common. Recurrence is most rapid in the younger child.

Tibia Vara

Tibia vara, or Blount disease, is a growth disorder involving the medial portion of the proximal tibial growth plate that produces a localized varus deformity [B]. The incidence is greater if the child is black, obese, has an affected family, and resides in certain geographical locations such as the southeastern part of United States. The cause is unknown but it has been theorized that in susceptible individuals mechanical stress damages the proximal medial growth plate, thus converting physiologic bowlegs into tibia vara.

Evaluation Two clinical patterns of tibia vara are seen. Radiographs in early infantile tibia vara may be difficult to differentiate from physiologic bowing.

The metaphyseal–diaphyseal angle is often used. This angle [D] shows considerable overlap between physiologic and tibia vara cases. If the angle exceeds 15°, tibia vara is likely. Differentiation is made by following radiographs made every 3–6 months. Physiologic varus usually improves after the child's second birthday. Tibia vara progresses and shows diagnostic metaphyseal changes.

Bone scan is seldom necessary but will show increased uptake on the medial side of the proximal tibial physis [C].

MRI studies show considerable deformation, which might be helpful for complex deformity management.

Langenskiöld stages These are stages of the disease [E] with transition from one to the next over time.

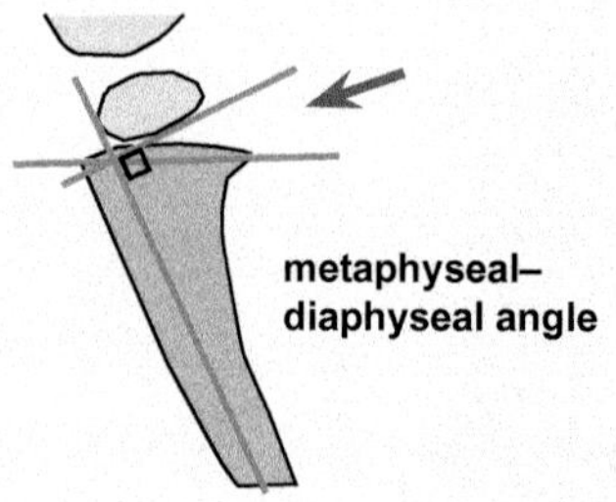

D The metaphyseal–diaphyseal angle This angle (red arrow) is commonly measured.

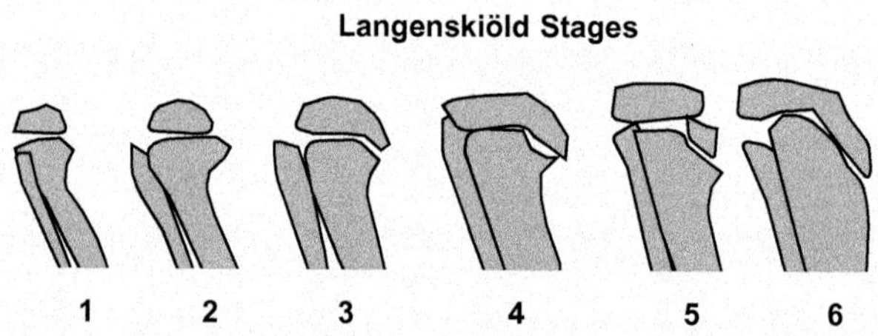

E Langenskiöld classification This classification is commonly used but sometimes difficult to apply.

Management Treatment is based on the stage of tibia vara [E, previous page] and the age of the child.

Bracing Mild deformities may resolve without treatment, so the beneficial effect of the brace is uncertain. Often braces are used to treat stage 1 and 2 disease. If treatment is elected, order a long-leg brace with a fixed-knee that incorporates valgus loading. The brace should be worn during active play and at nighttime.

Operative Correction Operative correction may be achieved by an osteotomy or by initiating asymmetrical growth to correct the deformity. This asymmetrical growth may be achieved by a permanent hemiepiphysiodesis or by a reversible stapling procedure.

Osteotomy in the child If tibia vara progresses or is first seen in stages 3 and 4, osteotomy is indicated. Perform the osteotomy before age 4 years if possible [A]. Deformities of stages 5 and 6 are more complex and may require a double-level osteotomy to correct both the genu varum and the articular incongruity. Also assess the shape of the distal femur as varus or valgus deformity may contribute to the deformity. Medial tibial torsion is also a common associated deformity. Correct the varus and torsion by a simple closing wedge with rotation or by an oblique osteotomy. Correct the thigh-foot angle to about +10 degrees and overcorrect the varus to about 10 degrees of valgus. Use a sterile tourniquet so the entire limb can be seen to ensure appropriate correction. Release the anterior compartment fascia to reduce the risk of a compartment syndrome. Fix the osteotomy with crossed pins and supplement the fixation with a long-leg cast.

Hemistapling may be an alternative to osteotomy for stage 2 or 3 deformities.

Physeal bridge resection Rarely, a physeal bridge is suspected in unilateral involvement in mid to late childhood. CT or MRI studies confirm the presence of the bridge. Resect the bridge, fill the defect with fat, and correct the tibial deformity by osteotomy.

Surgery in the adolescent Operative correction in the older child or adolescent is usually complicated by obesity. Stabilize the osteotomy with an external fixator. External fixation provides adequate immobilization without need for a cast and allows the option to adjust alignment during the postoperative period [B].

Stapling Stapling is a convenient method for correction. The disadvantages are the larger scar, the risk of staple extrusion, and a second operation for staple removal. The advantage is simplicity. The staples (usually two) are placed, the patient carefully followed, and when the deformity is corrected the staples are removed. If the staples are placed extraperiosteal, growth can be expected to resume. The zone system is commonly used to determine the need for correction. A zone 3 deformity may be an indication for stapling. A rebound often occurs after staple removal, undoing some correction, so overcorrect slightly in anticipation of this common problem, especially in children younger than 12 years of age.

Hemiepiphysiodesis With accurate timing, hemiepiphysiodesis has several advantages. The scar is short and the procedure simple and definitive. Bowen has developed a table to aid in timing [C]. Careful follow-up is essential because if the deformity appears to be destined for overcorrection, arresting the entire epiphysis becomes necessary.

Timing The timing of the stapling is not critical. When correction is achieved, the staples are removed. Timing of epiphysiodesis is critical, and tables have been developed to help estimate the appropriate timing.

Prognosis The prognosis depends upon the severity, stage, and treatment. Recurrence of varus and increasing shortening are common during childhood. Persisting articular deformity often leads to degenerative arthritis in adult life.

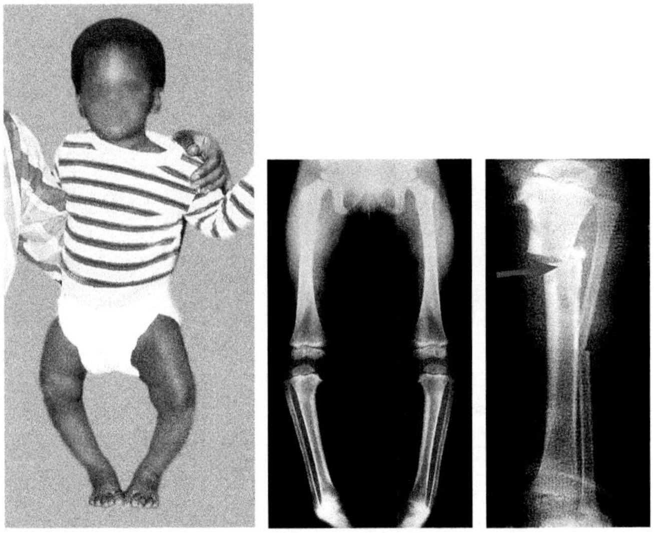

A Infantile tibia vara This disease is usually bilateral and may cause deformity that requires correction by osteotomy (red arrow).

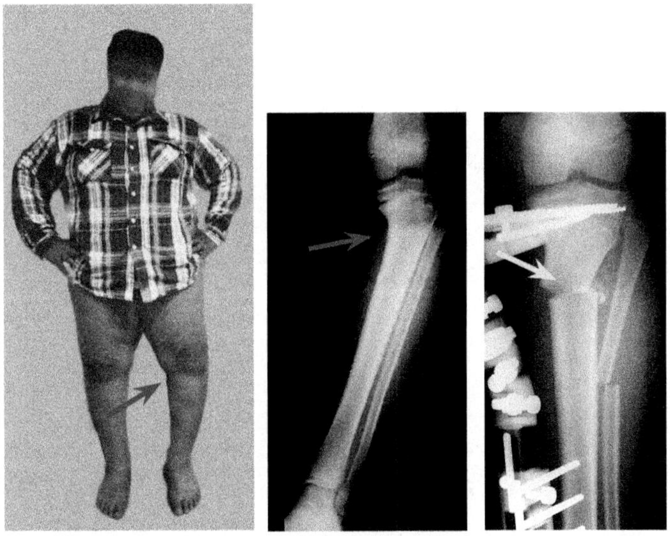

B Adolescent tibia vara This form is often unilateral (red arrows) and usually requires operative correction. External fixation is often an excellent choice in operative correction (yellow arrow).

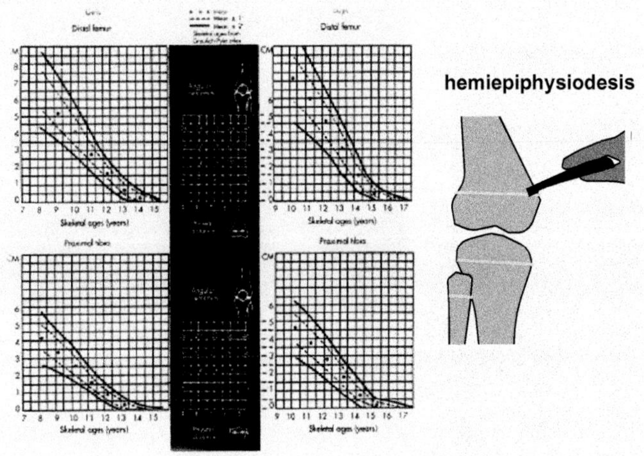

C Chart for timing hemiepiphysiodesis This chart was created to time correction of angulatory deformities. From Bowen (1985).

Level	Normal	Deformity
Terms	Version within ± 2 SD mean	Torsion >2 SD from mean
Tibia	Tibial version	Tibial torsion Internal (ITT) External (ETT)
Femur	Femoral version Anteversion Retroversion	Femoral torsion Internal (IFT) External (EFT)

A Terminology of rotational variations Normal variations and deformities are described by different terms.

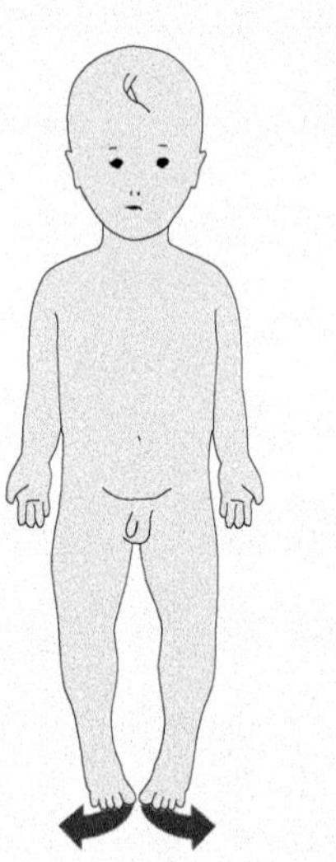

B Lower limb laterally rotates with age Both the femur and tibia laterally rotate with growth. Femoral anteversion declines and tibial version becomes more lateral.

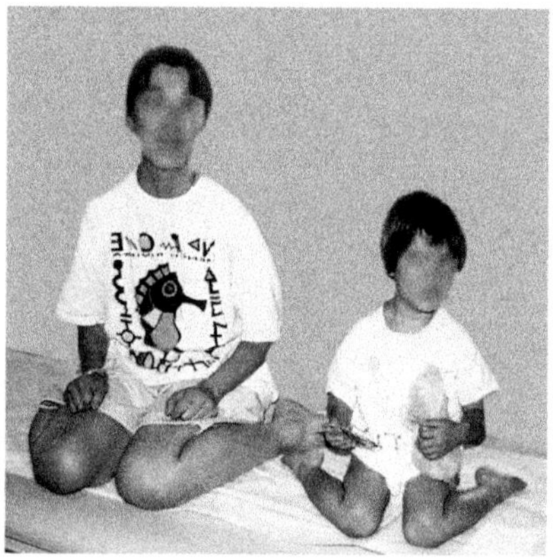

C Internal femoral torsion affecting mother and child Evaluation of the parent often reveals a rotational pattern similar to that present in the child.

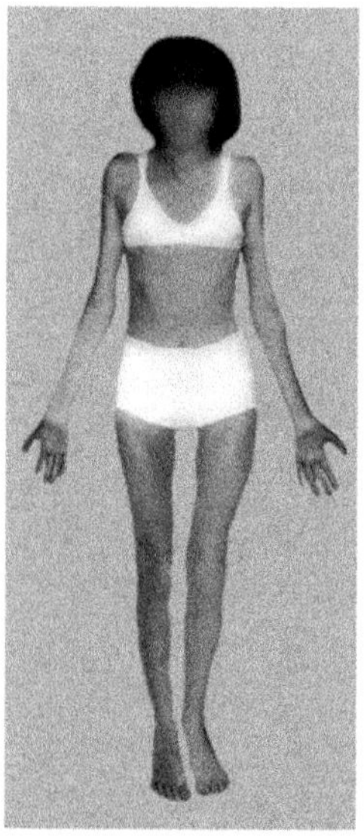

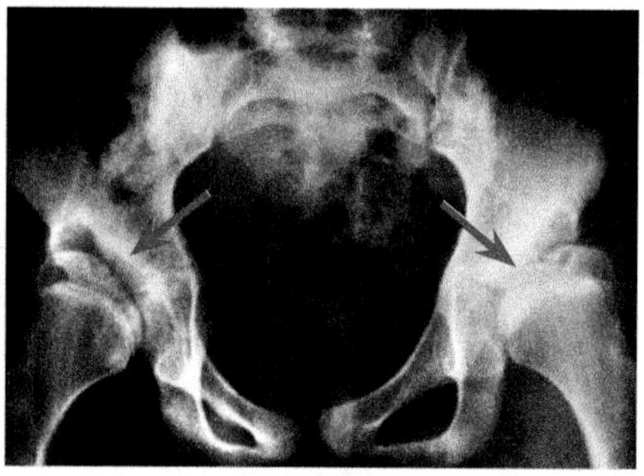

D Asymmetrical hip rotation requires further evaluation This 12-year-old girl was seen for in-toeing. The rotational profile was abnormal, showing asymmetry of hip rotation. A radiograph of the pelvis showed severe bilateral hip dysplasia (arrows). Operative correction of the hip dysplasia was performed.

Torsion

Torsional problems of in-toeing and out-toeing often concern parents and frequently prompt a variety of treatments for the child. Management of torsional problems is facilitated by clear terminology, an accurate diagnosis, a knowledge of the natural history of torsional deformity, and an understanding of the effectiveness of management options.

Terminology

Version describes normal variations in limb rotation [A]. Tibial version is the angular difference between the axis of the knee and the transmalleolar axis. The normal tibia is laterally rotated. Femoral version is the angular difference between the transcervical and transcondylar axes. The normal femur is anteverted.

Torsion describes variation beyond ±2 standard deviations (SD) from the mean and is considered abnormal and described as a "deformity." Internal femoral torsion (IFT) or antetorsion, and external femoral torsion (EFT) or retrotorsion, describe abnormal femoral rotation. Internal tibial torsion (ITT) and external tibial torsion (ETT) describe abnormal tibial rotation.

Torsional deformity may be simple, involving one level, or complex, involving multiple segments. Complex deformities may be additive or compensating. Thus, internal tibial torsion and internal femoral torsion are additive. In contrast, external tibial torsion and internal femoral torsion are compensatory.

Normal Development

The lower limb rotates medially during the seventh fetal week to bring the great toe to the midline. With growth, femoral anteversion declines from about 30° at birth to about 10° at maturity [B]. Values for anteversion are higher in the female and in some families [C]. With growth, the tibia laterally rotates from about 5° at birth to a mean of 15° at maturity. Because growth is associated with lateral rotation in both the femoral and tibial segments, medial tibial torsion and femoral antetorsion in children improve with time. In contrast, lateral tibial torsion usually worsens with growth.

Evaluation

Although the diagnosis of torsional deformities can be made by the physical examination alone, the history is helpful in excluding other problems and assessing extent of disability.

History Inquire about the onset, severity, disability, and previous treatment of the problem. Obtain a developmental history. A delay in walking may suggest a neuromuscular disorder. Is there a family history of a rotational problem? Often rotational problems are inherited, and the status of the parent foretells the child's future.

Screening examination Screen to rule out hip dysplasia and such neurological problems as cerebral palsy.

Rotational profile The rotational profile provides the information necessary to establish the level and severity of any torsional problem. Record the values in degrees for both right and left sides. Evaluate in four steps:

Observe the child walking and running. Estimate the foot progression angle (FPA) during walking [A, next page]. This is the angular difference between the axis of the foot and the line of progression. This value is usually estimated by observing the child walking in the clinic hallway. Estimate the average degree of in-toeing or out-toeing. A minus value is assigned to an in-toeing gait. In-toeing of –5° to –10° is mild, –10° to –15° moderate, and more than –15° severe. Ask the child to run. The child with femoral antetorsion may show an "eggbeater" running pattern with the legs flipping laterally during the swing phase.

Assess femoral version by measuring hip rotation [B, next page]. Measure external rotation (ER) and internal rotation (IR) with the child prone, the knees flexed to a right angle and the pelvis level. Assess both sides at the same time. Internal rotation is normally less than 60°–70°. If hip rotation is asymmetrical, evaluate with a radiograph [D].

Quantitate tibial version by assessing the thigh-foot angle (TFA) [D]. With the child prone and the knee flexed to a right angle, the TFA is the angular difference between the axis of the foot and the axis of the thigh. The TFA measures the tibial and hindfoot rotational status. The TMA is the angular difference between the transmalleolar axis and the axis of the thigh. This is a measure of tibial rotation. The difference between the TMA and the TFA is a measure of hindfoot rotation. The normal range of both the TFA and TMA is broad, and the mean values increase with advancing age. For these measurements, positioning of the foot is critical. Allow the foot to fall into a natural position. Avoid manual positioning of the foot, as this is likely to cause errors in assessment.

Assess the foot for forefoot adductus. The lateral border of the foot is normally straight. Convexity of the lateral border and forefoot adduction are features of metatarsus adductus. An everted foot or flatfoot may contribute to out-toeing. Include both in the rotational profile.

From the screening examination and rotational profile, establish the level and severity of the torsional deformity [C].

Special Studies

Order special imaging studies if hip rotation is asymmetrical or if the rotational problem is so severe that operative correction is being considered. In general, special imaging to document rotational problems is not very useful. Before operative correction, image severe antetorsion to rule out hip dysplasia and to measure the degree of femoral antetorsion. Measurements can be made by CT scans or biplane radiographs. Antetorsion usually exceeds 50° in children whose condition is severe enough to require operative correction.

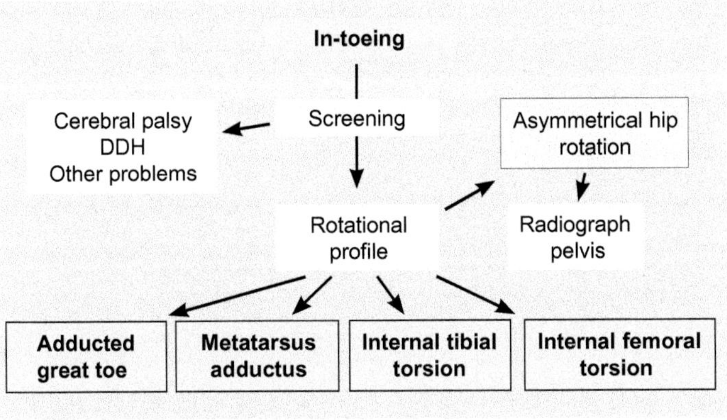

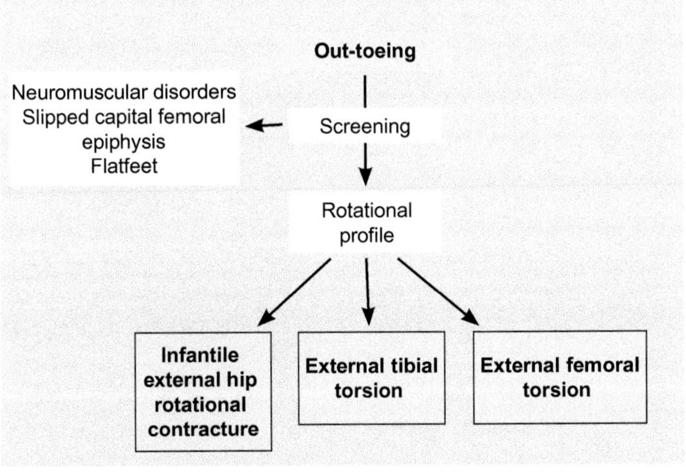

C Flowcharts for assessment of in-toeing and out-toeing By using the screening examination and the rotational profile, the diagnosis can usually be readily established.

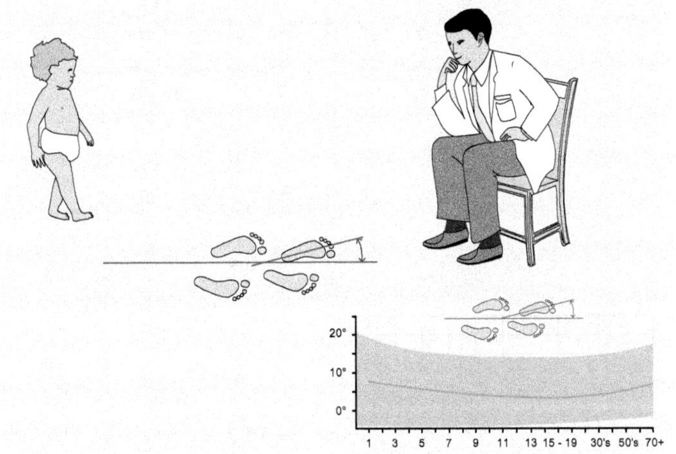

A Foot progression angle The foot progression angle is estimated by observing the child walking. The normal range is shown in green.

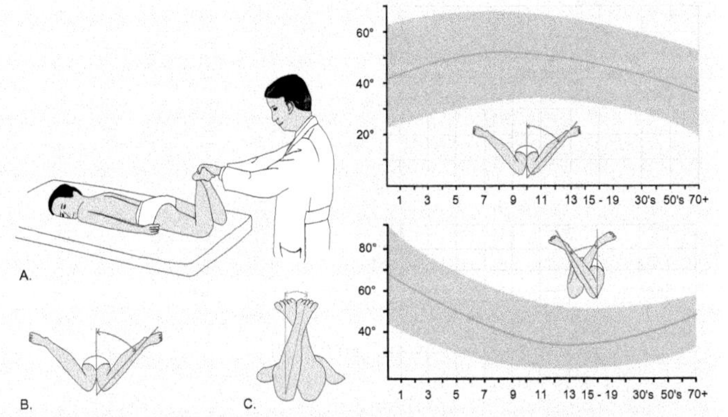

B Hip rotation Hip rotation is assessed with the child prone (A). Internal rotation (B) and external rotation (C) are measured. Normal ranges are shown in green.

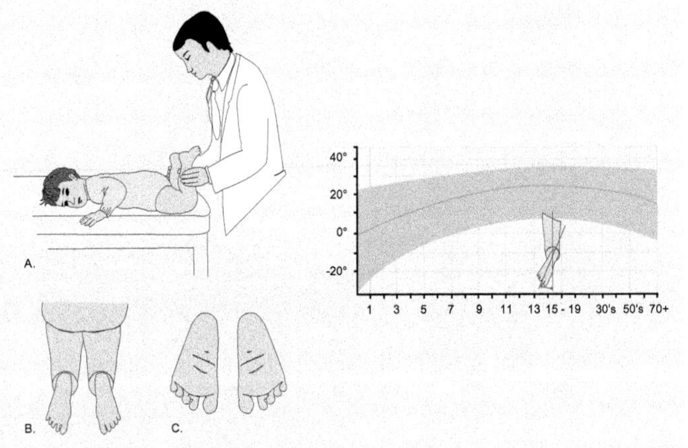

D Assessing rotational status of tibia and foot The rotational status of the tibia and foot are best assessed by evaluating the child in the prone position (A), allowing the foot to fall into a natural resting position. The thigh-foot axis (B) and shape of the foot (C) are readily determined. The range of normal is shown in green.

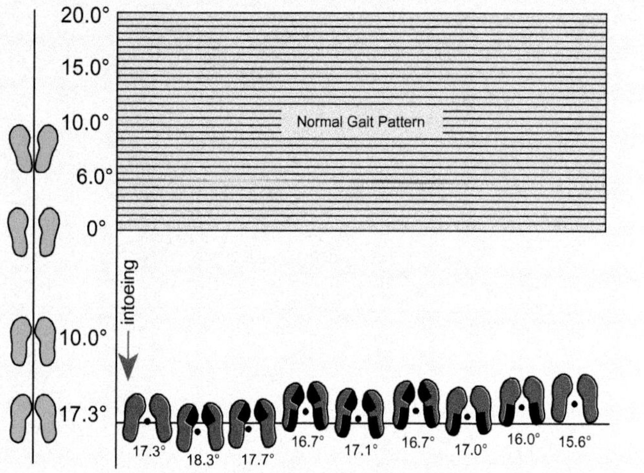

A Ineffectiveness of shoe wedges Various wedges were placed (shown in black). Mean values for in-toeing for each wedge and for unwedged controls are shown. Redrawn from Knittle and Staheli (1976).

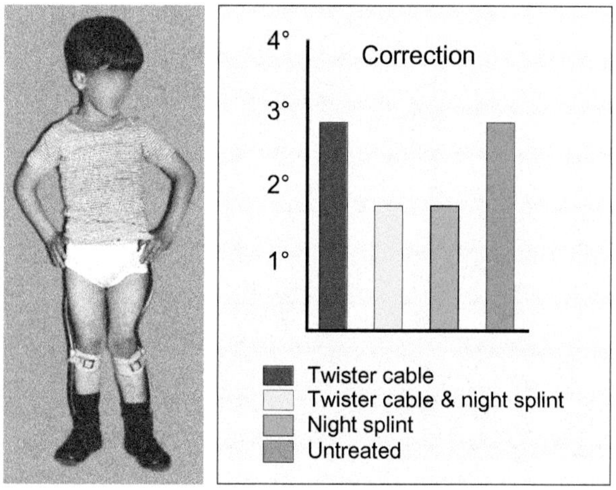

B Lack of effectiveness of twister cables The chart compares the effectiveness of various "treatments" and the untreated child with antetorsion. These interventions made no difference in the measured femoral anteversion before and after treatment. From Fabry et al. (1973).

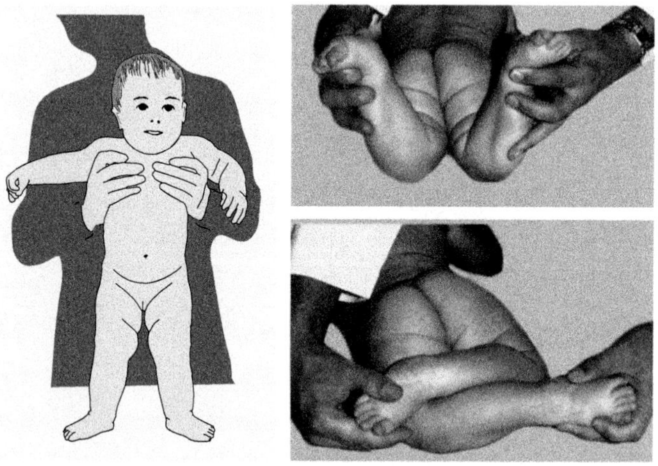

C Physiologic infantile out-toeing Out-toeing in early infancy is usually due to a lateral rotation contracture of the hips. In this infant, medial rotation is limited to about 30° (upper photograph), whereas lateral rotation is about 80° (lower photograph). This results in a lateral rotation of the limb (drawing), which resolves spontaneously.

Management Principles

The first step is establishing a correct diagnosis. In managing rotational problems, the most common management challenge is dealing effectively with the family. Because the lower limbs laterally rotate with time, in-toeing spontaneously corrects in the vast majority of children. Thus, simply waiting to allow this spontaneous resolution is best for the child. Attempting to control the child's walking, sitting, or sleeping positions is impossible. Such attempts only create frustration and conflict between the child and parent.

Shoe wedges or inserts are ineffective [A]. Likewise, daytime bracing with twister cables only limits the child's walking and running activities [B]. Night splints that laterally rotate the feet are better tolerated and do not interfere with the child's play, but probably have no long-term benefit.

Thus, observational management is best. The family needs to be convinced that only observation is appropriate. This requires careful evaluation, education, reassurance, and follow-up. The family should be informed that only rarely does a torsional problem persist. Less than 1% of femoral and tibial torsional deformities fail to resolve and may require operative correction in late childhood. The need for rotational osteotomy is rare, and the procedure is effective.

Infant

Out-toeing may be due to flatfeet with heel valgus or, more commonly, due to a lateral rotation contracture of the hips or a combination of both. In-toeing may be due to an adducted great toe, forefoot adductus, or internal tibial torsion.

Lateral hip rotational contracture Because the hips are laterally rotated in utero, lateral hip rotation is normal. When the infant is positioned upright, the feet may turn out [C]. This may worry the parents. Often only one foot turns out, usually the right. The turned-out foot is the more normal one. The opposite limb, the one that is considered normal by the parents, often shows metatarsus adductus or medial tibial torsion.

Adducted great toe The adducted great toe has been described both as a spastic abductor hallucis and as a "searching toe." This is a dynamic deformity due to a relative overpull of the abductor hallucis muscle that occurs during stance phase [D]. This may be associated with adduction of the metatarsals. The condition resolves spontaneously when maturation of the nervous system allows more precision in muscle balance around the foot. No treatment is required.

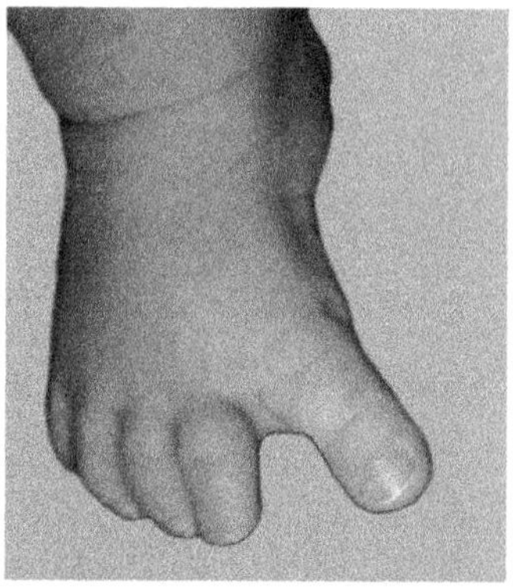

D Searching toe This is a dynamic deformity due to overactivity of the abductor hallucis muscle.

Forefoot adductus describes a spectrum of foot deformities characterized by a medial deviation of the forefoot of different degrees [A]. The prognosis is clearly related to stiffness. The condition is detailed in Chapter 9.

Metatarsus adductus Flexible deformities occur from intrauterine crowding. Like other deformations, they resolve spontaneously with time. Most resolve within the first year and the rest over childhood. Manage with observation and reassurance [B]. Braces, casting, special shoes, or exercises are not necessary.

Metatarsus varus Rigid forefoot adductus tends to persist. This rigid form is uncommon compared with metatarsus adductus. The deformity is characterized by stiffness with a crease on the sole of the foot. The natural history is for incomplete spontaneous resolution. The deformity produces no functional disability and is not the cause of bunions. It produces a cosmetic problem, and when severe, a problem with shoe fitting.

Be sure to distinguish the rare skewfoot. Recall that the skewfoot occurs in loose-jointed children and is characterized by marked forefoot adductus and hindfoot valgus.

Most parents want the deformity corrected. Correct with serial long-leg casts starting at about 6 months of age [B]. Apply the casts at 1–2-week intervals until the deformity is corrected. In children over 2 years of age, cast correction is sometimes effective but is more difficult for the child and families to accept.

Operative correction is very rarely appropriate, as the metatarsus varus produces no functional disability or secondary deformities.

Toddler

In-toeing is most common during the second year, usually noticed when the infant begins to walk. This in-toeing is due to internal tibial torsion, metatarsus adductus, or an adducted great toe.

Internal tibial torsion ITT is the most common cause of in-toeing. It is often bilateral [C]. Unilateral ITT is most common on the left side [D]. Observational management is best. Fillauer or Denis Browne night splints are commonly prescribed, but have no long-term value; resolution occurs with or without treatment. Avoid daytime bracing and shoe modifications because they can slow the child's running and may harm the child's self-image.

Correction occurs spontaneously but often requires 1–2 years. Inform the family about the time required for correction in years, not weeks or months.

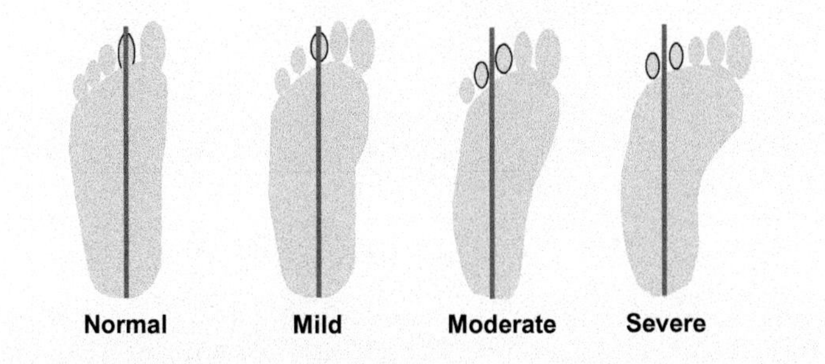

A Grading severity of forefoot adductus Project a line that bisects the heel. Normally it falls on the 2nd toe. The projected line falls through toe 3 in mild, between toes 3–4 in moderate, and between toes 4–5 in severe deformity. From Bleck (1983).

	Adductus	Varus
0 – 6 Months	Observation	Observation
6 – 24 Months	Observation	Cast treatment
24+ Months	Observation as necessary	May try casting

B Management of adductus and varus Manage these problems based on age and stiffness.

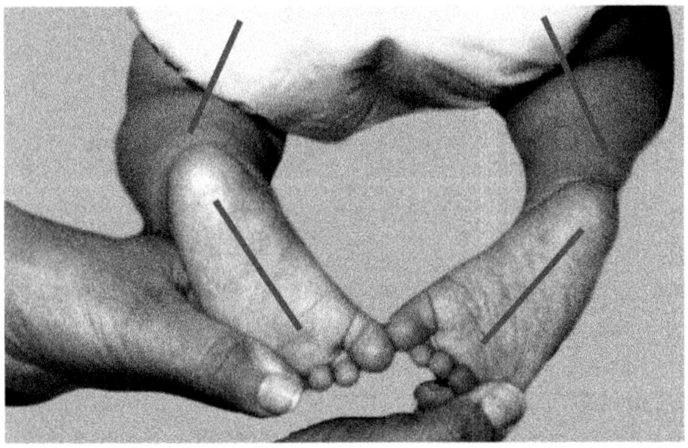

C Bilateral internal tibial torsion The thigh-foot angles are negative (red lines) for both legs.

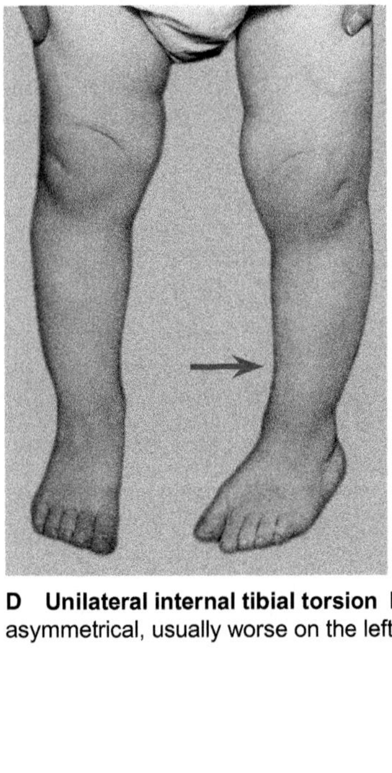

D Unilateral internal tibial torsion Medial tibial torsion is often asymmetrical, usually worse on the left side (arrow).

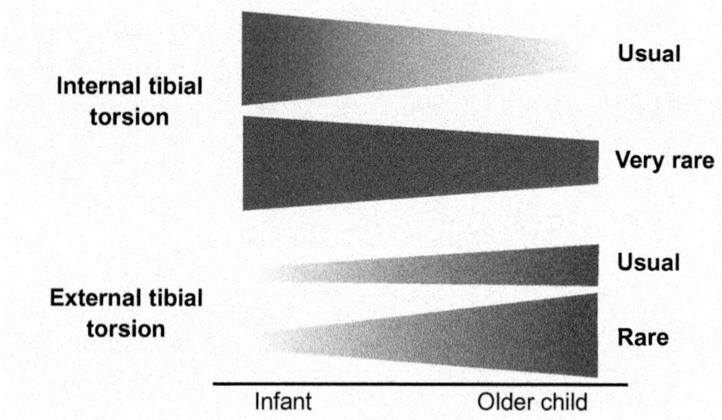

A Comparison of natural history of internal and external tibial torsion As the tibia laterally rotates with growth, internal torsion improves and external torsion may worsen. Torsion severe enough to require tibial rotational osteotomy is more common with lateral torsional deformities.

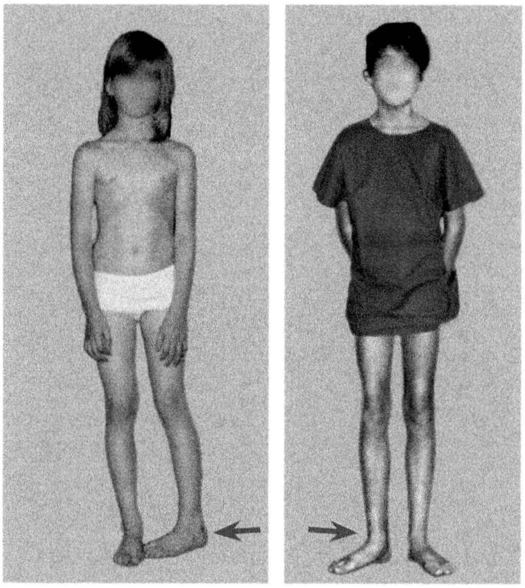

B Persisting tibial torsion Rotational deformities do not always resolve with time. These girls show persisting tibial torsion (arrows), which caused enough disability to require tibial rotational osteotomy for correction.

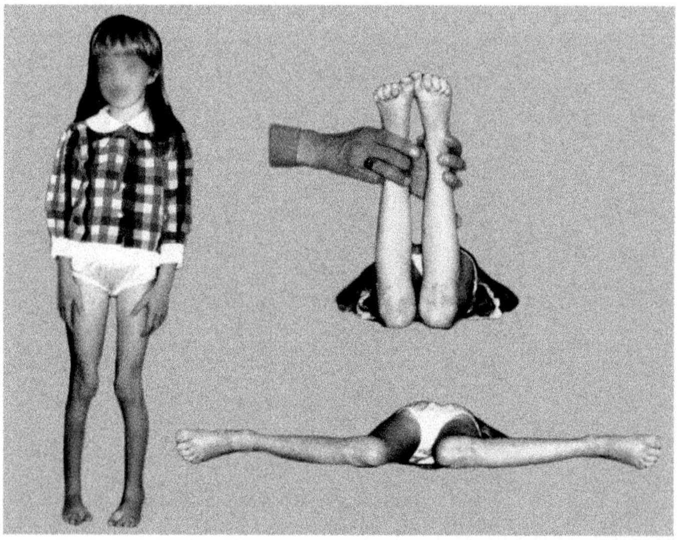

C Medial femoral torsion This girl has medial femoral torsion. Her patella face inward on standing. Her lateral rotation is 0° (upper) and her internal rotation is 90° (lower).

Child

In-toeing in childhood is commonly due to femoral antetorsion and rarely to persisting internal tibial torsion. In late childhood, out-toeing may be due to external femoral torsion or external tibial torsion. The natural history is to externally rotate with growth, often correcting internal tibial torsion and making external tibial torsion worse [A].

Internal tibial torsion is less common than external tibial torsion in the older child. ITT may also require operative correction if the deformity persists and produces a significant functional disability and cosmetic deformity in the child over 8 years of age [B]. Operative correction may be indicated if the thigh-foot angle is internally rotated more than 10°.

External tibial torsion Because the tibia normally rotates laterally with growth, ITT usually improves but ETT becomes worse with time [A and B, right, and A, next page]. ETT may be associated with knee pain. This pain arises in the patellofemoral joint and is presumably due to malalignment of the knee and the line of progression. This malalignment is most pronounced when ETT is combined with IFT. The knee is internally rotated and the ankle externally rotated, both out of alignment with the line of progression, producing a "malalignment syndrome." This condition produces an inefficient gait and patellofemoral joint pain.

Femoral antetorsion or internal femoral torsion is usually first seen in the 3–5 year age groups and is more common in girls [C]. Mild residual deformity is often seen in the parents of affected children. The child with MFT sits in the "W" position, stands with the knees medially rotated ("kissing patella"), and runs awkwardly ("egg-beater"). Internal hip rotation is increased beyond 70°. IFT is mild if the internal hip rotation is 70°–80°, moderate if 80°–90°, and severe if 90+°. External hip rotation is reduced correspondingly, as the total arch of rotation is usually about 90°–100°.

Femoral antetorsion usually is most severe between 4 and 6 years of age and then resolves [D]. This resolution results from a decrease in femoral anteversion and from a lateral rotation of the tibia. In the adult, femoral antetorsion does not cause degenerative arthritis and rarely causes any disability.

Femoral antetorsion is not affected by nonoperative treatment. Persistence of severe deformity after the age of 8 years may necessitate correction by a femoral rotational osteotomy.

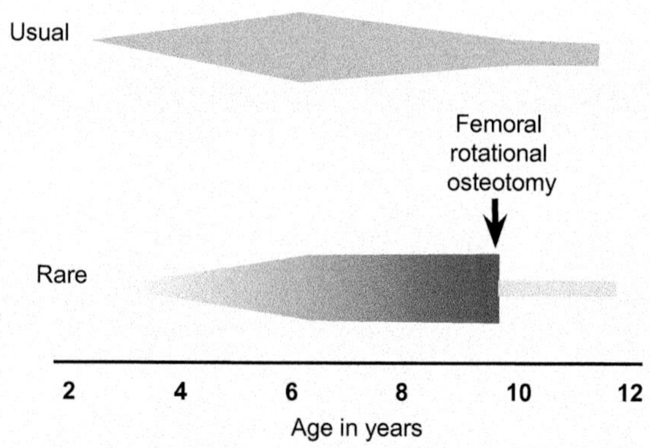

D Clinical course of femoral antetorsion Femoral antetorsion becomes more clinically apparent during infancy and early childhood. The deformity is usually most severe between about 4 and 6 years of age. Resolution occurs regardless of common treatments. Rarely, the deformity is severe and fails to improve and thus requires rotational osteotomy for correction.

Femoral retrotorsion (external femoral torsion) may be of greater significance than commonly appreciated. Retrotorsion is more common in patients with slipped capital femoral epiphysis. Presumably, the shear force on the physis is increased. Retrotorsion is associated with increased degenerative arthritis and an out-toeing gait. The gait problem is not sufficiently severe to warrant operative correction.

Operative Correction

Rotational osteotomy is effective in correcting torsional deformities of the tibia or femur [B]. Osteotomy is indicated only in the older child, over 8–10 years of age, who has a significant cosmetic and functional deformity, and with a single deformity with measures falling beyond the normal 2 SD range. The child's problem should be sufficiently severe to justify the risks of the procedure. These procedures should not be considered "prophylactic."

Femoral correction Femoral rotational osteotomy is best performed at the intertrochanteric level. At this level, healing is rapid, fixation is most secure, and scarring is least obvious and, should malunion occur, least noticeable. Usually rotational correction of about 50° is required.

Tibial correction Tibial rotational osteotomy is best performed at the supramalleolar level [B]. Correct rotation to bring the thigh-foot angle to about 10°–15°.

Rotational Malalignment Syndrome

This syndrome usually includes external tibial and internal femoral torsion. The axis of flexion of the knee is not in the line of progression. Patellofemoral problems of pain and, rarely, dislocation follow.

Manage most conservatively. Very rarely is operative correction necessary. Correction is a major undertaking, as it usually requires a 4-level procedure (both femoral and tibia). The site of the tibial osteotomy may be distal (most safe) or proximal. Proximal osteotomy just above the tibial tubercle has been reported.

Rarely, rotational malalignment is associated with severe patellofemoral disorders such as congenital dislocations [C]. Correction is complex and may require both osteotomy and soft tissue reconstructions.

Prognosis

The long-term effects of rotational deformity have shown that external rotational deformities are much more likely to be associated with disability than those from internal torsion.

Internal tibial torsion This deformity is rarely seen in the older child. It has not been found to be associated with any significant problems. Mild deformity may enhance sprinting by improving push-off.

External tibial torsion Degenerative changes in the knee, osteochondritis dissecans, and patellofemoral instability have been associated with external tibial torsion. External tibial torsion is the rotational deformity most likely to require operative correction. A combination of obesity, flatfoot, and external tibial torsion has been associated with foot pain in adolescence. External tibial torsion is a common secondary deformity seen in paralytic conditions such as myelodysplasia.

Femoral antetorsion Adults with mild to moderate antetorsion have no functional disability as compared with controls. No association between antetorsion and osteoarthritis of the hip has been found.

Femoral retrotorsion Retrotorsion may increase the risk of slipped capital femoral epiphysis and has been associated with degenerative arthritis of the hip.

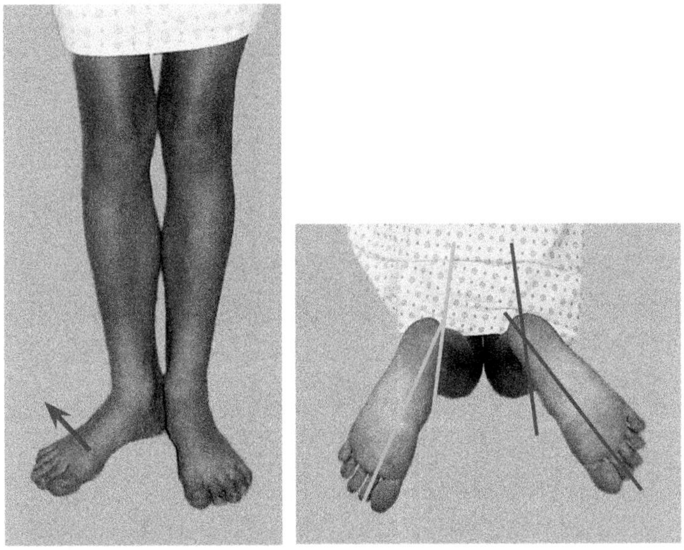

A External tibial torsion External tibial torsion is often unilateral. When asymmetrical, it is usually worse on the right side (red arrow). Note that the thigh-foot angle is more external on the right (red lines).

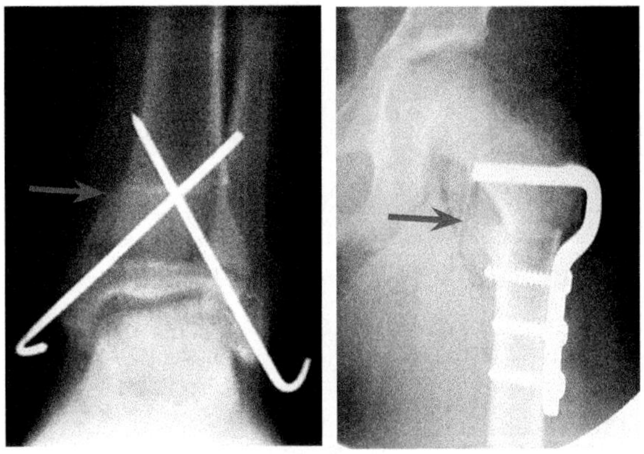

B Rotational osteotomy Rotational osteotomies are usually performed at the supramalleolar tibial or intertrochanteric femoral levels (red arrows). Fix tibial osteotomies with crossed transcutaneous pins and a long-leg cast. Fix femoral osteotomies with pins and a cast or a blade-plate.

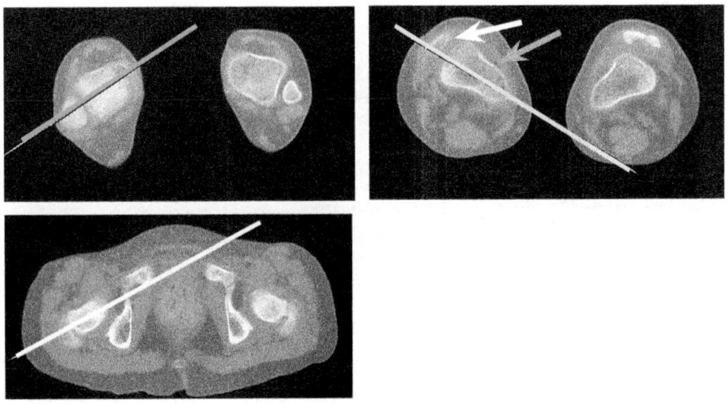

C Rotational malalignment with patellar dislocations This CT study is of a child with a dislocated patella (white arrow) displaced from the normal position (orange arrow). Note the rotational malalignment with lateral tibial torsion (blue line), the medial rotation of the axis of the knee (yellow line), and femoral antetorsion (white line).

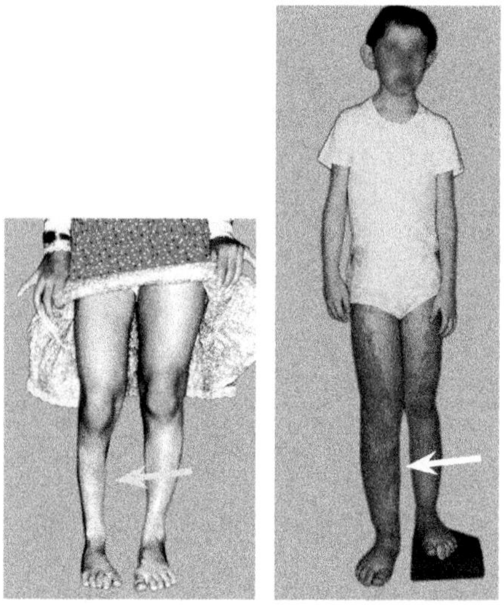

A Leg length differences This girl has a short right leg due to weakness secondary to poliomyelitis (yellow arrow). The boy has overgrowth of the right leg (white arrow) due to Klippel-Weber-Trenaunay syndrome.

Category	Short	Long
Congenital	Aplasia Hypoplasia Hip dysplasia Clubfoot	Hyperplasia
Neurogenic	Paralysis Disuse	Sympathectomy
Vascular	Ischemia Perthes disease	AV fistular
Infection	Physeal injury	Stimulation
Tumors	Physeal involvement	Vascular lesions
Trauma	Physeal injury Malunion	Fracture stimulation Distraction

B Causes of limb length discrepancy The common causes of short or long limbs.

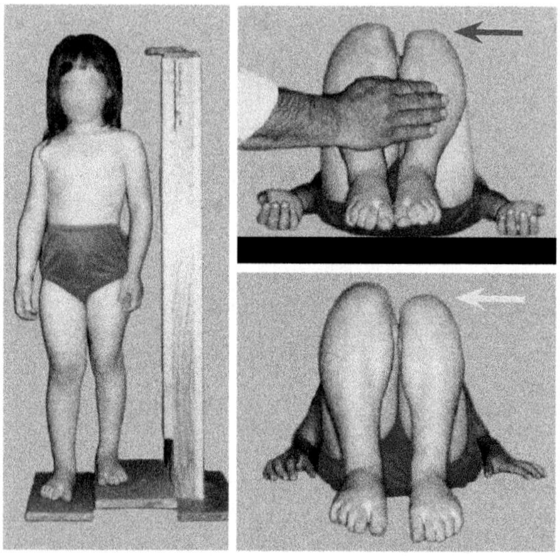

C Leg length inequality In this child, the right lower leg is hypertrophied. Note that the tibia is longer and the diameter greater. The left leg is more proportional in size to the rest of the body. The left limb is shorter both in the femur and tibia. Compare femoral lengths with the feet above the surface (red arrow). Compare tibial lengths with the feet on the surface (yellow arrow).

Leg Length Inequality

Leg length inequality, or *anisomelia,* may be structural [A] or functional. Functional anisomelia is secondary to joint contractures, producing an apparent discrepancy in length. Structural discrepancies may occur at any site in the limb or pelvis. Often only discrepancies of the tibia or femur are measured. The height of the foot and pelvis should be included in calculating the total disparity. Discrepancies of 1 cm or more are considered significant.

Etiology

The causes of anisomelia are numerous [B]. Minor discrepancies are seen in clubfeet, hip dysplasia, and Perthes disease. Major differences are seen in tibial, fibular, or femoral agenesis.

Natural History

The course of anisomelia is determined by the cause. The inhibition or acceleration that causes progressive forms of anisomelia varies according to the etiology. Growth inhibition from congenital defects is usually constant and makes predicting the final disparity feasible. Inhibition or acceleration from vascular, infectious, or neoplastic disorders are variable. For example, growth acceleration may be associated with chronic diaphyseal osteomyelitis. The acceleration occurs only when the infection is active.

Gait

The effect on gait depends on the magnitude of the discrepancy and the age of the patient. Children compensate for discrepancies by flexing the knee on the long side or by standing in equinus on the shortened limb. These compensations level the pelvis. Discrepancies are compensated by altered function. The long limb may be circumducted during the swing phase or by "vaulting" over the long limb during the stance phase. This vaulting results in a rise and fall of the body and consumes more energy than a normal gait.

Adverse Effects

The adverse effects of anisomelia have been overstated. Limb length difference in childhood does not lead to an increased risk of structural scoliosis or back pain in adults.

Evaluation

During evaluation, calculate the projected height of the patient and the degree of shortening at skeletal maturity if untreated. This evaluation requires a screening examination, a search for the cause, clinical and radiographic assessment of severity, and a determination of bone age. Serial evaluations are necessary during growth to improve the accuracy of the evaluation. From the history, determine if the child has been injured or has experienced any musculoskeletal diseases.

Screening examination Note any asymmetry and alterations in body proportions. For toddlers examine for developmental hip dysplasia. Does the asymmetry involve only the lower limbs? Is the long side the normal or abnormal side? Sometimes overgrowth makes the long side the abnormal one. Is it a hemihypertrophy or hemihypoplasia? Hemihypertrophy [A right] is important to recognize because it is sometimes associated with Wilm's tumor. The finding of hemihypertrophy should prompt an abdominal ultrasound evaluation. Hemihypoplasia is usually due to hemiparesis from cerebral palsy. Often these underlying problems are more significant than the length discrepancy itself. Observe the child walking. Is equinus, vaulting, circumduction, or abductor lurch present? Assess the abnormal limb to determine the site or sites of the discrepancy. Are the feet of equal length? Are the tibial and femoral segments equal? Are the forearms of equal length? Are any associated abnormalities present? Is joint motion symmetrical? Assess to determine whether the difference is in the femur, tibia, or a combination [C].

Clinical measures of discrepancy Assess leg length difference by placing blocks of known thickness under the short side until the pelvis is level. The patient will often sense when symmetry is established. By this method, all segments, including foot and pelvis, are assessed.

Imaging methods Image to measure discrepancies and determine any associated bone or joint deformities. Radiographic measures include the teleroentgenogram with a single exposure or orthodiagrams requiring multiple exposures on the same film. The orthodiagrams may be full length on a 36-inch film or telescoped on a 17-inch film [A]. For the infant and young child, order a teleroentgenogram because it provides an excellent screen for other problems such as hip dysplasia, it requires only one exposure, and it does not require patient cooperation. Enough serial studies should be made to provide adequate documentation to accurately predict the discrepancy at maturity and to time the epiphysiodesis. These need not be done yearly. If the discrepancy is detected in the infant, obtain the baseline study early and repeat at about 3, 6, and 9 years of age.

Bone age Bone age is the most inaccurate of the measurements. Often measurements are given with a ±2 year qualification. The standard for assessment is the Gruelich-Pyle atlas. It is wise to sample bone ages over a period of several years and average any differences from the chronological age to improve reliability.

Body height at skeletal maturation The projected height at skeletal maturation is sometimes useful in planning correction of anisomelia. Shortening is more feasible for the tall individual, whereas lengthening may be more acceptable for those of short stature. The estimation can be made by comparing the child's height with the bone age to determine a percentile. This percentile is projected to maturity to estimate adult height.

Calculating discrepancy at maturation The discrepancy at maturation is the sum of the current discrepancy and the discrepancy accumulated during the period of remaining growth. The current discrepancy is assessed by clinical and radiographic measures. The discrepancy created by remaining growth must be calculated based on the percentage of growth retardation (or acceleration).

Minimal acceptable height (MAH) The MAH is the shortest stature that would be acceptable to the family. This will be based on racial, social, cultural, individual, and family differences. As a starting point for discussion, set the MAH at 2 SD below the mean value, or about 65 inches for men and 59 inches for women [B]. Establishing the MAH involves an integration of complex issues such as the value the family gives to preservation of height, balanced with the increased risks of limb lengthening over shortening.

Management Principles

The objective of management is to level the pelvis by equalizing extremity length without imposing excessive risk, morbidity, or height reduction. The severity of the discrepancy determines the general approach to management.

Severity Degrees of shortening can be categorized to aid in planning management. These values are influenced by the minimal acceptable height as determined during evaluation. For severe discrepancies, start with lengthening. Assess progress and then consider epiphysiodesis to complete the correction.

Lifts Lifts may be useful in discrepancies greater than 2–3 cm [C]. Lifts cause problems for the child. They make the shoe heavier and less stable and are usually a source of embarrassment. Lifts make a clear statement, "I have a disability," which may be harmful to the child's self-image and status among piers. Because no immediate or late harmful effect of uncompensated anisomelia has been shown, the lift should improve function enough to compensate for inherent problems of wearing a lift. Walking without the lift will not damage the child. Lifts may be applied inside the shoe or on the heel. Make the lift as inconspicuous and lightweight as possible. More in-shoe correction can be placed in a high-top shoe. Consider placing one centimeter inside and another centimeter on the heel. Order tapered lifts when possible, as less bulk means a lighter, more stable and less conspicuous lift. To further reduce lift size, order a lift that will leave the correction about 2 cm less than the disparity.

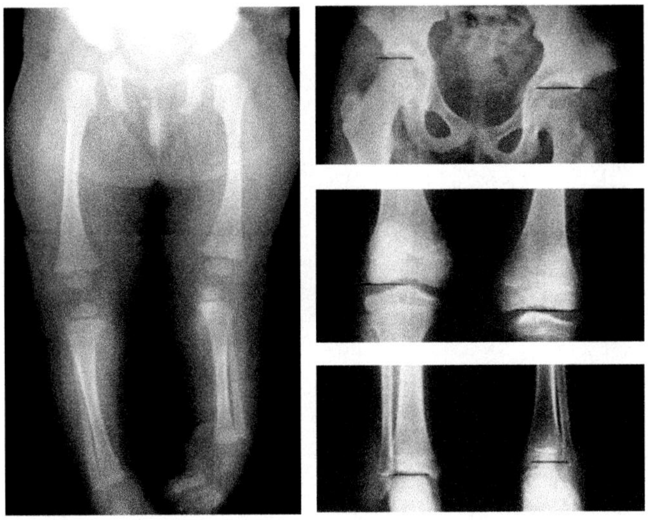

A Radiographic measures The long radiograph (left) is best for young children. The orthodiagram (right) is more accurate for older children.

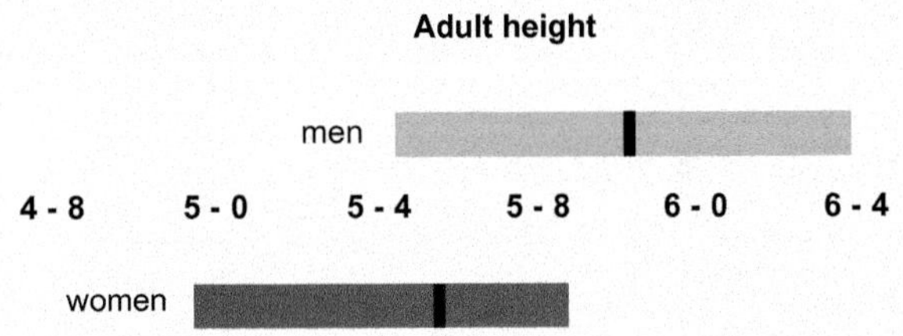

B Distribution of normal adult height The mean value is shown in black with the range of ±2 SD shown in blue for men and red for women.

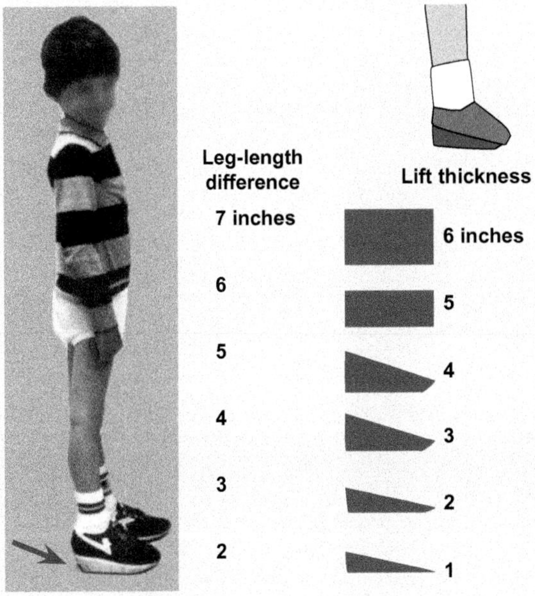

C Shoe lifts Attempt to use wedges to minimize size and weight. For large discrepancies, block lifts are necessary. Maintain correction below the actual discrepancy to minimize disability related to the lift.

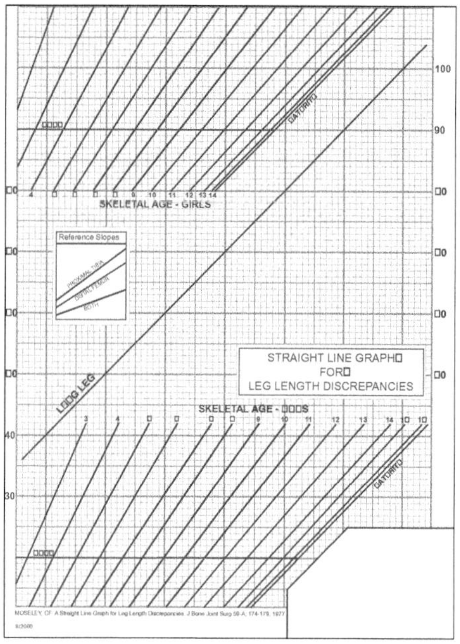

A Moseley straight-line graph This method utilizes graphic presentation of data to calculate the age for epiphysiodesis.

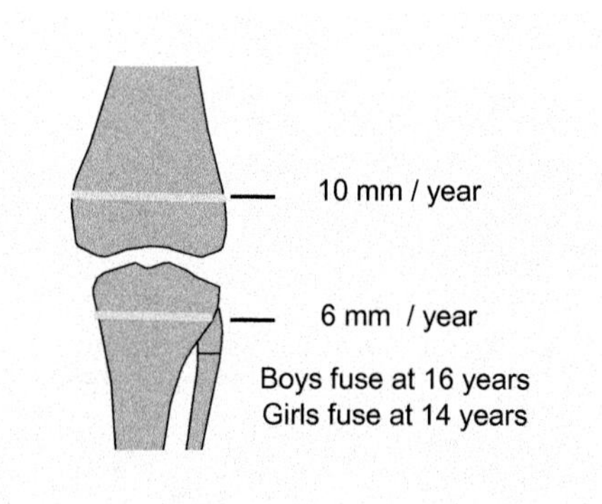

B Arithmetic method of predicting effect of epiphysiodesis The growth rate per year for the lower femur and upper tibia are shown.

LOWER LIMB Multiplier for BOYS

Age (yr + mo)	*M*	*Age (yr + mo)*	*M*
Birth	5.080	7 + 6	1.520
0 + 3	4.550	8 + 0	1.470
0 + 6	4.050	8 + 6	1.420
0 + 9	3.600	9 + 0	1.380
1 + 0	3.240	9 + 6	1.340
1 + 3	2.975	10 + 0	1.310
1 + 6	2.825	10 + 6	1.280
1 + 9	2.700	11 + 0	1.240
2 + 0	2.590	11 + 6	1.220
2 + 3	2.480	12 + 0	1.180
2 + 6	2.385	12 + 6	1.160
2 + 9	2.300	13 + 0	1.130
3 + 0	2.230	13 + 6	1.100
3 + 6	2.110	14 + 0	1.080
4 + 0	2.000	14 + 6	1.060
4 + 6	1.890	15 + 0	1.040
5 + 0	1.820	15 + 6	1.020
5 + 6	1.740	16 + 0	1.010
6 + 0	1.670	16 + 6	1.010
6 + 6	1.620	17 + 0	1.000
7 + 0	1.570	Mature Length = L ¥ M	

LOWER LIMB Multiplier for GIRLS

Age (yr + mo)	*M*	*Age (yr + mo)*	*M*
Birth	4.630	6 + 0	1.510
0 + 3	4.155	6 + 6	1.460
0 + 6	3.725	7 + 0	1.430
0 + 9	3.300	7 + 6	1.370
1 + 0	2.970	8 + 0	1.330
1 + 3	2.750	8 + 6	1.290
1 + 6	2.600	9 + 0	1.260
1 + 9	2.490	9 + 6	1.220
2 + 0	2.390	10 + 0	1.190
2 + 3	2.295	10 + 6	1.160
2 + 6	2.200	11 + 0	1.130
2 + 9	2.125	11 + 6	1.100
3 + 0	2.050	12 + 0	1.070
3 + 6	1.925	12 + 6	1.050
4 + 0	1.830	13 + 0	1.030
4 + 6	1.740	13 + 6	1.010
5 + 0	1.660	14 + 0	1.000
5 + 6	1.580		

Modified from Dror Paley et al., *JBJS Am* 2000

C Lower limb multipliers Use these charts to predict lower limb lengths for boys at girls at the end of growth. Courtesy Paley et al. (2000).

Timing of Correction

The usual objective of management is to correct the leg length discrepancy to within 1.5 cm of the opposite side, with the long leg remaining as the longer leg. Because of its simplicity, effectiveness, and safety, epiphysiodesis remains the most effective means of correcting discrepancies between 2 and 5 cm.

The timing of epiphysiodesis determines the degree of correction, and five methods of timing are currently used.

The simplistic method is useful for giving a rough estimate of the discrepancy at maturation from discrepancies of congenital origin. This is based on the assumption that the growth retardation is consistent. For example, a child with a congenital discrepancy of 3 cm at age 2 years has reached roughly half of projected adult height. Thus, at skeletal maturation, the discrepancy is likely to be about 6 cm.

The straight-line graph method of Moseley requires a special graph for each patient [A]. The method is graphic and has the advantage of averaging the bone ages.

The arithmetic method is based on average growth rates and chronological age. On average, the distal femur contributes 3/8 inch of growth per year, and the proximal tibia contributes 1/4 inch per year [B]. Girls complete growth at 14 and boys at 16 years of age. Use this method for long-term planning.

The Paley multiplier method allows prediction of eventual discrepancy and the appropriate time for correction by a contralateral epiphysiodesis. This timing is performed in steps:

Predict the disparity at maturation Apply the appropriate formula based on whether the deformity is congenital or acquired to determine the disparity at maturation. This makes use of the multiplier charts that are different for boys and girls [C].

Determine the timing for epiphysiodesis Apply a special formula to calculate the time for correction.

Mosca approach This method combines key elements of the arithmetic and multiplier methods.

Principles It is assumed that in the vast majority of acquired arrests, the arrest is total and the effect can be calculated by the arithmetic method.

Be aware that a contralateral epiphysiodesis will only arrest the progressively increasing disparity and not reduce the disparity. Dealing with the existing disparity requires accepting the current disparity, adding another level to the epiphysiodesis, or performing a shortening or lengthening procedure.

Calculate disparity at maturity Determine the current discrepancy. Level the pelvis by placing blocks of known thickness under the foot of the short leg. Make a standing radiography of the pelvis. From this study, measure the difference in level of the femoral heads. Combine the block height and the radiographic measures to establish the total leg length difference. This difference includes the disparity in length of the femur, tibia, and foot. Determine the difference at maturity by multiplying this measured difference with the multiplier factor (M) [C].

Calculate age for epiphysiodesis Use the arithmetic method [B] to determine the appropriate age for the epiphysiodesis. To increase the accuracy of timing, consider adjusting growth potential numbers slightly based on the height of the child and family. If the family is tall, the distal femur may grow 11 mm instead of 10 mm per year. Likewise, if the family is short, this growth may be only 8 or 9 mm.

Example In a child of average height with a calculated 3 cm disparity at maturation, perform a distal femoral epiphysiodesis at age 13 years for a boy or age 11 years for a girl.

Correction

Plan management based on age of diagnosis, severity, projected height at maturity, and other special factors [C].

Bone shortening is a relatively safe and effective method of correcting discrepancies in the patient beyond the age when correction by epiphysiodesis is possible. Closed shortening procedures are now the standard [A].

Stapling as a means of achieving an epiphysiodesis is appropriate only when calculating the appropriate timing for an epiphysiodesis is not possible due to difficulties in reading bone age and plotting growth.

Epiphysiodesis is the best method to correct most discrepancies between 2 and 5 cm. The traditional method leaves a long scar. Newer percutaneous methods use either a curette [B] or a drill to remove the growth plate.

Lengthening as a means of correcting anisomelia has been practiced for 90 years. During the past two decades, the worldwide application of a 50-year-old method has reduced the risks and made the procedure more effective [D]. This increased effectiveness is primarily due to the improved osteogenesis achieved by applying biological principles established through research.

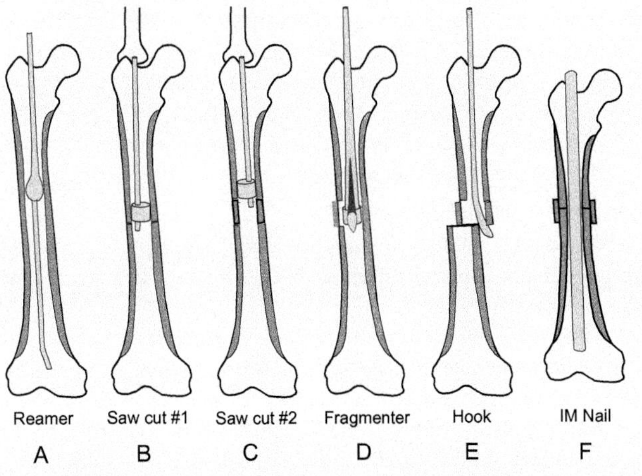

A Closed femoral shortening A segment of femur is removed by a saw placed down the medullary canal from above. A segment is divided, split, and displaced, then the femur is fixed with an intramedullary nail. From Winquist (1986).

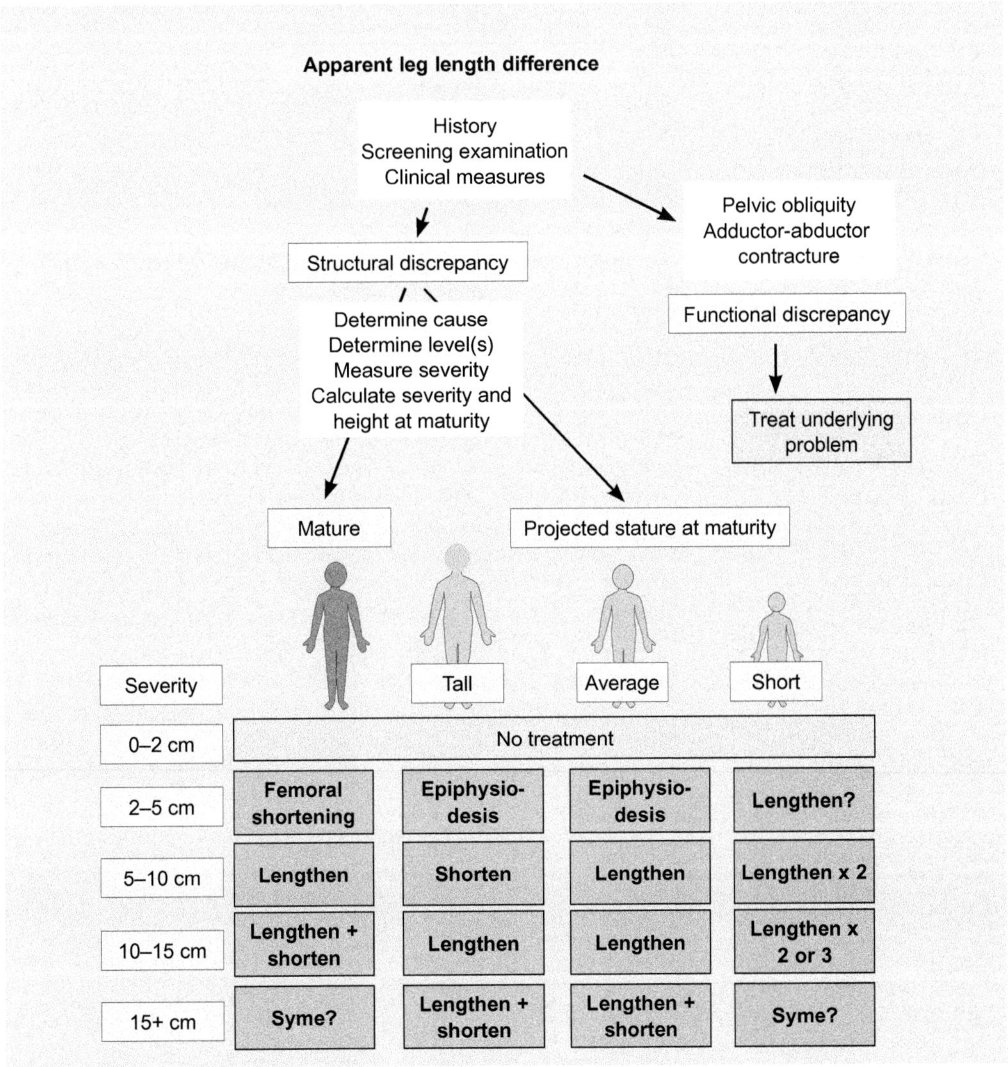

C Management flowchart for leg length inequality Management is based on the age of diagnosis, severity, and projected height at skeletal maturity.

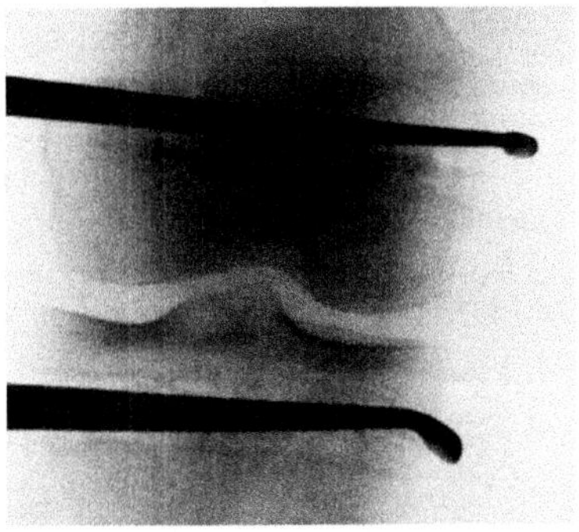

B Epiphysiodesis Growth plates are removed with a cannulated drill supplemented with a curette.

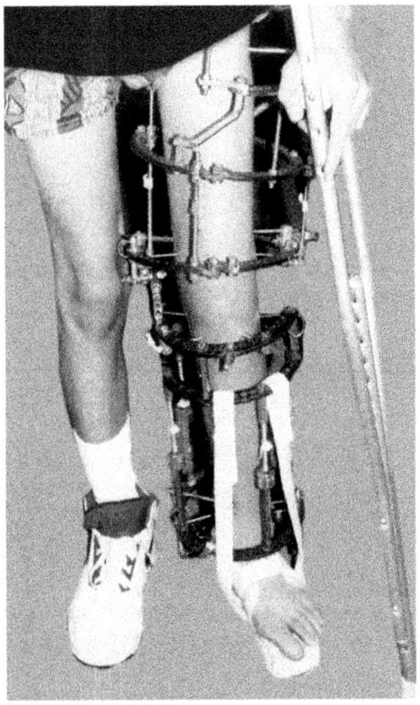

D Ilizarov lengthening

Lower Limb Deficiencies

Lower limb deficiencies are rare deformities. The diagnosis and evaluation were covered in Chapter 2. Management of lower limb deficiencies is complex, requiring correcting length equalization, stabilizing unstable joints, and correcting angular and rotational deformity. Prudent management requires a balanced approach, balancing cosmetic and functional outcomes against risks and costs of surgery.

Principles of Management

Diagnosis Establish an accurate diagnosis. Refer to a children's limb deficiency clinic when available. Refer to a geneticist. Consider other problems.

Family distress Deal with the family's shock and guilt. Be positive. Most children can have a relatively normal childhood and can become independent and productive adults.

Planning Plan a management strategy. Tailor the plan to address the unique deformities of the child and social and cultural values of the family.

Family preferences Be prepared to deal with the family's preference to lengthening over amputation, even for deformities best managed by conversion and prosthetic fitting. Be prepared for the impact of the Internet, support groups, and input from other parents on decision making.

Support groups Encourage the family to discuss management with others in support groups and medical centers.

Growth Be prepared for the effect of growth.

Amputations This procedure is well-tolerated in children, but peer and family issues often complicate management.

Pain Children rarely have phantom pain after amputation.

Greater demands Children impose greater physical demands on prosthetics.

Dealing with Deformity

Preserve length and growth plates.

Stabilize the proximal joints when possible.

Save the knee joint if possible.

Complex Be prepared to deal with problems other than limb deficiency, as deformities are often complex.

Length Estimate roughly the anticipated magnitude of shortening at maturity to plan management [A].

Anticipate lengthening to roughly 20%–25% of the bone length with each lengthening.

Perform disarticulations rather than transosseous amputations when possible to prevent diaphyseal overgrowth.

Coordinate operative and prosthetic management thoughtfully.

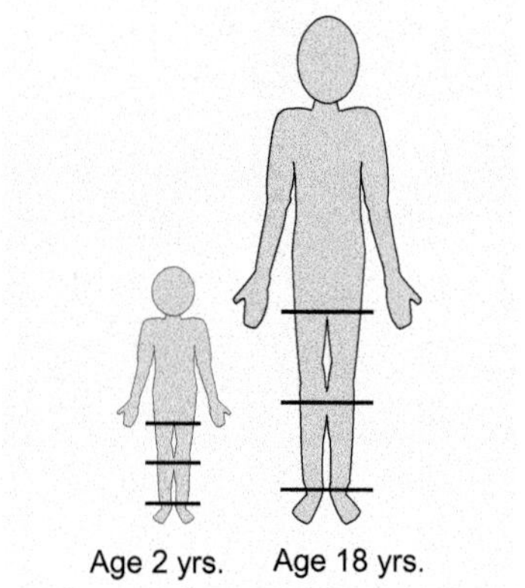

A Growth in congenital deficiencies Note that the percentage shortening of the limb remains constant throughout growth for congenital deficiencies.

Tibial Deficiency

Tibial deficiency is a congenital hypoplasia or aplasia of the tibia. Classify the deformity based on the extent of loss [B]. This deficiency may be genetic. Refer to a geneticist for a consultation and counseling. Management is based on the adequacy of the upper tibial segment.

Adequate Upper Tibial Segment

Centralize the fibula under the tibia and disarticulate the ankle at about one year of age. Fit the child with a Syme prosthesis.

Inadequate Upper Tibial Segment

Best management is disarticulation of the knee and prosthetic fitting in late infancy or early childhood.

Femoral Deficiency

Congenital femoral deficiency (CFD) includes a spectrum of deformities that may be associated with fibular deficiency [A, next page]. Some divide the condition into proximal defects (proximal femoral focal deficiency, or PFFD) and defects that involve the shaft of the femur [B, next page].

Natural History

The normal and abnormal sides remain proportionately the same throughout growth. The limb length inequality is the most obvious source of problems. Less obvious, but often significant, are hip and knee joint instability. Less significant is an external rotation deformity of the femur.

Evaluation

Study the shape of the acetabulum, the shape of the proximal ossification of the femur, and the length of the femur. Classify the deformity traditionally [C, next page] or as simply *short* or *too short*.

Deformity

PFFD includes a number of limb deformities. Consider each as part of general management.

Length Length is a major problem. Calculate the estimated discrepancy at maturity to guide management. Base the management decision on severity.

Hip joint Predict hip status based on the volume of the acetabulum. A poor acetabulum suggests that the hip will be unstable during lengthening. Mild degrees of dysplasia are correctable. Be aware that an unstable hip joint jeopardizes the success of femoral lengthening.

Proximal femur A bulbous shape of the upper femur suggests that the proximal femur is complete, but with a varus deformity and slow ossification. In contrast, a pointed and sclerotic upper femur suggests a more severe deficiency. Perform arthrography early to determine the pathology [D, next page]. Correct the varus early to enhance ossification. Congenital absence of the cruciate ligaments is common, and requires knee stabilization during femoral lengthening.

Timing of Correction

Correct proximal femoral deformity during the first year. Fit with temporary prosthesis by age 2 years. Staged lengthenings may be started as early as the second year. Delay rotational plasties until about age 4 years.

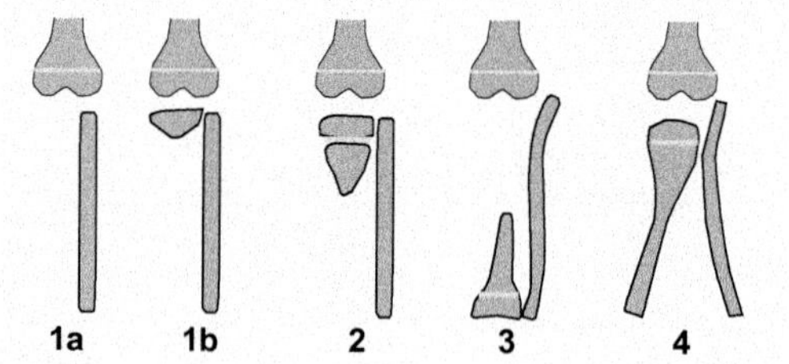

B Tibial deficiency classification Based on Jones, Barnes, and Lloyd-Roberts (1978).

Fibular Deficiency

Fibular deformities [E] are the most common of the lower limb deficiencies. They occurs sporadically and seldom have a genetic basis.

Pathology

There is partial or complete absence of the fibula [F]. A fibrous analogue may replace the osseous fibula. Fibular shortening causes lateral ankle instability. Tibial deformities may include shortening, anterior bowing, and valgus deformity. Foot deformities include the absence of the lateral portions of the foot, talocalcaneal fusions, and ankle equinus.

Natural History

Shortening is progressive but remains proportionally shortened compared to the opposite, normal side. Ankle instability results in deformity and pain in the second decade. Knee valgus may cause disability. Disability from shortening is proportional to severity.

Management

Classify the type of deformity. Calculate roughly the expected shortening at skeletal maturation. Operative management is largely determined by the extent of foot deficiencies and ankle instability. Managing the deformity is often less difficult than effectively dealing with the family.

Dealing with the family Families often have difficulty accepting Syme amputation and prosthetic management, even for severe deformities. Families often wish to delay a decision in the hope that new technology will make amputation unnecessary, or delay until the child can participate in the decision. Families often use electronic communication with other families and may elect to visit centers where complex reconstructive procedures are offered. If the family cannot make a decision, provide a special prosthesis that can incorporate the foot while the decision is being made.

Operative management Plan amputation late in the first year just before the infant would normally stand and walk. Perform a Syme or Boyd procedure. The value of resection of the fibular analogue is controversial. Correct significant tibia vara to facilitate prosthetic fitting and walking. Lengthening is best delayed until midchildhood. A shoe lift may be necessary before lengthening. Make the lift light, least intrusive, and about one inch less in height than is necessary to level the pelvis.

Genu valgum is a common associated deformity. If significant, correct by a medial distal femoral stapling in late childhood or a distal femoral osteotomy.

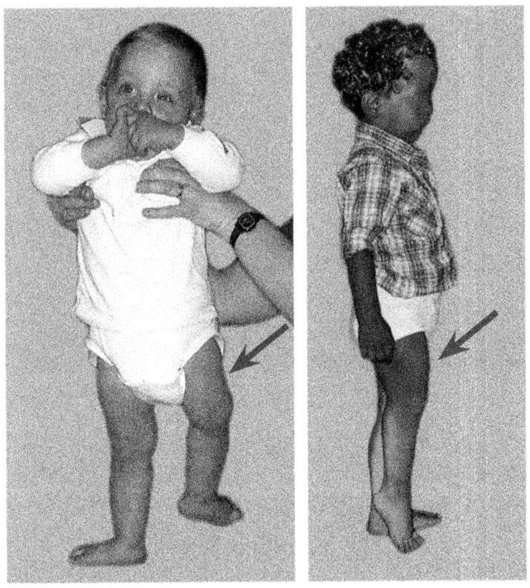

A Congenital femoral deficiency Note the shortening and lateral rotation.

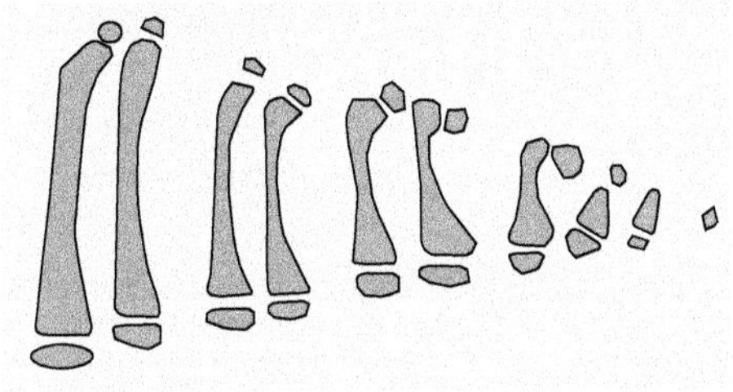

B Spectrum of the congenitally short femur This figure shows the wide variation in deformities included in this classification. Based on Hamanishi (1980).

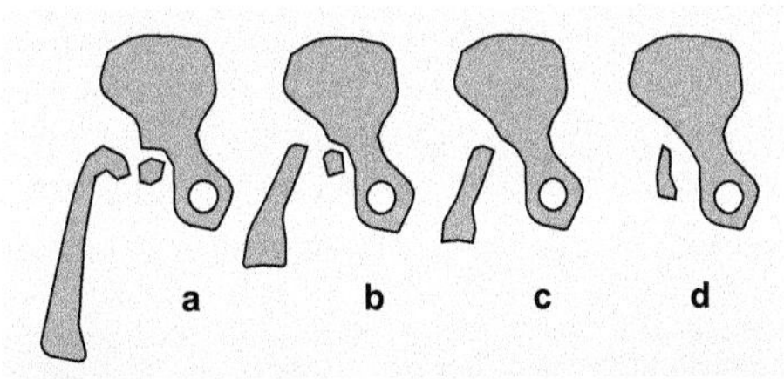

C Aiken's classification of proximal femoral focal deficiency (PFFD).

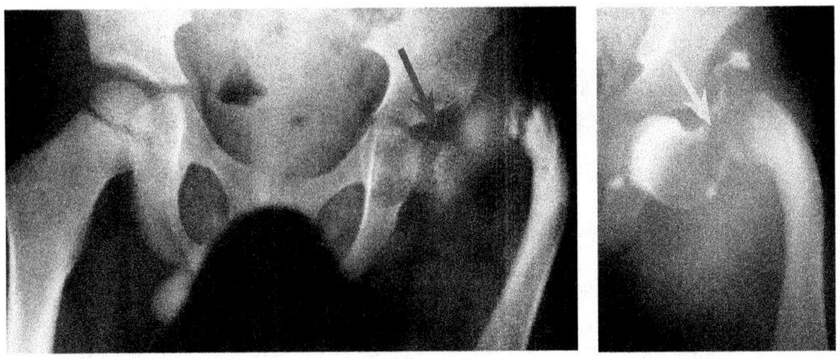

D PFFD type b Note the well-developed acetabulum (red arrow). The arthrogram shows the unossified femoral neck (yellow arrow) and severe varus.

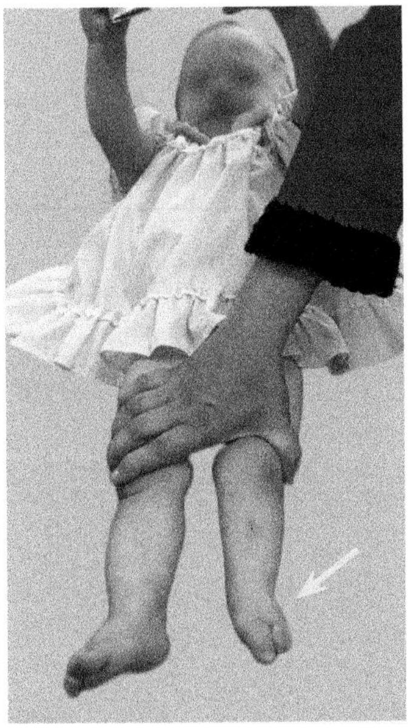

E Foot deformity with fibular deficiency The foot deformity cannot be corrected.

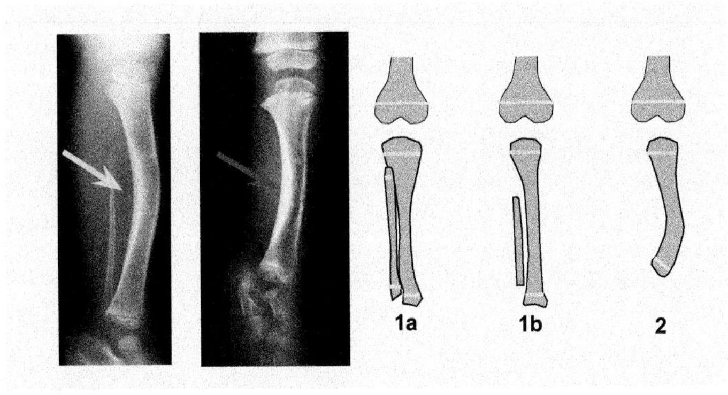

F Fibular deficiency classification Clinical examples of type 1b (yellow arrow) and type 2 (red arrow). From Achterman and Kalamchi (1979).

LIMP

Sutherland DH, Olshen R, Cooper L, Woo SLY: The development of mature gait. J Bone Joint Surg.1980, 62-A:336–353.

LEG ACHES

Naish JM, Apley J. Growing pains: a clinical study of non-arthritic limb pain in children. Arch Dis Child. 1951;26:134-140.

TORSION

Delgado ED, Schoenecker PL, Rich MM, Capelli AM. Treatment of severe torsional malalignment syndrome. J Pediatr Orthop 1996:16:484.

Fuchs R, Staheli LT. Sprinting and intoeing. Journal of Pediatric Orthopedics,1996; 16(4): 489-91.

Staheli LT, Corbett M, Wyss C, King H. Lower-extremity rotational problems in children. Normal values to guide management. Journal of Bone & Joint Surgery 1985; 67(1)A: 39-47.

GENU VALGUM and VARUM

Davids JR, Blackhurst DW, Allen BL. Radiographic evaluation of bowed legs in children. J Pediatr Orthop 2001 Mar-Apr;21(2): p257-63.

Davids JR, Blackhurst DW, Allen Jr BL. Clinical evaluation of bowed legs in children. J Pediatr Orthop B 2000 Oct;9(4): p278-84.

Heath CH, Staheli LT. Normal limits of knee angle in white children--genu varum and genu valgum. J Pediatr Orthop. 1993 Mar-Apr;13(2):259-62.

Vankka E, Salenius P. Spontaneous correction of severe tibiofemoral deformity in children. Acta orthop. scand. 53:567-570, 1982.

BLOUNT DISEASE

Blount WP. Tibia vara. Osteochondrosis deformans tibiae. J Bone Joint Surg. 1937;19:1-29.

Blount WP, Clarke GR. Control of bone growth by epiphyseal stapling; a preliminary report. J Bone Joint Surg Am. 1949;31:464-78.

Gushue DL, Houck J, Lerner AL. Effects of childhood obesity on three dimensional knee joint biomechanics during walking. J Pediatr Orthop. 2005;25:763-8.

Langenskiöld A. Tibia vara; (osteochondrosis deformans tibiae); a survey of 23 cases. Acta Chir Scand. 1952;103:1-22.

Levine AM, Drennan JC. Physiological bowing and tibia vara. The metaphysealdiaphyseal angle in the measurement of bowleg deformities. J Bone Joint Surg Am.1982;64:1158-63.

Rab GT. Oblique tibial osteotomy for Blount's disease (tibia vara). J Pediatr Orthop. 1988;8:715-20.

Smith SL, Beckish ML, Winters SC, Pugh LI, Bray EW. Treatment of late-onset tibia vara using Afghan percutaneous osteotomy and Orthofix external fixation. J Pediatr Orthop. 2000;20:606-10.

van Huyssteen A, Hastings C, Olesak M, Hoffman E. Double-elevating osteotomy for late-presenting infantile Blount's disease. J Bone Joint Surg Br. 2005;87:710-5.

Westberry DE, Davids JR, Pugh LI, Blackhurst D. Tibia vara: results of hemiepiphyseodesis. J Pediatr Orthop B. 2004;13:374-8.

OSTEOCHONDROSIS

Osgood R. Lesions of the tibial tubercle occurring during adolescence. Boston Med and Surg J.1903;148:114-7.148114 1903.

Schlatter C. Verletzungen des schnabelförmigen Fortsatzes der oberen Tibiaepiphyse. Beitr Klin Chir.1903;38:874-87.38874 1903.

CONGENITAL DISLOCATION of the KNEE

Curtis B, Fisher RL. Congenital hyperextension with anterior subluxation of the knee: Surgical management and long term observations. J Bone Joint Surg. 1969 51-A:255-69.

CONGENITAL DISLOCATION of the PATELLA

Stanisavljevic S, Zemenick G, Miller D. Congenital, irreducible, permanent lateral dislocation of the patella. Clinical Orthopaedics & Related Research 1976 (116): 190-9.

POPLITEAL CYST

Wilson PD, Eyre-Brook AL, Francis JD. A clinical and anatomical study of the semimembranosus bursa in relation to popliteal cyst. J Bone Joint Surg. 1938 20-A:963–984.

BIPARTITE PATELLA

Scapinelli R: Blood supply of the human patella: Its relation to ischaemic necrosis after fracture. J Bone Joint Surg. 1967, 49-B:563-570.

LOWER LIMB LENGTH DISCREPANCY

Anderson, M.; Messner, M. B.; and Green, W. T.: Distribution of lengths of the normal femur and tibia in children from one to eighteen years of age. J. Bone and Joint Surg., 46-A: 1197-1202, Sept. 1964.

Canale ST, Russell TA, Holcomb RL. Percutaneous epiphysiodesis: experimental study and preliminary clinical results. J Pediatr Orthop. 1986 Mar-Apr;6(2):150-6.

Green WT, Wyatt GM, Anderson M: Orthoroentgenography as a method of measuring the bones of the lower extremities. J Bone Joint Surg 1946;28:60-65.

Greulich WW, Pyle SI: Radiographic Atlas of Skeletal Development of the Hand and Wrist, 2nd edition. Stanford, CA: Stanford University Press, 1959.

Gross RH: Leg length discrepancy: How much is too much? Orthopedics 1978;1:307-310.

Gurney B, Mermier C, Robergs R, Gibson A, Rivero D. Effects of Limb-Length Discrepancy on Gait Economy and Lower-Extremity Muscle Activity in Older Adults. J Bone Joint Surg Am. 2001;83:907–915.

Ilizarov GA. Transosseous Osteosynthesis. Theoretical and Clinical Aspects of the Regeneration and Growth of Tissue. Springer-Verlag, Berlin, 1992.

Little DG, Nigo L, Aiona MD. Deficiencies of current methods for the timing of epiphysiodesis. J Pediatr Orthop. 1996 Mar-Apr;16(2):173-9.

Moseley CF: A straight-line graph for leg-length discrepancies. J Bone Joint Surg Am 1977;59:174-179.

Paley D, Bhave A, Herzenberg JE, Bowen JR. Multiplier Method for Predicting Limb-Length Discrepancy. J Bone Joint Surg Am, 2000 Oct 01;82(10):1432-1432.

Phemister DB. Operative arrestment of longitudinal growth of bones in the treatment of deformities. J. Bone and Joint Surg. 15:1-13, 1933.

Song KM, Halliday SE, Little DG: The effect of limb-length discrepancy on gait. J Bone Joint Surg Am 1997;79:1690-1698.

Westh RN, Menelaus MB: A simple calculation for the timing of epiphyseal arrest: A further report. J Bone Joint Surg Br 1981;63:117-119.

Winquist RA. Closed intramedullary osteotomies of the femur. Clin Orthop Relat Res. 1986 Nov;(212):155-64\ Nordsletten L, Holm I, Steen H, Bjerkreim I. Muscle function after femoral shortening osteotomies at the subtrochanteric and mid-diaphyseal level. A follow-up study. Arch Orthop Trauma Surg. 1994;114(1):37-9.

HEMIMELIA

Achterman C, Kalamchi A. Congenital deficiency of the fibula. Journal of Bone & Joint Surgery -British Volume 1979; 61-B(2): 133-7.

Aitken GT. Proximal femoral focal deficiency. A congenital anomaly. Subcommittee on Child Prosthetics Problems Committee on Prosthetics Research and Development, Division of Engineering of the National Research Council, National Academy of Sciences, 1968.

Frantz CH, O'Rahilly R. Congenital skeletal limb deficiencies. J. Bone Joint Surg. 43A:1202-1210, 1961.

Gillespie R, Torode IP. Classification and management of congenital abnormalities of the femur. J Bone Joint Surg (Br) 1963; 65(557-68).

Jones D, Barnes J, Lloyd-Roberts GC. Congenital aplasia and dysplasia of the tibia with intact fibula. J Bone Joint Surg (Br) 1978;60:31-9.

Stevens, C. A., Moore, C. A. Tibial hemimelia in Langer-Giedion syndrome--possible gene location for tibial hemimelia at 8q. Am. J. Med. Genet. 85: 409-412, 1999.

BOWING

Andersen KS. Congenital pseudarthrosis of the leg. Late results. Journal of Bone & Joint Surgery - American Volume 1976;58(5):657-62.

Ghanem I, Damsin JP, Carlioz H. Ilizarov technique in the treatment of congenital pseudarthrosis of the tibia. J Pediatr Orthop 1997:17:685.

Johnston CE. Congenital pseudarthrosis of the tibia: results of technical variations in the charnley-williams procedure. J Bone Joint Surg Am 2002 Oct;84-A(10): p1799-810.

Keret D, Bollini G, Dungl P, Fixsen J, Grill F, Hefti F, Ippolito E, Romanus B, Tudisco C, Wientroub S. The fibula in congenital pseudarthrosis of the tibia: the EPOS multicenter study. European Paediatric Orthopaedic Society (EPOS). J Pediatr Orthop B 2000 Apr;9(2): p69-74.

Ohnishi I; Sato W; Matsuyama J; Yajima H; Haga N; Kamegaya M; Minami A; Sato M; Yoshino S; Oki T; Nakamura K. Treatment of congenital pseudarthrosis of the tibia: a multicenter study in Japan. J Pediatr Orthop. 2005;25:219-24.

Pappas AM. Congenital posteromedial bowing of the tibia and fibula. Journal of Pediatric Orthopedics 1984; 4(5): 525-31.

Romanus B; Bollini G; Dungl P; Fixsen J; Grill F; Hefti F; Ippolito E; Tudisco C; Wientroub S. Free vascular fibular transfer in congenital pseudoarthrosis of the tibia: results of the EPOS multicenter study. European Paediatric Orthopaedic Society (EPOS). J Pediatr Orthop B. 2000;9:90-3.

FOOT

CHAPTER 9

Developmental variations of the foot are common. Thus, they are a frequent source of concern to the family and a common reason for referral to an orthopedist.

Development

Growth

The lower limb bud forms by about 4 weeks of gestation, and the foot develops over the next 4 weeks [A]. The foot achieves its adult length earlier than the rest of the body [B]. Half of the adult length of the foot is achieved between 12 and 18 months of age. By comparison, half of adult height is achieved at 2 years, and half of the lower limb length by 3 to 4 years of age. Rapid foot growth requires frequent shoe changes in infancy and childhood.

Arch Development

The longitudinal arch of the foot develops with advancing age [C]. The flatness of the infant's foot is due to a combination of abundant subcutaneous fat and joint laxity common in infants. This joint laxity allows flattening of the arch when the infant stands, and the fatty foot further obscures the longitudinal arch.

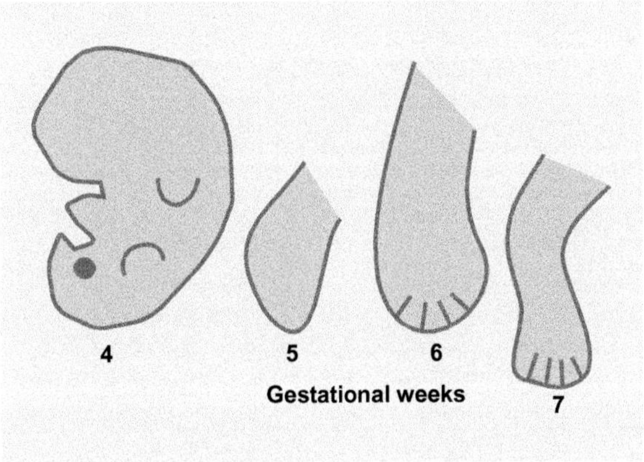

A Fetal foot development The limb bud appears by about 4 weeks of gestation and the foot is well formed by about 7 weeks.

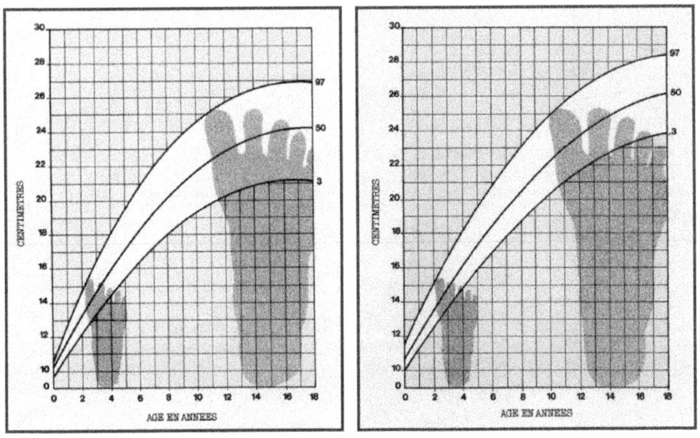

B Foot growth Dimeglio charts show the growth of the foot for girls (left) and boys (right). Note that growth of the foot slows earlier than growth in stature.

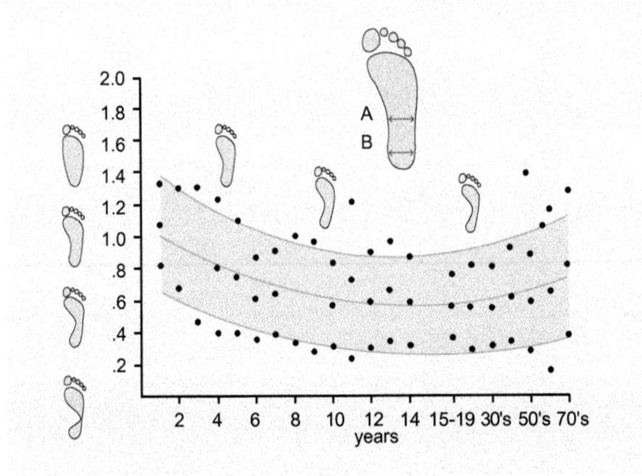

C Arch development The longitudinal arch develops with growth in childhood. Note the wide range of normal. Flatfeet fall within the normal range. From Staheli et al. (1987).

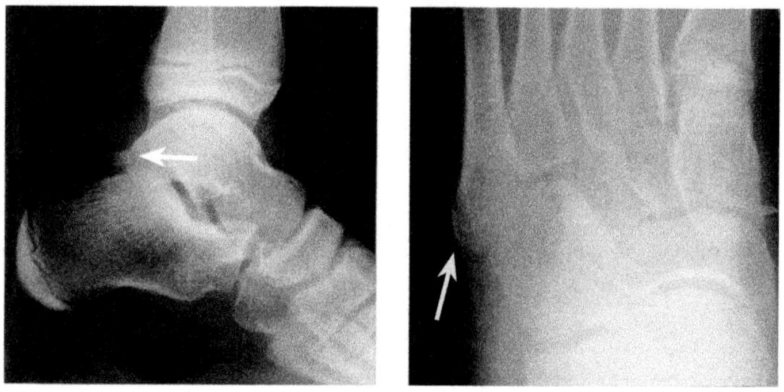

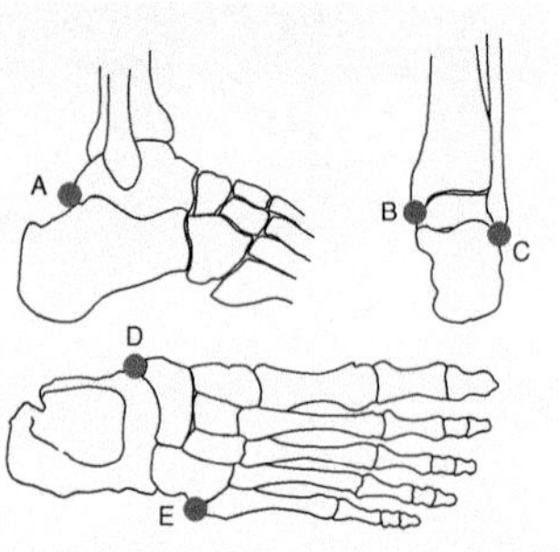

A Common accessory ossification centers about the foot (A) Os trigonum (white arrow), (B) medial malleolar ossicle, (C) lateral malleolar ossicle, (D) accessory navicular (often painful), and (E) os vesalianum. An apophysis may be confused with an accessory ossicle (yellow arrow).

Normal Variability

Accessory centers of ossification are common about the foot [A]. Most fuse with the primary center and become part of the parent ossicle. Others remain as separate ossicles, usually attached to the parent bone by cartilage or fibrous tissue. These ossicles are clinically important because they may be confused with a fracture, and they may become painful when the syndesmosis or synchondrosis is disrupted. Such disruptions commonly involve the accessory navicular and an ossicle inferior to the lateral malleolus.

Foot in Systemic Disorders

Evaluation of the foot is a useful aid in diagnosing constitutional disorders. For example, polydactylism is seen in chondroectodermal dysplasia. Dysplastic nails are found in the nail–patella syndrome.

Nomenclature

To clarify this discussion, terms describing joint motion versus those describing deformities are defined separately [B]. The anatomical position is considered neutral. Often deformity is designated simply by describing the motion and adding the term *deformity* behind it. Thus, the subtalar joint fixed in inversion is referred to as an *inversion deformity*. Note that the description of great toe position is inconsistent with standard terminology. The reference point is the center of the foot rather than the center of the body. Thus, the position of the great toe toward the midline of the body is referred to as *abduction*.

Both bones and joints may be deformed. For example, medial deviation of the neck of the talus occurs in clubfeet. This contributes to the adduction deformity. Joint deformity is usually due to stiffness with fixation in a nonfunctional position. Limit the use of the terms varus and valgus to describe deformities.

Site	Motion	Deformity
Ankle joint	Flexion	Equinus
	Extension	Calcaneus
Subtalar joint	Inversion	Heel varus
	Eversion	Heel valgus
Midtarsal joint	Adduction	Adductus
	Abduction	Abductus
	Flexion	Cavus deformity
	Extension	Rocker-bottom
	Pronation	Pronation deformity
	Supination	Supination deformity
Great toe	Abduction	Hallux varus
	Adduction	Hallux valgus
	Flexion	Flexion deformity
	Extension	Extension deformity
Toes	Flexion	Flexion deformity
	Extension	Extension deformity

B Nomenclature for normal joint motion and deformity Joint motion and deformity should be described independently.

Evaluation

Family History

Foot shape often runs in families [C]. If the deformity is present in an adult, inquiry about disability may help in managing the child's problem.

Screening Examination

Perform a screening examination. Look at the back for evidence of a spinal dysraphism that may account for a cavus foot. Assess joint laxity [D], as this may be a cause of flexible flatfeet.

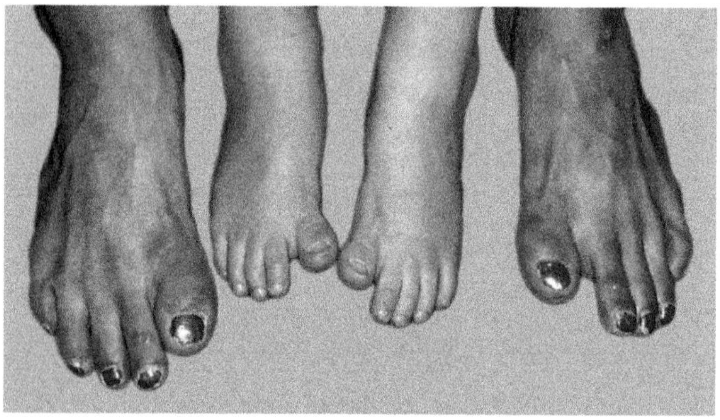

C Familial hallux varus Note the same deformity in the mother's and daughter's feet.

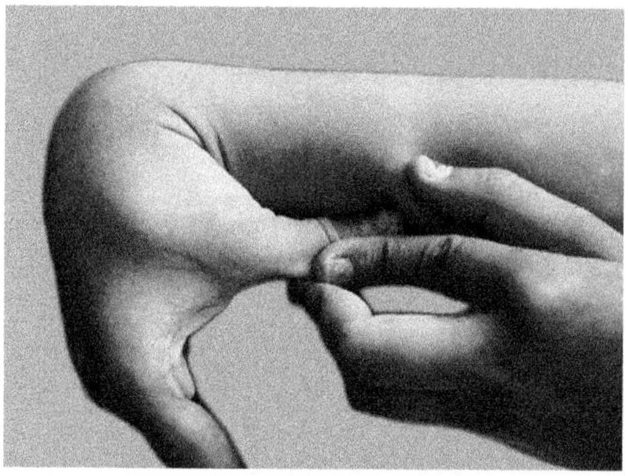

D Generalized joint laxity This child's thumb is easily opposed to the forearm. The child also has a flexible flatfoot.

Foot Examination

The diagnosis of most foot disorders can be made by physical examination. Bones and joints of the foot have little overlying obscuring soft tissue, thus deformity and swelling are easily observed. Furthermore, localization of the point of maximum tenderness (PMT) is readily established.

Observation

Observe the skin on the sole of the foot for signs of excessive loading [A and B]. Excessive loading that causes calluses is not normal in children. Common sites of excessive loading include the metatarsal heads, the base of the fifth metatarsal, and under the head of the talus. The deformities that cause the calluses are likely to cause pain in adolescence.

Observe the foot with the child standing. Note the alignment of the heel. Heel valgus is common. Note the height of the longitudinal arch. Next, ask the child to toe stand. A longitudinal arch is established in the child with a flexible flatfoot [C]. With the child seated and the foot unweighted, a longitudinal arch also appears in the child with a flexible flatfoot.

Range of Motion

Estimate the range of motion of the toes and the subtalar and ankle joints. Estimate subtalar joint mobility by the range of inversion and eversion motion. Assess ankle motion both with the knee flexed and extended and with the subtalar joint in neutral alignment [D]. Dorsiflexion to at least 20° with the knee flexed and to 10° with the knee extended should be possible.

Palpation

By palpation, determine if any tenderness is present. Determining the PMT is especially helpful in the foot because much of the foot is subcutaneous. The PMT is often diagnostic or at least helpful in making decisions regarding imaging.

Imaging

Whenever possible, radiographs of the feet should be taken with the child standing [E]. If radiographs are indicated, order AP and lateral projections. If subtalar motion is limited, an oblique view of the foot should be added to rule out a calcaneonavicular coalition. The ankle can be evaluated with AP and lateral radiographs. Order a "mortise" view if a problem such as an osteochondritis dissecans of the talus is suspected. Other special views such as flexion–extension studies may be helpful. Compare the radiographs to published standards for children. The normal range is broad and changes with age [F]. CT scans are useful in evaluating the subtalar joint for evidence of a talocalcaneal coalition. Bone scans are useful in confirming the diagnosis of an osteochondrosis, such as Freiberg disease. The scan will be abnormal before radiographic changes are present. MRI is useful for evaluating tumors.

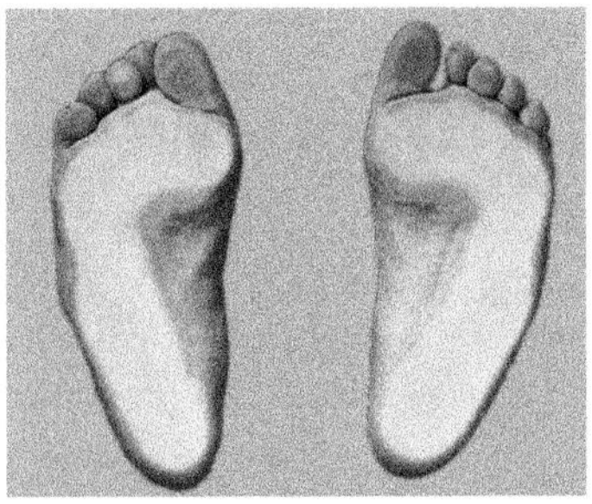

A Sole contact area Note the broad even weight distribution on the soles of these normal feet. Child is standing on a glass surface.

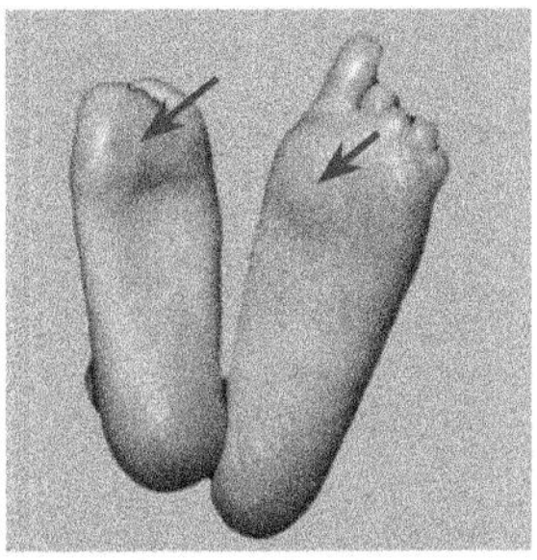

B Examine the sole for signs of excessive loading Note the calluses under the metatarsal heads of both feet in this child with congenital toe malformations.

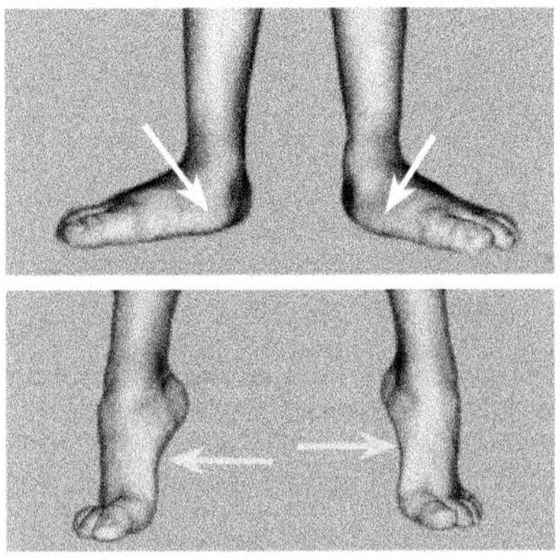

C Flexible flatfeet The longitudinal arch absent on standing (white arrows) appears on toe standing (yellow arrows).

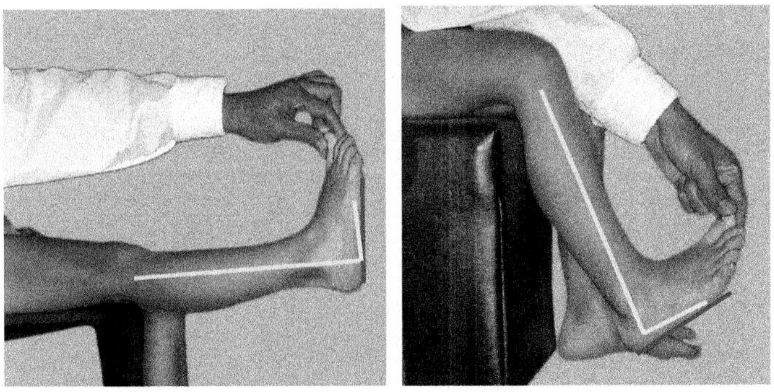

D Assessing ankle dorsiflexion Right angle (yellow) is neutral position. Assess dorsiflexion (red lines) with the knee extended and flexed to determine site and severity of triceps contractures.

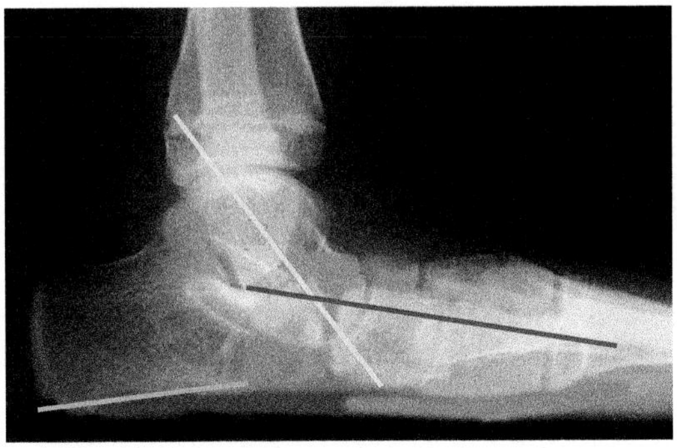

E Standing radiographs Standing radiographs allow the most consistent evaluation. In the adolescent with a skewfoot deformity, the talar inclination (yellow line), metatarsal axis (red line), and calcaneal pitch (orange line) are readily measured.

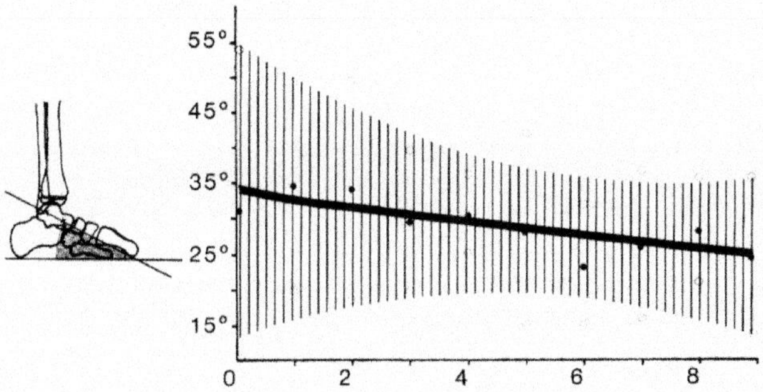

F Inclination of the talus by age The shaded area represents two standard deviations above and below the mean (heavy line). Note that the values change with age and that the normal range is very broad. From Vander Wilde et al. (1988).

Category	Disorder
Trauma	Fracture Sprain Soft tissue injury Overuse syndrome
Infections	Osteomyelitis Septic arthritis Nail puncture wound Ingrown toenail
Arthritis	Degenerative Juvenile rheumatoid Pauciarticular arthritis
Osteochondritis	Freiberg disease Köhler disease Sever disease
Impingement pain	Os trigonum syndrome Anterior tarsal compression
Syndesmosis disruptions	Accessory navicular Lateral malleolar ossicle Medial malleolar ossicle
Idiopathic disorders	Osteochondritis dissecans Tarsal tunnel syndrome Reflex sympathetic dystrophy
Deformities	Bunion Bunionette Tarsal coalition Skewfoot Flatfoot with Achilles contracture Calcaneal prominence Cavus foot Recurrent clubfoot

A Classification of foot pain The causes of foot pain can be placed in categories for classification and diagnosis.

Foot Pain

Foot pain in children is common and varied [A and B]. During the first decade of life, foot pain is usually due to traumatic and inflammatory problems, such as injuries and infections, and is seldom due to deformity. During the second decade, foot pain is often secondary to deformity.

The cause of the foot pain can often be determined by the history and physical examination. Determining the PMT is especially useful about the foot because the structures are subcutaneous and easily examined [C]. This localization often allows a presumptive diagnosis.

Trauma

Stress–occult fractures Fractures without trauma history are not uncommon in infants and young children. They may be considered as part of the toddler fracture spectrum. Fractures of the cuboid, calcaneus, and metatarsal bones can be best identified by bone scans.

Tendonitis–fasciitis Repetitive microtrauma is a common source of heel pain in children. This is most common about the os calcis either at the attachment of the heel-cord or the plantar fascia.

Infections

Infections of the foot are relatively common. Septic arthritis commonly affects the ankle and occasionally other joints of the foot. Osteomyelitis may occur in the calcaneus and other tarsal bones. Infection may be hematogenous or iatrogenic (heel sticks for blood sampling) or result from penetrating injuries.

Nail puncture wounds Nail puncture wounds are common injuries [A and B, next page] that may be complicated by osteomyelitis [C, next page]. About 5% of nail penetrations become infected, but less than 1% develop osteomyelitis. Puncture wounds under the metatarsal are more likely to be caused by *Pseudomonas* septic arthritis. Infections in the heel are commonly from *Staphylococcus* or *Streptococcus*.

Initial management Examine the foot and remove any protruding foreign material. Probing the wound will be unpleasant and unrewarding. Update tetanus immunization. Inform the family about the risk of infection and the need to return if signs of infection occur. Usually infections will show signs several days after the injury and include increasing discomfort, swelling on the dorsum of the foot, and fever.

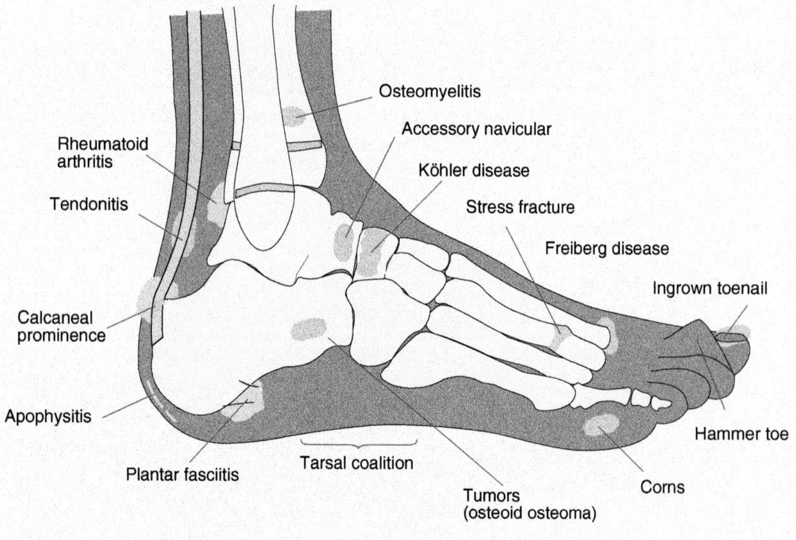

B Foot pain localization Because the foot is largely subcutaneous, localization of the tenderness will often aid in establishing the diagnosis.

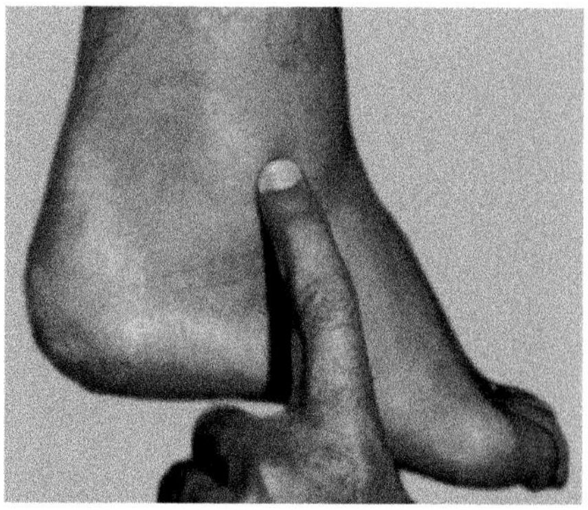

C Point of maximum tenderness The ankle is swollen and tenderness is present just anterior to the distal fibula, typical of a sprain.

Management of infection Culture the wound and obtain an AP radiograph of the foot to serve as a baseline. The time of onset of signs of an infection suggests the infecting agent. If the interval between penetration and infection is 1 day, the organism is likely to be *Streptococcus*. If the interval is 3–4 days, *Staphylococcus* is most likely, and if a week, *Pseudomonas*. Children with *Pseudomonas* infections were usually wearing shoes at the time of the penetration. Operative debridement and drainage are indicated in all *Pseudomonas* infections. Drainage is also indicated in all infections that fail to improve promptly with antibiotic treatment.

Ingrown toenails Ingrown toenails [D] are common infections resulting from a combination of anatomical predisposition, improper nail trimming, and trauma. Injury or constricting shoes or stockings may initiate the infection. In children prone to developing this problem, the nail is abnormal, often showing a greater lateral curvature of the nail into the nailbed.

Management of early infections Choose treatment based on the severity of the inflammation. Mild irritation requires only proper trimming of the nail and properly fitting shoes. Nails should be trimmed at right angles. Avoid trimming the nail to create a convex end. Instruct the family to trim the nail to create a concave end that leaves the nail edges extending beyond the skin to prevent recurrent ingrowth. Elevate the soft tissue from the nail plate with a wisp of cotton. Avoid forceful packing. Repeat this several times if necessary to lift the inflamed soft tissue from the nail plate. If inflammation is more severe, rest, elevation, protection from injury, soaking to clean and promote drainage, and antibiotics may be necessary.

Management of late infections Persistent severe lesions require operative management. The hypertrophic chronic granulation tissue is excised, and removal of the lateral portion of the nail together with a portion of the nail matrix may be necessary to prevent recurrence.

Pauciarticular Arthritis

Pauciarticular arthritis may present with foot pain in the infant or young child. A limp, limited ankle or subtalar motion, and swelling for more than 6 weeks' duration suggests this diagnosis [E]. In contrast with septic arthritis, pauciarticular arthritis looks like it should hurt more than the child reports. The pain is often minimal.

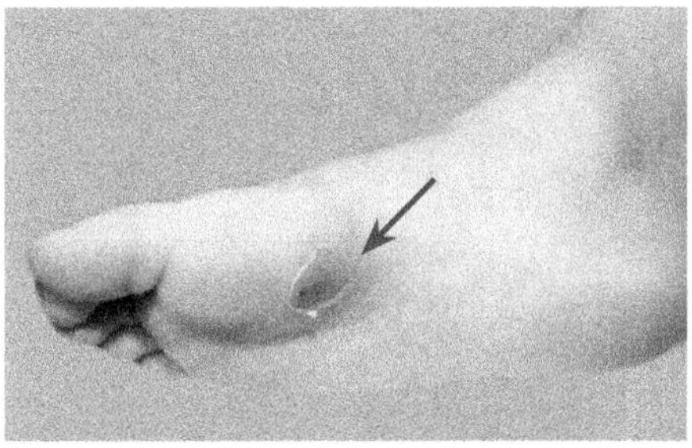

A Nail puncture wound Erythema and a puncture wound (arrow) show the site of nail entry. Swelling is most prominent on the dorsum of the foot.

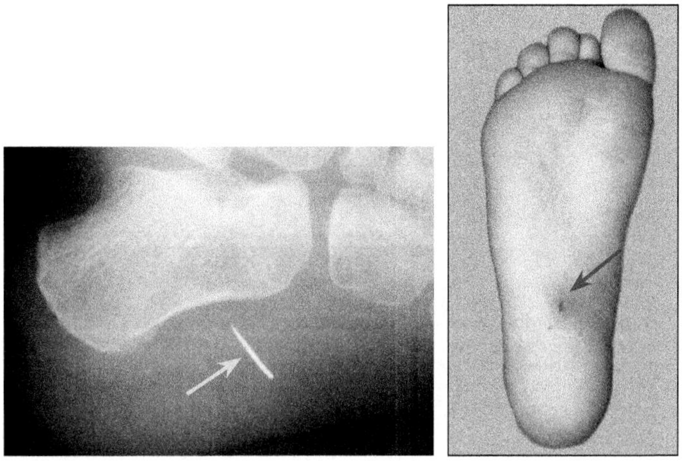

B Needle penetration into heel Radiograph (left) shows broken needle. Photograph (right) shows site of entry of needle and surrounding inflammation.

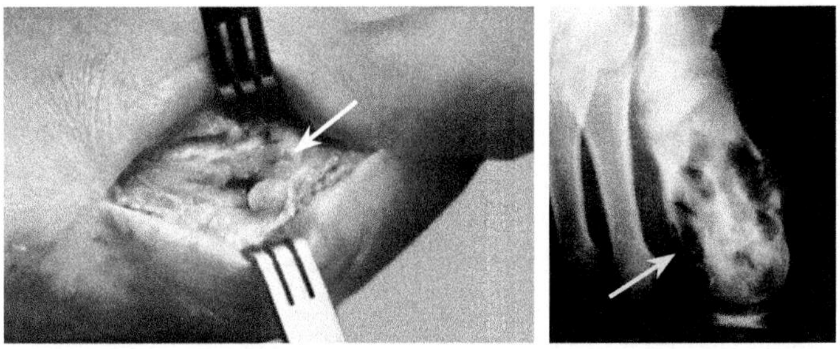

C Chronic osteomyelitis A nail puncture wound through a shoe was followed by this infection that involved the bone and joint (white arrow). The joint was destroyed. Chronic osteomyelitis of the first metatarsal (yellow arrow) is evident in the radiograph.

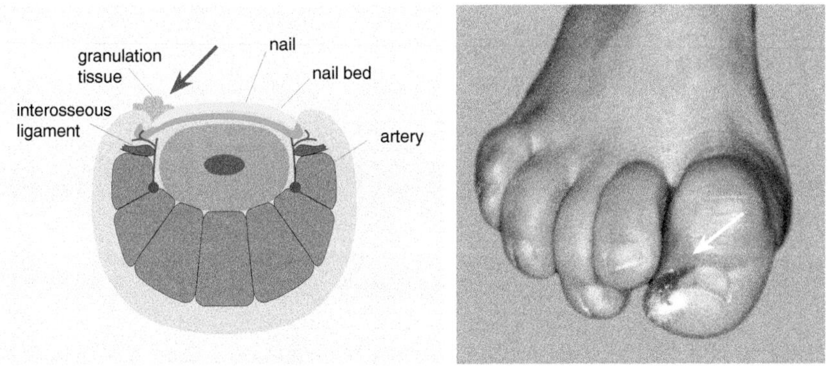

D Ingrown toenails Inflamed soft tissue around the ingrown nail (red arrow). Photograph shows typical clinical appearance (white arrow).

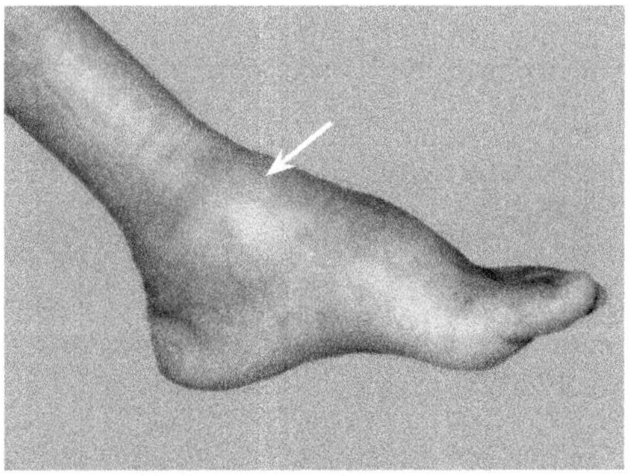

E Arthritis of the ankle This child has pauciarticular arthritis affecting the ankle.

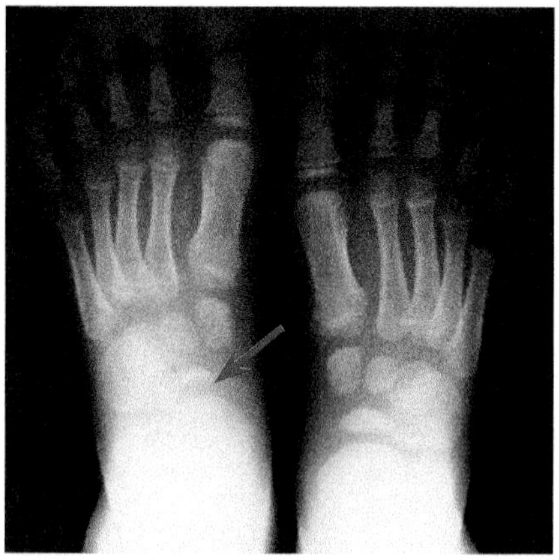

A Köhler disease in a 5-year-old boy The tarsal navicular of the left foot is sclerotic (arrow) and the site of tenderness.

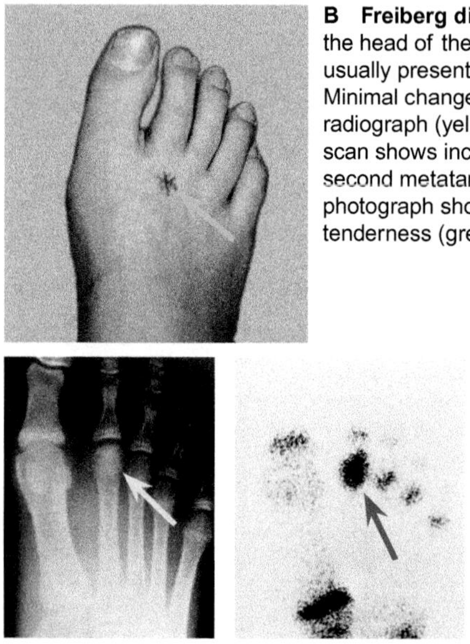

B Freiberg disease Tenderness over the head of the second metatarsal is usually present in Freiberg disease. Minimal changes are present in the radiograph (yellow arrow), and the bone scan shows increased uptake over the second metatarsal head (red arrow). The photograph shows the point of maximum tenderness (green arrow).

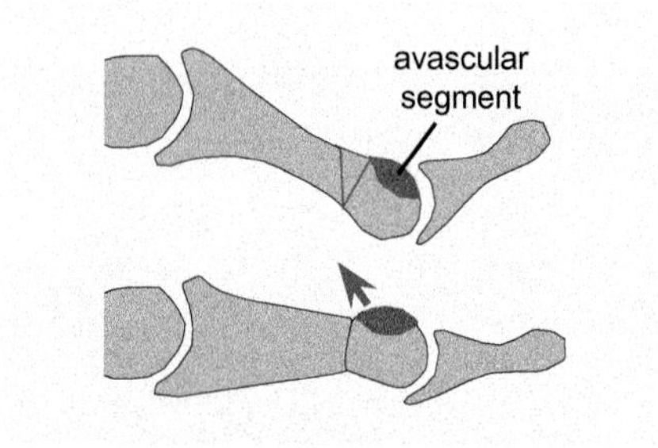

C Metatarsal osteotomy for pain due to Freiberg deformity This procedure moves the avascular segment of the metatarsal head away from the joint.

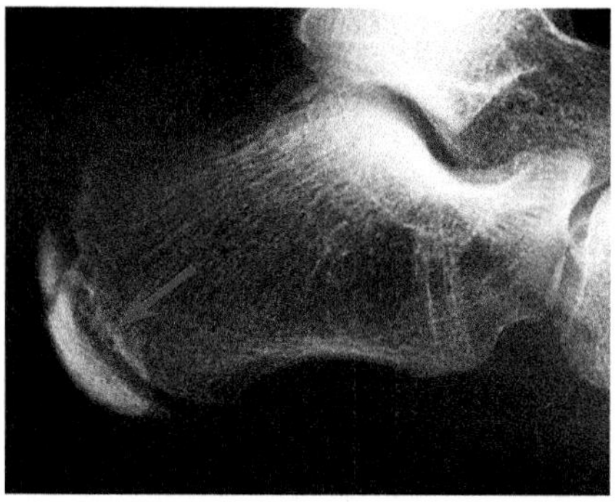

D Calcaneal apophysis In the normal child, this apophysis often shows sclerosis and fragmentation.

Osteochondritis

Köhler disease Tarsal navicular osteochondritis, also known as Köhler disease, is an avascular necrosis most common in boys between 3 and 10 years of age [A]. It also occurs uncommonly in girls 2 to 4 years of age. The disease produces inflammation, localized tenderness, pain, and a limp. Radiographic changes depend on the stage of the disease. The navicular first shows collapse and increased density. Patchy deossification follows. Finally, the navicular is reconstituted. Because healing occurs spontaneously, only symptomatic treatment is necessary. If pain is a significant problem, immobilize the foot in a short-leg walking cast for 6–8 weeks to reduce inflammation and provide relief of pain. Long-term follow-up studies show no residual disability.

Freiberg disease Metatarsal head osteochondritis, also known as Freiberg disease or infraction, is an idiopathic segmental avascular necrosis of the head of a metatarsal. It most commonly occurs in adolescent girls, 13–18 years, and involves the second metatarsal. Pain and localized tenderness [B] are common. If the patient is seen early, a bone scan will show increased uptake and establish the diagnosis. Later, radiographs will show irregularity of the articular surface, sclerosis, fragmentation, and finally reconstitution. Residual overgrowth and articular irregularity may lead to degenerative changes and persistent pain. Treat with rest and immobilization to reduce inflammation. An orthosis to unweight the involved metatarsal head, sole stiffeners to reduce motion of the joint, and even a short-leg walking cast may be useful. For severe persisting pain, operative correction may be necessary. Options include joint debridement, excisional arthroplasty (proximal phalanx), interposition arthroplasty using the tendon of the extensor digitorum longus, and dorsiflexion osteotomy [C] of the metatarsal (often the best choice).

Sever disease or calcaneal apophyseal osteochondrosis is commonly diagnosed by heel pain and radiographic features of fragmentation and sclerosis of the calcaneal apophysis. These radiographic changes occur commonly in asymptomatic children [D]. This condition resolves with time. Most heel pain in children is due to inflammation of the attachment of the plantar fascia or heel-cord.

Impingement Pain

Os trigonum syndrome Compression of the ossicle in dancers often causes foot pain.

Mid tarsal impingement Mid foot pain is sometimes due to compression of articular margins often secondary to tarsal coalitions or heel-cord contracture [E].

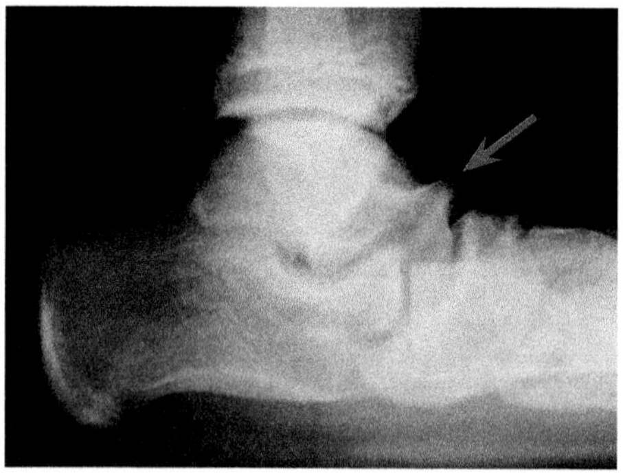

E Impingement This is talar beaking associated with a tight heel-cord and impingement.

Syndesmosis Disruption

Disruption of the syndesmosis between the primary ossicle and a secondary center of ossification (accessory ossicle) is a common cause of pain in the feet of children and teenagers. This disruption is the equivalent of a stress injury of the cartilaginous or fibrous attachment. It becomes painful and tender [A] unless healing is complete. The condition commonly recurs.

Accessory navicular is an accessory ossification center on the medial side of the tarsal navicular that occurs in about 10% of the population and remains as a separate ossification center in about 2%. They are classified into three types [B]. Type 1 is seldom symptomatic. Type 2 is most likely to have pain from disruption of the synchondrosis. Disruptions are common during late childhood and adolescence and are probably due to repetitive trauma. This disruption causes pain and localized tenderness. Type 3 causes a prominence that, if large, may cause irritation of the overlying skin.

Manage pain with a short-leg cast or splint. If the pain persists, excision of the accessory navicular may be necessary. Simply excise the ossicle and a portion of the elongated primary navicular through a longitudinal split in the fibers of the posterior tibial tendon [C]. Avoid the more extensive Kidner procedure, which requires rerouting the tendon and does not improve the outcome.

Malleolar ossicles Ossification centers occur below the medial and lateral malleoli. Persisting ossicles under the lateral malleolus are most likely to be painful [D]. Manage first by cast immobilization. Rarely, excision or stabilization by internal fixation is necessary.

Idiopathic Disorders

Tarsal tunnel syndrome Foot pain, Tinel's sign over tarsal tunnel, dysesthesias, and delayed nerve condition suggest this diagnosis. This syndrome differs in children. Typically, the child is female, walks with the foot in varus, may elect to use crutches, and often requires operative release.

Reflex sympathetic dystrophy This syndrome usually affects the lower limb in girls [E]. Consider this diagnosis when the foot is swollen, stiff, cool, and generally painful. A history of injury is common. Pain assessment by the child is exaggerated and does not match the history or physical findings. See Chapter 3 for management.

Foot Deformities

Foot deformities may cause pain due to pressure over bony prominences [F] or to altered mechanics of the foot. Pain from deformity is usually not difficult to recognize.

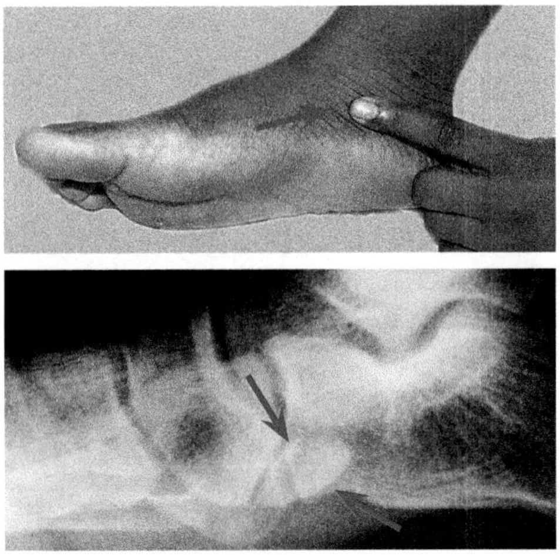

A Accessory navicular The accessory navicular is located on the medial aspect of the foot (arrows). It often produces a prominence and is sometimes painful.

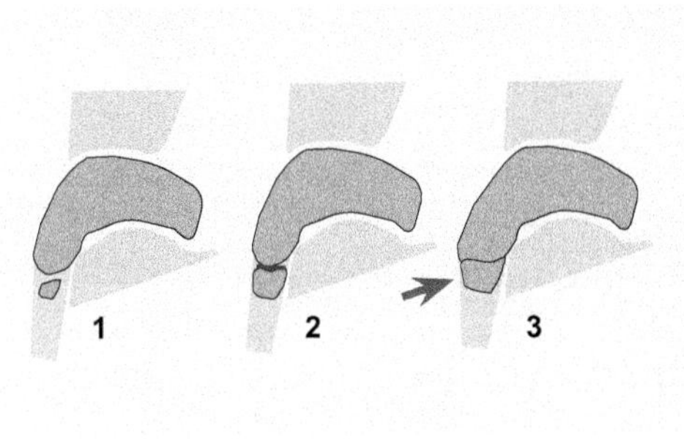

B Classification of accessory navicular Type 2 with disruption of the synchondrosis (red arc) and type 3 producing a prominence (arrow).

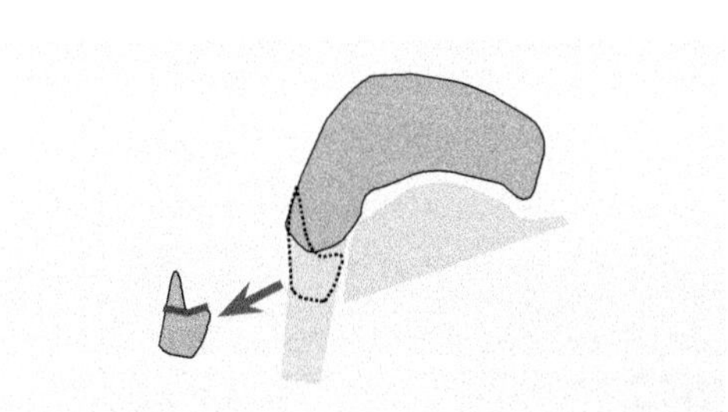

C Excision of accessory navicular The painful type 2 ossicle is removed, leaving the tendinous posterior tibial tendon attached to the navicular (arrow).

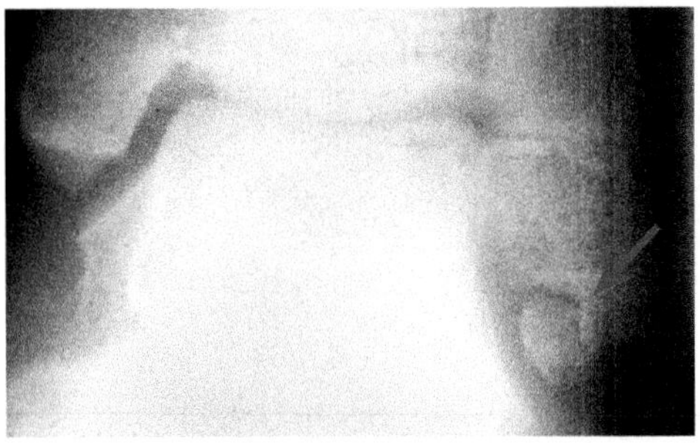

D Lateral malleolar ossicle This ossicle was painful, not improved by casting, and eventually required fusion with screw fixation.

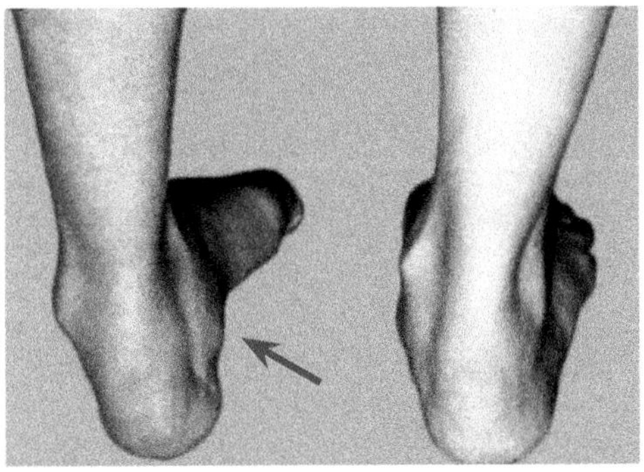

E Reflex sympathetic dystrophy The varus deformity of the left foot is due to reflex sympathetic dystrophy.

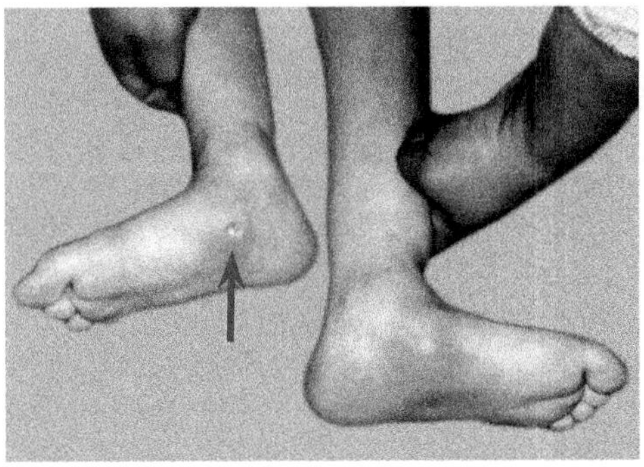

F Foot deformities in a child with spina bifida Prominence of the head of the talus caused skin breakdown in the foot with diminished sensation.

Toe Deformities	Disorders
Polydactyly	Chondroectodermal dysplasia Carpenter syndrome Otopalatodigital syndrome
Syndactyly	Apert syndrome
Metatarsal hypoplasia	Achondrogenesis Brachydactyly syndrome
Broad toe	Acromesomelic dysplasia

A Syndromes associated with toe deformities

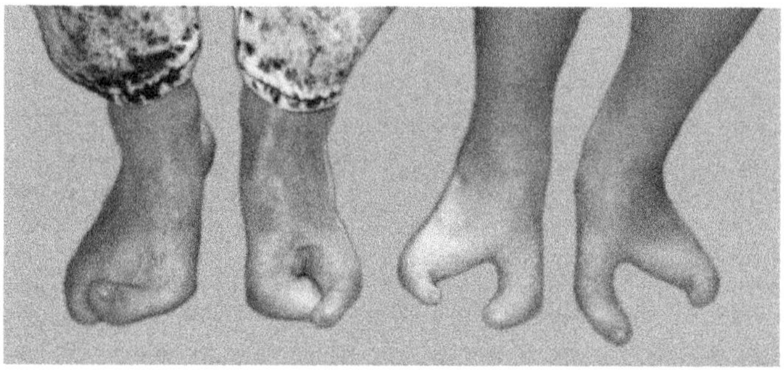

B Cleft foot deformity These deformities are present in both the father and the son. The major problems are difficulties with shoe fitting and the unusual appearance.

Toe Deformities

Generalized Disorders

If a toe deformity is found, carefully examine the hands and feet of the child and of the parents. These deformities are sometimes manifestations of a generalized disorder [A].

Cleft Foot Deformity

This rare deformity is transmitted as an autosomal dominant trait, is usually bilateral, and often involves the hands and feet [B]. A noninherited form is less common and is often unilateral. If it causes shoe-fitting problems, correct in late infancy or childhood by osteotomy and soft tissue approximation.

Microdactyly

Small toes are often found in Streeter dysplasia and may be secondary to intrauterine hypotension, causing insufficient circulation to the toes [C]. No treatment is required.

Syndactyly

Syndactyly is most common between the second and third toes, is usually bilateral and often familial. Fusion of the toes produces no functional disability and treatment is unnecessary. Look for some underlying problem if it involves more than two locations.

Polydactyly

Polydactyly or supernumerary digits are common [D]. They are most common in girls and in blacks and are sometimes inherited as an autosomal dominant trait. Most involve the little toe and duplication of the proximal phalanx with a block metatarsal or wide metatarsal head. Excise the extra digit late in the first year when the foot is large enough to make excision simple and before the infant is aware of the problem. Plan the procedure to minimize the scar, establish a normal foot contour, and avoid disturbing growth. Central duplications often cause permanent widening of the foot. Poor results are more likely for great toe duplications with persistent hallux varus and complex deformities [E and F].

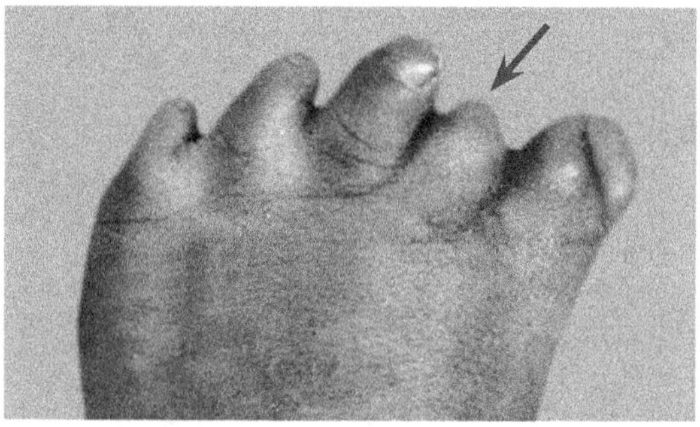

C Microdactyly

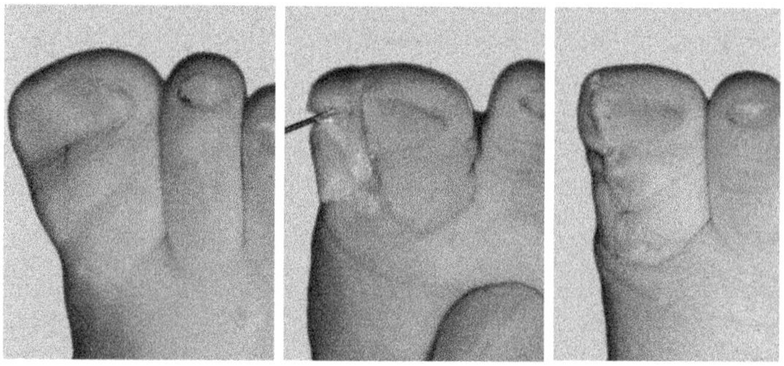

D Excision of bifid great toe Half of the toe is removed. Excision of complex polydactyly is sometimes difficult.

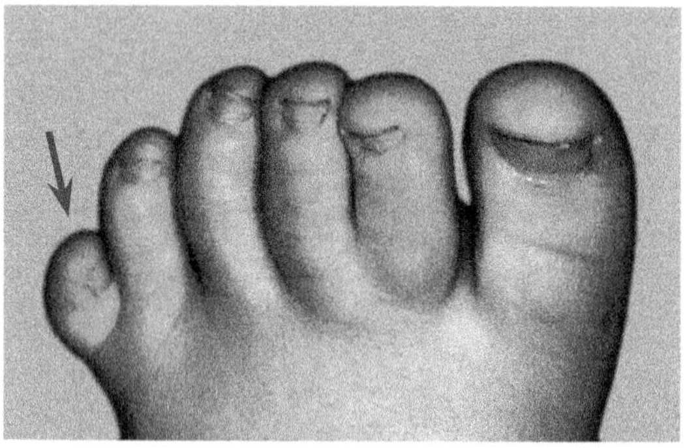

E Polydactyly Polydactyly causes a cosmetic and shoe-fitting problem. Excision of the accessory toe is appropriate late in the first year.

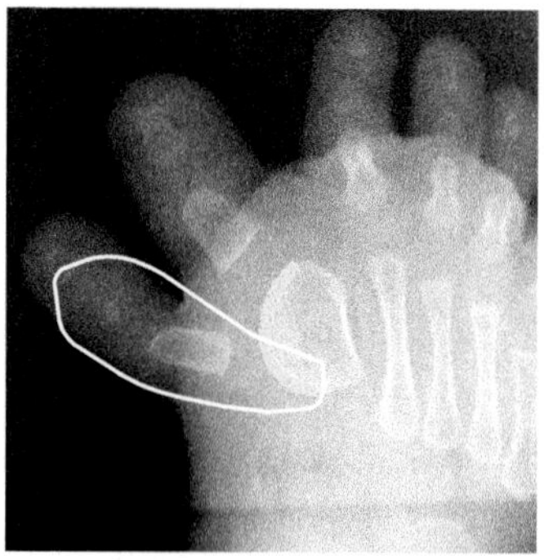

F Bracket epiphysis Toe deformities may be complex. In this case, the metatarsal epiphysis (yellow arc) is continuous for both toes. Excise the accessory digit and the adjacent portion of the growth plate.

Curly Toes
Curly toes [A] are common in infancy and produce flexion and rotational deformities of the lesser toes. The deformity nearly always resolves spontaneously. Rarely, flexor tendonectomy is required for those that persist beyond age 4 years.

Claw Toes
Claw toes are usually associated with a cavus foot and are often secondary to a neurologic problem. Correction is usually part of the management of the cavus foot complex.

Hammer Toes
Hammer toes are secondary to a fixed flexion deformity of the proximal interphalangeal (PIP) joint [B]. The distal joint may be fixed or flexible. The condition is often bilateral, familial, and most commonly involves the second toes and less frequently the third and fourth. Operative correction is indicated in adolescence if the deformity produces pain or shoe-fitting problems. Correct by releasing the flexor tendons and fusing the PIP joint.

Mallet Toes
Mallet toes are due to a fixed flexion deformity of the distal interphalangeal (DIP) joint. These deformities are uncommon.

Overlapping Toes
Overlapping toes are common. Overlapping of the second, third, and fourth toes usually resolves with time. Overlapping of the fifth toe is more likely to be permanent [C] and cause a problem with shoe fitting. Overlapping of the fifth toe is often bilateral and familial. If overlapping becomes fixed, persists, and causes shoe-fitting problems, operative correction is appropriate. Correct with the Butler soft tissue alignment procedure [D]. This involves a double racket-handle incision, lengthening of the extensor tendon, releasing the joint contracture, and skin repair with the toe translated to a more plantar and lateral position.

Hypertrophy
Hypertrophy [E] is seen in children with Proteus syndrome, neurofibromatosis, or vascular malformation, or it can occur as an isolated deformity. Most show abnormal accumulation of adipose tissue, and some show endoneural and perineural fibrosis and focal neural and vascular proliferation. Management is difficult. Epiphysiodesis, debulking, ray resection, and through-joint amputations are often necessary. Recurrence is frequent, and several procedures are often required during childhood to facilitate shoe fitting.

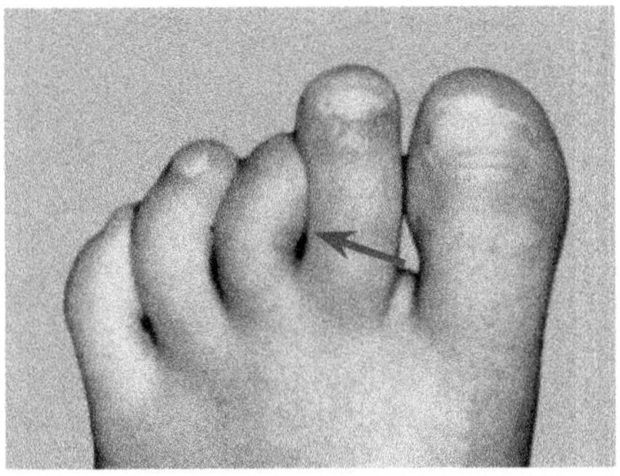

A Curly toes This deformity may involve one or more toes and usually resolves spontaneously.

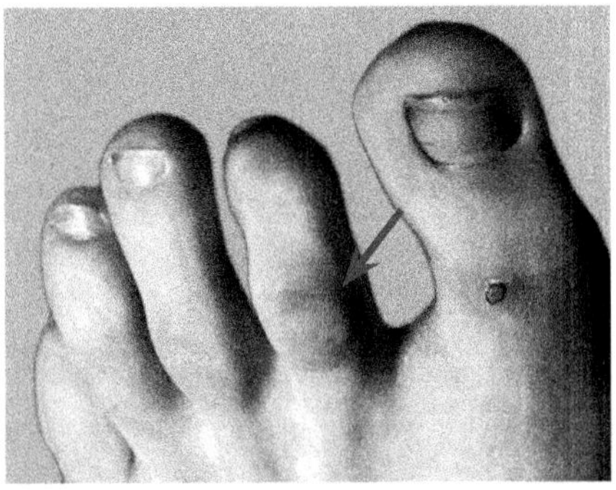

B Hammer toe The fixed flexion deformity of the PIP joint of the second toe causes a callus (arrow) to form over the toe.

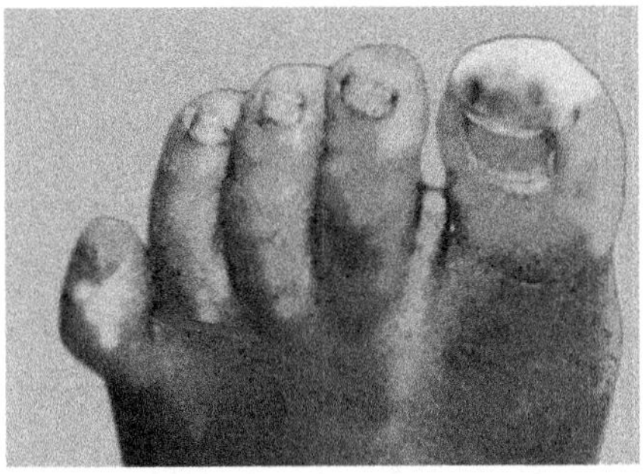

C Overlapping toe This overlapping fifth toe persisted and required operative correction.

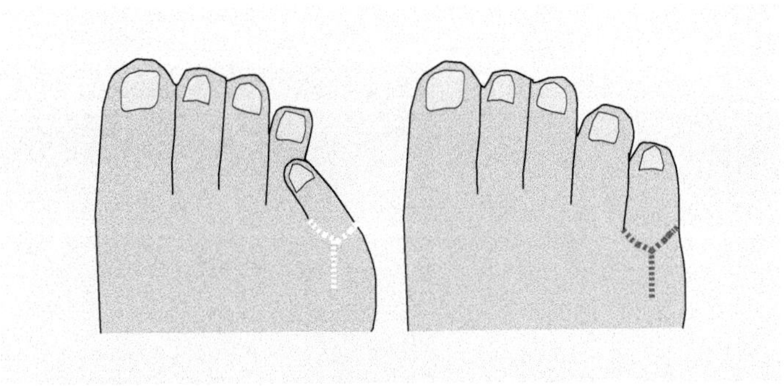

D Operative correction of overlapping toe Through a bucket handle incision (white line) lengthen the extensor tendon and capsule, correct the deformity, and close the skin, maintaining the correction (red line).

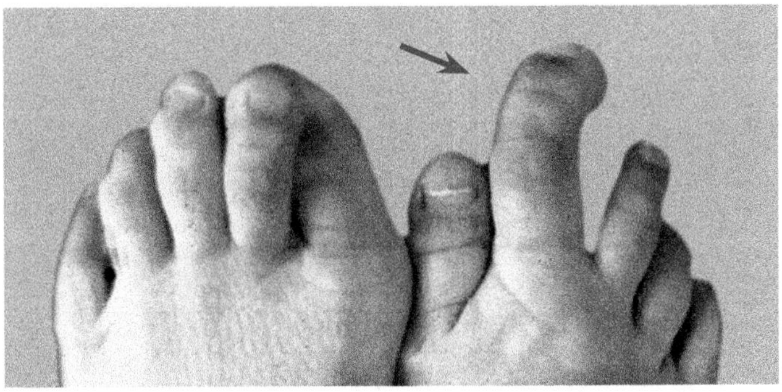

E Hypertrophy Overgrowth may cause severe shoe-fitting problems and require resection, epiphysiodesis, or amputation.

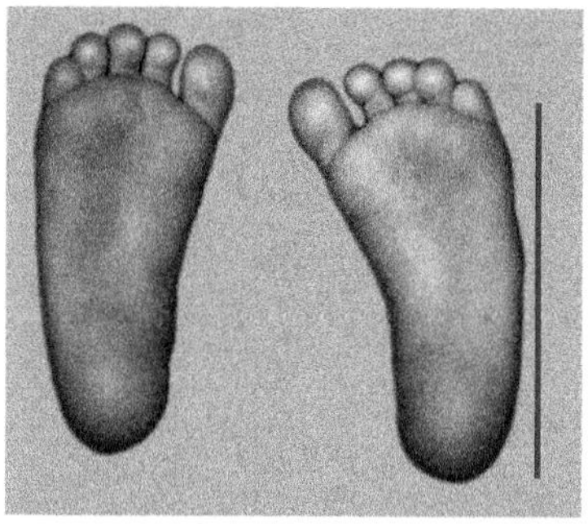

A Metatarsus adductus A convexity of the lateral border of the foot (red line) is the most consistent feature of this deformity.

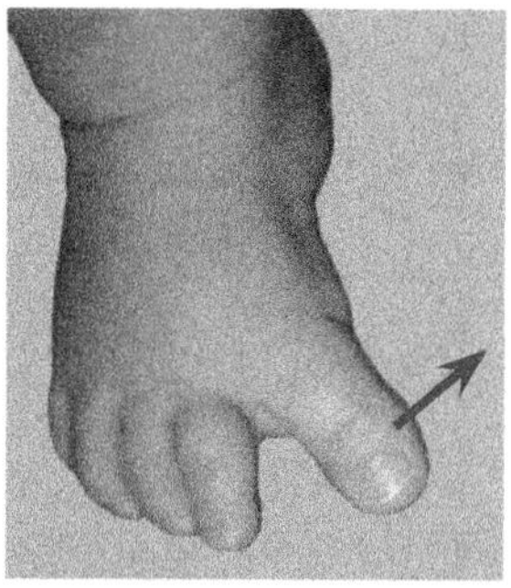

B Great toe abduction This is a dynamic deformity that resolves with time.

Type	Etiology	Comment
Metatarsus adductus	Late intrauterine, positional deformity	Common form 90% resolve spontaneously
Metatarsus varus	Earlier onset, intrauterine position?	Often rigid Cast correction necessary
Skewfoot	Familial Generalized joint laxity	Hindfoot valgus Abduction midfoot Adduction forefoot Treatment difficult
Abducted great toe	Unknown	Dynamic deformity Resolves spontaneously

C Types of forefoot adductus and varus deformities The differential diagnosis of metatarsus adductus should include the rigid, nonresolving form, and the skewfoot.

Forefoot Adductus

Metatarsus Adductus and Varus

Adductus of the forefoot is the most common foot deformity. It is characterized by a convexity to the lateral aspect of the foot [A] or a dynamic abduction of the great toe [B]. The deformities fall into four categories [C].

Metatarsus adductus is a common intrauterine positional deformity. Because it is associated with hip dysplasia in 2% of cases, a careful hip evaluation is essential. Metatarsus adductus is common, flexible, benign, and resolves spontaneously.

Metatarsus varus is an uncommon rigid deformity that often persists and requires cast correction. Metatarsus varus does not produce disability and does not cause bunions, but it does produce cosmetic and occasionally shoe-fitting problems.

Skewfoot is discussed on the next page.

Great toe abduction is a dynamic deformity due to overactivity of the great toe abductor. It is sometimes called a "searching toe." The condition improves spontaneously. No treatment is required.

Management

Evaluate by performing a screening examination, test for stiffness, and consider the child's age [D]. Manage metatarsus adductus by documentation and observation [E].

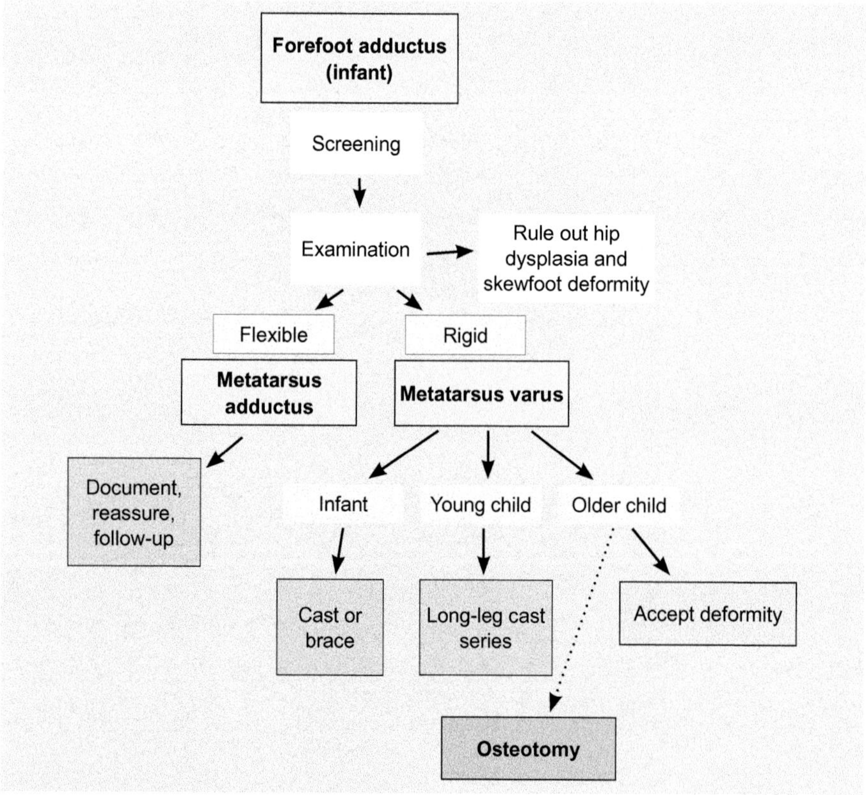

D Steps in managing forefoot adductus

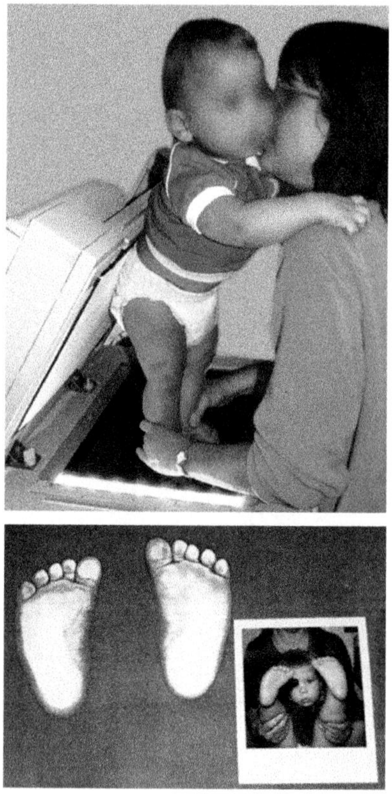

E Imaging the adducted foot The infant's foot shape is recorded on a copy machine. The printout from the copy machine is compared to a photograph.

Manage metatarsus varus by serial casting [A and B] or bracing. Long-leg bracing is useful in the toddler. Serial casting is most effective. The deformity yields much more rapidly when the cast is extended above the flexed knee.

The following technique is useful to about age 5 years. Apply a short-leg cast first. As the cast sets, mold the forefoot into abduction and the hindfoot in slight varus-inversion. Finally, while holding the short-leg cast in neutral rotation and with the knee flexed about 30°, extend the cast to include the thigh. This long-leg cast allows both walking and effective correction.

In the older child, it may be best to accept the deformity, as it does not cause disability. If operative correction is selected, correct by opening wedge cuneiform and closing wedge cuboid osteotomies. Avoid attempting correction by capsulotomy or metatarsal osteotomies, as early and late complications are frequent.

Skewfoot

Skewfoot, *Z-foot,* and *serpentine foot* are all terms given to a spectrum of complex deformities. This deformity includes hindfoot plantarflexion, midfoot abduction, and forefoot adduction [D]. A tight heel-cord is usually present in symptomatic cases. Skewfeet are seen in children with myelodysplasia; they are sometimes familial but are usually isolated deformities. There is a spectrum of severity. Some practitioners describe overcorrected clubfeet as skewfeet. Idiopathic skewfeet may persist and cause disability in adolescence and adult life.

Manage idiopathic skewfeet in young children by initial serial casting, correcting the forefoot adductus while carefully avoiding any eversion stress on the hindfoot. Document the effect of growth on the deformity. Most will persist. Plan correction in late childhood with heel-cord lengthening and osteotomies. Lengthen the calcaneus and medial cuneiform by opening wedge osteotomies [C].

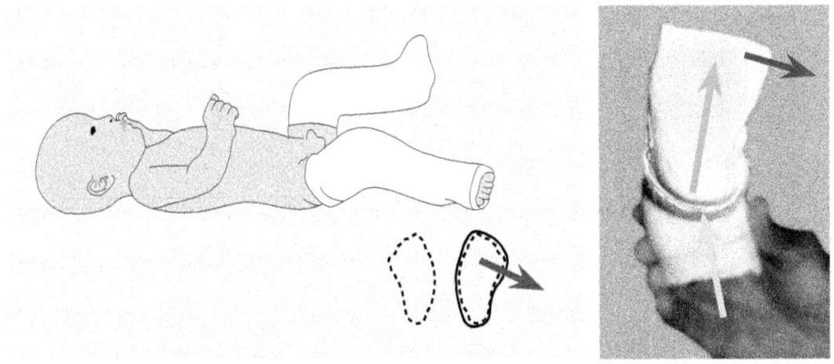

A Long-leg cast for metatarsus varus This treatment of metatarsus varus is most effective, as the flexed knee provides control of tibial rotation. Using the thigh portion of the cast as a point of fixation (yellow arrow), the foot is laterally rotated (green arrow) and abducted (red arrow) to achieve the most effective correction.

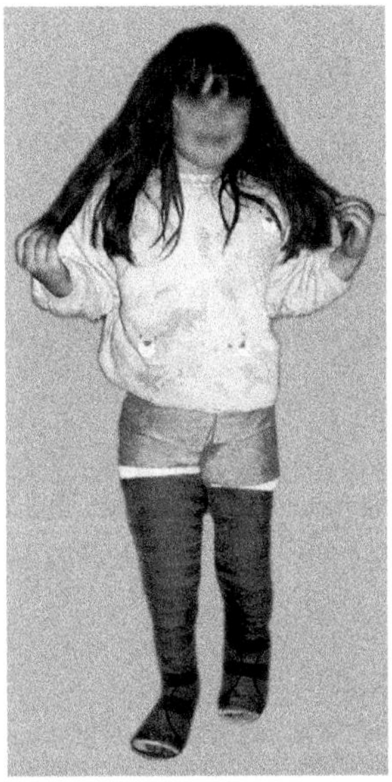

B Cast treatment of metatarsus varus This child with a persisting stiff deformity was corrected using these long-leg casts. The knee is flexed to about 30° to control rotation. The foot is abducted in the casts. The casts are changed every 2–3 weeks until correction is completed.

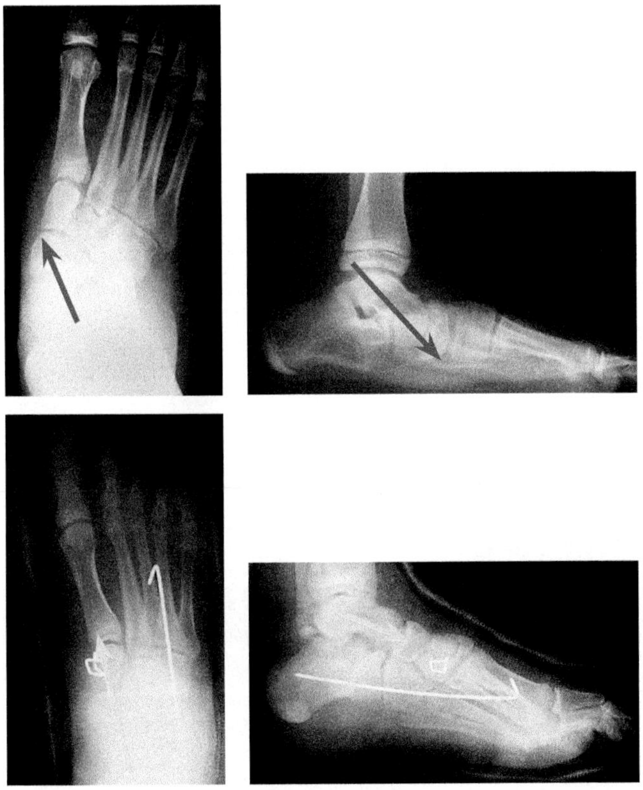

C Sequence of correction of skewfoot Calcaneal and cuneiform osteotomies and a heel-cord lengthening were performed. Note the changes in talar alignment between the preoperative (red arrows) and postoperative (yellow arrows) radiographs.

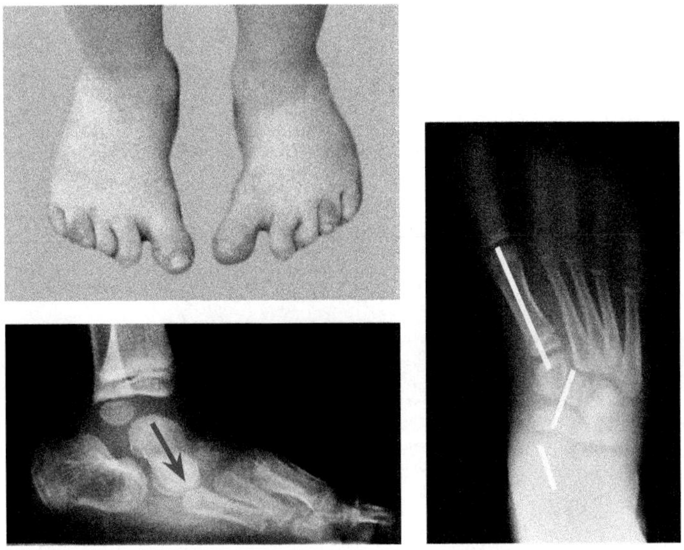

D Skewfoot deformity Note the forefoot adduction in the photograph, the plantar flexed talus (red arrow), and the Z alignment (white lines).

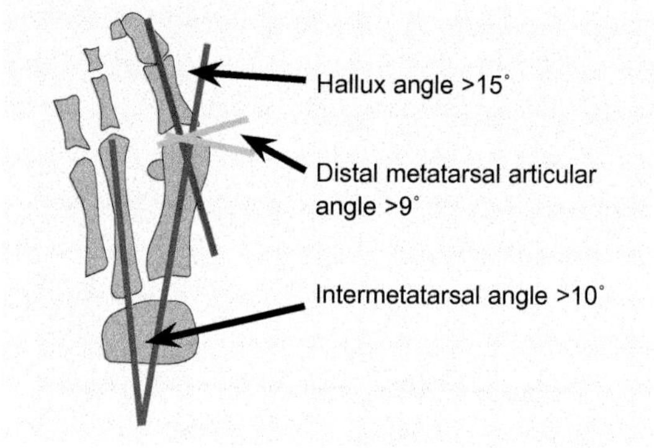

A Measurements for bunion assessment These values are usually present in bunion deformity.

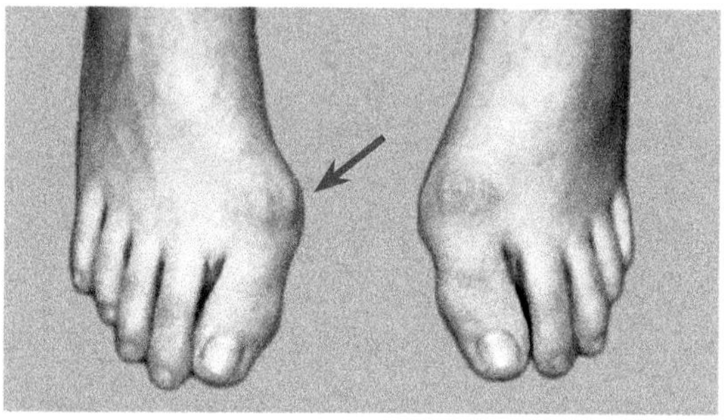

B Moderate bunion deformities The bunion is a prominence over the head of the first metatarsal. The left bunion (arrow) is most prominent here, and both are relatively moderate. Usually no active treatment is required for bunions of this severity.

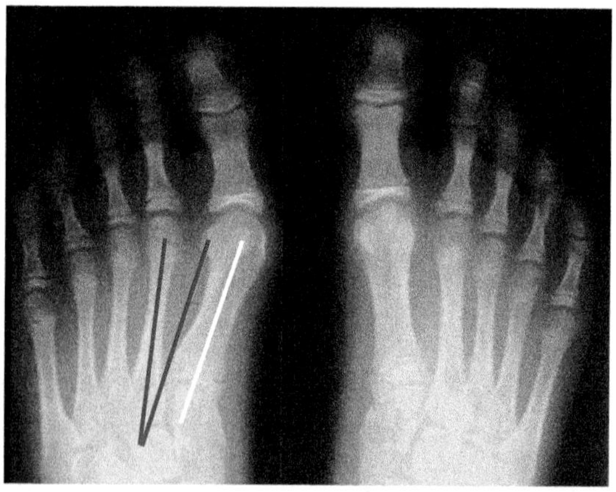

C Metatarsus primus varus An increased intermetatarsal angle (between red lines) is present in metatarsus primus varus. The hallux valgus is a secondary deformity.

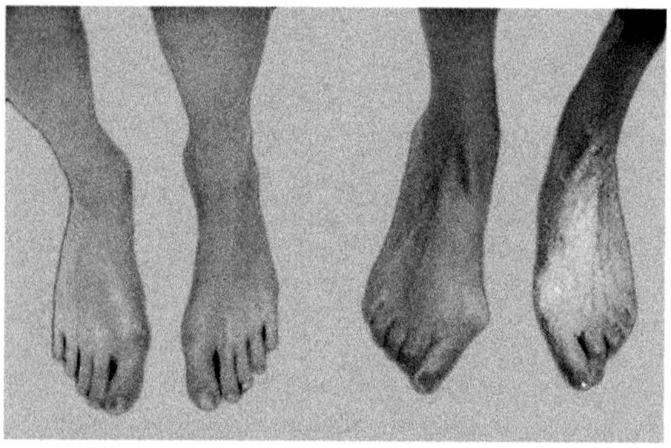

D Familial bunions Both mother and daughter have bunions.

Bunions

A bunion is a prominence of the head of the first metatarsal [A]. It is most common in girls. In children, it is usually due to metatarsus primus varus, a developmental deformity characterized by an increased intermetatarsal angle [B] that exceeds about 9° between the first two rays. Over time, the medial cuneiform becomes more trapezoid in shape and the metatarsal phalangeal joint subluxated. Hallux valgus is a secondary deformity aggravated by wearing shoes, as the great toe must be positioned in valgus to fit within a shoe. The normal hallux valgus angle is <15°. The combination of primary and secondary deformities causes the typical adolescent bunion [C].

Bunions are often familial [D] and may occur in children with neuromuscular disorders [E]. Other factors may include pronation of the forefoot, joint laxity, and pointed shoes. Bunions are uncommon in barefoot populations.

Evaluation Look for evidence of joint laxity, heel-cord contracture, pes planus, or other skeletal defects. Is the toe rotated? Is there a family history of bunions? If considering operative correction, order AP and lateral standing radiographs. Measure the intermetatarsal angle. Measure the distal metatarsal articular angle (DMAA). This is normally less than 8°. Is the metatarsal–phalangeal joint subluxated? Is the cuneiform–metatarsal articulation oblique? Note the relative lengths of the first and second rays.

Management Attempt to delay operative correction until the end of growth to reduce the risk of recurrence.

Shoes Encourage girls to avoid shoes with pointed toes and high heels, as they aggravate the deformity and increase discomfort.

Splints For nighttime use, splints may be effective but are difficult to use because of the required duration of management.

Operative Correction Correct bunions when symptoms are unacceptable and nonsurgical measures fail. Be aware that bunion correction in the child is complicated by the effects of growth and varied pathology.

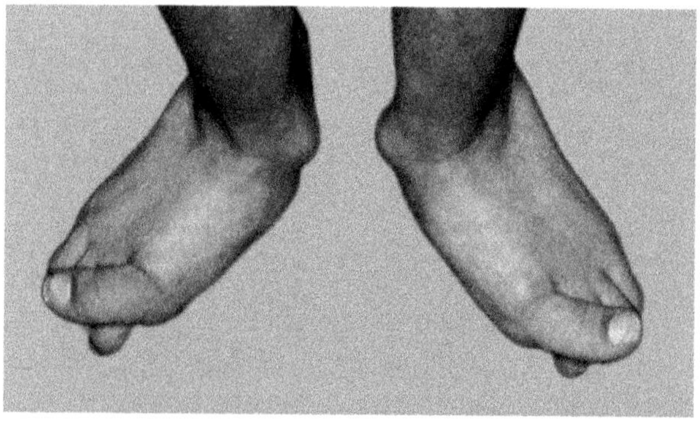

E Severe hallux valgus in cerebral palsy Note the absence of metatarsus primus varus and any prominence of the metatarsal head.

Dorsal Bunion

The uncommon dorsal bunion [A] is due to an elevation of the first metatarsal. This elevation is caused by an imbalance between a stronger tibialis anterior and peroneus longus muscle. It is most common in operatively treated clubfeet. This can be corrected by a plantar flexion osteotomy of the medial cuneiform or metatarsal and muscle-balancing procedures.

Bunionette

Bunionette (tailor's bunion) is a painful bony prominence on the lateral side of the fifth metatarsal head, often associated with an inflamed thickened bursa and callus formation. These deformities are developmental and involve an increased metatarsophalangeal angle of the fifth toe and an increased intermetatarsal angle between the fourth and fifth toes. Management often requires a metatarsal osteotomy for correction.

Hallux Rigidus

This is a degenerative arthritis of the first metatarsal phalangeal joint due to repetitive trauma, which causes stiffness, limited dorsiflexion, and pain. Manage by protecting the joint with a shoe stiffener. If severe and persistent, correct by a dorsiflexion osteotomy [B] to move the arc of motion into more extension, improving functional motion and reducing discomfort.

Short Metatarsal

Shortening of one or more metatarsals may be due to a developmental abnormality as part of a generalized disorder or from trauma, infection, or tumors. It may the result of a premature growth plate closure that is bilateral and familial. Severe shortening may cause metatarsalgia and a cosmetic disability. Rarely, the deformity is severe enough to justify operative correction. This can be done by a single-stage lengthening technique [C] or by gradual distraction histiogenesis.

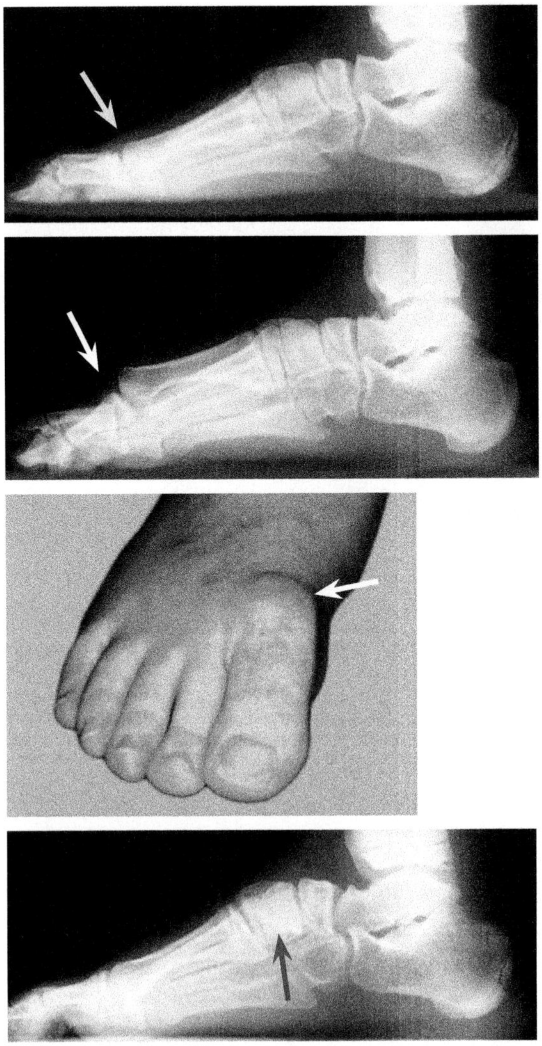

A Dorsal bunion This child's bunion developed between the ages of 14 (yellow arrow) and 18 years (white arrows). The deformity was corrected by a plantar closing wedge osteotomy (red arrow) and lateral transfer of the anterior tibialis and transfer of the flexor hallucis longus to the first metatarsal.

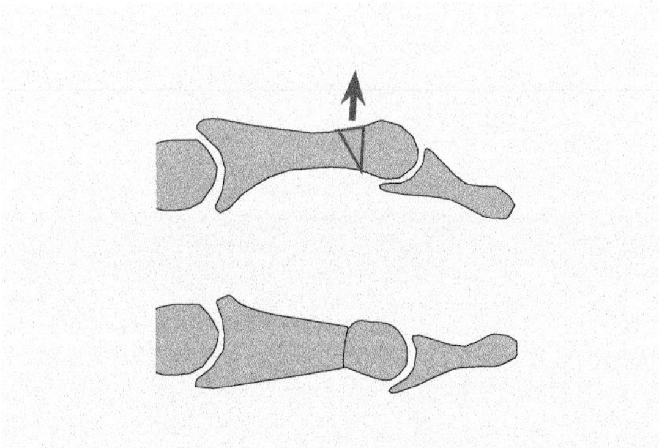

B Dorsal osteotomy for hallux rigidus A dorsal closing wedge osteotomy moved the arc of motion of the metatarsal phalangeal joint into a position for improved function.

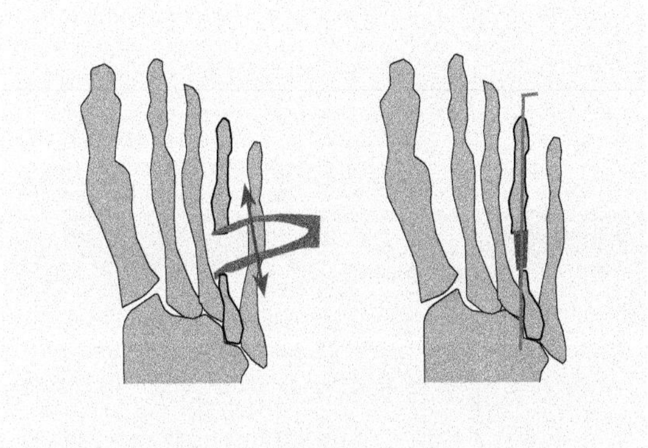

C Technique of metatarsal lengthening This one-stage lengthening is described by Baek and Chung (1998).

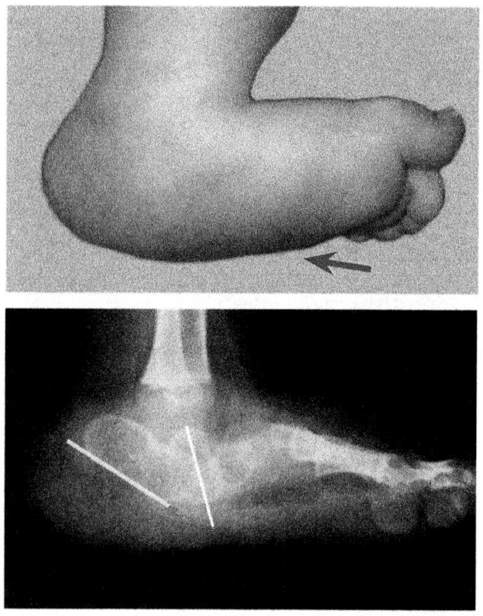

A Vertical talus Note the convexity to the sole of the foot (red arrow) and the near vertical orientation of the talus on the radiograph (white line) and the plantarflexion of the calcaneus (yellow line).

Type	Comment
Distal arthrogryposis	Mild
Amyoplasia	Rigid
Myelodysplasia	Rigid
Syndrome	Rigid
Genetic	Variable

B Vertical talus associations This deformity usually occurs as part of a generalized problem.

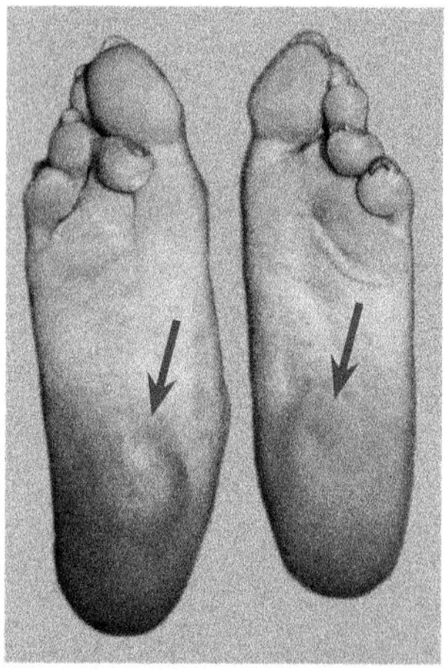

C Vertical talus in an adult Note the prominences on the sole of the foot causing calluses and pain with walking.

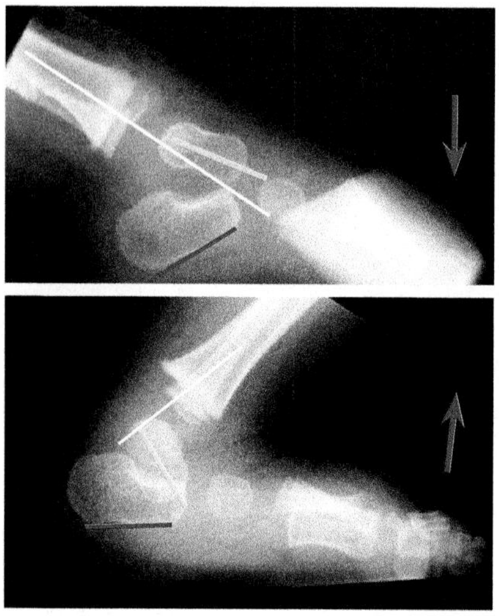

D Plantarflexed talus These radiographs were taken with the ankle in plantarflexion (upper) and then in dorsiflexion (lower). Note that on the extension view, the talus (yellow line) aligns with the first ray. On the plantarflexion view, the calcaneus becomes dorsiflexed. This study shows that the foot is flexible and consistent with a deformity due to hypermobility of the talus and not a stiff foot as seen in the vertical talus.

Vertical Talus

The vertical talus is the most severe and serious pathologic flatfoot. It is a congenital deformity that produces not only flattening but an actual convexity of the sole of the foot [A].

Etiology

Vertical talus is usually associated with other conditions such as myelodysplasia and arthrogryposis [B].

Evaluation

Differentiate the stiff vertical talus from the benign plantar-flexed talus due to hypermobility.

Clinical The foot is stiff, with contractures of both the dorsiflexors and plantarflexors. The head of the talus projects into the plantar aspect of the foot, producing the convexity of the sole. Look at the parents' feet for evidence of a genetic etiology [C].

Imaging The diagnosis is suggested by a lateral radiograph of the foot showing the vertical orientation of the talus [A]. The calcaneus is also plantarflexed. The vertical talus may be confused with flexible oblique talus, a different condition. Make the differentiation by studying lateral plantarflexion and dorsiflexion radiographs of the foot [D]. The vertical talus will show stiffness and fixation in contrast to the flexible oblique talus, which shows a freely mobile mid- and hindfoot. Note especially the mobility of the calcaneus. If the calcaneus is fixed in plantarflexion in both views of the foot, the diagnosis is vertical talus.

Management

Correct during the first year.

Serial casts Apply serial casts to stretch out the skin and the anterior soft tissues.

Anterior release Through a transverse incision [E] release the contracted ankle capsule and the talonavicular and calcaneocuboid joints. Place a K wire to secure the reduced navicular.

Posterior release Through a second transverse incision, lengthen the heel-cord and release the ankle capsule. Dorsiflex the foot to neutral. Immobilize in a long-leg cast.

Severe deformity In a more severe deformity in the untreated older child or for recurrent deformity, it may be necessary to resect the navicular and perform a subtalar fusion.

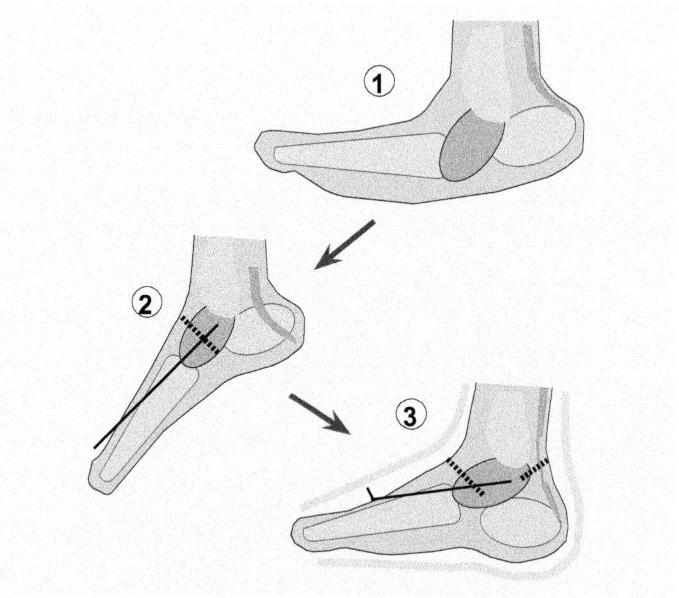

E Operative correction The foot before the procedure with a plantarflexed navicular (1). An anterior release reduces the talus (2). A posterior release allows the foot to be dorsiflexed to a neutral position (3).

Clubfoot

Clubfoot (CF) is a complex congenital deformity that includes components of equinus, cavus, adductus, varus, and internal rotation [A]. Clubfoot is also referred to as *talipes equinovarus* (TEV). It occurs in about 1 in 1000 births, is bilateral in half the cases, and affects males more frequently.

Etiology

The cause of clubfeet is multifactorial. In affected families, clubfeet are about 30 times more frequent in offspring than for the general population. Fetal ultrasound screening shows the deformity in the first trimester [B]. Clubfoot can be associated with other congenital abnormalities such as neural tube defects (spina bifida) , anomalies of the urinary or digestive system, and other musculoskeletal abnormalities as seen in arthrogryposis. The clubfoot deformity can have different causes, as evidenced by the variability of expression and response to management.

Mild or positional clubfoot is a late intrauterine deformity (see Chapter 1) and corrects rapidly with cast treatment. At the other end of the severity spectrum, severe clubfoot behaves like a disruption, having an origin earlier in fetal life and requiring operative correction. Severe clubfoot is seen in conditions such as arthrogryposis [C]. Classic or idiopathic clubfoot is a multifactorial disorder, is relatively common, and occupies the middle range of the severity spectrum.

Pathology

The pathology of clubfoot is typical of a dysplasia. The tarsals are hypoplastic. The talus is most deformed; the size is reduced and the talar neck is shortened and deviated in a medial and plantar direction. The navicular articulates with the medial aspect of the neck of the talus due to the abnormal shape of the talus. The relationship of the tarsals are abnormal. The talus and calcaneus are parallel in all three planes. The midfoot becomes more medially displaced, and the metatarsals are adducted and plantarflexed. In addition to the deformities of cartilage and bone, the ligaments are thickened and the muscles hypoplastic. This results in a generalized hypoplasia of the limb with shortening of the foot and smallness of the calf [D]. Because the hypoplasia primarily involves the foot, limb length discrepancy is usually less than 1 cm. The foot is small, and split size shoes are often required. The amount of foot shortening is proportional to the severity of the clubfoot.

Natural History

Untreated, clubfoot produces considerable disability [E]. The dorsolateral skin becomes the weight-bearing area. Calluses form and walking becomes limited.

Operatively treated clubfeet are often stiff, weak, and may be in varus. These problems often cause considerable disability in adult life.

Clinical Features

The diagnosis of clubfoot is not difficult and is seldom confused with other foot deformities. Sometimes severe metatarsus varus is confused with clubfoot, but the equinus component of clubfoot makes the differentiation clear. The presence of a clubfoot should prompt a careful search for other musculoskeletal problems.

Examine the back for evidence of dysraphism, the hips for dysplasia, and the knees for deformity. Perform a screening neurologic examination. Note the size, shape, and flexibility of the feet. Take radiographs of the spine or pelvis only if abnormalities are found on physical examination. Clubfoot is not associated with developmental hip dysplasia or spinal deformity.

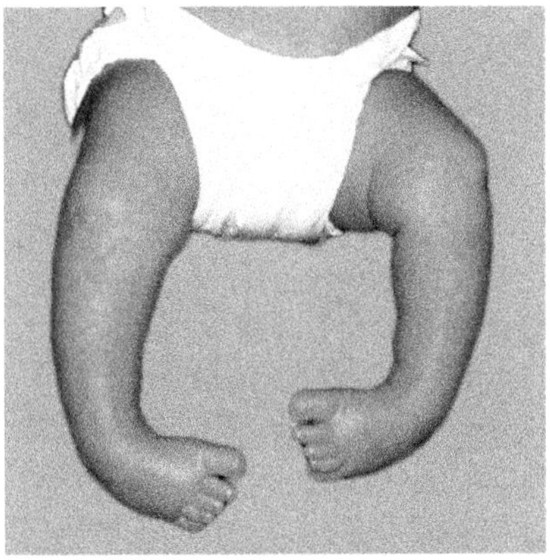

A Typical appearance of bilateral clubfeet The deformity includes equinus, cavus, adductus, varus, and internal rotation.

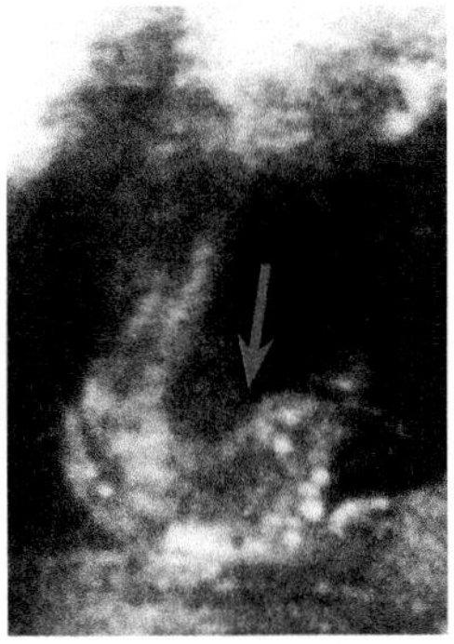

B Clubfoot on ultrasound at 16 weeks

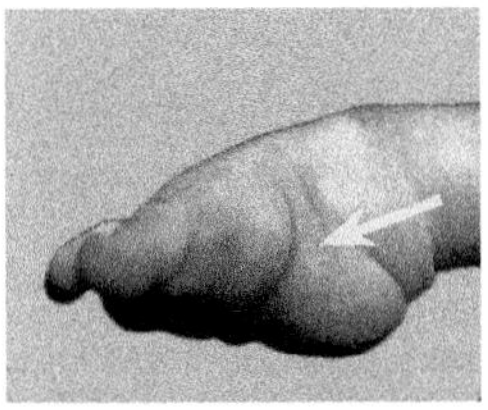

C Severe clubfoot Note the prominent medial crease (arrow).

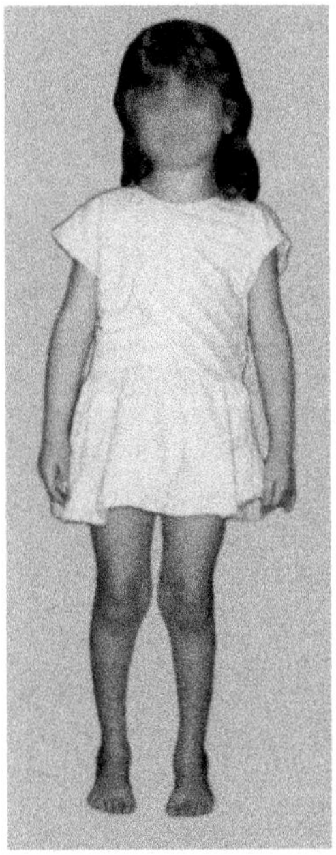

D Reduction in leg size (Left) This girl with bilateral clubfeet has bilateral calf hypoplasia. (Below) The left clubfoot is more severe (red arrow) and is significantly shorter than the right foot with mild deformity. The degree of hypoplasia parallels the severity of the clubfoot deformity.

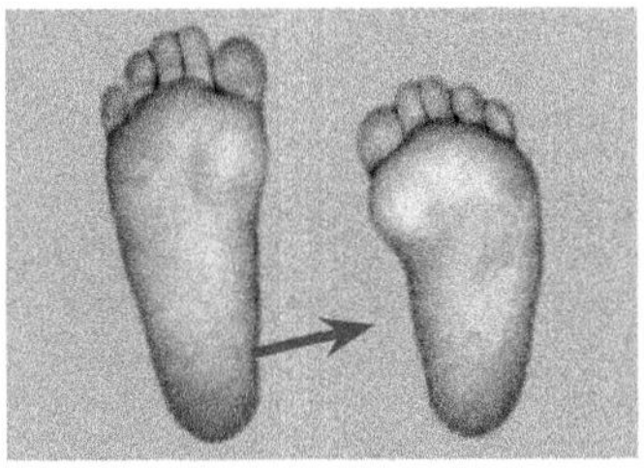

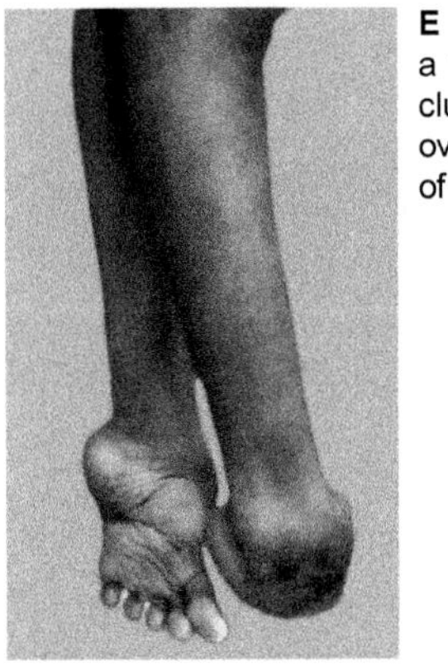

E Untreated clubfeet These are the feet of a 13-year-old Cambodian boy with untreated clubfeet. A large callus and bursa have formed over the site of weight bearing on the dorsum of each foot.

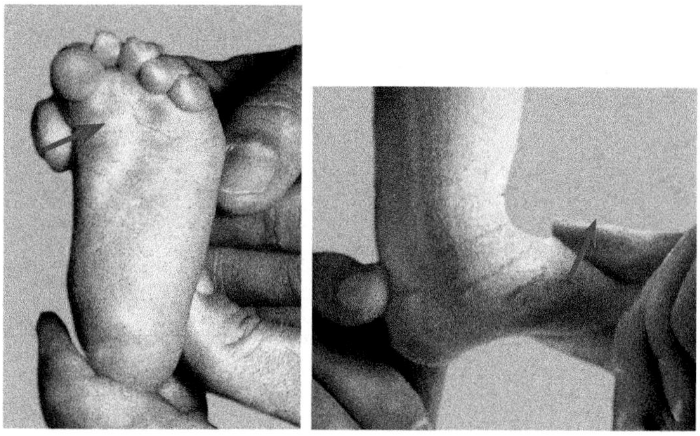

A **Testing flexibility** Assessing flexibility is a good way to determine the severity of the clubfoot.

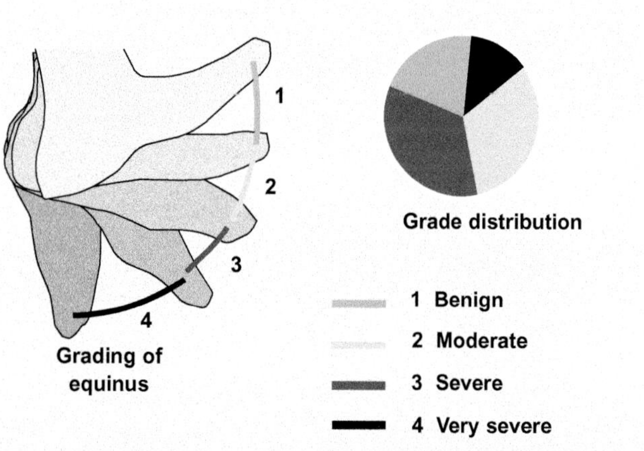

B **Dimeglio classification** Clubfoot stiffness in equinus (shown here), varus, rotation, and adduction are assessed. The sum of these scores is used to establish severity. The distribution of clubfeet into the four grades of severity are shown in the pie chart. Based on Dimeglio et al. (1995).

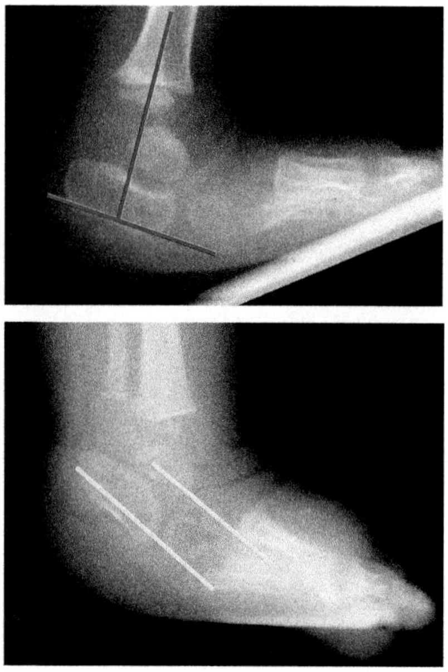

C **Radiographic evaluation of clubfoot** On a maximum dorsiflexion radiograph, measure the tibial calcaneal angle (red lines). On resting or standing radiographs, note the parallelism between the axes of the talus and calcaneus (yellow lines).

Note the degree of stiffness of the foot [A] and compare the size of the foot with the uninvolved foot. Marked differences in foot length suggest that the deformity is severe and foretell the need for operative correction. Document the components of the clubfoot deformity, the equinus, cavus, heel varus, forefoot adductus, and medial rotation.

Equinus is due to a combination of a plantar flexed talus, posterior ankle capsular contracture, and shortening of the triceps.

Cavus is due to a contracture of the plantar fascia with plantar flexion of the forefoot on the hindfoot.

Varus results from inversion of the subtalar joint.

Adductus and medial rotation are due to medial deviation of the neck of the talus, medial displacement of the talonavicular joint, and metatarsus adductus. Tibial rotation is normal.

Classification

A number of classifications for clubfoot have been proposed.

Etiologic classification This is based on the possible causes of clubfoot and include several types.

Positional clubfeet are flexible and thought to result from intrauterine position late in gestation. These resolve quickly with serial casting.

Idiopathic clubfeet include the classic forms with an intermediate degree of stiffness. They are multifactorial in etiology.

Teratologic clubfeet are associated with arthrogryposis, meningomyelocele, and other generalized disorders. These feet are very stiff and difficult to manage.

Pirani classification This classification is becoming widely used. It provides a numeric score based on three midfoot and three hindfoot features. Each is considered as normal, moderately abnormal, or severe abnormal. Make scores periodically during management to assess progress.

Midfoot scores are based on the lateral border, medial crease, and talar head coverage.

Hindfoot scores are based on the posterior crease, equinus rigidity, and the heel configuration.

Dimeglio classification This classification is based on stiffness. Range of motion in equinus, adduction, varus, and medial rotation are then given points. The sum of these points establishes the severity [B].

Imaging Studies

Radiographs, ultrasound, and MRI imaging are rarely used or necessary for assessment. Because active treatment usually occurs during early infancy, when ossification is incomplete, the value of radiographic studies is limited. Furthermore, because Ponseti management does not utilize radiographs, radiography is becoming less widely used than in the past. Ultrasound studies may become more widely used in the future. Radiographs become increasingly valuable with increasing age [C]. The common measures are as follows:

Tibial calcaneal angle in maximal dorsiflexion is a measure of equinus. To fall into the normal range, the angle should be >10° above a right angle.

Lateral talocalcaneal angle is a measure of varus. Parallelism is a sign of residual heel varus.

AP calcaneocuboid alignment provides an assessment of the severity of the midfoot adduction and varus.

Navicular position Dorsal displacement of the navicular is a sign of malalignment of the midtarsal joints.

The value of radiographs is uncertain because long-term studies suggest that triceps strength, foot mobility, and plantar loading as measured clinically are more significant than static radiographic measures in assessing outcomes.

Routine screening radiographs of the pelvis are not necessary in children with clubfoot. Provide the same screening as for any normal child.

Management

The objective of management of clubfoot is to correct the deformity and retain mobility and strength. The foot should be plantigrade and have a normal load-bearing area. Secondary objectives include the ability to wear normal shoes, satisfactory appearance, and avoidance of unnecessarily complicated or prolonged treatment. The clubfoot is never fully corrected. When compared with a normal foot, all clubfeet show some residual stiffness, shortening, or deformity.

Management trends are influenced by data that suggest that maintaining mobility and triceps strength are more important than judging outcomes on radiographic criteria. Current trends favor early cast treatment [A], Ponseti approach [C], customized procedures [B], and a greater focus on function and less on deformity.

Idiopathic clubfeet Start treatment as soon as possible after birth. Several approaches are used [C].

Ponseti management This approach has recently become the standard approach in most of the world. This management includes manipulation and casting to correct the deformities in an orderly sequence. Correct the cavus, rotate the foot from under the talus, and finally correct the equinus. Usually a percutaneous tenotomy is performed to facilitate equinus correction. Sometimes a transfer of the anterior tibialis (AT) is performed in early childhood. Rotational splinting is an essential part of management. Flexibility and strength are maintained with this approach.

French management (Dimeglio) emphasizes prolonged intense manipulations and splinting.

Traditional management usually includes initial casting and then one of several techniques for operative correction. Make the correction during the first year of life. Tailor the extent of the procedure to the severity of deformity [B]. Prevent recurrent deformity with night splinting.

Arthrogrypotic clubfeet Reduce the deformity by initial casting using the Ponseti technique. Individualize management depending upon the response. It may be necessary to perform percutaneous lengthenings of the flexor hallucis longus, the posterior tibialis, and the heel-cord, then return to the casting sequence. In others, a posterior mediolateral release may be necessary to correct deformity not resolved by casting.

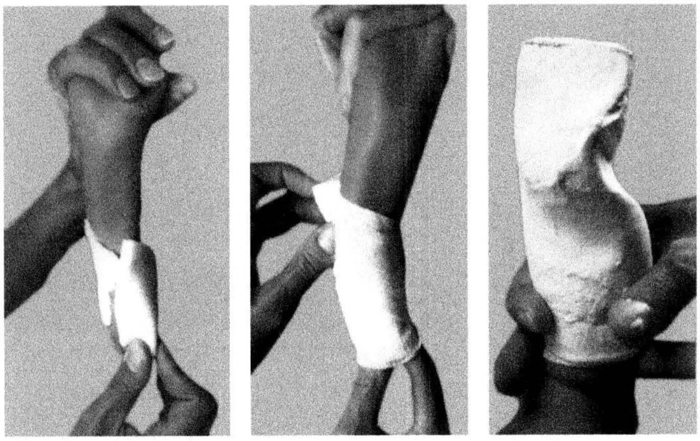

A Initial management with corrective casts Cast treatment is helpful in correcting or reducing clubfoot deformity. Padding is first applied. The short-leg portion is applied first as shown. This was extended to become a long-leg cast to make it more effective.

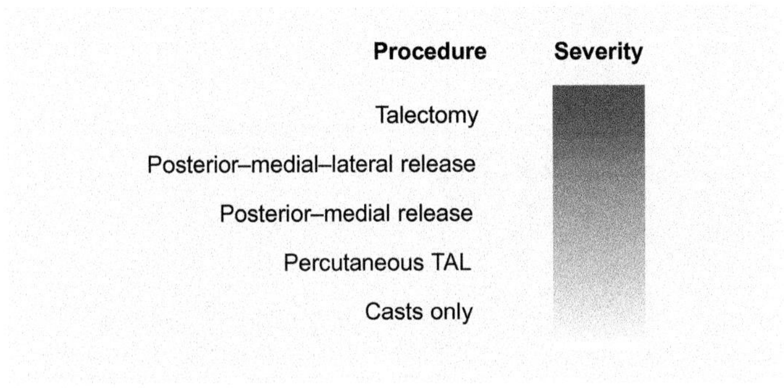

B Relating clubfoot severity to management Clubfoot management is often related to the severity of the clubfoot.

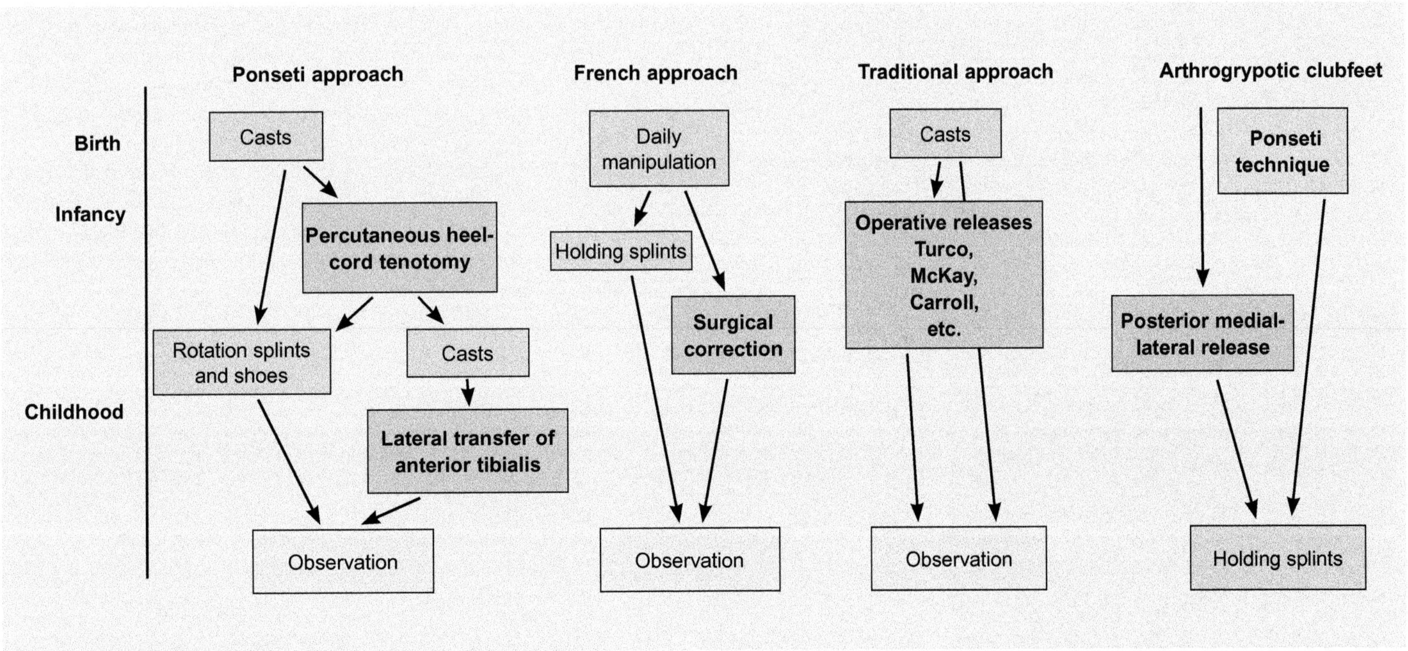

C Approaches to management of clubfeet

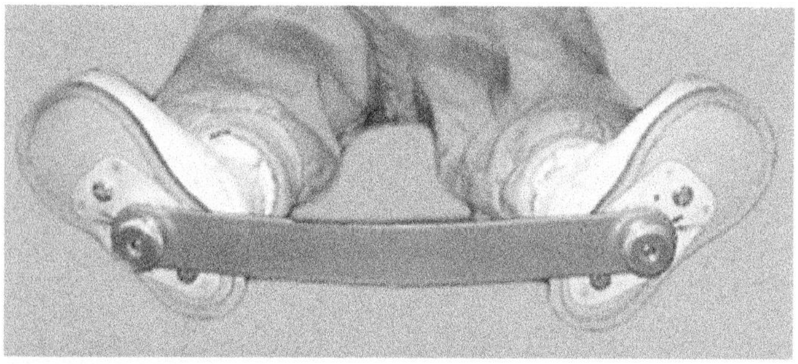

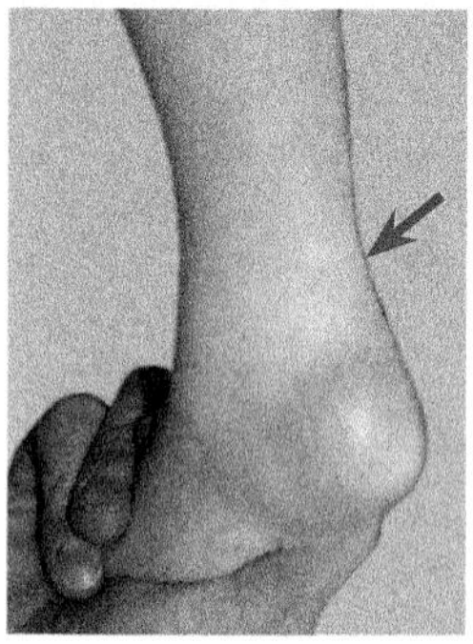

A Ponseti management This child had serial casting, a percutaneous tenotomy (arrow), and an excellent outcome with a flexible, strong, plantigrade foot.

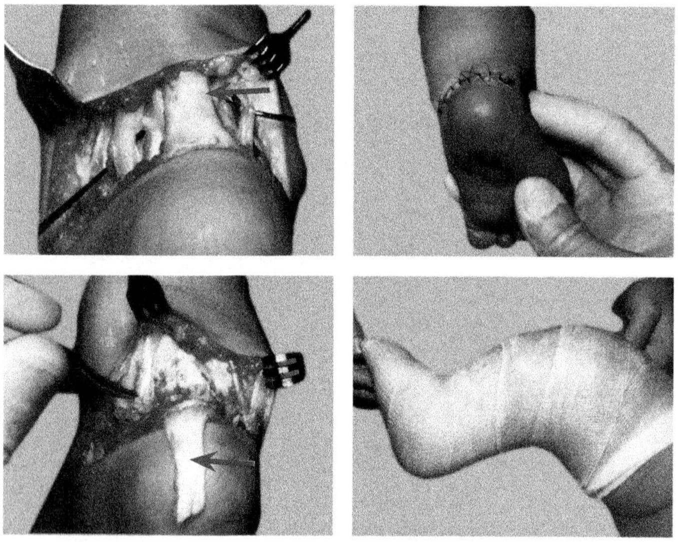

B Operative correction This posterior release includes lengthening of the heel-cord (arrows) and opening of the joint capsule. Immobilization is provided by a long-leg cast.

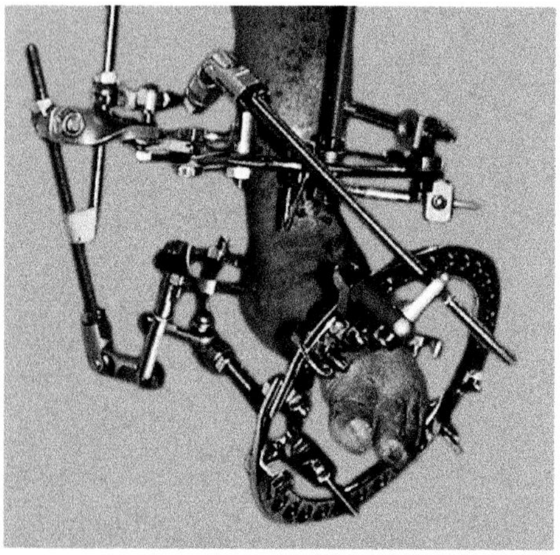

C Ilizarov frame This is an effective method of correcting severe deformity in the older child.

Uncommon forms of clubfoot These occur in infants who have some underlying problem.

Non-idiopathic clubfeet These are clubfeet that occur in apparently normal infants but behave differently. These individuals have hypermobility and, with conventional treatment, may show overcorrection such as heel valgus. These overcorrections are less likely to occur with Ponseti management [A] than with conventional management.

Syndrome associated clubfoot This is the classic clubfoot that occurs in arthrogryposis and meningomyelocele. Typically, these clubfeet are more difficult to correct and recurrence is more likely. Individualize management. Start with the Ponseti approach. If correction is not progressing at a satisfactory rate, consider a limited posteromedial release. Perform the releases subcutaneously; the casting may be resumed. Complete the correction by a posterior mediolateral release later in the first year [B]. Be aware that recurrence is more likely and more difficult to control than seen with idiopathic clubfoot.

Complications Are common in clubfoot management. They may be early or late. Recurrence is the most common early complication.

Recurrence Nearly half of clubfeet that are treated operatively recur and require additional treatment. Correct recurrent deformities with casts. Avoid repeated major operative procedures. Plan a final bony correction at the end of growth. Complications of this treatment are common.

Stiffness may result from excessive articular pressure during treatment, compartment syndromes complicating surgery, internal fixation, avascular necrosis of the talus, and operative scarring.

Weakness of the triceps jeopardizes function. Overlengthening and repeated lengthening procedures increase this risk.

Varus deformity commonly causes excessive plantar pressure over the base of the fifth metatarsal.

Overcorrection with a valgus hindfoot is common following operative correction. This is most likely in children with excessive joint laxity. Correction is challenging.

Salvage procedures These procedures may be necessary in special situations.

Talectomy Some surgeons perform an initial resection of the talus in teratologic clubfeet as a primary procedure or more likely for salvage when other treatment fails.

External fixator Severe deformity in older children is sometimes best managed with the Ilizarov frame [C]. Use the frame to stretch soft tissues to achieve gradual correction. Be aware that recurrent deformity is a common and difficult problem. Provide postoperative splinting using an AFO. Position the foot in dorsiflexion to prevent recurrent deformity. This splint is important, but recurrence is still common.

Bony corrections In severe clubfeet with recurrent deformity, delay recorrection until the end of growth. When possible, correct with osteotomies rather than arthrodeses to preserve what little joint motion remains. Bone procedures performed at the end of growth provide correction that is most likely to be permanent.

Ponseti Clubfoot Management

The Ponseti approach to management of clubfeet has been refined over a period of 50 years, has been shown to produce excellent long-term results, and is becoming the management standard throughout the world.

Management

This management shows 90+% success in idiopathic clubfoot, and is also appropriate for other forms of clubfoot. Correction is achieved by manipulation and cast correction in a definite sequence. A percutaneous heel-cord tenotomy corrects equinus, and prolonged night-time bracing is essential to prevent recurrence. The technique for correction involves specific steps.

Understand pathology The idiopathic clubfoot [A] is due to a medial displacement of the mid and forefoot around the head of the talus [B]. In addition, a cavus deformity is present [C] with plantarflexion of the first ray. The initial step is correction of the cavus.

Cavus correction This correction is achieved by dorsiflexion of the first ray. This a brief manipulation [D and E] followed by casting the forefoot in supination [F].

Adduction and varus correction This correction requires several casts applied 3–7 days apart. With the finger over the head of the talus, the mid and forefoot are abducted and externally rotated [G]. The foot is then immobilized in a long-leg cast with maximum correction [H]. Note that the foot requires an extreme position to achieve correction.

Equinus correction A percutaneous tenotomy [I] is nearly always performed to fully correct the equinus component. A holding cast is applied for about a month following the procedure.

Brace treatment This step is often the most difficult as night bracing [J] is required until the child is age 3–5 years. Without bracing, expect recurrence. This requires skill in dealing with the family.

Anterior tibial transfer Some children require this procedure [K] to correct the muscle balance about the foot. This procedure is performed in early childhood.

Results

More than 90% of children can expect to have an excellent result. The foot is plantigrade, mobile, and strong. The results are far superior to those achieved by surgery with the traditional posteromedial release procedure. The surgically corrected feet usually become painful during adolescence or early adult life.

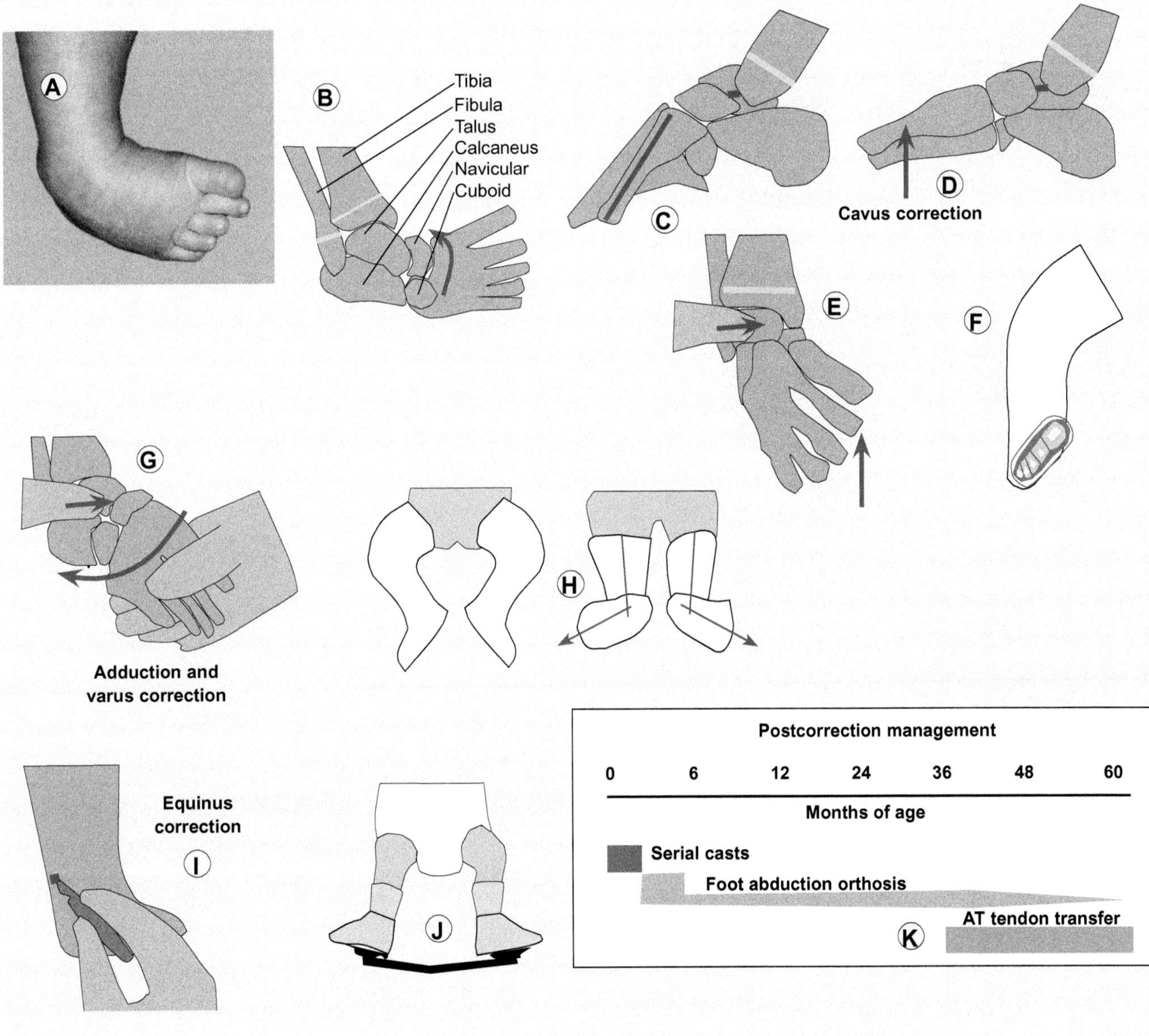

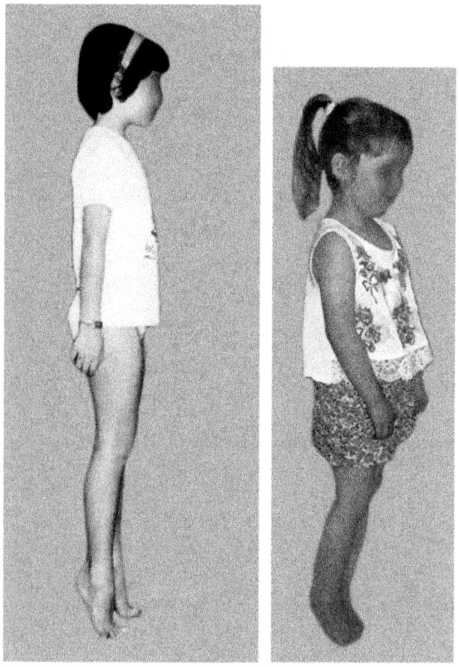

A **Idiopathic toe walking** These girls have contractures of the gastrocnemius, causing an equinus gait.

Category	Diagnosis
Congenital	Clubfoot
Idiopathic	Gastrocnemius contracture Accessory soleus muscle Generalized triceps contracture
Neurologic	Cerebral palsy Poliomyelitis
Myogenic	Muscular dystrophy
Functional	Habitual toe walking
Behavioral	Autism

B **Toe walking classification** This classification includes the common causes of an equinus gait.

Toe Walking

Toe walking, or *equinus gait,* may occur in otherwise normal children [A] or in children with underlying disorders [B].

Secondary Toe Walking

Equinus is common in children with a variety of other primary problems [B]. Toe walking is often seen in children with autism or those with developmental delay.

Accessory soleus is a rare congenital deformity in which the body of the soleus muscle extends to the ankle. This produces equinus and a fullness on the medial side of the ankle. Operative lengthening may be necessary.

Idiopathic Toe Walking

Idiopathic toe walking (ITW) in infants and young children is uncommon and not associated with a heel-cord contracture. It may be an early sign of autism.

Etiology The cause is unknown but the problem appears to be familial. Examination of the parents often demonstrates some asymptomatic tightness of the heel-cord.

Natural history The condition is always bilateral and present when the toddler begins to walk. The contracture develops over the first few years, limiting ankle dorsiflexion. Later in childhood, the condition appears to improve spontaneously. Heel-cord contracture may increase the risk of overuse syndromes and the development of a symptomatic flatfoot with heel valgus, and lateral column shortening may occur during the second decade.

Clinical features include an onset with the initiating of walking, variable toe walking, altered shoe wear [C], reduction in ankle dorsiflexion, and a normal neurological examination. The diagnosis is made by the history and physical examination [E]. Laboratory studies are seldom necessary. The diagnosis is made by exclusion.

Management is controversial.

Nonoperative Traditionally, physical therapy, casting, bracing, and Botox injections have been recommended. Temporary improvement is often followed by recurrent equinus. These treatments are unlikely to affect the long-term outcome. If nonoperative treatment is undertaken, the least disruptive option is the articulated AFO with plantarflexion block [D].

Heel-cord lengthening Correct persisting deformity by lengthening of the heel-cord after the age of 4. Percutaneous or open procedures are effective. Immobilize in a short-leg walking cast for 4 weeks following the procedure. Recurrence is rare.

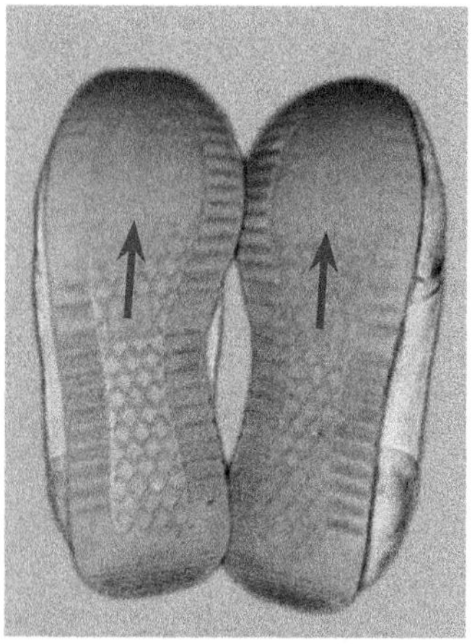

C **Shoe wear on toes only** These shoes show typical wear patterns with loss of sole tread only on the toe regions (arrows).

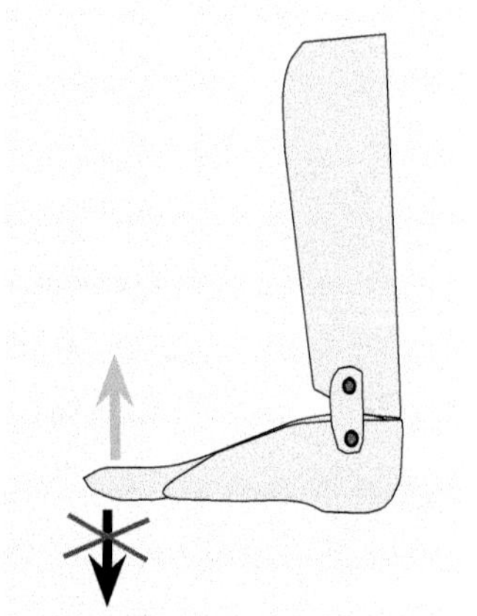

D **Plantarflexion block brace** This molded articulated ankle-foot orthosis (AFO) allows free dorsiflexion but blocks plantarflexion.

Feature	ITW	Other causes
Extent	Localized	Generalized
Initiation of walking	Before 18 months of age	Often delayed
Location	Bilateral	May be unilateral
Onset	With walking	Anytime
Natural history	Improves during childhood	Most progress
Developmental delay	Sometimes	Often

E **Differentiating features** These features are helpful in differentiating idiopathic toe walking (ITW) from other causes.

Flatfoot

The flatfoot (FF), or *pes planus,* is a foot with a large plantar contact area. The flatfoot is often associated with a valgus heel and a reduction in height of the longitudinal arch. Flatfeet are classified as physiologic or pathologic [E]. Physiologic flatfeet are flexible, common, benign, and a variation of normal. Pathologic flatfeet show some degree of stiffness, often cause disability, and usually require treatment. Ankle valgus, as seen in myelodysplasia and poliomyelitis, may be confused with a flatfoot deformity. Foot valgus is in the subtalar joint. Make the differentiation radiographically.

Flexible Flatfoot

The flexible flatfoot, or physiologic flatfoot, is present in nearly all infants, many children, and about 15% of adults. Flatfeet often run in families [A]. Flatfeet are most common in those who wear shoes, are obese, or have generalized joint laxity [B]. There are two basic forms. Developmental flatfeet occur in infants and children as a normal stage of development [C]. The hypermobile flatfoot persists as a normal variant. Two studies of military populations have shown that the flexible flatfoot does not cause disability and, in fact, is associated with a reduction in stress fractures.

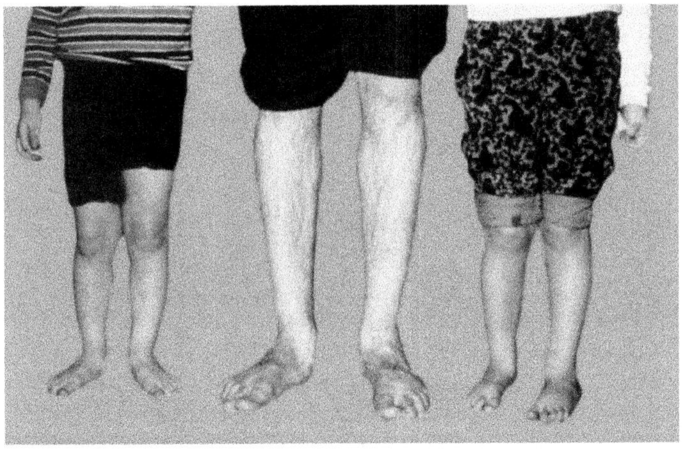

A Familial flatfeet Each member of this family had flexible flatfeet. None were symptomatic. Demonstrating the flatfoot in the asymptomatic adult provides reassurance for the parents.

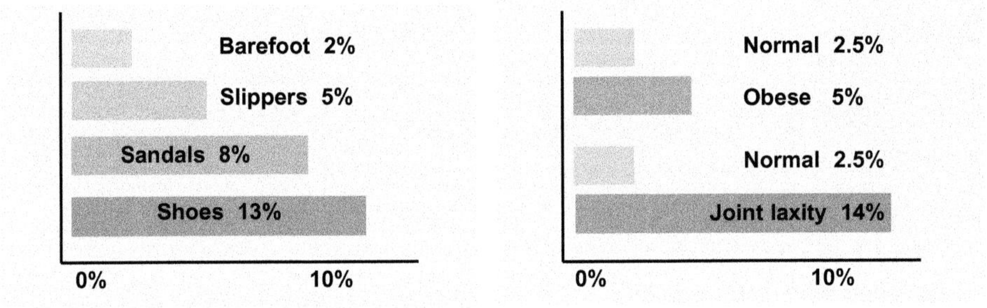

B Associations of flexible flatfoot These studies from India demonstrate that flatfeet are more common in adults who wore shoes as children, the obese, and those with joint laxity. From Roe and Joseph (1993).

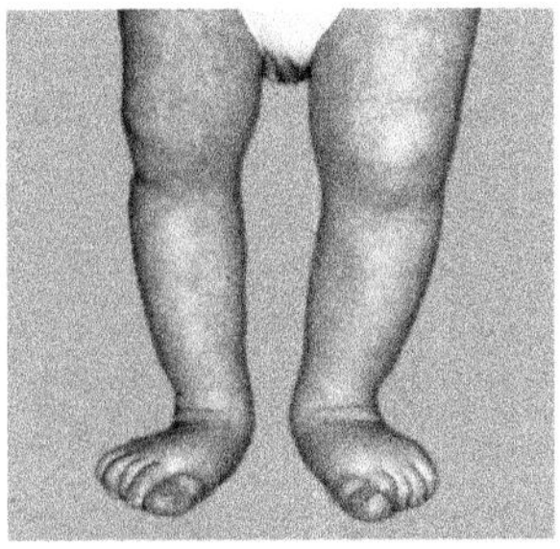

C Developmental flatfoot Most infants and many children have flatfeet. Infants' flatfeet are often due to their thick subcutaneous plantar fatpad and joint laxity.

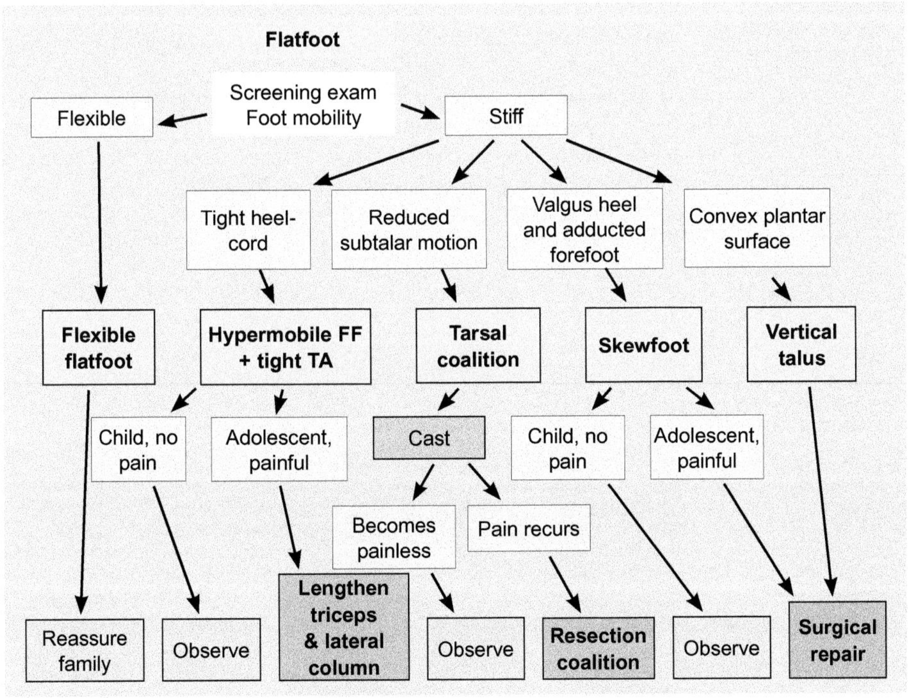

D Flatfoot management This algorithm outlines the evaluation and management of flatfeet.

Category	Disorder
Flexible flatfoot	Developmental flatfoot
	Hypermobile flatfoot
	Calcaneovalgus foot
Pathologic flatfoot	Hypermobile flatfoot + tight heel-cord + lateral tibial torsion + obesity
	Tarsal coalitions Talocalcaneal Calcaneonavicular
	Neurogenic flatfoot
	Severed posterior tibialis tendon
	Vertical talus

E Classification of Flatfeet Flatfeet are categorized into flexible (or physiologic) and pathologic types.

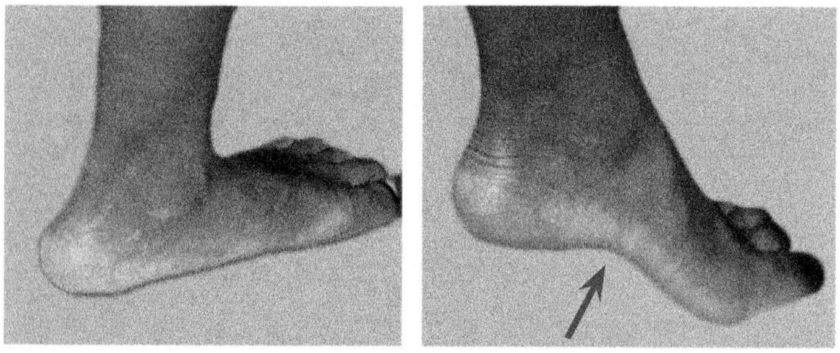

A Arch develops on toe standing This is a characteristic finding in flexible flatfeet.

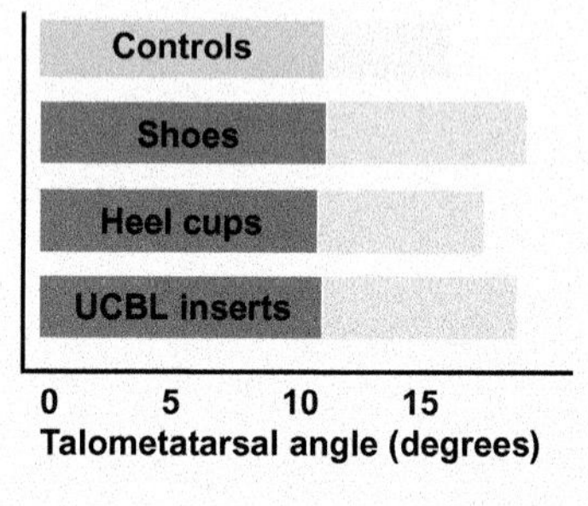

B Effect of shoe modifications in flatfeet This prospective, controlled study compared arch development with various treatments. No difference was found. Talarmetatarsal angles before (light shade) and after (dark shade) treatment. From Wenger et al. (1989).

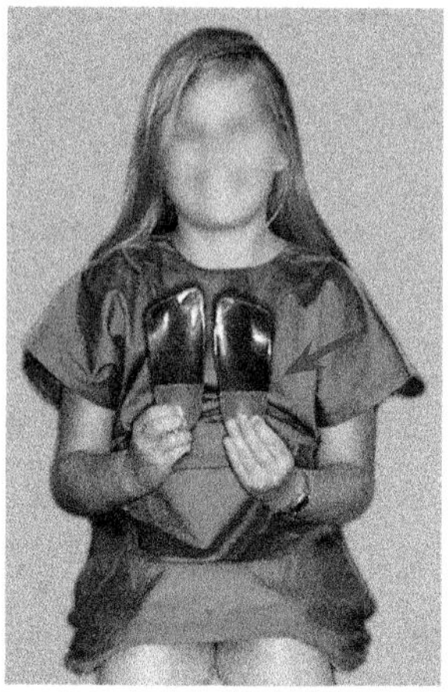

C Orthotics can be discarded This girl was pleased when she was told she could discard the orthotics. Plastic inserts are uncomfortable and make the child feel abnormal.

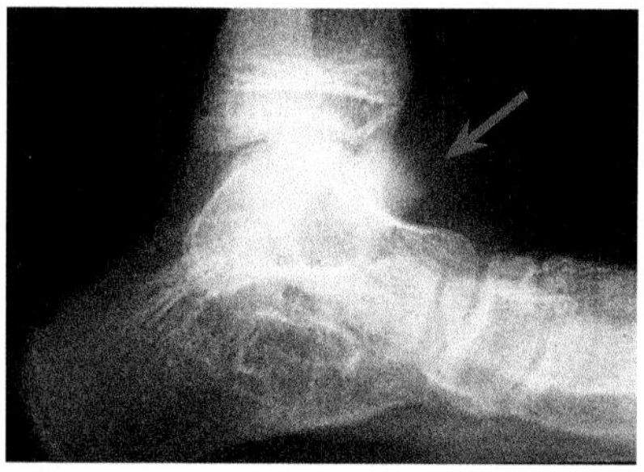

D Extrusion of silastic implant This implant was placed in a child with flexible flatfeet.

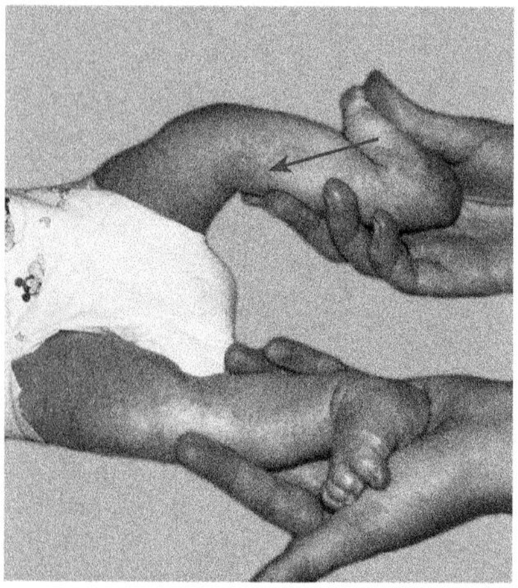

E Calcaneovalgus deformity This is a positional deformity that requires no treatment.

Evaluation Evaluate to establish a diagnosis [D, previous page]. The screening examination may show generalized joint laxity. On standing, the foot appears flat and the heel may show mild valgus. The arch reappears when the child toe stands or the foot is unweighted [A]. Subtalar and ankle motions are full. Radiographs are unnecessary.

Management The flexible flatfoot requires no treatment, as it has been shown that the condition is not a source of disability. Shoe modifications or inserts [B and C] are ineffective, expensive, result in a bad experience for the child, and may adversely affect the individual's self-image. Operative intervention to create an arch by blocking subtalar motion may establish an arch, but expose the child to the risks of an operation [D], perhaps months of postoperative discomfort, and may possibly, because of damage to the subtalar joint, cause degenerative arthritis of the subtalar joint in adult life.

Interventions Do not impose interventions on the child to "satisfy" the parent. Provide reassurance and make copies of the parent education material (see page 290) to show the grandparents and other family members. If the family insists that something be done, encourage the use of flexible shoes, limitation of excess weight, and a healthy lifestyle for the child.

Calcaneovalgus Deformity

This congenital deformity is due to intrauterine crowding, producing both calcaneus and valgus [E]. The condition may be confused with a vertical talus. Differentiation is made by determining the degree of stiffness. The calcaneovalgus foot is very flexible and the calcaneus lies in dorsiflexion. This condition is associated with developmental hip dysplasia, which should be ruled out by a careful examination of the hips. Because the calcaneovalgus flatfoot is a positional deformity, it resolves spontaneously. Treatment is not required.

Hypermobile Flatfoot and Heel-Cord Contracture

Heel-cord contractures cause an obligatory heel valgus, altered tarsal motion, lateral column shortening, and a painful pathologic flatfoot.

Evaluation The patient is usually in the second decade and has vague activity-related foot pain. The foot is flat on standing and the heel-cord is contracted. The foot cannot be dorsiflexed beyond neutral with the knee extended and the subtalar joint inverted to neutral [F]. Radiographs often show excessive plantarflexion of the talus. This condition is often confused with simple hypermobile flatfoot and inappropriately called a symptomatic flexible flatfoot.

Management Lengthen the contracture of the triceps. If the soleus is contracted, lengthen the heel-cord. If only the gastrocnemius is contracted, perform a recession. Most cases have secondary shortening of the lateral column and require a calcaneal lengthening.

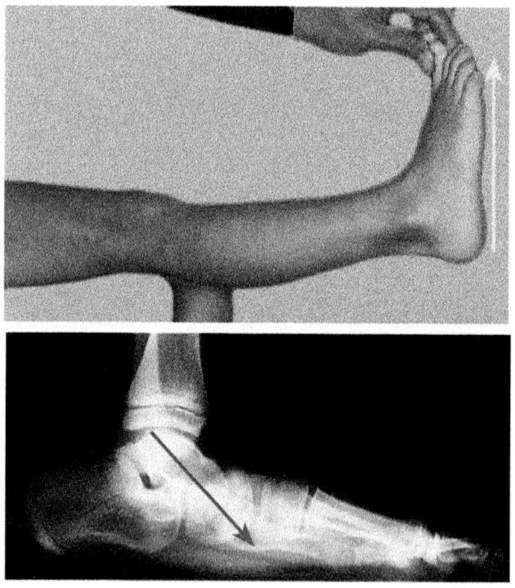

F Heel-cord contracture with flexible flatfoot This child with a flexible flatfoot also has a heel-cord contracture. Note that the foot cannot be dorsiflexed above a neutral position with the knee extended and the subtalar joint in neutral (yellow arrow) and that the foot shows plantarflexion of the talus (red arrow).

Tarsal Coalitions

Coalitions are fusions between tarsal bones that cause a loss of inversion and eversion motion. They are often familial, may be unilateral or bilateral, and occur in both sexes equally. Coalitions may involve more than one joint. The fusion imposes increased stress on adjacent joints and sometimes causes degenerative arthritis, pain, and peroneal spasm. These symptoms usually develop during early adolescence. Often coalitions remain silent. Treatment is indicated only for intractable pain, not the mere existence of a coalition. Two common forms are present.

Calcaneonavicular (C-N) Coalitions

C-N coalitions are most common and sometimes identified on a lateral radiograph [A] but are readily shown by an oblique radiograph of the foot [B]. The coalition may be composed of bone, cartilage, or fibrous tissue. Incomplete coalitions may show only narrowing or irregularity of the calcaneonavicular articulation.

Manage symptomatic coalitions with a trial of immobilization [F]. Apply a short-leg walking cast for 4 weeks. The pain should disappear. If pain recurs soon after removal, operative correction is usually necessary. Resect the coalition and interpose extensor hallucis brevis muscle to prevent recurrence.

Talocalcaneal (T-C) Coalitions

T-C coalitions usually involve the middle facet of the subtalar joint. Conventional radiographs are often normal, but sometimes the C-sign of Lateur may be present [C]. A special calcaneal or Harris view may show the fusion. The coalition is best demonstrated by CT scans of the foot [D].

Manage symptomatic coalitions with a trial using a short-leg cast. If pain recurs, consider operative resection. Assess the size of the coalition by CT imaging. Resection is likely to fail if coalitions exceed 50% of the joint. Technical problems are common [E]. Heel valgus may be increased by resection. Sometimes a calcaneal lengthening will be needed to correct this component. Outcomes for resection of subtalar coalitions are much less predictable than for the more common calcaneonavicular fusions. Advise the family of the potential for an unsatisfactory result and the possibility that additional procedures may be necessary.

Other Coalitions

Other coalitions may occur at the talonavicular and naviculocuneiform joint. More extensive coalitions may be present in children with clubfeet, fibular hemimelia, and proximal focal femoral deficiencies. Pain and stiffness of the subtalar joint may occur with arthritis, tumors, and articular fractures. Consider these uncommon causes of pain if calcaneonavicular and talocalcaneal fusions are ruled out by radiography.

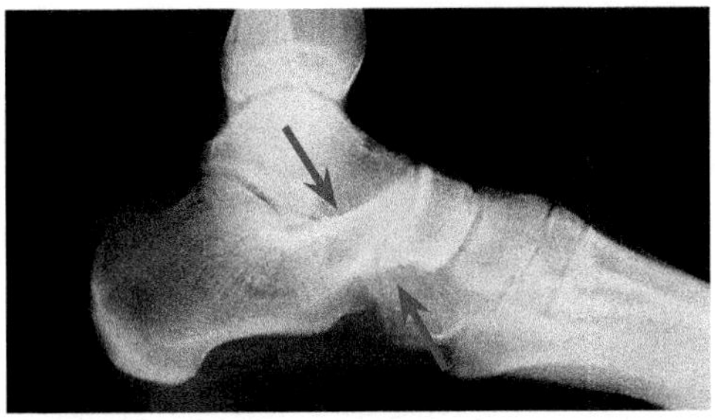

A "Ant-eater sign" The calcaneonavicular coalition is seen in lateral radiographs with this characteristic feature (arrows).

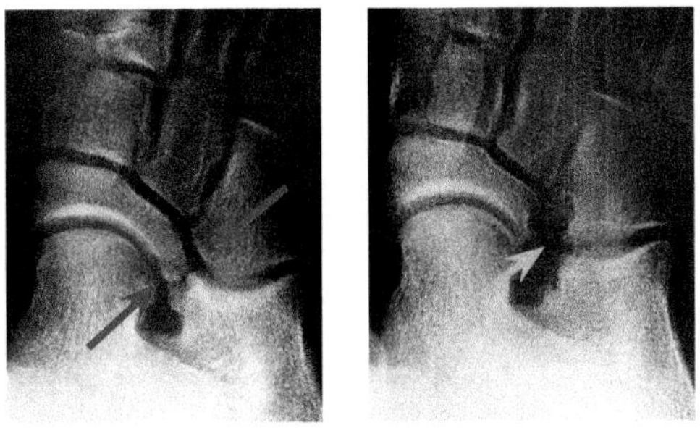

B Calcaneonavicular coalition This C-N coalition is readily seen on oblique radiographs of the foot before resection (red arrows). Surgical resection (orange arrow) reduced discomfort and restored motion.

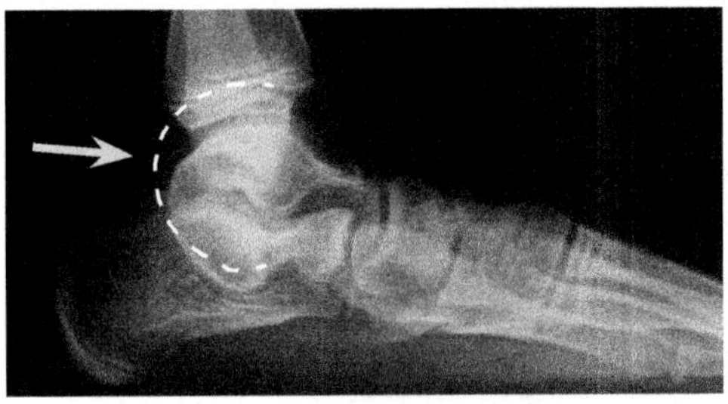

C C-sign of Lateur The *C-sign of Lateur* (arrow) is often present with subtalar coalitions.

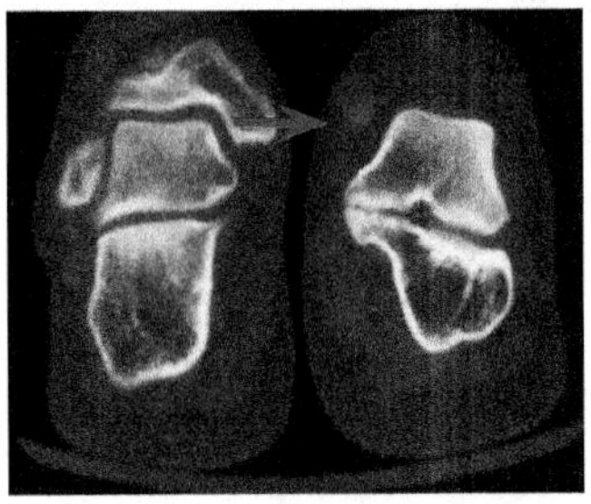

D Subtalar coalition The middle facet subtalar coalition (arrow) is readily identified by CT imaging.

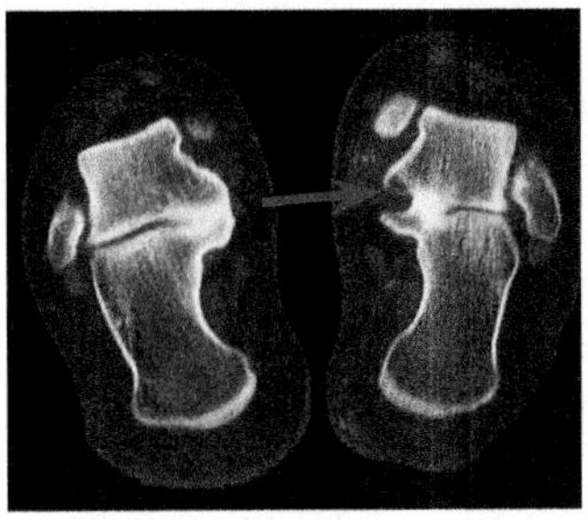

E Failed resection This resection failed because the coalition was not fully resected.

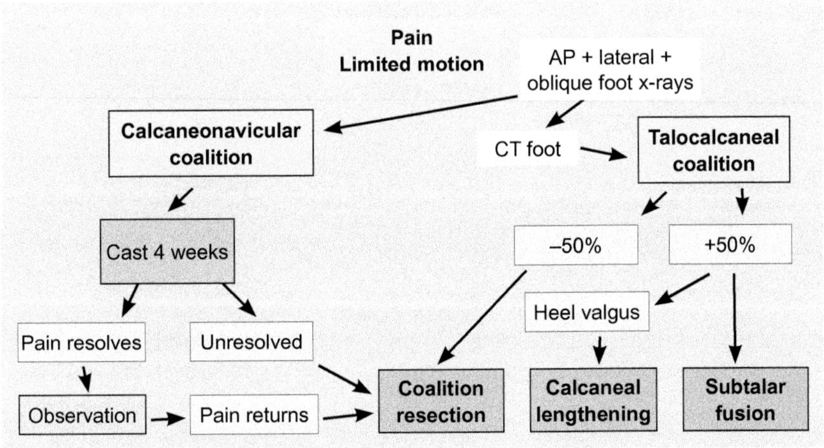

F Flowchart for managing tarsal coalitions

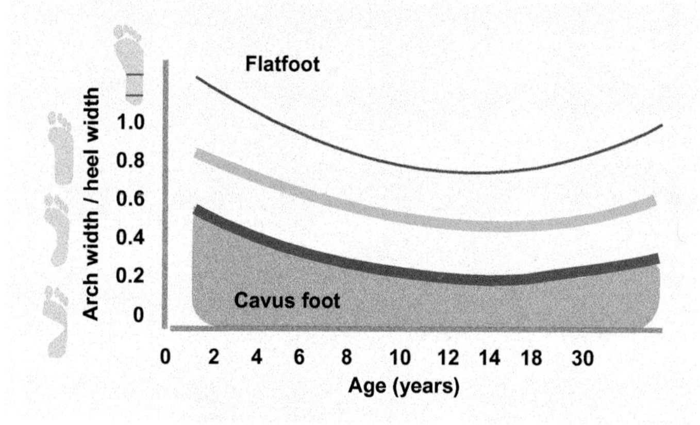

A Normal values for foot contact area Contact area is described by the ratio of the arch width to the heel width. The mean value (green line), and two standard deviation levels for a low arch (blue line) and a high arch (red line) are shown. A foot is considered to have a cavus deformity if the arch contact area falls outside the ±2 SD level (light red area).

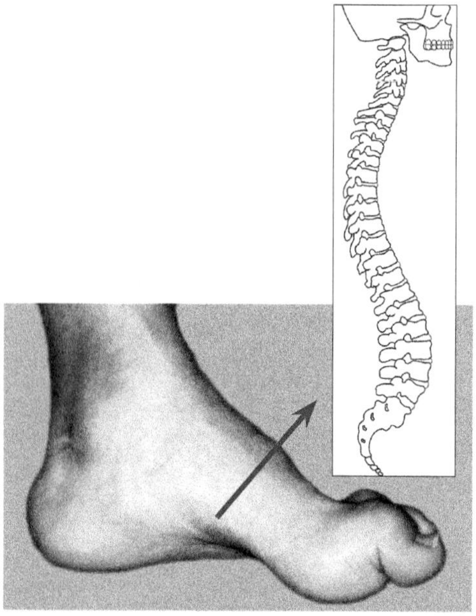

B Cavus—think spine The high arch should prompt an evaluation of the spine.

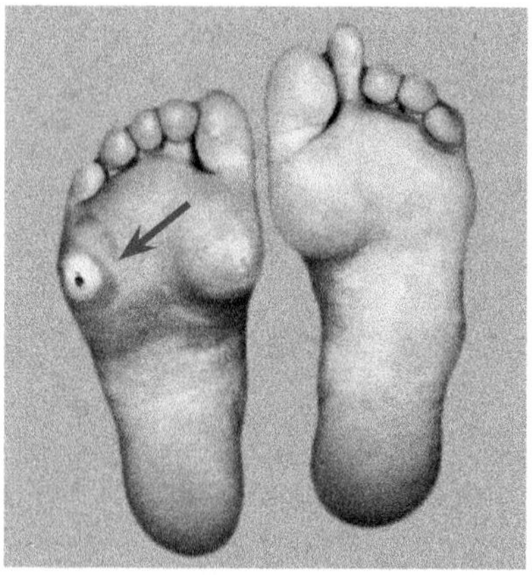

C Skin irritation with cavus deformity The cavus deformity increases the load on the metatarsal heads. If sensation is poor, as in the child with spina bifida, skin breakdown (arrow) is common.

Cavus Deformity

A cavus foot is characterized by increased height of the longitudinal arch and is often associated with clawing of the toes and heel varus [B]. Cavus is most often physiological. It is simply the extreme end of the spectrum of normal variability of the shape of the longitudinal arch. This physiologic form is often familial. Pathologic forms of cavus deformity are usually neurogenic or myopathic.

Physiologic Cavus

This deformity falls outside the normal range of ±2 SD in arch height [A]. Often a parent's feet have a high arch. The parent often volunteers that they have a "good" (high) arch. In fact, these parents are more likely to have pain than those with normal or low arches. The cavus is usually bilateral, with an onset in infancy. They may also have calluses under the metatarsal heads. The child's musculoskeletal and neurologic screening examinations are normal, and clawing of the toes is absent. This is a diagnosis of exclusion. Occasionally, the teenager will complain of metatarsal pain. This is best managed by shock-absorbing shoeware and, if necessary, a soft shoe insert to unload the metatarsal heads.

Pathologic Cavus

Pathologic cavus is usually secondary to a neuromuscular disorder causing muscle imbalance. A major objective of management is to determine the underlying cause of the deformity.

Evaluation The neuromuscular disorders causing cavus deformities are often familial, so the family history is important. Look at the parents' feet. Sometimes they may claim their feet are normal when they are clearly deformed. Perform a careful screening examination of the child. Examine the musculoskeletal system for other problems. Look for midline skin lesions over the spine [B]. A careful neurologic examination is essential. Check muscle strength. Examine the foot, noting the severity of the cavus, degree of rigidity, and presence of clawing of the toes and skin changes under the metatarsal heads [C]. Standing radiographs of the feet are useful in documenting the type and severity of the deformity. Special studies such as spine radiographs for spinal dysraphism, electromyography (EMG), DNA blood tests for Charcot–Marie–Tooth (CMT) disease, nerve conduction velocity measurements, and CPK determination for muscular dystrophy assessment may be necessary. Consultation with a neurologist may be appropriate. Establish the etiology of the cavus deformity [D].

Natural history Because of the reduced area of plantar contact, deformity, and rigidity, cavus feet often cause considerable disability.

Category	Type	Etiology
Physiologic	Cavovarus	Familial
Pathologic	Cavovarus	Clubfoot residual cavus Idiopathic Neuromuscular disease Friedreicht ataxia Charcot-Marie-Tooth Spinal dysraphism
	Calcaneocavus	Spina bifida Poliomyelitis Overlengthened heel-cord

D Classification of cavus deformity This classification includes the majority of causes of cavus feet. Pathologic cavus is often associated with neurologic disorders.

Types of Cavus Deformities

Congenital cavus is a rare deformity that may be due to intrauterine constraint or fixed deformity [A]. Assess the effect of growth.

Calcaneocavus results from weakness of the triceps. There is an increase in the calcaneal pitch, and a cavus deformity. Correct muscle imbalance, if possible. This deformity is seen in poliomyelitis [B], in spina bifida, and following overlengthening of the triceps.

Cavovarus is the most common form. Muscle imbalance results in plantarflexion of the forefoot, inversion of the hindfoot, and a mild increase in the calcaneal pitch. This deformity is seen in CMT disease. Clawing of the toes is often seen.

Management

Follow a flowchart to manage [D]. The teenager will often complain of difficulty in fitting shoes, calluses over the claw toes and under the metatarsal heads, pain, and instability causing recurrent ankle sprains.

Mild deformity Order shock-absorbing footwear and soft molded shoe inserts to broaden the load-bearing area of the foot.

Moderate or severe deformity This requires operative correction. Operations improve muscle balance, flatten the arch to broaden the weight-bearing surface, and correct toe deformity.

Flexible deformities or those in young children are best managed by a plantar medial release and appropriate tendon transfers. If performed during childhood, recurrence can occur.

Fixed deformities require correction in two stages. First, perform a soft tissue release, as described above. Follow this by osteotomies to correct bony deformity and tendon transfers to balance the foot. In most cases, perform a calcaneal osteotomy [C] for calcaneocavus deformity and a dorsiflexion medial cuneiform osteotomy for cavovarus correction. Avoid arthrodesis whenever possible to maintain mobility and reduce the risk of degenerative arthritis of adjacent joints.

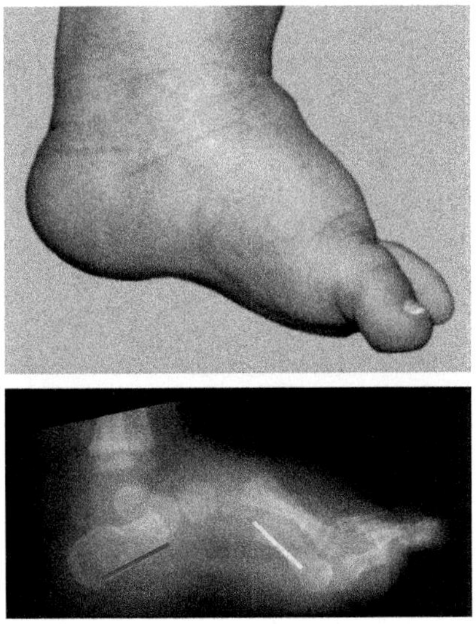

A Congenital cavus This deformity gradually resolved during the first two years of growth. Note the calcaneal pitch (red line) and first metatarsal (yellow line) alignments.

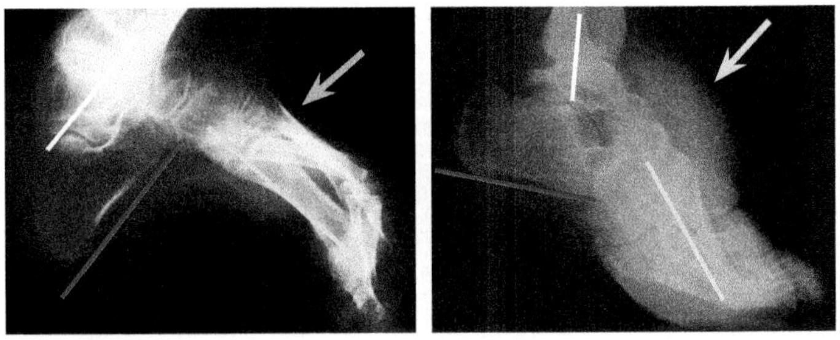

B Hindfoot and forefoot cavus deformity Note the severe hindfoot cavus (orange arrow) secondary to weakness of the triceps from poliomyelitis. Note the forefoot cavus (yellow arrow). The white lines show the tibial axis, the red lines the calcaneal pitch, and the yellow lines the first metatarsal axis.

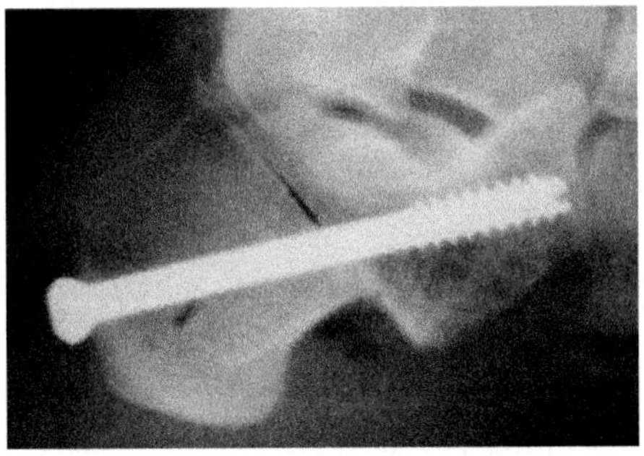

C Calcaneocavus deformity This patient underwent a calcaneal dorsal displacement osteotomy to effectively reduce the cavus deformity.

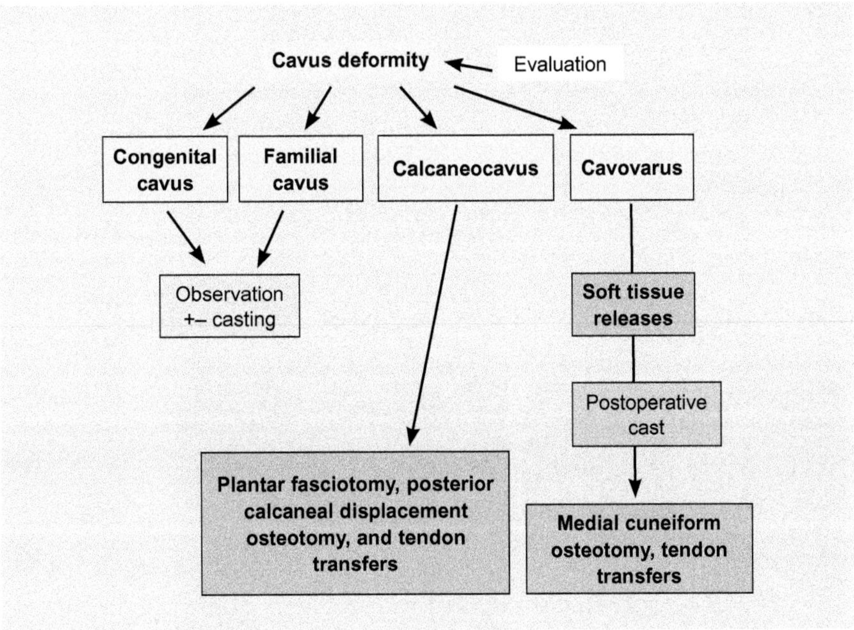

D Cavus management flowchart From Mosca (2000).

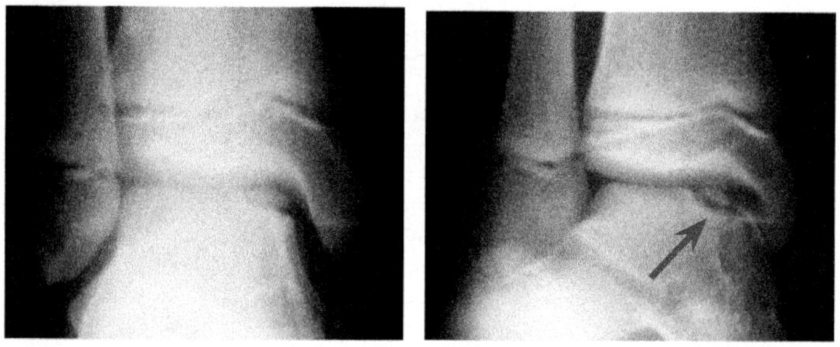

A **Osteochondritis dissecans of the talus** Most can be diagnosed with conventional radiographs. Note that the lesion is best seen on the mortise view (red arrow). The degree of displacement can be demonstrated by CT or MRI studies.

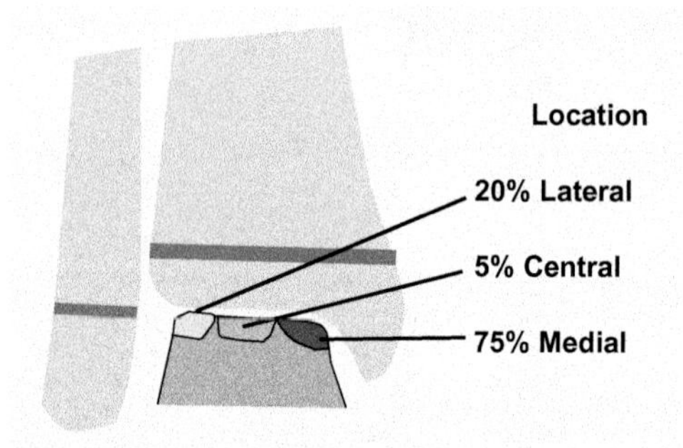

B **Location of osteochondritis dissecans of the talus** This is the distribution in children. From Letts et al. 2003, JPO.

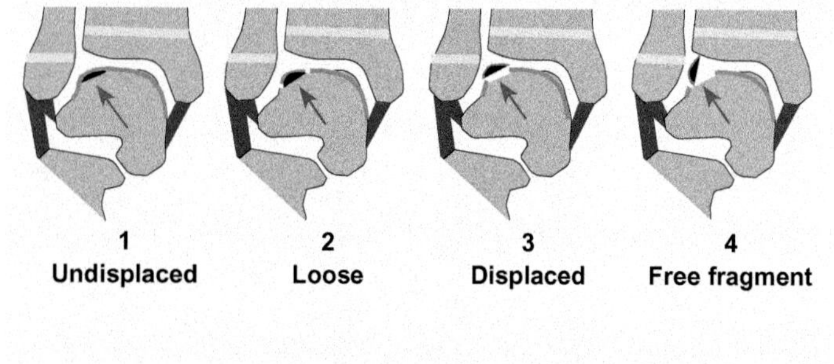

C **Classification of osteochondritis dissecans of the talus** This Berndt and Hartly classification is based on Giguera et al. (1998).

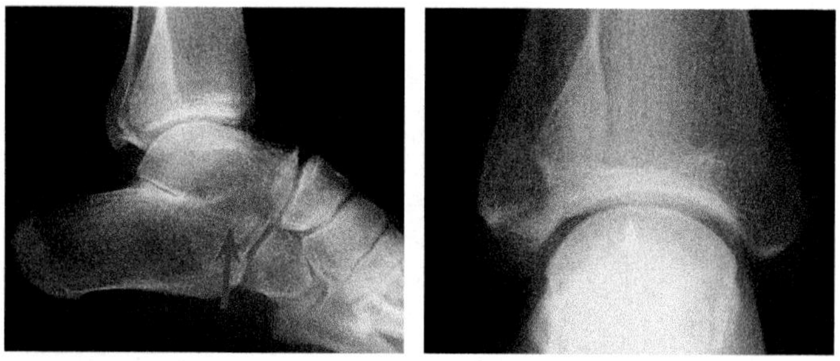

D **Ball-and-socket ankle** Note the subtalar fusion (red arrow) and the spherical shape of the ankle (yellow arrow).

Osteochondritis Dissecans of the Talus

These lesions are segments of avascular bone that occur most commonly on the anterolateral and posteromedial aspects of the talar dome. The talus is the third most common site after the knee and elbow and accounts for about 4% of all lesions. Medial lesions are usually due to a variation of ossification. Lateral lesions often secondary to trauma and are more serious. Vascular variations and genetic factors may contribute. Often lesions occur with no trauma history. In children, the gender incidence is about equal. The onset may occur late in the first decade but is most common during the teen years.

Clinical Features

Ankle pain, swelling, stiffness, and a trauma history suggest this diagnosis.

Imaging Order standard radiographs of the ankle supplemented with lateral plantar flexion and dorsiflexion views. The mortis view may show the lesion best [A]. CT and MRI may be helpful to assess the extent of the lesion and cartilage status if operative management is being considered. Most lesions are medial [B].

Classification Lesions are classified into four categories [C].

Stage 1 Subchondral osteonecrosis. Lesion is undisplaced and stable.

Stage 2 The lesion is demarcated from the talus, but stabilized by the articular cartilage.

Stage 3 The lesion is loose with disruption of the articular cartilage, but the lesion is not grossly displaced.

Stage 4 The fragment becomes a loose body in the joint.

Management

Manage most lesions in children with limitation of activity and immobilization. Lateral, sclerotic lesions that are separated are most likely to require surgery.

Stage 1 and 2 lesions Manage with activity modification, non-steroidal antiinflammatory drugs (NSAIDs), and time. Consider immobilizing in a short-leg cast for 4 to 6 weeks. Manage persisting type 2 lesions with retrograde drilling.

Stage 3 lesions Manage by reduction and immobilization of the fragment. The options for stabilization include bioabsorbable implants, bone pegs, wires, or screws.

Stage 4 lesions Approach by arthroscopy or with the aid of a transmalleolar osteotomy. Excise small fragment. Treat larger lesions with excision, curettage, and cancellous grafting. For very large lesions, consider mosaicplasty using autogenous osteocartilaginous grafts taken from the non-weight-bearing cartilage of the ipsilateral knee.

Prognosis

Good to excellent results are expected for type 1 and 2 lesions. Medial lesions do less well than lateral lesions. Lesions that result in loss of the articular cartilage often lead to osteoarthritis and the need for ankle fusion or replacement.

Ball-and-Socket Ankle

Ball-and-socket ankle is a rare deformity associated with conditions such as extensive tarsal coalitions [D], congenital shortening of the lower limb, absent digital rays, and aplasia or hypoplasia of the fibula. It is thought to be an acquired deformity secondary to limitation of movement of the subtalar and midtarsal joints. The deformity is usually completely developed by about five years of age. It causes little or no disability, and no treatment is required.

Tumors of the Foot

The tumors that involve the foot are typical of other locations [A]. The majority are cysts [B]. Some tumors, such as dysplasia epiphysialis hemimelica [C], are unique to the limbs. They are rarely malignant [D].

Calcaneal Prominence

This deformity is seen in adolescence, is often bilateral, and is thought to be related to irritation from shoewear [E]. Manage most cases with thoughtful shoe selection. Rarely, exostectomy is required. Operative results are often poor.

Accessory Soleus

This is a rare variation in the soleus causing a swelling just medial to the Achilles tendon. The mass is smooth, round, and nontender, and grows proportionately with the foot. No treatment is required.

Plantar Fibromatosis

This is a rare tumor with a characteristic location on the anteromedial portion of the heel pad [F]. Because recurrence following resection is common, and many resolve spontaneously, observational management is usually indicated.

Subungal Exostosis

This is a benign bone tumor of the distal phalanx occurring beneath or adjacent to the nail [G]. This rare tumor occurs in late childhood or adolescence and most commonly affects the great toe. Its characteristic location and radiographic appearance establish the diagnosis. Manage by careful and complete excision to avoid recurrence.

Benign tumors	Malignant tumors
Osteochondromata	Osteogenic sarcoma
Enchondromas	Ewing sarcoma
Simple bone cysts	Synovial sarcoma
	Fibromatosis

A Foot tumors These are the tumors that are common but not unique to the foot.

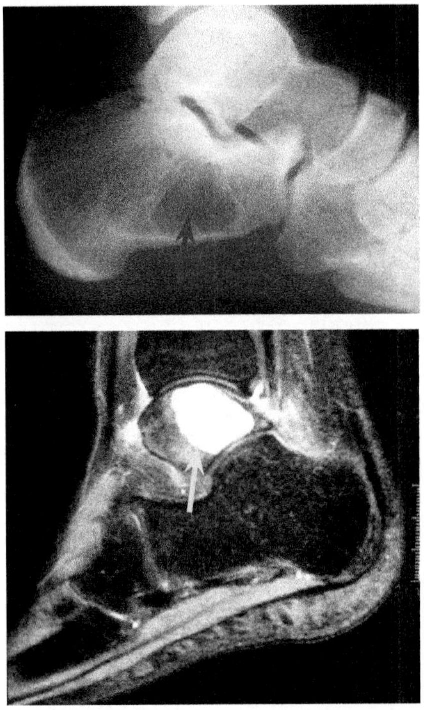

B Cysts Cysts most commonly affect the calcaneus (red arrow) and may often be identified by a lateral radiograph. Others, such as this cyst of the talus (yellow arrow), are best shown by MRI and CT scans.

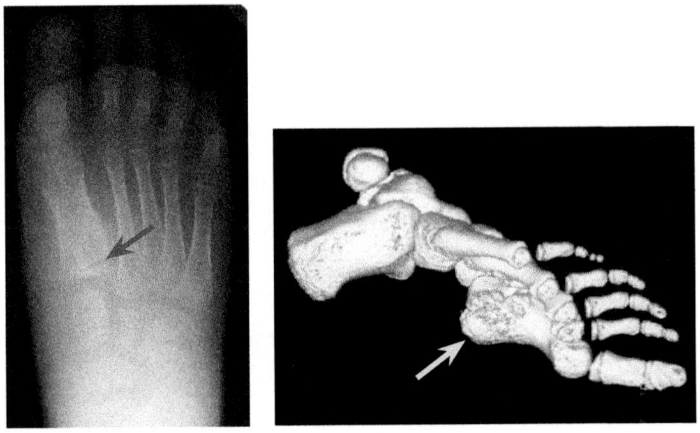

C Dysplasia epiphysialis hemimelica Note the lesion on a radiograph (red arrow) and how well it is demonstrated on a CT reconstruction (yellow arrow).

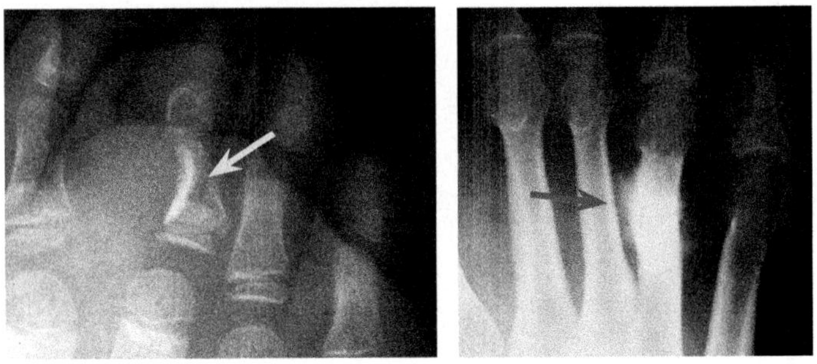

D Malignant tumors These include lesions such as desmoid tumors (yellow arrow) and osteogenic sarcoma (red arrow).

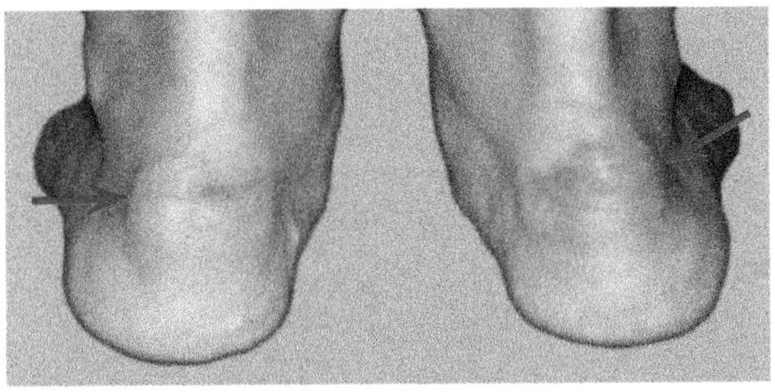

E Calcaneal prominences This teenage girl has bilateral prominences with some discomfort.

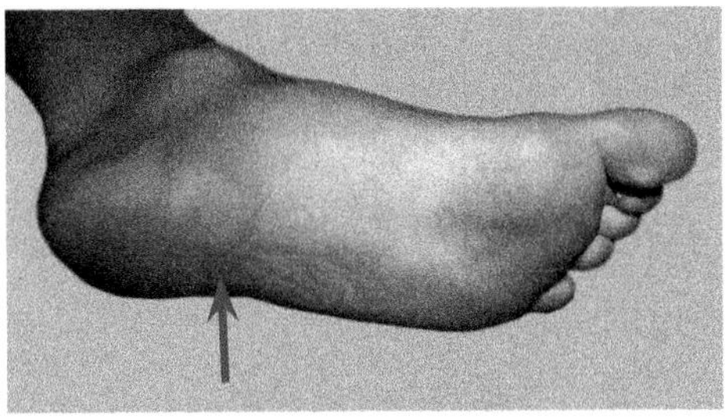

F Plantar fibromatosis

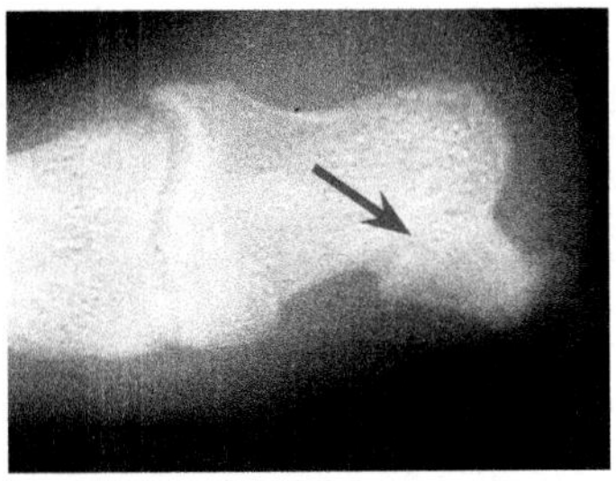

H Subungal exostosis

TOE DEFORMITY

Aikin OF. The treatment of hallux valgus: a new operative procedure and its results. Medical Sentinel 33:678, 1925.

Albuisson J, Isidor B, Giraud M, Pichon O, Marsaud T, David A, Le Caignec C, Bezieau S. Identification of two novel mutations in Shh long-range regulator associated with familial pre-axial polydactyly. Clin. Genet. 79: 371-377, 2011.

Chang CH, Kumar SJ, Riddle EC, Glutting J. Macrodactyly of the foot. J Bone Joint Surg 84-A:1189-94, 2002.

Cockin J. Butler's operation for an over-riding fifth toe. J Bone Joint Surg. 50-B(1):78-81 1968.

Furniss D, Critchley P, Giele H, Wilkie AOM. Nonsensemediated decay and the molecular pathogenesis of mutations in SALL1 and GLI3. Am. J. Med. Genet. 143A:3150-3160, 2007.

Girdlestone GR. Journal of the Chartered Society of Physiotherapy, 32, 167, 1947.

Lichtblau S. Section of the abductor hallucis tendon for correction of metatarsus adductus varus deformity. Clin Orthop. 110:227–232, 1975.

McBride ED. A conservative approach to bunions. J Bone Joint Surg. 10-B:737, 1928.

Peterson HA, Newman SR. Adolescent bunion deformity treated with double osteotomy and longitudinal pin fixation of the first ray. J Pediatr Orthop. 13(1):80-4, 1993.

Radhakrishna U, Blouin J-L, Mehenni H, Patel UC, Patel MN, Solanki JV, Antonarakis SE. Mapping one form of autosomal dominant postaxial polydactyly type A to chromosome 7p15-q11.23 by linkage analysis. Am. J. Hum. Genet. 60: 597-604, 1997.

Shea KG, Mubarak SJ, Alamin T. Preossified longitudinal epiphyseal bracket of the foot: treatment by partial bracket excision before ossification. J Pediatr Orthop 21(3):360-5, 2001.

Taylor RG. The treatment of claw toes by multiple transfers if flexor into extensor tendons. J Bone Joint Surg. 33-B(4):539-542, 1951.

Umm-e-Kalsoom BS, Kamran-ul-Hassan NS, Ansar M, Ahmad W. Genetic mapping of an autosomal recessive postaxial polydactyly type A to chromosome 13q13.3-q21.2 and screening of the candidate genes. Hum. Genet. 131: 415-422, 2012.

FOREFOOT

Kite JH. Congenital metatarsus varus: report of 300 cases. J Bone Joint Surg 32-A:500, 1950.

HINDFOOT

Alvarado DM, McCall K, Aferol H, Silva MJ, Garbow JR, Spees WM, Patel T, Siegel M, Dobbs MB, Gurnett CA. Pitx1 haploinsufficiency causes clubfoot in humans and a clubfoot-like phenotype in mice. Hum. Molec. Genet. 20:3943-3952, 2011.

Anderson RJ. The presence of an astragaloschaphoid bone in man. J. Anat. Physiol. 14:452–455, 1879.

Browne D. Modern methods of treatment of club-foot. Br. Med. J. Sep:570-572, 1937.

Cowell HR. Extensor brevis arthroplasty. J. Bone Joint Surg. 52-A:820, 1970.

Crim J, Kjeldsberg K. Radiographic diagnosis of tarsal coalition. Am. J. Roentgenol. 18:323–328, 2004.

Evans D. Relapsed clubfoot. J Bone Joint Surg. 43-B:722, 1961.

Ezra E, Hayek S, Gilai AN, Khermosh O, Wientroub S. Tibialis anterior tendon transfer for residual dynamic supination deformity in treated club feet. J Pediatr Orthop B 9(3):207-11, 2000.

Giannini S, Ceccarelli F, Vannini F, Baldi E. Operative treatment of flatfoot with talocalcaneal coalition. Clin Orthop 411:178-87, 2003.

Grogan DP, Gasser SI, Ogden JA. The painful accessory navicular: a clinical and histopathological study. Foot Ankle 10:164, 1989.

Kite JH. The Clubfoot. New York, Grune & Stratton, 1964.

Leonard MA. The inheritance of tarsal coalition and its relationship to spastic flat foot. J. Bone Joint Surg. 56-B: 520-526, 1974.

Lichtblau S. A medial and lateral release operation for clubfoot: a preliminary report. J Bone Joint Surg. 55-A:377, 1973.

McKay DW. New concept of and approach to clubfoot treatment. Section II. Correction of the clubfoot. J Pediatr Orthop 3:10, 1983.

Ponseti IV. Congenital club foot: the results of treatment. J Bone Joint Surg. 45-A:2610, 1963.

Raikin S, Cooperman DR, Thompson GH. Interposition of the split flexor hallucis longus tendon after resection of a coalition of the middle facet of the talocalcaneal joint. J. Bone Joint Surg. 81-A:11–19, 1999.

Swiontkowski MF, Scranton PE, Hansen S. Tarsal coalitions: long-term results of surgical treatment. J. Pediatr. Orthop. 3:287–292, 1983.

Turco VJ. Surgical correction of the resistant clubfoot: one stage posteromedial release with internal fixation. J Bone Joint Surg 53-A:477, 1971.

Wilde PH, Torode IP, Dickens DR, Cole WG. Resection for symptomatic talocalcaneal coalition. J. Bone Joint Surg. 76-B:797–801, 1994.

Zadek J, Gold AM. The accessory tarsal scaphoid. J Bone Joint Surg. 30-A:1948, 1948.

MIDFOOT

Dwyer FC. Osteotomy of the calcaneum for pes cavus. J. Bone Joint Surg. 41-B:80, 1959.

Echarri JJ, Forriol F. The development in footprint morphology in 1851 Congolese children from urban and rural areas, and the relationship between this and wearing shoes. J Pediatr Orthop B 12(2):141-6, 2003.

Harris RI, Beath T. Hypermobile flat-foot with short tendo achillis. J Bone Joint Surg. 30-A:116-140, 1948.

Hibbs RA. An operation for "clawfoot". JAMA 73:1583, 1919.

Jahss MH. Tarsometatarsal truncated-wedge arthrodesis for pes cavus and equinovarus deformity of the fore part of the foot. J. Bone Joint Surg. 62-A:713, 1980.

Japas LM. Surgical treatment of pes cavus by V-osteotomy: preliminary report. J. Bone Joint Surg. 50-A:927, 1968. Méary R. Le pied creux essentiel. Symp Rev Chir Orthop. 53:389, 1967.

Lamy L, Weissman L. Congenital convex pes planus. J Bone Joint Surg 21:79, 1939.

Mazzocca AD, Thomson JD, Deluca PA, Romness MJ. Comparison of the posterior approach versus the dorsal approach in the treatment of congenital vertical talus. J Pediatr Orthop 21(2): p212-7, 2001.

Mosca VS. Calcaneal lengthening for valgus deformity of the hindfoot. Results in children who had severe, symptomatic flatfoot and skewfoot. J Bone Joint Surg. 77-A:500, 1995.

Peterson HA. Skewfoot (forefoot adduction with heel valgus). J Pediatr Orthop 6:24-30, 1986.

Ragab AA, Stewart SL, Cooperman DR. Implications of subtalar joint anatomic variation in calcaneal lengthening osteotomy. J Pediatr Orthop 23(1): p79-83, 2003.

Staheli LT, Chew DE, Corbett M. The longitudinal arch: A survey of eight hundred and eighty-two feet in normal children and adults. J Bone Joint Surg. 69-A:426-428, 1987.

Steindler A. Stripping of the os calcis. J. Orthop. Surg. 2:8, 1920. Harris RI, Beath T. Etiology of peroneal spastic flat foot. J Bone Joint Surg 1948 30-B:624-634.

van der Wilde R, Staheli LT, Chew DE, et al. Measurements on radiographs of the foot in normal infants and children. J Bone Joint Surg 1988;70A:407-415.

Ward CM, Dolan LA, Bennett DL, Morcuende JA, Cooper RR. Long-term results of reconstruction for treatment of a flexible cavovarus foot in Charcot-Marie-Tooth disease. J. Bone Joint Surg. 90(12)-A:2631-42, 2008.

Wenger DR, et al. Corrective shoes and inserts as treatment for flexible flatfoot in infants and children. J Bone Joint Surg. 71-A:800, 1989.

ANKLE

Alberktsson B, Rydholm A, Rydholm U. The tarsal tunnel syndrome in children. J Bone Joint Surg 64-B:215-217, 1982.

Grogan DP, Walling AK, Ogden JA. Anatomy of the os trigonum. J Pediatr Orthop 10:618, 1990.

Lamb D. The ball and socket ankle joint: a congenital abnormality. J Bone Joint Surg. 40-B:240-3, 1958.

Silfverskiöld N. Reduction of the uncrossed two-joints muscles of the leg to one-joint muscles in spastic conditions. Acta Chir Scand. 56:315-30, 1924.

Strayer LM. Recession of the gastrocnemius. J Bone Joint Surg. 32-B:671, 1950.

OSTEOCHONDROSIS

Borges JL, Guille JT, Bowen JR. Köhler's bone disease of the tarsal navicular. J. Pediatr. Orthop. 15:5:596-598, 1995.

Freiberg AH. Infarction of the second metatarsal bone. J Bone Joint Surg. 8:257, 1926.

Köhler A. Uber eine haufige bisher anscheinend unbekannte Erkrankung einzelner kindlicher Knowchen. Munchen Med Wochenschr 55:1923, 1908.

Sever JW. Apophysitis of the os calcis. NY State J Med. 95:1025–1029, 1912.

Waugh W. The ossification and vascularization of the tarsal navicular and their relation to Köhler disease. J Bone Joint Surg. 40-B:765, 1958.

TUMOR

Landon GC, Johnson KA, Dahlin DC. Subungual exostosis. J Bone Joint Surg. 61-A:256, 1979.

INFECTION

Jacobs RF, McCarthy RE, Elser JM. Pseudomonas osteochondritis complicating puncture wounds of the foot in children: a 10-year evaluation. J. Infect Dis. 160:657-661, 1989.

Winograd AM: A modification in the technique of operations for ingrown toenails. JAMA 92:229, 1929.

CHAPTER 10

Knee and Tibia

This chapter addresses disorders of the knee and tibia. In all age groups, knee problems account for more than one-fourth of musculoskeletal complaints. In children, knee complaints are substantially less common but increase in frequency during the teen years. Osteomyelitis and osteogenic sarcoma develop more often about the knee than at any other site, thought to be due to the rapid growth rate of the distal femoral and upper tibial physes.

Development

Nomenclature

The fully extended knee is the neutral or zero position. The normal range of motion extends from neutral to about 140°, with most activities performed in the 0°–65° segment of the flexion arc. In the child, hyper-extension of up to 10°–15° is normal [A]. The difference between active and passive motion is termed *lag.*

Hyperextension, if associated with stiffness, is called a recurvatum deformity. Restricted motion is described by specifying the arc of motion. For example, a stiff knee may be described as having an "arc of motion from 20 to 55 degrees." The arc of motion in hyperextension is preceded by a minus sign. A child with a hyperextension deformity may have a range from –20° to 30°, giving a 50-degree arc of motion.

The knee angle is the thigh–leg angle or femoral–tibial angle (see Chapter 8). Changes in the knee angle that represent normal variations are physiological and cause bowlegs or knock-knees. Deformities, those falling outside the normal range (±2 SD) and those due to pathological processes, are termed genu varum or genu valgum.

Normal Development

The knee develops as a typical synovial joint during the first two fetal months. The secondary centers of ossification for the distal femur form between the sixth and ninth fetal months and for the upper tibia between the eighth fetal and first postnatal months. The patella ossification center appears between the second and fourth years in girls and the third and fifth years in boys.

Developmental Variations

Variations of ossification or development may cause confusion in assessing radiographs.

Bipartite patella is due to an accessory ossification center of the patella that usually occurs in the superior–lateral corner [B].

Fibrocortical defects are usually insignificant developmental variations that are most common about the knee. They are eccentric and show sclerotic margins and radiolucent centers. They resolve spontaneously [C].

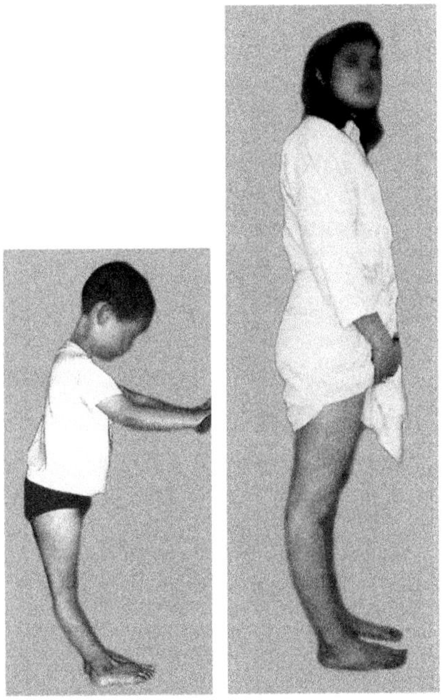

A Hyperextension deformities of the knee The boy's knees hyperextend due to generalized joint laxity. The girl's have a hyperextension deformity due to a knee injury with loss of knee flexion.

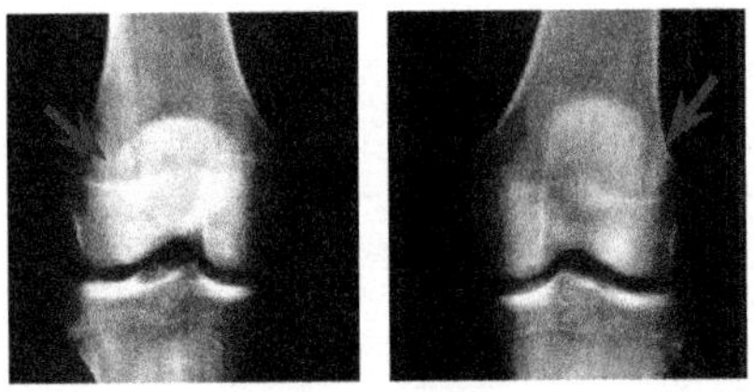

B Bilateral bipartite patellae Secondary centers may appear on both knees. They are usually asymptomatic.

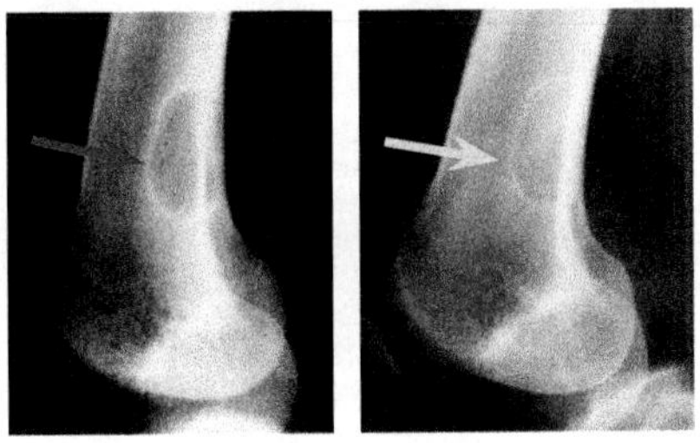

C Fibrocortical defect This is a typical large lesion in the distal femur (red arrow). Two years later, spontaneous healing has occurred (yellow arrow).

Clinical Feature	Disorder
Patellar hypoplasia	Nail–patella syndrome Beals syndrome Diastrophic dysplasia Neurofibromatosis
Genu varum	Rickets Achondroplasia TAR syndrome Metaphyseal dysplasia
Genu valgum	Rickets Morquio syndrome Poliomyelitis Ellis-Van Creveld syndrome
Genu recurvatum	Myelodysplasia Arthrogryposis Larsen syndrome
Flexion contracture	Arthrogryposis Pterygium syndrome Myelodysplasia
Patellofemoral disorders	Nail-patella syndrome Rubinstein-Taybi syndrome
Excessive joint laxity	Ehlers-Danlos syndrome

A Syndromes associated with knee deformity These are examples that illustrate the relationship of knee deformities in various generalized disorders.

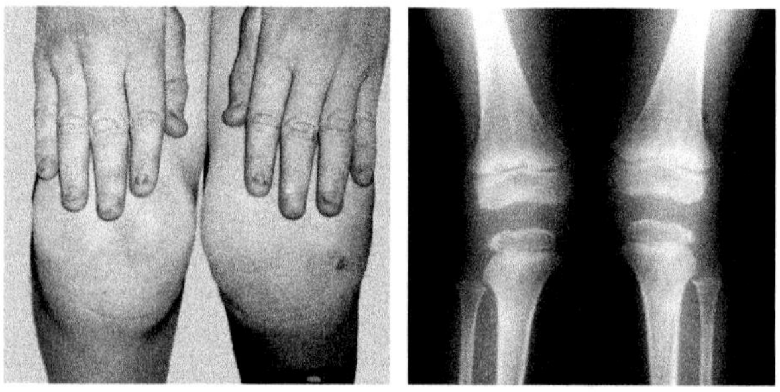

B Nail–patella syndrome Note the nail dysplasia and absence of the patella.

Evaluation

Evaluating the child's knee is different from evaluating the knee of the adult because disorders are more likely to be due to some underlying generalized dysplasia or to focal congenital or developmental deformity.

Screening Examination

Screen for some underlying abnormality [A], such as nail–patella syndrome [B]. Asymptomatic dislocation of the patella is common in Down syndrome. Dimpling over the knee is common in arthrogryposis. Recurvatum occurs in spina bifida and in arthrogryposis. Genu varum and valgum are common in ricketic disorders, and genu valgum is common in Morquio and Ellis-Van Creveld syndromes.

Physical Examination

The physical examination usually provides the diagnosis or at least the basis for ordering further studies.

General inspection Look for obvious deformity, check the knee angle, and perform a rotational profile [C].

Knee Observe the child standing and note symmetry, knee angle, position of patella, masses, joint effusion, muscle definition and atrophy [D], and signs of inflammation. Is there full extension or hyper extension?

Patellar tracking Ask the child to sit and slowly flex and extend the knee. Observe the tracking of the patella. Does it move in a linear fashion or displace laterally as the knee extends [E]? Repeat the examination with the hand on the patella as the knee is flexed both actively and passively. Does the patella move smoothly and track in the midline? Does the knee fully flex and extend?

Q angle is the angle formed by a line connecting the anterior superior iliac spine with the midportion of the patella and a second line from the patellar midpoint to the tibial tubercle. Normally, the enclosed angle is less than about 15°. Be aware that the Q angle has no direct relationship with knee pain or patellar instability.

Point of maximum tenderness Locate the PMT by systematically examining the entire knee and tibia. The PMT often establishes a working diagnosis [A, facing page].

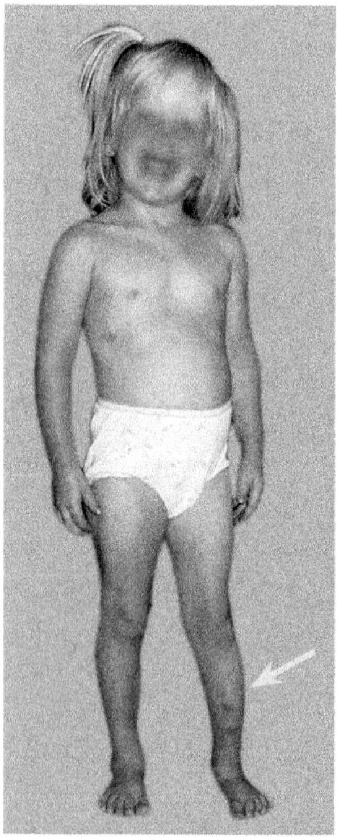

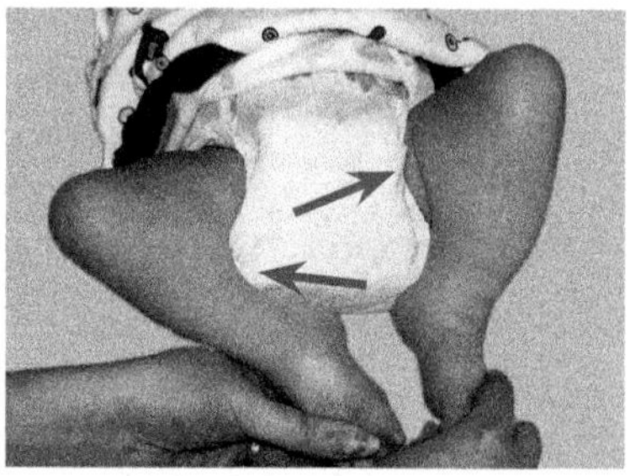

C Inspection The screening examination of this standing child shows the shortening and bowing of the left tibia (yellow arrow) and the café-au-lait spots of neurofibromatosis. Severe flexion contractures are present in the popliteal pterygium syndrome (red arrows).

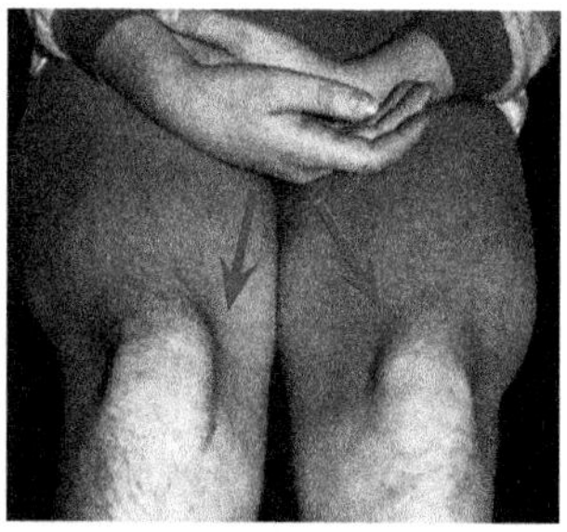

D Hypoplasia of the quadriceps Hypoplasia is a common dysplastic feature in patellofemoral disorders in children and adolescents (arrows).

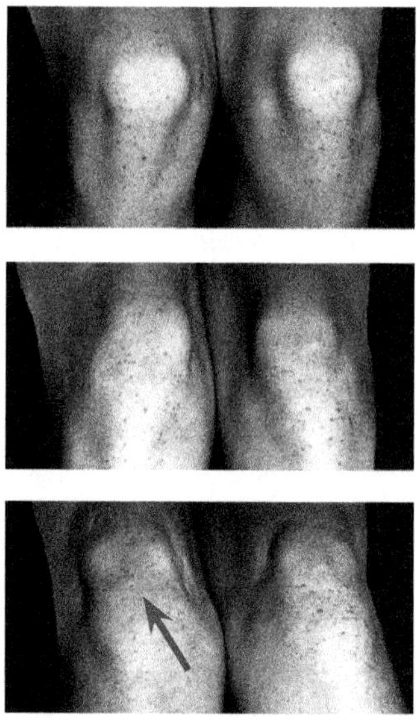

E Patellar tracking As the child slowly extends the knee, the patella normally tracks vertically. Lateral patellar displacement as the knee becomes fully extended (arrow) is described as "J" tracking.

Palpate to assess temperature, swelling, and tenderness. Is the affected knee warmer than the other knee? Is a joint effusion present [B]? Parapatellar fullness suggests a joint effusion. Evaluate any fullness by extending the knee, compressing the suprapatellar region, and checking for a fluid wave in the knee. A posttraumatic effusion is a sign of a significant intraarticular injury such as a torn peripheral meniscus, anterior cruciate ligament (ACL) injury, or osteochondral fracture. Do not confuse prepatellar swelling with an intraarticular effusion.

Manipulate to determine if the patella is displaceable. In loose-jointed children, the patella is very mobile and more likely to dislocate.

Patellar apprehension is elicited by extending the knee and attempting to displace the patella laterally [B]. Patients with recurrent dislocations who sense that this may cause the patella to dislocate may become apprehensive and may reach out to stop the examination.

Knee motion Is the arch of motion free and unguarded? Is crepitation or snapping present?

Lachman test Test anteroposterior laxity with this test. Flex the knee about 15°–20° and attempt to displace the tibia anterior in its relationship to the femur. Normally, a firm endpoint will be felt. Check for instability with varus and valgus stress [C]. With the knee flexed to a right angle, evaluate for anterior or posterior drawer signs.

Rotational instability test Test the pivot-shift for ACL injury and capsular laxity by extending the knee fully and apply valgus and internal rotation stress to demonstrate anterolateral tibial subluxation.

Perform the reverse pivot shift test by first flexing and externally rotating the knee. Next, extend the knee to demonstrate postero-lateral capsular laxity associated with PCL injury.

Imaging Studies

Special radiographic projects such as sunrise and notch views [D] may be useful. If conventional radiographs are not adequate, order special imaging studies [E].

Bone scans may be helpful in determining the location or activity of lesions. The study is sensitive but not specific.

MRI studies are overused and not appropriate for screening and are frequently overread, even in normal knees. They may be useful for ligamentous and meniscal injuries when correlated with clinical findings.

Ultrasound is useful for cysts and pre-patellar swelling evaluation.

Arthroscopy

Arthroscopy is essential for assessing meniscal injuries and for other ligamentous and osteochondral problems in children. It is less valuable for assessing pain.

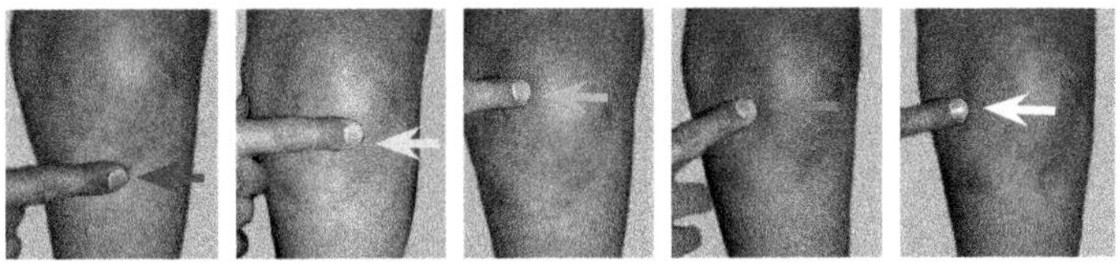

Arrow	PMT	Condition
Red	Tibial tubercle	Osgood-Schlatter disease
Yellow	Distal pole patella	Sinding-Larsen-Johansson syndrome
Green	Medial patellar margin	Patellar instability
Blue	Medial joint line	Meniscal lesion
White	Medial collateral ligament	Ligament injury

A Point of maximum tenderness Evaluate the PMT for common painful conditions about the knee.

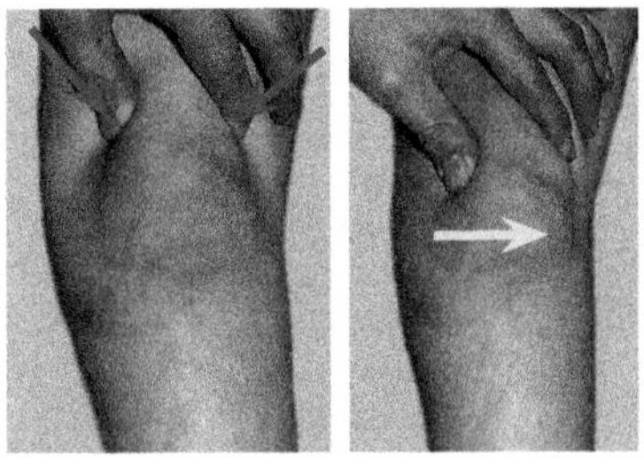

B Knee tests Compressing the suprapatellar bursa (red arrows) displaces any joint fluid into the joint to demonstrate an effusion. Displacing the patella laterally (yellow arrow) may elicit the patellar apprehension sign.

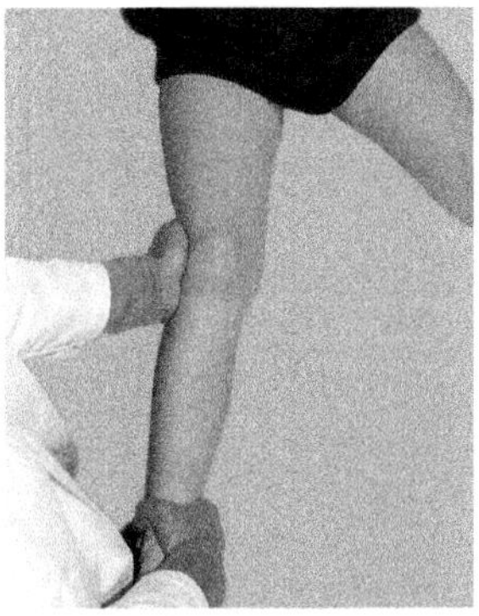

C Knee stability Test for medial lateral instability with the knee flexed to 30°. Test the opposite or normal knee to determine what is normal for the child.

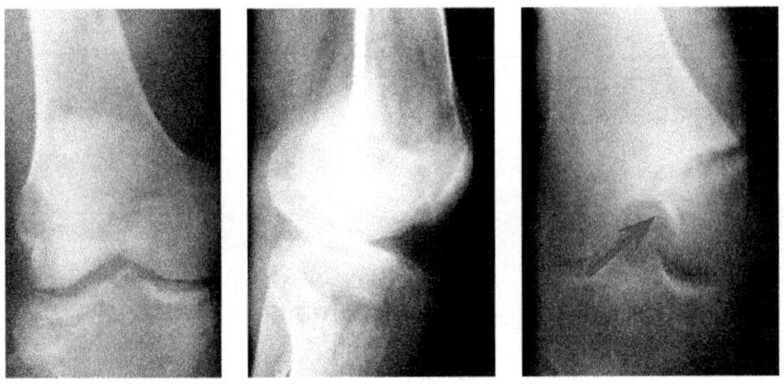

D Notch view The condylar fracture is seen only in the notch view (red arrow).

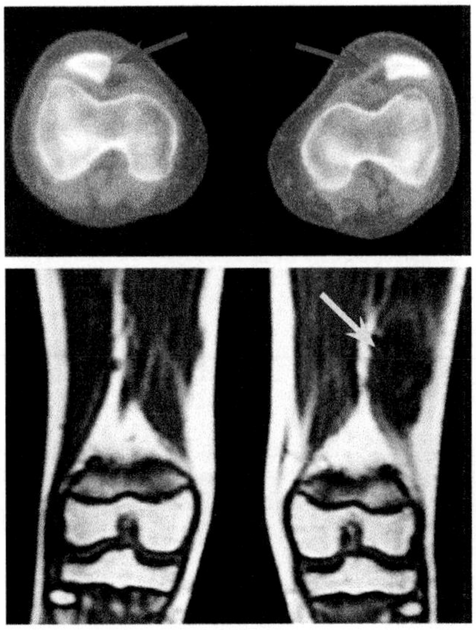

E Special imaging studies These special studies demonstrate lateral patellar positioning (red arrows), and a hemangioma by MRI (yellow arrow).

Category	Disorder
Referred	SCFE, other hip problems Spine disorders Tumors
Stress	Osgood-Schlatter disease Sinding-Larsen-Johansson syndrome Stress fractures Proximal tibia Patella Distal femur Medial collateral ligament
Bursitis	Prepatellar Pes anserina
Intraarticular	Meniscus Ligaments Osteochondritis dissecans
Tumors	Popliteal cyst Miscellaneous
Arthritis	Septic Pauciarticular Juvenile rheumatoid arthritis Rheumatoid spondylitis

A Classification of knee pain Knee pain has many causes. Some examples are listed.

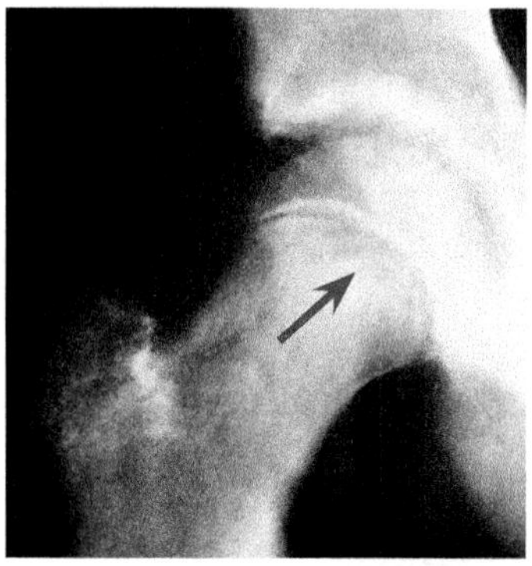

B Pitfalls in evaluating knee pain Referred pain can occur from this slipped capital femoral epiphysis. Note the subtle changes in the proximal metaphysis (arrow) consistent with a preslip.

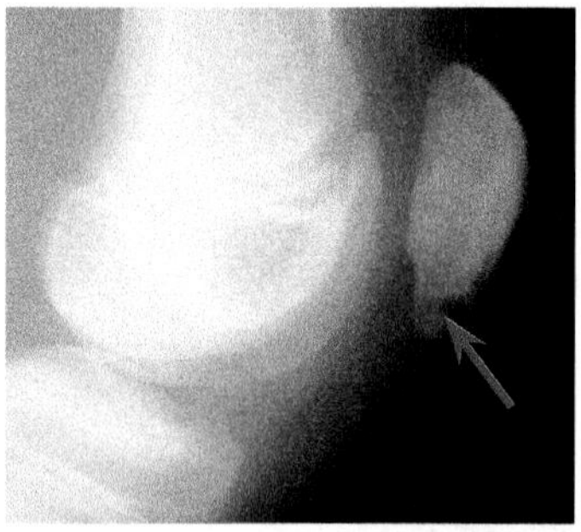

C Sinding-Larsen-Johansson syndrome Note the separate lesion of the distal pole of the patella. This should be differentiated from the uncommon type of bipartite patella involving the inferior pole of the patella.

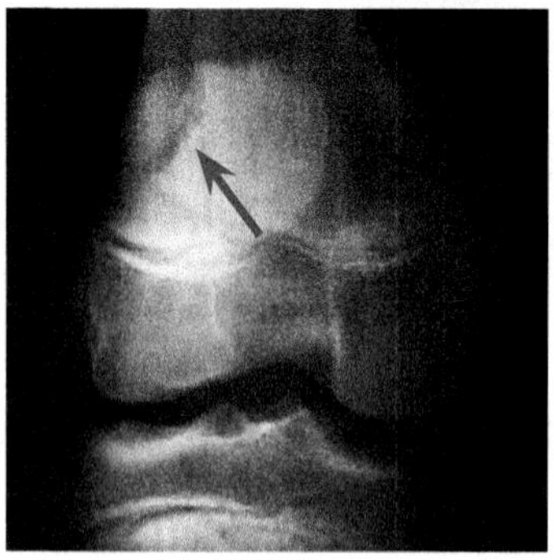

D Bipartite patella Note the separate ossicle on the superolateral aspect of the patella, consistent with a type III lesion. This lesion was painful.

Knee Pain

Knee pain is a common presenting complaint [A].

Referred Pain

First consider the possibility of referred pain from slipped capital femoral epiphysis [B], the spine, or from a tumor.

Sinding-Larsen-Johansson Disorder

Sinding-Larsen-Johansson syndrome is a traction apophysitis of the distal pole of the patella [C]. The condition is most common in males at or before puberty. Resolution occurs in 6–12 months. Rest the knee to resolve the pain and tenderness. Quadriceps flexibility exercises are commonly prescribed. No residual disability has been reported.

Pes Anserina Bursitis

Inflammation of the pes anserina bursa causes pain and tenderness over the hamstring tendon insertions on the posterior medial aspect of the upper tibial metaphysis. Evaluate for lower extremity malalignment. This uncommon condition occurs during the teen years. Manage the bursitis with rest and nonsteroidal antiinflammatory medications.

Medial Collateral Ligament Pain

Medial collateral ligament pain is an overuse condition causing pain and tenderness over the medial collateral ligament. This ligament lies on the posteromedial aspect of the knee at or above the joint line.

Bipartite Patella

Accessory centers of ossification of the patella [D] may produce a bipartite patella. These variations are classified into three types [E]. The separate ossicle is attached to the body of the patella by fibrous or cartilaginous tissue. Trauma may disrupt this attachment, and the ossicle then becomes painful. The disruption may heal with rest. In others, healing fails to occur and the ossicle remains chronically painful. Small painful ossicles may be removed. Larger ossicles should be fixed with a screw to the patella and grafted to promote union.

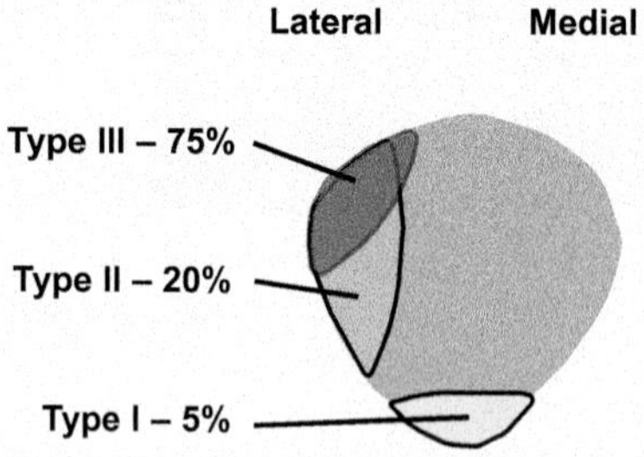

E Classification of bipartite patellae These variations occur on the lateral and inferior aspects of the patella. Note the common type III involves the superior-lateral aspect of the patella. From Saupe (1921).

Osgood-Schlatter Disease

Osgood-Schlatter disease (OSD) is a traction apophysitis of the tibial tubercle due to repetitive tensile microtrauma. It occurs between ages 10 and 15 years, with the onset in girls about 2 years before that in boys. OSD is usually unilateral and occurs in 10–20% of children participating in sports. OSD is associated with patella alta.

Cause

The condition is due to a differential growth rate between bone and soft tissues. Whether this association is a cause or the result of OSD is not known. The tibial tubercle may be enlarged on the asymptomatic side. OSD may be associated with patella alta.

Clinical Findings

Clinical findings will demonstrate swelling and localized tenderness over the tibial tubercle [A] and no other abnormalities. Order a radiograph if the condition is unilateral or atypical. Radiographs usually show soft tissue swelling and fragmentation of the anterior apophysis.

Natural History

OSD resolves with time in most children [B]. In about 10% of knees, some residual prominence of the tibial tubercle or persisting pain from an ossicle may cause problems.

Manage

Manage based on severity of discomfort. Modify activities, use NSAIDs, and use a knee pad to control discomfort. If OSD is severe or persists, apply a knee immobilizer for 7–10 days to relieve inflammation. Injection of steroids is not recommended. Quadriceps and hamstring flexibility exercises are the most useful treatment.

Managing the family To reduce apprehension, consider referring to ODS as a *disorder or condition* rather than a *disease* when discussing the problems with the patient and family. Make certain that they are aware that resolution is usually slow, often requiring 12–18 months.

Persisting disability from tenderness and tubercle prominence may be sufficient to require excision of the ossicle and prominence [C].

Complications are rare and include growth arrest with recurvatum deformity and rupture of patellar tendon or avulsion of the tibial tubercle.

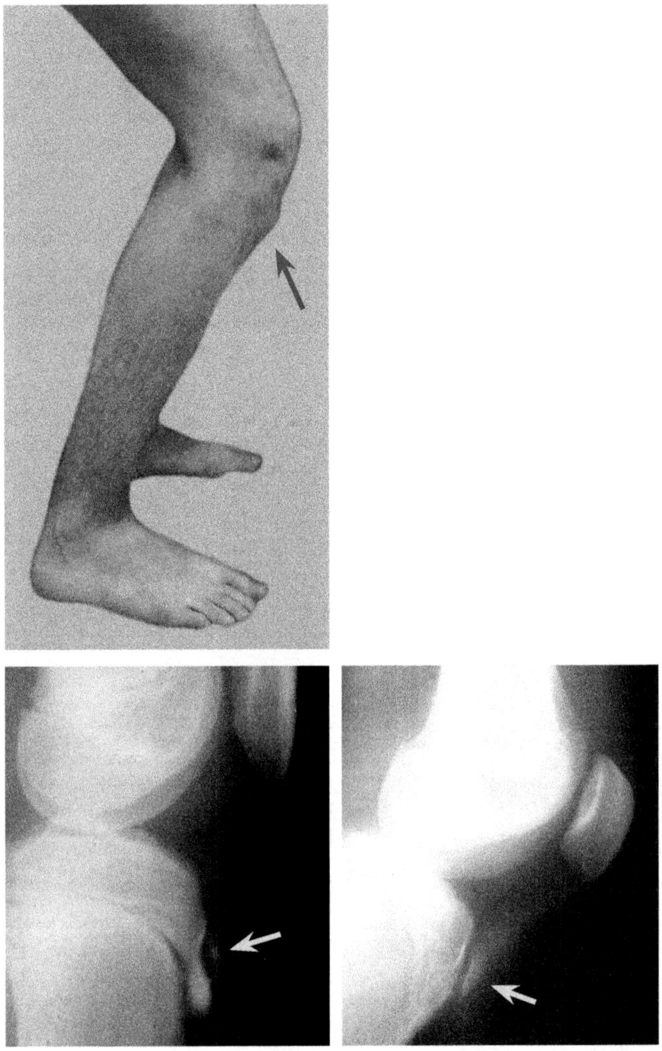

A Osgood-Schlatter disease Note the prominence and the ossification over the tibial tubercle (red arrows). Persisting tenderness over an ossicle in the mature knee (yellow arrows) is an indication for excision.

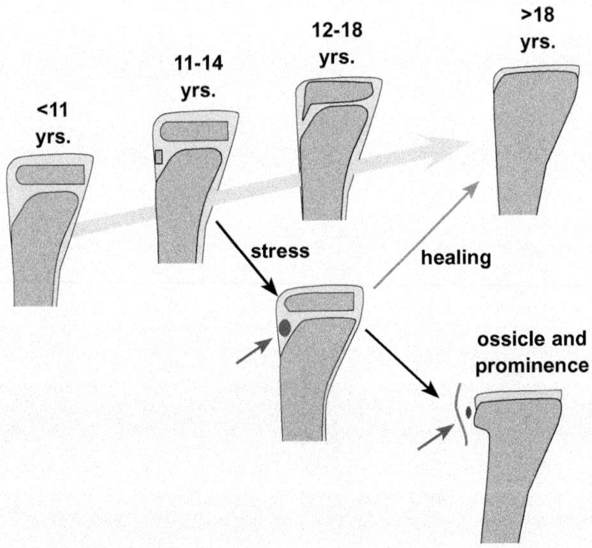

B Natural history of OSD The normal development of the apophysis is shown by the green arrow. Excessive traction (red) of the patellar tendon causes inflammation. Usually this process heals (blue arrow). In some cases, inflammation and a separate ossicle persist (red arrows). Based on Flowers and Bhadreshwar (1995).

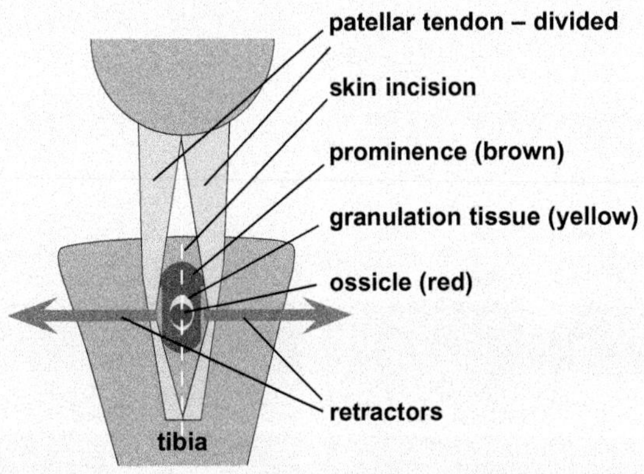

C Excision of the ossicle and prominence The procedure is performed through a midline incision to the ossicle and prominence. Sometimes inflammatory granulation tissue is present in active lesions.

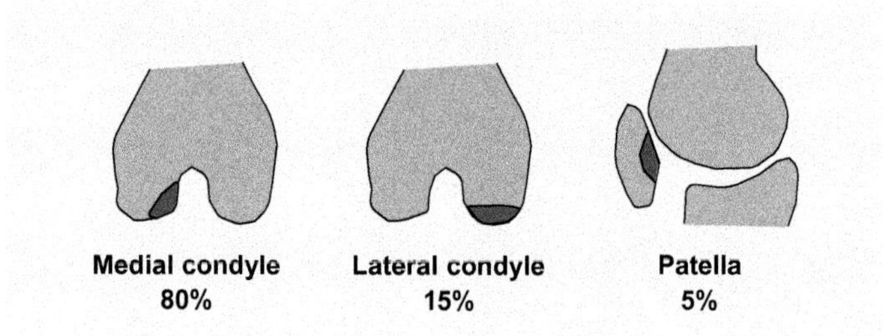

A Sites of knee involvement Most lesions occur on the posterolateral aspect of the medial femoral condyle.

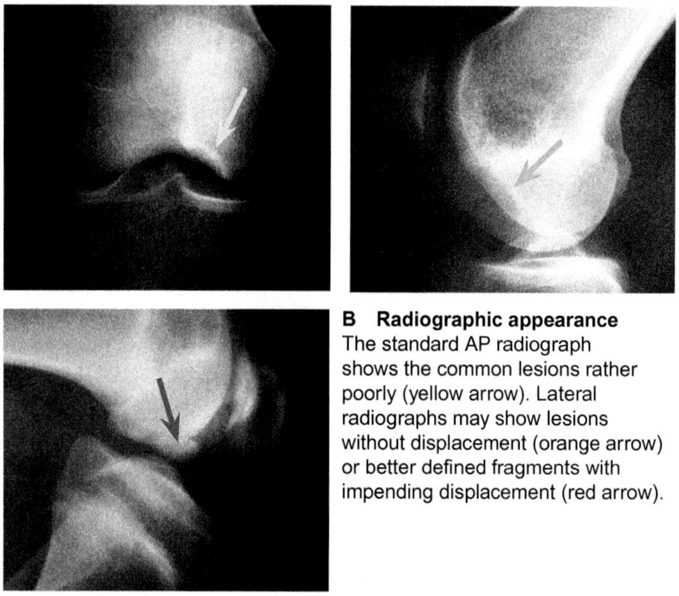

B Radiographic appearance The standard AP radiograph shows the common lesions rather poorly (yellow arrow). Lateral radiographs may show lesions without displacement (orange arrow) or better defined fragments with impending displacement (red arrow).

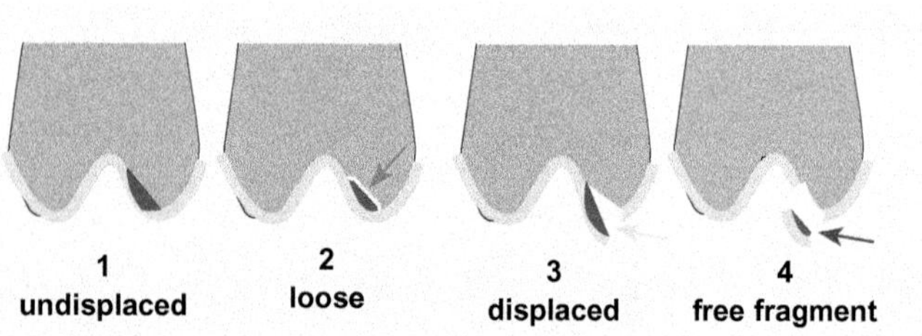

C Classification of osteochondritis dissecans The lesion (red) may be undisplaced or be loosely in place (blue arrow). Displacement may be partial (yellow arrow) or complete (red arrow), allowing the fragment to be free in the joint .

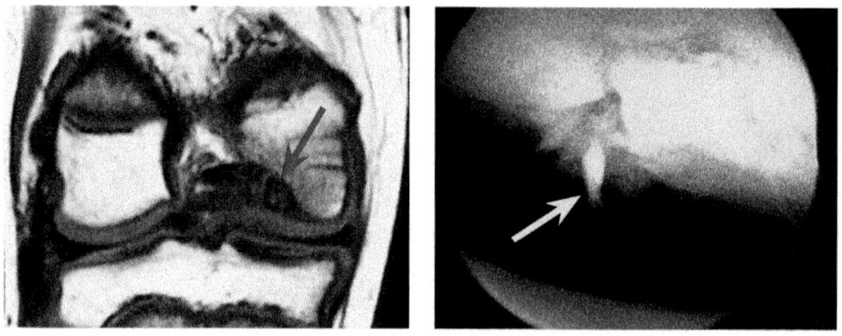

D Imaging MRI demonstrates a large defect (red arrow) with intact cartilage. Arthroscopy shows a lesion with overlying irregular cartilage (yellow arrow).

Osteochondritis Dissecans

Osteochondritis dissecans (OCD) is an idiopathic lesion of subchondral bone that may resolve spontaneously. Progressive lesions may involve the overlying articular cartilage. These lesions are most common about the knee, usually involving the lateral aspect of the medial femoral condyle [A]. Patellar lesions usually occur later than those of the condyles.

Cause

The cause is multifactorial with trauma, vascular insufficiency, and genetics being factors. OCD lesions are associated with lateral tibial torsion, genu varum and valgum, and meniscal lesions.

Clinical Findings

Juvenile OCD occurs in children 5–15 years of age, with an average age of onset between 11 and 14 years. Boys are more commonly affected. Symptoms include pain, a mild effusion, or later mechanical symptoms. Because most lesions involve the posterolateral aspect of the medial femoral condyle, they are best shown by a notch view [B]. Classify lesions based on degree of displacement [C]. Sometimes the displacement can be appreciated only on MRI or arthroscopy [D].

Irregular ossification of the lateral femoral condyle may be a normal variation of ossification and not osteochondritis dissecans. These variations are often bilateral and found incidentally when radiographs of the knee are made. They do not cause pain or effusion, and are nontender.

Natural History

Small lesions in children or early adolescence often resolve without treatment. Larger lesions, older age, and a weight-bearing location are more likely to displace and cause joint damage and eventual osteoarthritis. Aggressive treatment of these lesions is appropriate.

Management

Management depends upon the site, size, patient's age, and classification of the lesion.

Type 1 and 2 lesions Manage with activity modification, isometric exercises, and a knee immobilizer. Manage based on symptoms rather than on radiographic appearance. Radiographic healing takes many months.

Type 3 lesions Manage by drilling and stabilizing with K wires [E] or absorbable pins.

Type 4 lesions Manage small lesions by excision. Replace large lesions or those involving the weight-bearing areas and fix internally if adequate subchondral bone exists on the fragment.

Prognosis

Up to 90% of small lesions in juvenile OCD may heal spontaneously. Lesions with an onset later, especially large lesions in weight-bearing regions of the knee, require aggressive treatment. Management is not always successful, and osteoarthritis may occur in adult life.

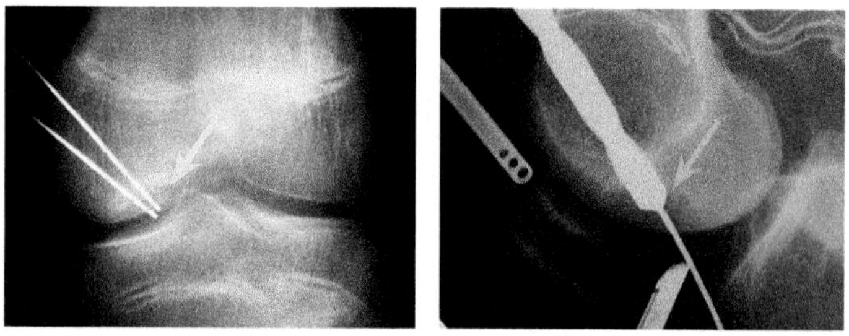

E Operative treatment The lesion may be drilled and fixed with K wires (yellow arrow). A large drill may be required for larger lesions (orange arrow).

Anterior Knee Pain

Anterior knee pain is common during the second decade and may occur in up to a third of adolescents. This pain may be associated with some underlying patellofemoral malalignment or may be idiopathic, occurring in normal individuals.

Structural Anterior Knee Pain

Pain associated with some knee dysplasia is more serious and often requires operative correction.

Evaluation Identify the underlying dysplastic features, such as lateral tibial torsion, genu valgum, patella alta, quadriceps hypoplasia, lateral tether, shallow sulcus, or excessive joint laxity. Consider imaging the patellofemoral joint with a CT scan to rule out patellar malpositioning [A].

Management Manage first with NSAIDS and isometric exercises. During the first visit, introduce the possible need for a realignment procedure [B]. Identify and, if possible, quantitate the severity of each dysplastic feature. Correct obvious manageable deformities early. In other cases, the decision is difficult. For example, bilateral double-level osteotomies are necessary to correct severe rotational malalignment. Thoughtfully place the operative incision [C].

Idiopathic Anterior Knee Pain

This pain is common among teenagers, especially girls, and is often associated with a period of rapid growth. The pain is often activity related, is poorly localized, and may cause disability. It has been described as the *headache of the knee*. About one-third of these patients have features of the MMPI found in individuals with nonorganic back pain. Its natural history is one of spontaneous improvement over a period of years.

Diagnosis This pain involves a history of discomfort after sitting; pain with exercise, walking down stairs, or with sitting and squatting; a crunching sound with walking up stairs; and/or a sense of giving way with jumping or running. Often it is most prominent in the morning or after sitting and improves with time and warm up. When asked to localize the pain, the patient will often grab the entire front of the knee (grab sign).

Cause The causes are numerous and often associated with muscle imbalance. Aggravating factors may be poor training and shoeware.

Management Prescribe NSAIDS, isometric exercises, activity modification, and reassurance. Sometimes applying ice reduces discomfort. Sometimes a knee sleeve with a patellar cutout seems to help. Avoid arthroscopy and lateral release procedures.

Rehabilitation After the acute phase has passed, the patient should establish flexibility and strength before gradually resuming full activity. Stretching should be painfree.

Prevention Suggest warm up and stretching before activity, and avoiding activities that cause pain. This may require modification of activities by substituting others that are less stressful for the knee.

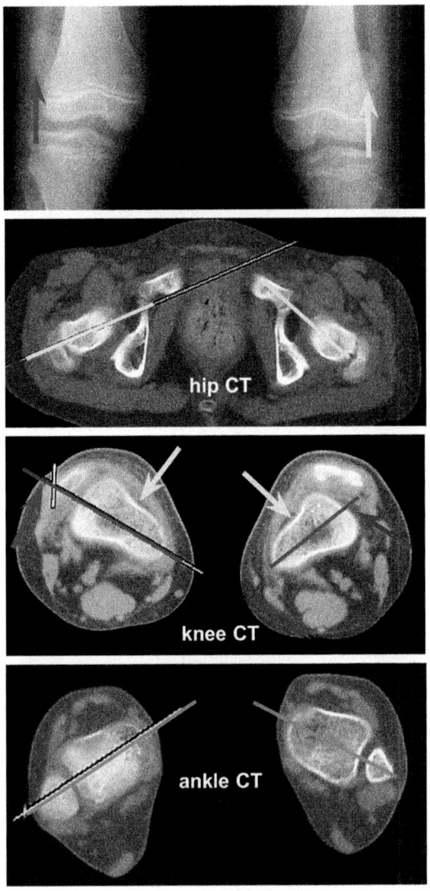

A Severe rotational malalignment syndrome This child had habitual dislocations at age 5 years. Realignment was performed on the worse left side. She was not seen again until age 10 years. At that time, shown here, she was asymptomatic. Her left patella was subluxated and right patella dislocated. The child has severe rotational malalignment, as demonstrated by CT scans. Note that the bicondylar axis is medially rotated 30° (yellow lines). This results in 60° of anteversion (red lines) and about 75° of lateral tibial torsion (blue lines). Note the displaced patella (red arrows) and the shallow condylar grooves (yellow arrows). It was elected not to attempt operative repair because rotational osteotomies of both femora and tibiae and realignment would be necessary. The chance of success was considered too poor to justify the magnitude of the procedures. This case demonstrates the complex pathology of some types of congenital development patellofemoral disorders.

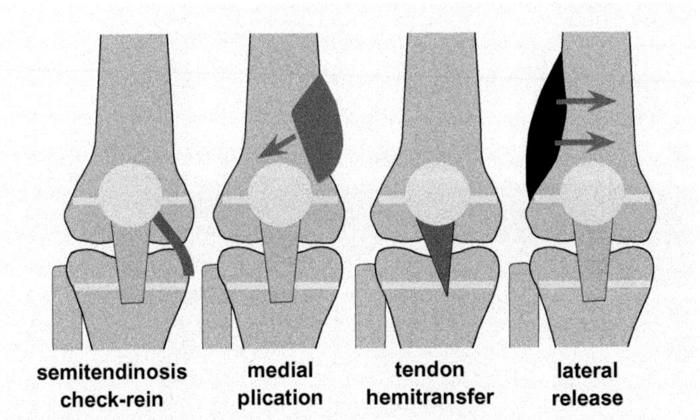

B Components of operative repair These components are usually combined to correct all dysplastic features. The lateral release alone is usually inadequate.

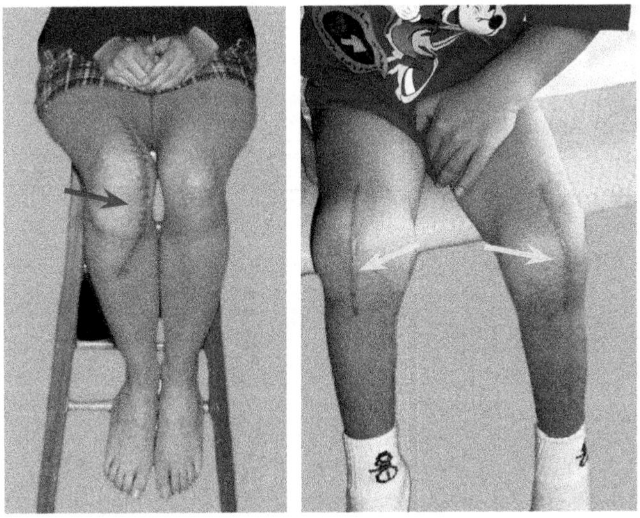

C Operative knee scars Knee scars cause considerable disability (red arrow). A midline vertical incision is optimal for extensive realignment procedures (yellow arrows).

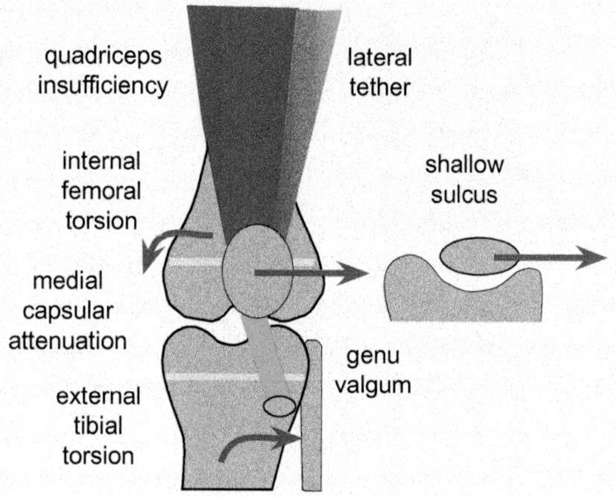

Condition	Effect
Femoral and tibial torsion	Increases Q angle Overall limb management
Genu valgum	Increases Q angle
Condylar hypoplasia	Promotes lateral subluxation or dislocation
Patella alta	Results in less lateral stability
Quad insufficiency	Produces imbalance in quadriceps
Med. cap. attenuation	Inadequate medial check-rein
VL contracture	Tethers patella laterally

A Factors contributing to patellofemoral instability These factors combine to increase the risk of patellar subluxation or dislocation.

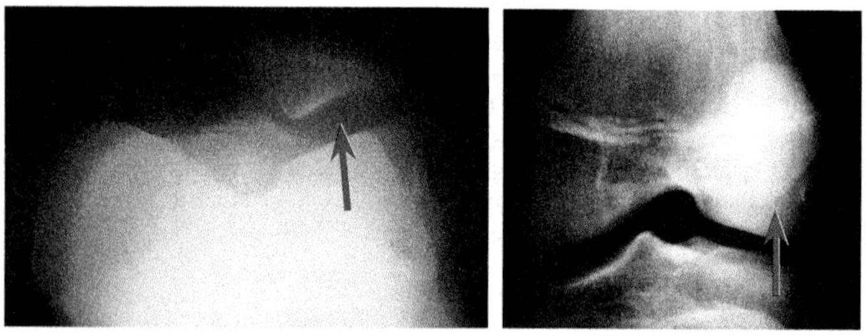

B Patellar hypoplasia This deformity was part of the nail–patella syndrome.

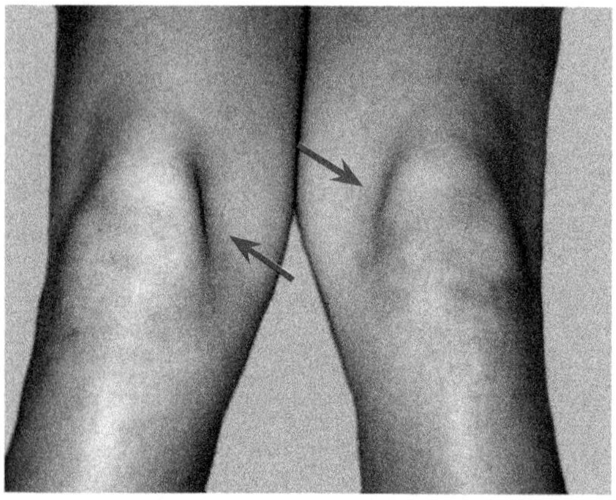

C Quadriceps hypoplasia Note the loss of delineation of the VMO. The hypoplasia and weakness contribute to patellar instability.

Patellofemoral Disorders

Many factors may contribute to patellofemoral instability [A].

Systemic Disorders

Patellofemoral instability is more common in children with (1) knee dysplasias, such as occurs in nail–patella syndrome [B], Rubinstein–Taybi syndrome, and Turner syndrome and (2) conditions with increased joint laxity such as Down syndrome. These underlying conditions complicate management.

Congenital Dislocation

Congenital patellar dislocation is a rare condition that causes a progressive flexion, valgus, and tibial external rotational deformities of the knee. Reduce the dislocation and realign the quadriceps mechanism late in the first year. An extensive lateral release is often required.

Patellar Subluxation or Dislocation in Childhood

So-called *habitual* subluxation or dislocation is usually due to a dysplastic knee with contracture of the lateral portion of the quadriceps mechanism. This causes the patella to displace laterally whenever the knee is flexed. Early operative realignment is appropriate, but because the dysplastic features are severe, recurrence is common.

Traumatic Patellar Subluxation or Dislocation

Traumatic patellar dislocations cause an articular fracture. If the injury is severe, producing a tense hemarthrosis, arthroscopic evaluation may be appropriate.

Adolescent Recurrent Dislocation

Most recurrent dislocations occur in individuals with dysplastic knees. They may show generalized joint laxity, lateral tibial torsion, genu valgum, hypoplasia of the quadriceps [C], attenuation of the medial joint capsule, limited medial mobility of the patella, and abnormal patellar tracking. Observe the tracking of the patella as the patient slowly extends the knee. Lateral displacement of the patella as the knee nears full extension is described as *J tracking*. J tracking is a common finding. Sometimes the patella becomes subluxated with a sudden lateral shift. The patellar apprehension sign may also be positive. The patient becomes fearful that the patella will dislocate when the examiner applies lateral pressure to it. Radiographs may show lateral displacement of the patella [D].

Management Manage first by ordering quadriceps and hamstring flexibility and strengthening exercises. If the instability persists, operative correction is often necessary. Identify and correct each dysplastic component. In the growing child, often a lateral release, a medial plication, and a transfer of the semitendinosis to the patella are required. After growth is completed, reposition the tibial tubercle more medial and anterior to align and to optimize quadriceps alignment.

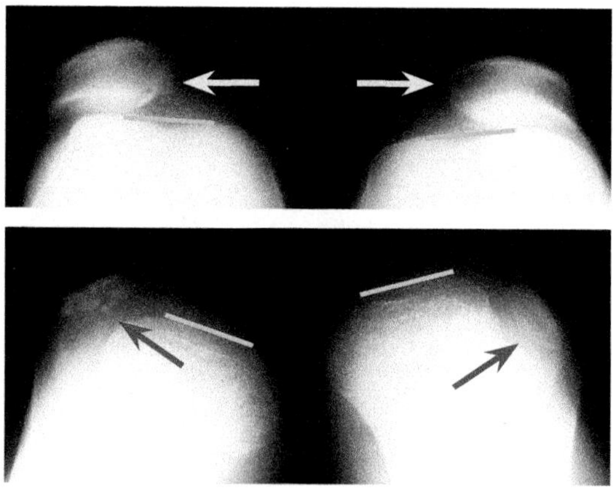

D Sunrise views These projections show subluxation (yellow arrows) and dislocations (red arrows) of the patella. Note the position of the anterior femoral articular surface (green lines).

Patellar Realignment

Perform patellar realignment to restore or improve the mechanical alignment of the quadriceps mechanism. Patellar realignment in childhood is complicated by the wide range of pathological elements. Lateral contracture, rotational and angular malalignment, condylar and patellar hypoplasia, muscle hypoplasia, and imbalance may be present either alone or in various combinations. Often realignment requires a combination of procedures [A], which is best accomplished through a direct anterior longitudinal incision. This allows intraoperative visualization of the pathology and tailoring of the repair to best correct the problems. Make certain at the end of the procedure that with passive flexion and extension of the knee the patella tracks vertically in the midline. Except for transfer of the tibial tubercle, these procedures may be performed in the growing child without the risk of growth arrest.

Lateral Release

Lateral contractures [B] are often present in congenital patellar dislocations or those that occur in infancy. In rare cases, very extensive, more proximal release is necessary. In others, a more limited release is adequate [C]. Be aware that lateral release is seldom indicated for most patellar instability cases. Excessive release may cause medial patellar dislocation from the loss of the normal lateral tether.

Medial Plication

Medial plication is necessary because of the attenuation of the medial capsule and the meniscofemoral ligament on the undersurface of the vastus medialis oblique (VMO) muscle that follows acute patellar dislocation [D]. This may be corrected by first reefing the medical capsule and then advancing the VMO over the quadriceps [E]. Avoid overcorrection, a common complication.

Hamstring Tenodesis

Tenodesis of the semitendinosis tendon into the patella creates a checkrein that is very effective in realignment [F and G]. Often this tenodesis is combined with a lateral release and medial capsular reconstruction.

Tibial Tubercle Transfer

This procedure is most commonly needed for the adolescent with malalignment that can be corrected by a distal procedure [H]. Perform the tibial tubercle rotational transfer through a longitudinal incision to allow correction of associated problems [I].

Patellar Tendon Hemitransfer

Patellar tendon hemitransfers are no longer done, as the procedure causes secondary problems due to a patellar tilt caused by the operation.

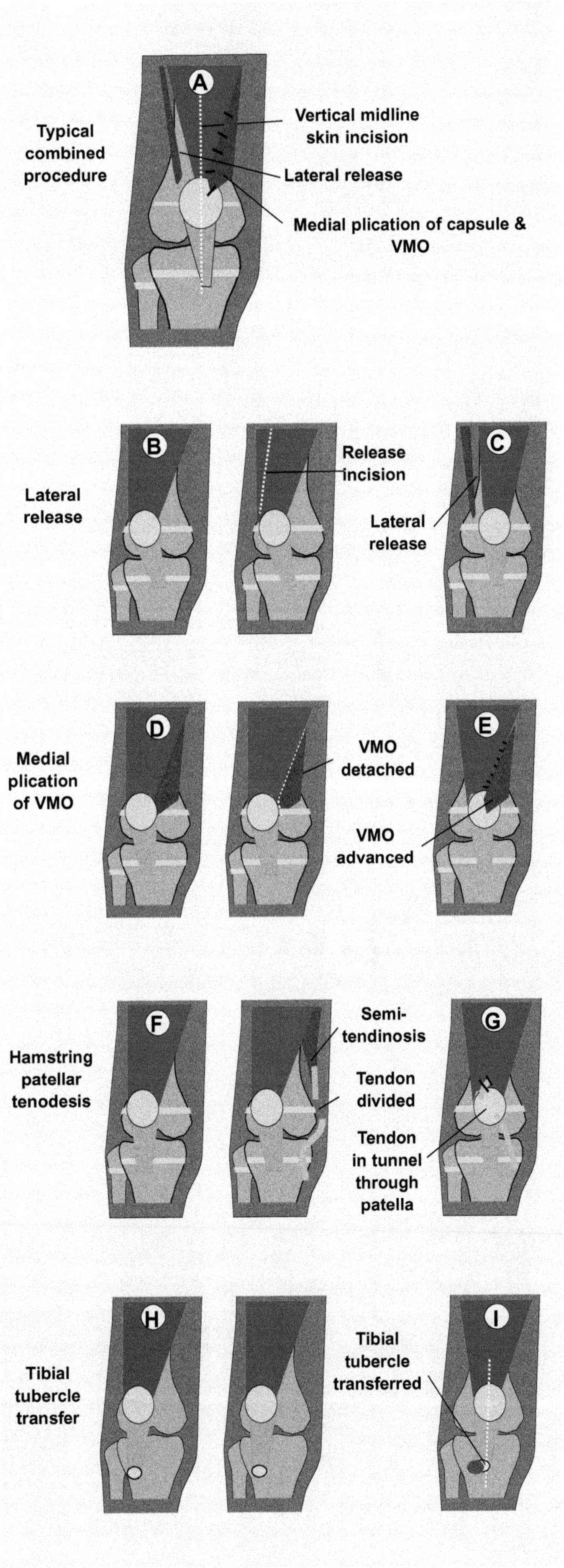

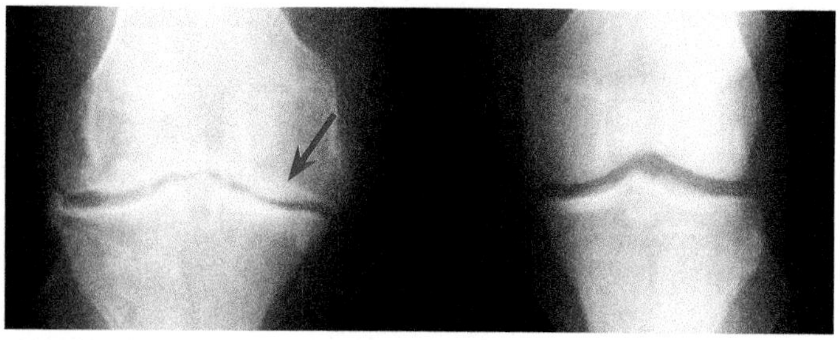

A Long-term effect of meniscectomy At age 13 years, this 29-year-old man had a total meniscectomy of the right knee. Note the degenerative changes compared to the unoperated knee.

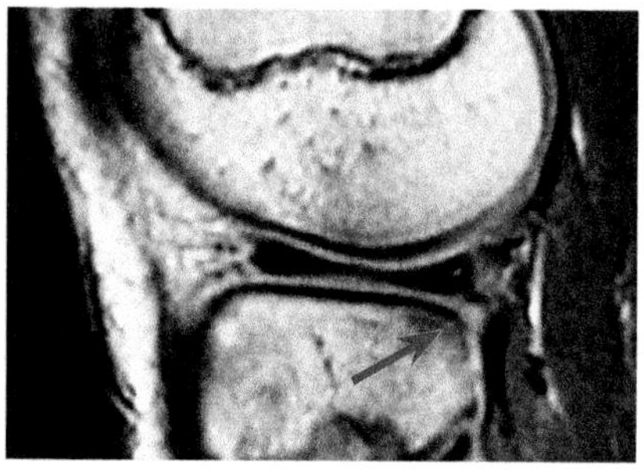

B Meniscal tear Note the meniscal tear on this MRI (arrow).

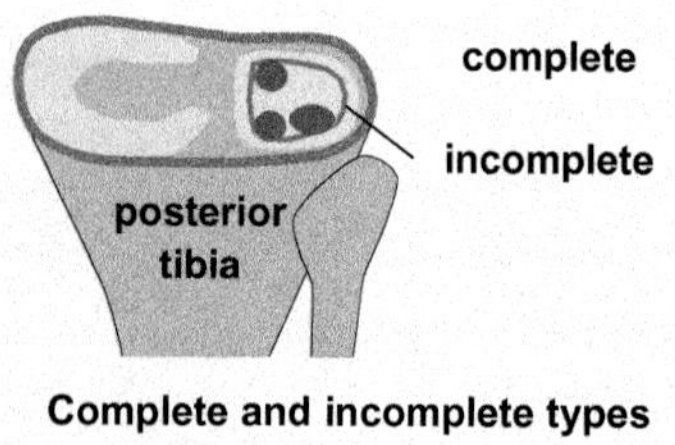

C Complete and incomplete types of discoid meniscus These menisci are fixed to the tibia both in front and back of the knee (brown spots). The most vulnerable site for injury is posterior (red spot). Based on Dickhaut and DeLee (1982).

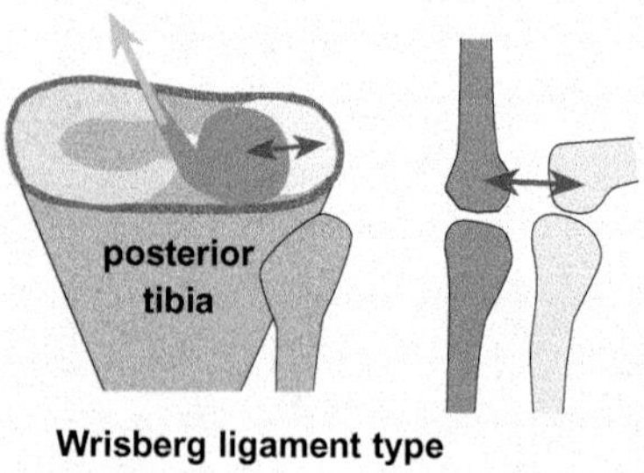

D Wrisberg ligament type of discoid meniscus The ligament is attached to the Wrisberg ligament (green arrow). This ligament (meniscofemoral ligament) attaches to the femur. With knee flexion and extension, the meniscus moves (red arrow) because it has no fixation to the tibia.

Intraarticular Disorders

Meniscal and ligamentous lesions are relatively rare in children but become more common during adolescence. The long-term consequences of early management can be profound [A].

Tears of Medial Meniscus

These lesions become more common during the teen years. Tears are usually peripheral and longitudinal—like in young adults [B]. Preserve the meniscus by repairing reducible outer third lesions. Perform a partial meniscectomy for inner third or comminuted lesions. Avoid total meniscectomy to preserve the stress shielding function of the meniscus.

Discoid Meniscus

Three types of discoid meniscus occur.

Complete and incomplete types are thicker than normal and cover all or part of the tibial surface [C].

Wrisberg ligament type is attached to the meniscofemoral ligament posteriorly [D]. This meniscus has no other fixation and is mobile. It is most likely to cause snapping and symptoms in the younger child. Because of its mobility, it may be caught between the femoral condyles and become torn or eroded.

Diagnosis Symptoms include pain, snapping or locking, loss of knee extension, and giving way. Tenderness and fullness may be present over the lateral joint line, and crepitation may be present with motion. In the young child, snapping may be the only complaint. Radiographs uncommonly show widening of the joint space [E]. MRI studies are usually diagnostic for complete or incomplete types but not useful for the Wrisberg ligament type. Arthroscopic confirmation should be delayed until operative treatment is considered necessary.

Management depends on the type, symptoms, and activity level of the child. Be conservative. Attempt to preserve the meniscus whenever possible. Total meniscectomy is the last resort. Long-term outcomes are poor due to premature osteoarthritis. Meniscoplasty is indicated for the meniscus with posterior attachments. Save as much meniscal periphery as possible.

Cruciate Ligament Deficiencies

Cruciate ligament insufficiency is seen in a variety of conditions in children.

Congenital deficiencies are common in fibular hemimelia and proximal focal femoral deficiencies. These deficiencies complicate limb lengthening procedures because of sagittal and rotational instability. Isolated absence of both anterior and posterior cruciate ligaments have been reported.

Acquired deficiencies occur from traumatic rupture of the ligament [F], attenuation associated with tibial spine fractures, and sometimes in association with diaphyseal femoral shaft fractures without known knee injury.

Management ACL tears are repaired in traumatic ruptures that cause disability, especially when associated with meniscal injuries.

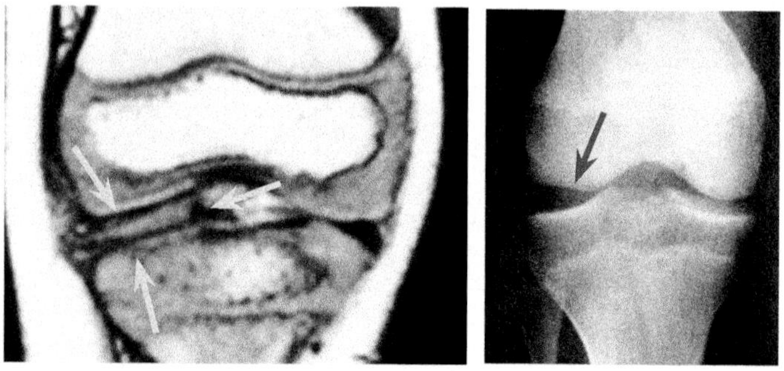

E Discoid lateral meniscus Note the widening of the lateral joint space (red arrow) and the bow-tie-shaped discoid meniscus on MRI (yellow arrows).

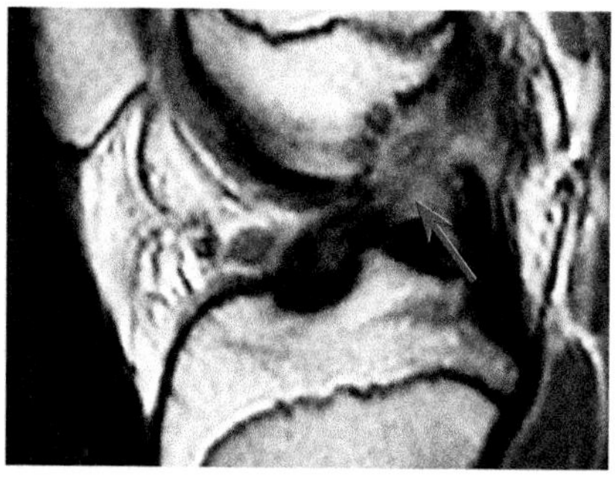

F Traumatic ACL tear in adolescent This 15-year-old boy has a tear in his ACL, as shown on the MRI.

Tumors of the Knee

Popliteal Cysts

These cysts are different in children than in adults. The cysts seldom communicate with the joint and are not related to intraarticular defects. The natural history is of spontaneous resolution.

Diagnosis is usually not difficult [A]. Most cysts are found by the parents through observation. The cysts are usually nontender, smooth, cystic to the touch, and located between the medial head of the gastrocnemius and the semitendinosis. Translumination demonstrates that the mass is a cyst. Ultrasound shows the lesion well, so that MRI is expensive and seldom necessary.

Management Reassure the family that the condition is benign and will resolve with time. If the family is still nervous, consider confirming the diagnosis by aspirating the cyst. Advise the family that the aspiration is only to confirm the diagnosis and not for treatment because the cyst will recur. Aspiration reassures the family that it is not cancer. Cysts resolve spontaneously over a period of several years. Resection is rarely indicated and is appropriate only for large painful cysts. Recurrence following resection is common.

Meniscal Cysts

Meniscal cysts are uncommon lesions that usually occur over the lateral aspect of the knee and may be associated with a meniscal tear. Image with ultrasound or by MRI [B]. Manage cyst decompression, debridement, and partial meniscectomy or repair, depending on the associated meniscal tear pattern.

Other Tumors

Hemangiomata These lesions infiltrate and thicken the synovium, making it subject to injury and bleeding [C]. The diagnosis can be made by aspirating blood from the joint and confirming by biopsy done concurrently with a synovectomy. Warn the family that recurrence during growth is likely.

Lipoma These tumors are subcutaneous, soft, and often poorly defined [D]. They may require removal if large.

Pigmental villonodular synovitis This knee joint tumor [D] is rare in children. It requires open or arthroscopic synovectomy.

Synovial chondromatosis This tumor is uncommon about the knee in children. It requires complete arthroscopic or open synovectomy.

Synovial sarcoma Most commonly occurs in the adolescent and may be confused with popliteal cyst. Typically, the tumor is deeply seated, painful, and tender, and the diagnosis is often delayed.

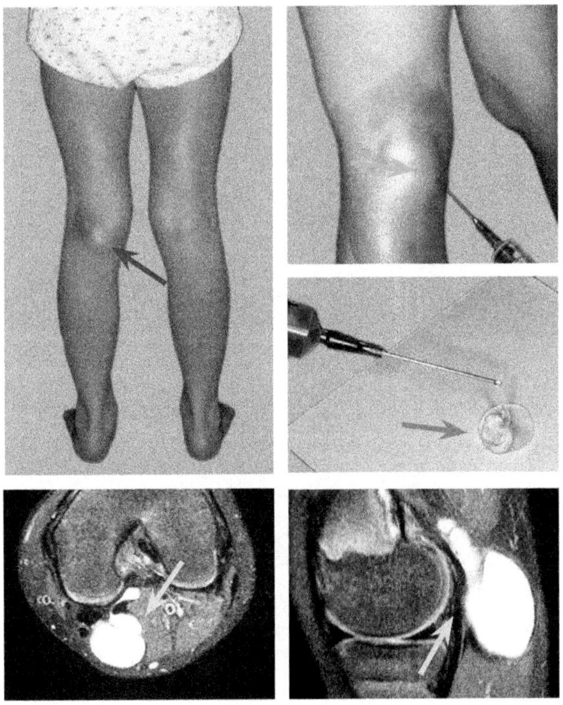

A Popliteal cyst Note the classic location (red arrow). Aspiration treatment (green arrow) removes viscous fluid (blue arrow) from within the cyst. In another case, note the MRI appearance (yellow arrows).

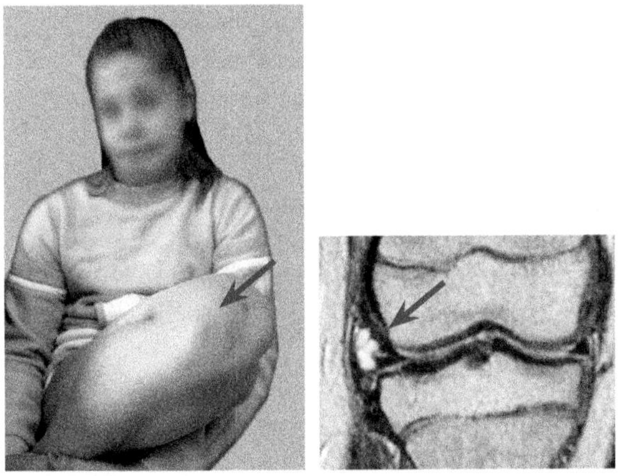

B Lateral meniscal cyst. Note cyst on physical examination and also on MRI.

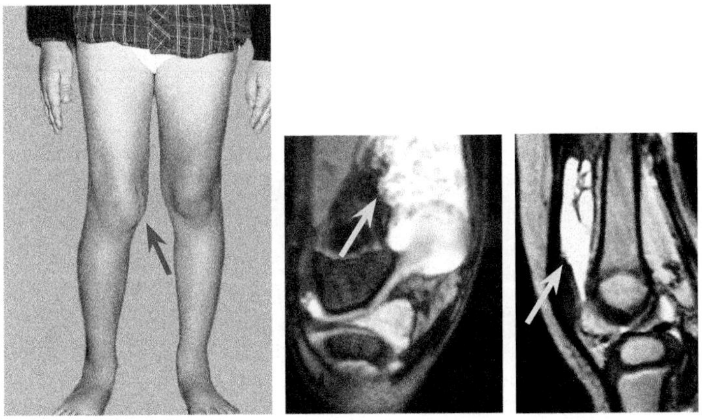

C Hemangiomata Intraarticular lesions may form within the joint and produce synovial swelling (red arrow). MRI imaging of other lesions show involvement in the adjacent soft tissues (yellow arrows).

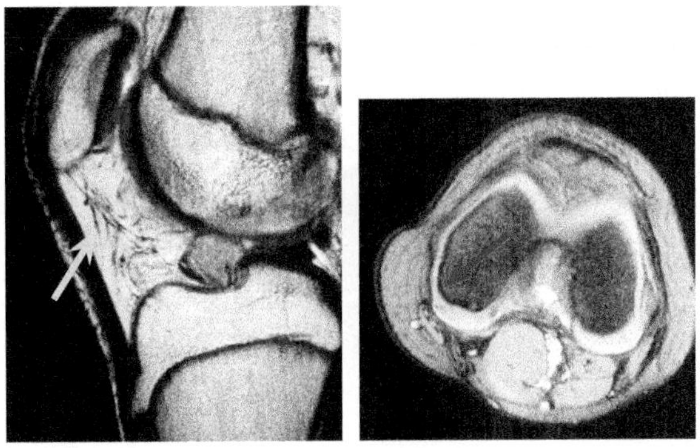

D MRI knee tumors Pigmental villonodular synovitis (yellow arrow) within the joint and the lipoma (red arrow) in typical subcutaneous location.

Knee Flexion and Extension Deformities

Knee flexion and extension deformities are common and disabling. They have many causes, including congenital contractures, deformities from neuromuscular disorders, trauma, and infection.

Congenital Hyperextension

This deformity is often associated with other conditions [A], such as arthrogryposis, spina bifida, developmental hip dysplasia, and clubfeet. In many cases, the child was born breech.

Pathology The pathology depends upon severity. In dislocated knees, fibrosis of the quadriceps muscle, absence of the suprapatellar pouch, and valgus deformity of the knee are often present.

Evaluation Look for other abnormalities. Make a radiograph of the pelvis to make certain the hips are not dysplastic or dislocated. Ultrasound or MRI imaging may be necessary to assess the knee. Grade the severity of the deformity [B].

Management Manage by gentle stretching and casting [C] or by using the Pavlik harness if the knee can be flexed to 60°. For knee dislocations, perform a quadriceps lengthening at about 1–3 months of age [D]. Immobilize in 45° of flexion to avoid skin problems. Apply serial casts to achieve about 90° of flexion. Maintain this correction for one month. Consider correction of other deformities, such as hip dislocations and clubfeet, concurrently.

If treatment is delayed [E], management is more difficult. Limited quadriceps lengthening may move the arc of motion into a more functional plane. In older children or adolescents, bony deformity may require flexion osteotomy to improve alignment.

Prognosis The outcome is primarily determined by severity [F]. The prognosis is generally better for unilateral cases and those not associated with some underlying syndrome.

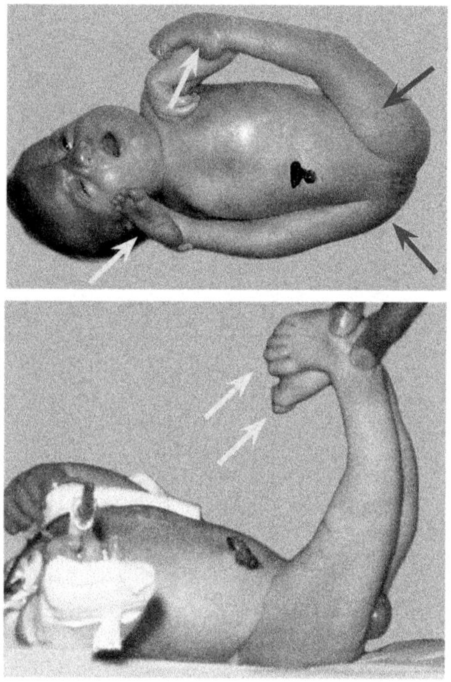

A Typical hyperextension deformity in the newborn This deformity is common in breech presentations and is often associated with other deformities such as dislocated hips (red arrows) and clubfeet (yellow arrows).

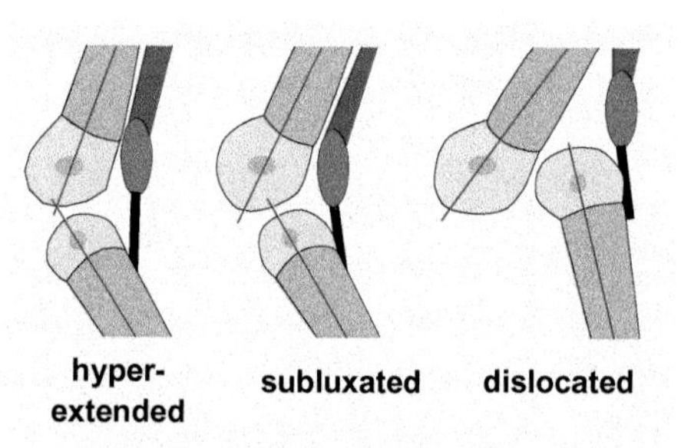

B Classification of extension deformities These deformities can be classified by severity. Based on Curtis and Fisher (1969).

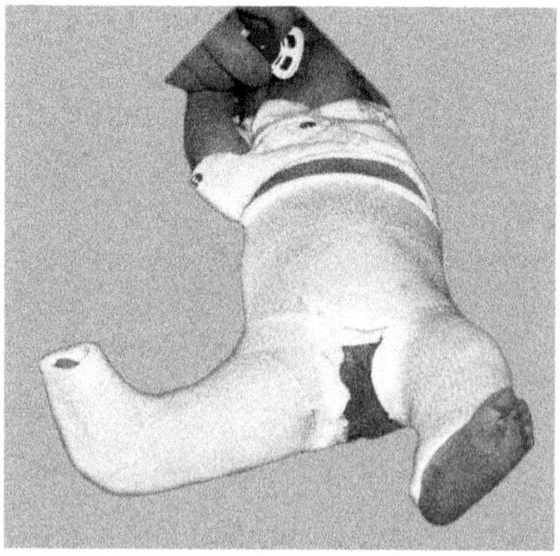

C Nonoperative management Serial cast correction is usually effective in hyperextended or subluxated hips.

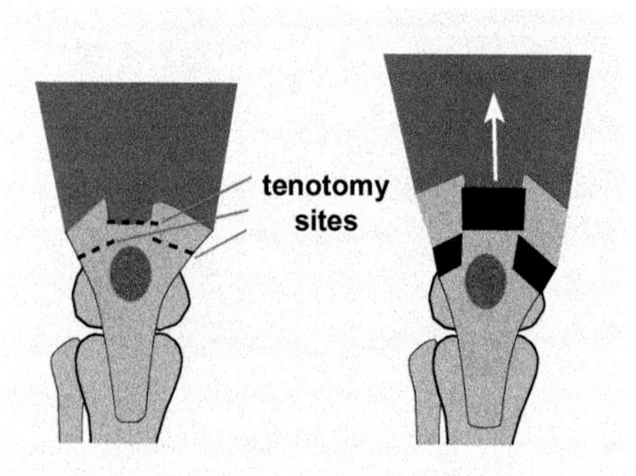

D Percutaneous quadriceps recession This procedure is performed in early infancy through a percutaneous approach with three incisions in the quadriceps mechanism. The infant is immobilized in a spica cast for 4–6 weeks. From Roy and Crawford (1989).

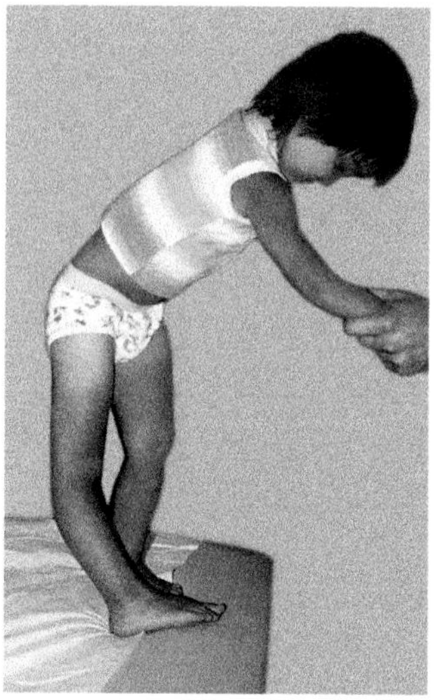

E Recurvatum during childhood This deformity has been present since birth. It causes the child considerable disability.

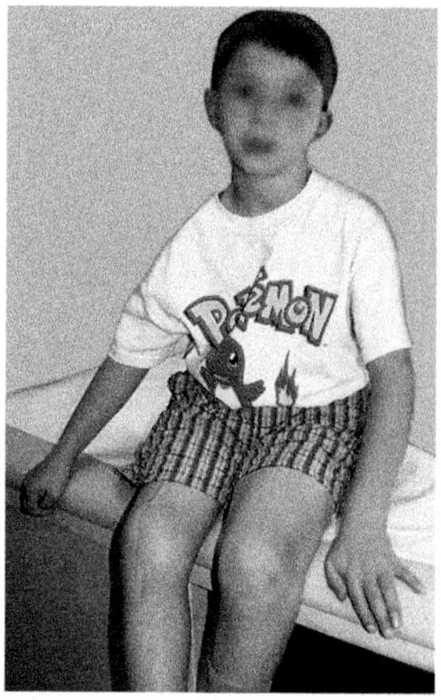

F Quadriceps lengthening This child had an open quadriceps lengthening of the right knee through a vertical midline approach.

Acquired Recurvatum Deformity

Bony deformity of the upper tibia usually results from trauma to the anterior proximal tibial physis [A]. This portion of the physis is vulnerable to arrest. Recurvatum has been reported following traction, spica cast immobilization, proximal tibial traction pin placement, femoral shaft fractures, and meningococcal infections.

Evaluation Make radiographs of the upper tibia with a true lateral study to assess articular inclination. Note that the tibia is usually inclined posteriorly by about 9°. Assess the status of the growth plate with MRI or CT scans.

Management Consider resection of physeal bars of the anterior tibia if two years of growth remain. At the end of growth, correct the deformity with a opening wedge osteotomy just proximal to the insertion of the patellar tendon [B].

Flexion Deformity

Congenital and acquired flexion contracture deformities are common in children with neuromuscular problems. Acquired deformities result from imbalance between the quadriceps and hamstrings. Flexion deformity is common in arthrogryposis [C], cerebral palsy [D], and myelodysplasia.

Correct deformities early by soft tissue procedures. Attempt to prevent recurrence by night splinting in extension. If recurrence occurs, regain correction by serial casting. If unsuccessful, try to delay correction until the end of growth, if possible. Then perform correction by a bony procedure.

Avoid correction by osteotomy during growth, as bone remodeling will result in the deformity recurring. Delay bony correction until the end of growth to provide a correction that is most likely to be permanent.

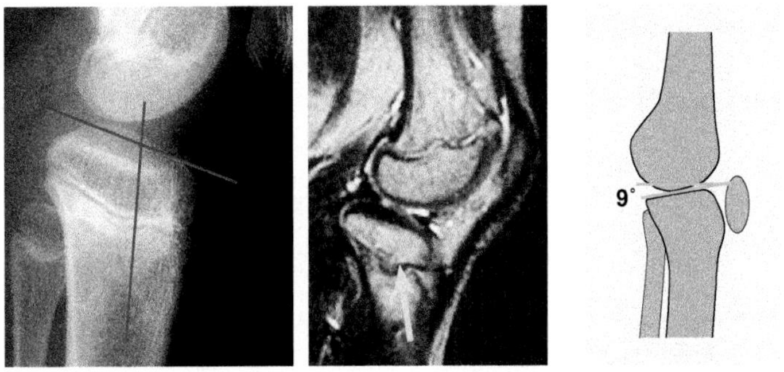

A Recurvatum from physeal injury Note the anterior inclination of the proximal tibia (red lines) and irregular physis on the MRI (yellow arrow). Normally, the tibial articular surface inclines posteriorly by about 9° (green lines).

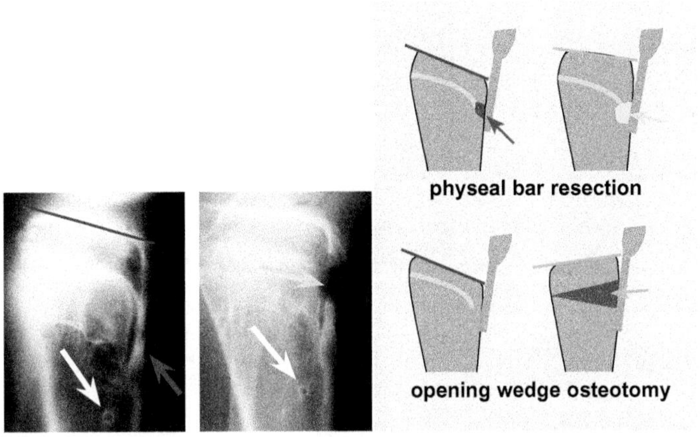

B Correction of physeal bar This child was treated with a proximal tibial pin (white arrows) causing a physeal bar (red arrow) and a secondary recurvatum deformity (red lines). This bar was resected and the defect filled with fat (yellow arrows). The established deformity at the end of growth can be corrected by an opening wedge osteotomy (green arrow) just proximal to the tibial tubercle.

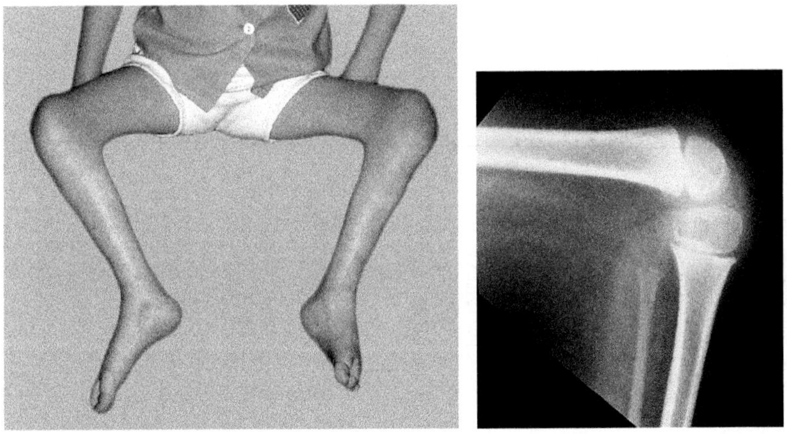

C Knee flexion in arthrogryposis This child was unable to walk because of the knee flexion contracture. Following correction by soft tissue releases and femoral shortening, the child became ambulatory.

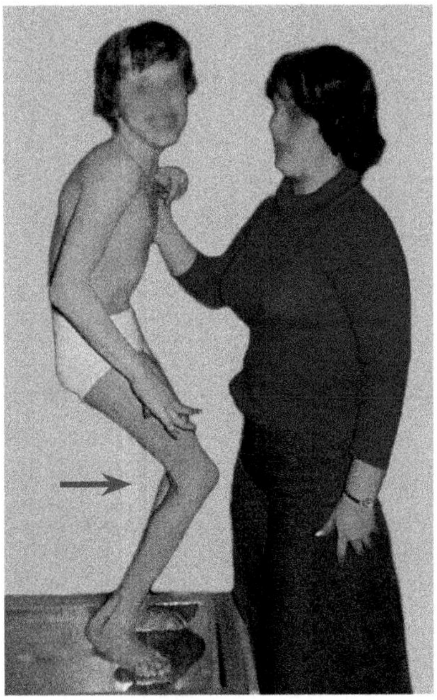

D Flexion deformity in cerebral palsy This is part of the crouch gait (red arrow).

Direction	Comment	Natural history
Lateral	Physiological in infancy	Resolves
Anterior	With other deformities	Persists
Posteromedial	Classic pattern	Resolves incompletely
Anterolateral	Pre-pseudarthrosis	Progressive deformity

A Patterns of tibial bowing The direction of the apex of the tibial bow determines the prognosis and management. Simple lateral bowing is benign, in contrast with anterolateral bowing, which often leads to pseudarthrosis of the tibia.

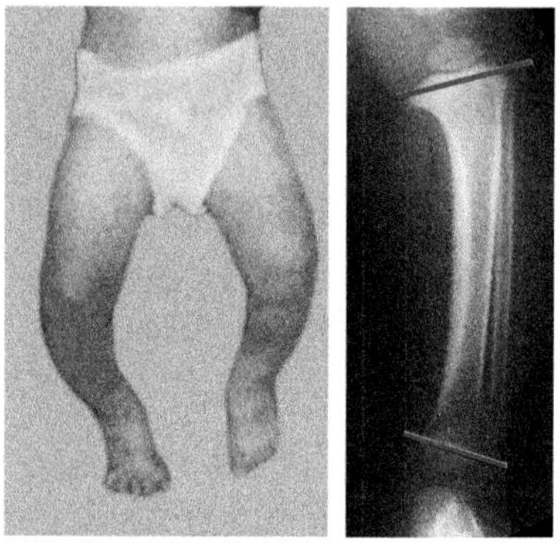

B Physiologic bowing This physiologic lateral tibial bowing resolves spontaneously in late infancy. Radiographs are usually not necessary.

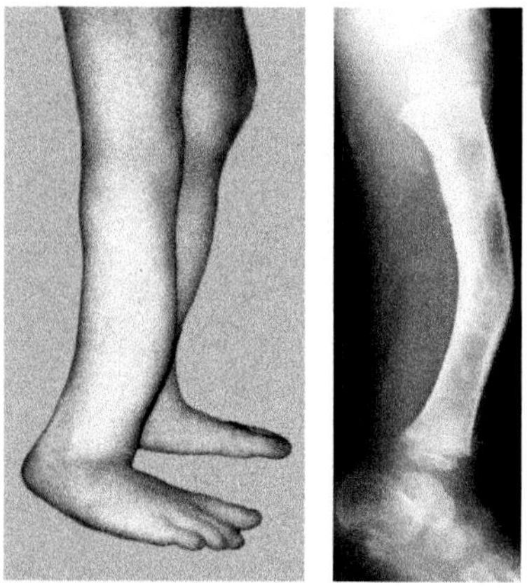

C Anterior bow in fibular deficiency.

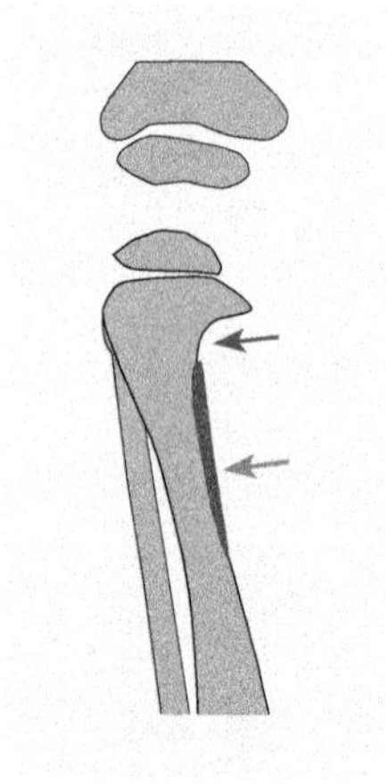

D Focal fibrocartilaginous dysplasia Note the lucency (red arrow) and the sclerosis (blue arrow).

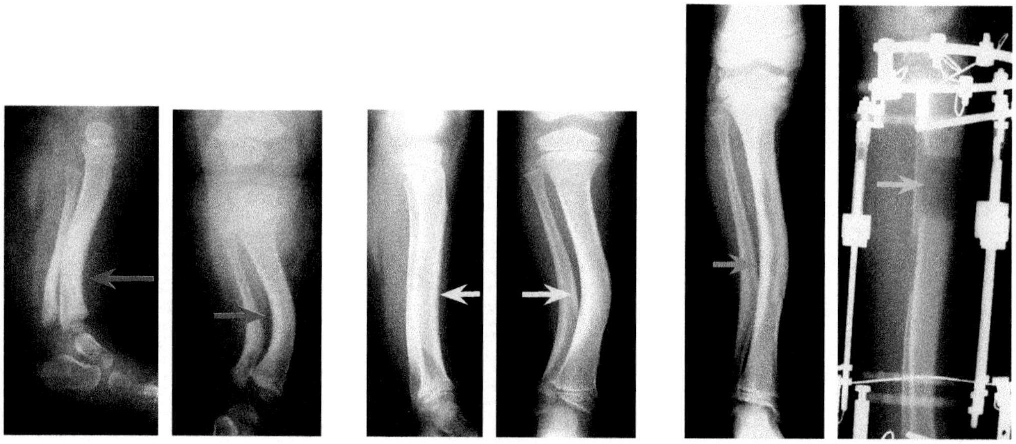

E Posteromedial tibial bowing This bow was present at birth (red arrows). The bowing improved gradually throughout childhood, as shown at age 3 years (yellow arrows) and 10 years (blue arrow). This is an unusually severe form with persistent bowing and shortening of 4.5 cm. The deformity was corrected by an osteotomy and lengthening (green arrow) with a circular frame at age 12 years.

Tibial Bowing

Tibial bowing is common and varied. The prognosis varies, depending upon the direction of the apex or convexity of the bowing [A].

Lateral Tibial Bowing

Lateral tibial bowing is common in infants and is simply a variation of normal [B]. The condition is usually mild, symmetrical, and unassociated with other problems. Reassure the family and provide a follow-up if necessary. Radiographs are usually unnecessary.

Anterior Tibial Bowing

Anterior bowing is often associated with fibular hemimelia [C]. Sometimes a dimple is present over the apex. Limb shortening is the major problem.

Focal Fibrocartilaginous Dysplasia

This rare deformity has a characteristic radiographic appearance [D]. The lesions tend to heal with growth.

Posteromedial Tibial Bowing

Posteromedial bowing [E] is a rare condition associated with a calcaneal deformity of the foot and mild limb shortening. The shortening is usually 2–4 cm at the end of growth. The condition may be due to abnormal intrauterine position. It is a common feature of fibular hemimelia. The calcaneal foot deformity resolves with time. The bowing improves with growth. Shortening tends to increase with time, and correction by epiphysiodesis or lengthening is often necessary.

Anterolateral Tibial Bowing

Anterolateral bowing is a serious form of tibial bowing [A]. The bowing may increase spontaneously and fracture at its apex. This leads to a pseudarthrosis of the tibia that is difficult to manage. Anteriolateral bowing is managed by protection with a cast or brace to prevent fracture or by operatively augmenting the bone strength to reduce the risk of fracture.

Pseudarthrosis of the Tibia

Pseudarthrosis of the tibia [A] results from a pathological fracture [B] that may occur before or after birth. It may be preceded by an anterolateral bowing of the tibia and is sometimes associated with neurofibromatosis. The pseudarthrosis occurs in the distal tibial diaphysis and can be graded by severity [C].

Management

Management is varied and depends on the severity of the condition and the success of previous treatments.

Brace Order a total contact orthoses to prevent progressive deformity and fracture.

Operative correction Several options are available [D].

Intramedullary fixation First, stabilize with an intramedullary (IM) rod and a graft to promote union [E].

Vascularized graft Consider this option if the IM fixation fails. Place a vascularized graft from the other fibula or immobilize with an Ilizarov device.

External fixation The Ilizarov fixator allows a segment of diaphysis to be transported. The pseudarthrosis is compressed while the proximal metaphysis is lengthened. If successful, union without sacrificing length is achieved. Consider grafting the distal docking site if union is delayed. Consider placing an IM rod to prevent recurrent deformity.

Amputation Union may not be achieved, even after several procedures. In other cases, only a tenuous union is obtained. The tibia is dysplastic and may refracture, and the leg is short and weak. The outcome is unsatisfactory, and amputation is necessary. The decision to amputate the limb is always difficult, and the decision is often delayed in a futile effort to save an unsalvageable limb. Delaying this decision harms the child.

Isolated Fibular Pseudarthrosis

Rarely, only the fibula is affected by the pseudarthrosis [B]. Consider bracing to prevent ankle and foot valgus. Operative management often is necessary with plate fixation, autogenous grafting, and ankle valgus correction. If the pseudarthrosis persists, create a synostosis between the distal fragment and the tibia to prevent further shortening.

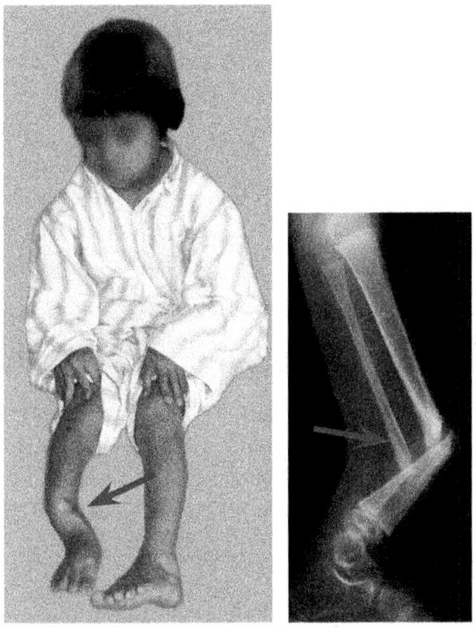

A Anterolateral bowing and pseudarthrosis of the tibia This girl has a pseudarthrosis of the right tibia (arrows).

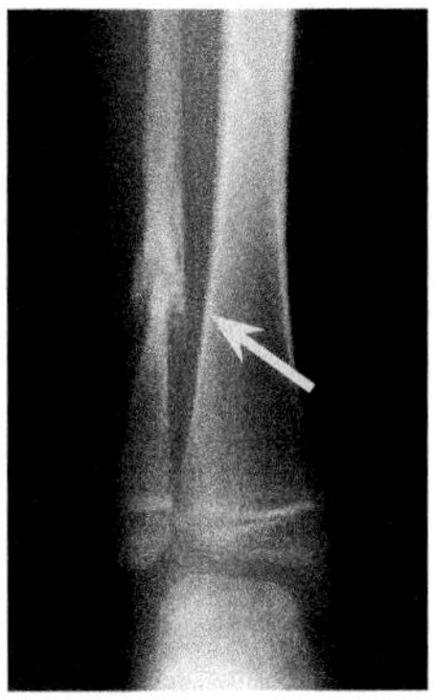

B Fibular pseudarthrosis

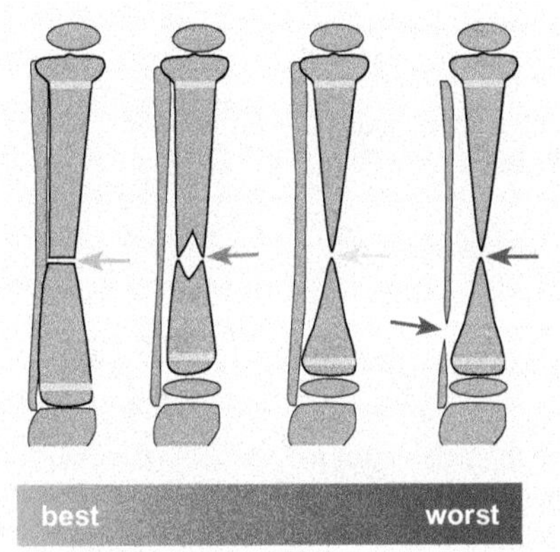

C Prognosis of tibial pseudarthrosis Outlook is best for simple pseudarthrosis (green arrow), cystic (blue arrow), sclerotic (yellow arrow), and worst for sclerotic type with pseudarthrosis of the fibula (red arrows).

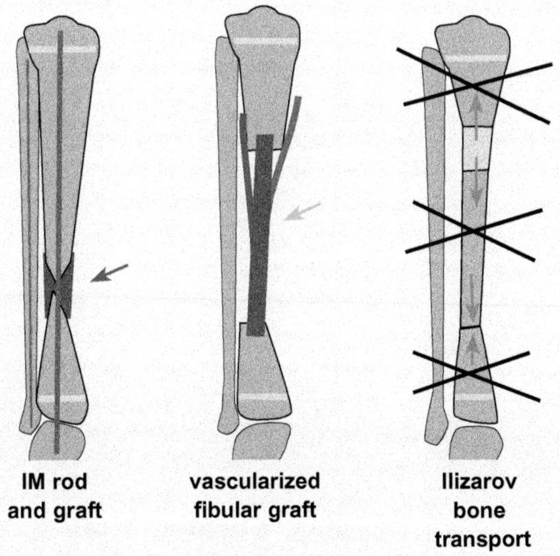

D Pseudarthrosis tibia treatment methods The most successful methods for treating this defect are the intermedullary rod and autogenous bone graft (red arrow), the vascularized fibular graft (green arrow), and the Ilizarov method with compression of the lesion and lengthening of the proximal tibia (blue arrows).

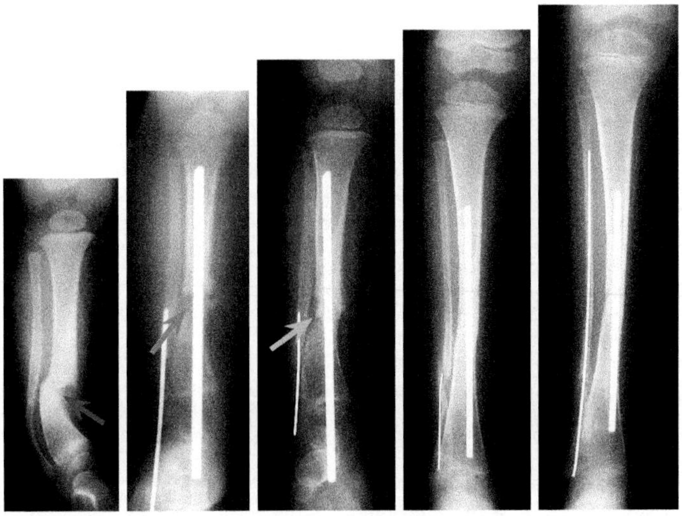

E Management by intramedullary fixation and grafting This infant was born with an anterolateral bow. He was managed in a clam-shell brace. While bathing without the brace, the infant fell and fractured the dysplastic tibia (red arrow). This was treated with IM rod fixation and grafting (blue arrow). Tenuous union was achieved (green arrow). The fibula remained unhealed at age 4 years, and ankle valgus developed. A distal tibial–fibular fusion was created to avoid further valgus from developing.

Ahn JH, Shim JS, Hwang CH, Oh WH. Discoid lateral meniscus in children: clinical manifestations and morphology. J Pediatr Orthop 2001 Nov-Dec;21(6): p812-6.

Anderson AF. Transepiphyseal replacement of the anterior cruciate ligament using quadruple hamstring grafts in skeletally immature patients. J Bone Joint Surg Am 2004 Sep;86-A Suppl 1(Pt 2): p201-9.

Aparicio G, et al. Radiologic study of patellar height in Osgood-Schlatter disease. J Pediatr Orthop 1997:17:63.

Beals RK, Buehler K. Treatment of patellofemoral instability in childhood with creation of a femoral sulcus. J Pediatr Orthop 1997:17:516.

Beguiristain JL, de Rada PD, Barriga A. Nail-patella syndrome: long term evolution. J Pediatr Orthop B 2003 Jan;12(1): p13-6.

Bensahel H, Souchet P, Pennecot GF, Mazda K. The unstable patella in children. J Pediatr Orthop B 2000 Oct;9(4): p265-70.

Bowen RE, Dorey FJ, Moseley C. Relative tibial and femoral varus as a predictor of progression of varus deformities of the lower limbs in young children. J Pediatr Orthop 2002 Jan-Feb;22(1): p105-11.

Bramer JA, Maas M, Dallinga RJ, te Slaa RL, Vergroesen DA. Increased external tibial torsion and osteochondritis dissecans of the knee. Clin Orthop 2004 May;(422): p175-9.

Bruce WD, Stevens PM. Surgical correction of miserable malalignment syndrome. J Pediatr Orthop 2004 Jul-Aug;24(4): p392-6.

Buckley SL, et al. Ligamentous instability of the knee in children sustaining fractures of the femur: a prospective study with knee examination under anesthesia. J Pediatr Orthop 1996:16.

Cameron JC, Saha S. External tibial torsion: an under recognized cause of recurrent patellar dislocation. Clin Orthop 1996:_328:177.

Choi IH, Kim CJ, Cho TJ, Chung CY, Song KS, Hwang JK, Sohn YJ. Focal fibrocartilaginous dysplasia of long bones: report of eight additional cases and literature review. J Pediatr Orthop 2000 Jul-Aug;20(4): p421-7.

Connolly B, et al. Discoid meniscus in children: magnetic resonance imaging characteristics. Can Assoc Radiol J 1996:47:347.

Dai L, Zhang W, Xu Y. Meniscal injury in children: long-term results after meniscectomy. Knee Surg Sports Traumatol Arthrosc 1997:5:77.

Davids JR, Blackhurst DW, Allen BL. Radiographic evaluation of bowed legs in children. J Pediatr Orthop 2001 Mar-Apr;21(2): p257-63.

Davids JR, Blackhurst DW, Allen Jr BL. Clinical evaluation of bowed legs in children. J Pediatr Orthop B 2000 Oct;9(4): p278-84.

De Greef I, Molenaers G, Fabry G. Popliteal cysts in children: a retrospective study of 62 cases. Acta Orthop Belg 1998:64:180.

Deie M, Ochi M, Sumen Y, Yasumoto M, Kobayashi K, Kimura H. Reconstruction of the medial patellofemoral ligament for the treatment of habitual or recurrent dislocation of the patella in children. J Bone Joint Surg Br 2003 Aug;85(6): p887-90.

Delgado ED, et al. Treatment of severe torsional malalignment syndrome. J Pediatr Orthop 1996:16:484.

Dobbs MB, Rich MM, Gordon JE, Szymanski DA, Schoenecker PL. Use of an intramedullary rod for treatment of congenital pseudarthrosis of the tibia. A long-term follow-up study. J Bone Joint Surg Am 2004 Jun;86-A(6): p1186-97.

Eilert RE. Congenital dislocation of the patella. Clin Orthop 2001 Aug;(389): p22-9.

Eilert RE. Dysplasia of the patellofemoral joint in children. Am J Knee Surg 1999:12:114.

Flowers MJ, Bhadreshwar DR. Tibial tuberosity excision for symptomatic Osgood-Schlatter disease. J Pediatr Orthop 1995:15:292.

Flynn JM, Kocher MS, Ganley TJ. Osteochondritis dissecans of the knee. J Pediatr Orthop 2004 Jul-Aug;24(4): p434-43.

Fraser RK, et al. Pes anserinus syndrome due to solitary tibial spurs and osteochondromas. J Pediatr Orthop 1996: 16:247

Ghanem I, Damsin JP, Carlioz H. Ilizarov technique in the treatment of congenital pseudarthrosis of the tibia. J Pediatr Orthop 1997:17:685.

Ghanem I, Wattincourt L, Seringe R. Congenital dislocation of the patella. Part II: orthopaedic management. J Pediatr Orthop 2000 Nov-Dec;20(6): p817-22.

Ghanem I, Wattincourt L, Seringe R. Congenital dislocation of the patella. Part I: pathologic anatomy.

Hallam PJ, Fazal MA, Ashwood N, Ware HE, Glasgow MM, Powell JM. An alternative to fixation of displaced fractures of the anterior intercondylar eminence in children. J Bone Joint Surg Br 2002 May;84(4): p579-82.

Hefti F, Bollini G, Dungl P, Fixsen J, Grill F, Ippolito E, Romanus B, Tudisco C, Wientroub S. Congenital pseudarthrosis of the tibia: history, etiology, classification, and epidemiologic data. J Pediatr Orthop B 2000 Jan;9(1): p11-5.

Hefti F, et al. Osteochondritis dissecans: a Mu Study of the European Pediatric Orthopedic Society. J Pediatr Orthop 1999:b 8:231.

Hirano A, Fukubayashi T, Ishii T, Ochiai N. Relationship between the patellar height and the disorder of the knee extensor mechanism in immature athletes. J Pediatr Orthop 2001 Jul-Aug;21(4): p541-4.

Hui JH, Chen F, Thambyah A, Lee EH. Treatment of chondral lesions in advanced osteochondritis dissecans: a comparative study of the efficacy of chondrocytes, mesenchymal stem cells, periosteal graft, and mosaicplasty (osteochondral autograft) in animal models. J Pediatr Orthop 2004 Jul-Aug;24(4): p427-33.

Ippolito E, Corsi A, Grill F, Wientroub S, Bianco P. Pathology of bone lesions associated with congenital pseudarthrosis of the leg. J Pediatr Orthop B 2000 Jan;9(1): p3-10.

Johnston CE. Congenital pseudarthrosis of the tibia: results of technical variations in the charnley-williams procedure. J Bone Joint Surg Am 2002 Oct;84-A(10): p1799-810.

Joseph B, Somaraju VV, Shetty SK. Management of congenital pseudarthrosis of the tibia in children under 3 years of age: effect of early surgery on union of the pseudarthrosis and growth of the limb. J Pediatr Orthop 2003 Nov-Dec;23(6): p740-6.

Keret D, Bollini G, Dungl P, Fixsen J, Grill F, Hefti F, Ippolito E, Romanus B, Tudisco C, Wientroub S. The fibula in congenital pseudarthrosis of the tibia: the EPOS multicenter study. European Paediatric Orthopaedic Society (EPOS). J Pediatr Orthop B 2000 Apr;9(2): p69-74.

King SJ, Carty HM, Brady O. Magnetic resonance imaging of knee injuries in children. Pediatr Radiol 1996:26:287.

Klingele KE, Kocher MS, Hresko MT, Gerbino P, Micheli LJ. Discoid lateral meniscus: prevalence of peripheral rim instability. J Pediatr Orthop 2004 Jan-Feb;24(1): p79-82.

Kocher MS, Mandiga R, Klingele K, Bley L, Micheli LJ. Anterior cruciate ligament injury versus tibial spine fracture in the skeletally immature knee: a comparison of skeletal maturation and notch width index. J Pediatr Orthop 2004 Mar-Apr;24(2): p185-8.

Kocher MS, Saxon HS, Hovis WD, Hawkins RJ. Management and complications of anterior cruciate ligament injuries in skeletally immature patients: survey of the Herodicus Society and The ACL Study Group. J Pediatr Orthop 2002 Jul-Aug;22(4): p452-7.

Kristiansen LP, Steen H, Terjesen T. Residual challenges after healing of congenital pseudarthrosis in the tibia. Clin Orthop 2003 Sep;(414): p228-37.

Lehman WB, Atar D, Feldman DS, Gordon JC, Grant AD. Congenital pseudarthrosis of the tibia. J Pediatr Orthop B 2000 Apr;9(2): p103-7.

Luhmann SJ. Acute traumatic knee effusions in children and adolescents. J Pediatr Orthop 2003 Mar-Apr;23(2): p199-202.

Maffulli N, et al. Knee arthroscopy in Chinese children and adolescents: an eight-year prospective study. Arthroscopy 1997:13:18.

McCall RE, Ratts V. Soft-tissue realignment for adolescent patellar instability. J Pediatr Orthop 1999:19:549.

McCarthy JJ, Betz RR, Kim A, Davids JR, Davidson RS. Early radiographic differentiation of infantile tibia vara from physiologic bowing using the femoral-tibial ratio. J Pediatr Orthop 2001 Jul-Aug;21(4): p545-8.

Mehlman CT, Rubinstein JH, Roy DR. Instability of the patellofemoral joint in Rubinstein-Taybi syndrome. J Pediatr Orthop 1998:18:508.

Meyer JS, et al. MRI of focal fibrocartilaginous dysplasia. J Pediatr Orthop 1995:15:304.

Miller TT, et al. Sonography of patellar abnormalities in children. AJR Am J Roentgenol 1998:171:739.

Muhammad KS, LA Koman, JF Mooney 3rd, BP Smith. Congenital dislocation of the knee: overview of management options. J South Orthop Assoc 1999:8:93.

Mukai S, Suzuki S, Seto Y, Kashiwagi N, Hwang ES. Early characteristic findings in bowleg deformities: evaluation using magnetic resonance imaging. J Pediatr Orthop 2000 Sep-Oct;20(5): p611-5.

O'Connor MA, Palaniappan M, Khan N, Bruce CE. Osteochondritis dissecans of the knee in children. A comparison of MRI and arthroscopic findings. J Bone Joint Surg Br 2002 Mar;84(2): p258-62.

Ogut T, Kesmezacar H, Akgun I, Cansu E. Arthroscopic meniscectomy for discoid lateral meniscus in children and adolescents: 4.5 year follow-up. J Pediatr Orthop B 2003 Nov;12(6): p390-7.

Pressman AE, Letts RM, Jarvis JG. Anterior cruciate ligament tears in children: an analysis of operative versus nonoperative treatment. J Pediatr Orthop 1997:17:505.

Romanus B, Bollini G, Dungl P, Fixsen J, Grill F, Hefti F, Ippolito E, Tudisco C, Wientroub S. Free vascular fibular transfer in congenital pseudarthrosis of the tibia: results of the EPOS multicenter study. European Paediatric Orthopaedic Society (EPOS). J Pediatr Orthop B 2000 Apr;9(2): p90-3.

Saciri V, Pavlovcic V, Zupanc O, Baebler B. Knee arthroscopy in children and adolescents. J Pediatr Orthop B 2001 Oct;10(4): p311-4.

Topoleski TA; Kurtz CA; Grogan DP. Radiographic abnormalities and clinical symptoms associated with patella alta in ambulatory children with cerebral palsy. J Pediatr Orthop 2000 Sep-Oct;20(5): p636-9.

Tudisco C, Bollini G, Dungl P, Fixen J, Grill F, Hefti F, Romanus B, Wientroub S. Functional results at the end of skeletal growth in 30 patients affected by congenital pseudarthrosis of the tibia. J Pediatr Orthop B 2000 Apr;9(2): p94-102.

Vahasarja V, et al. Axial radiography or CT in the measurement of patellofemoral malalignment indices in children and adolescents? Clin Radiol 1996:51:639.

Vahasarja V. Operative realignment of patellar malalignment in children. J Pediatr Orthop 1995:15:281.

Van Rhijn LW, Jansen EJ, Pruijs HE. Long-term follow-up of conservatively treated popliteal cysts in children. J Pediatr Orthop B 2000 Jan;9(1): p62-4.

Vitale MG; Guha A, Skaggs DL. Orthopaedic manifestations of neurofibromatosis in children: an update. Clin Orthop 2002 Aug;(401): p107-18.

Walker P, Harris I, Leicester A. Patellar tendon-to-patella ratio in children. J Pediatr Orthop 1998:18:129.

Washington ER 3rd, Root L, Liener UC. Discoid lateral meniscus in children. Long-term follow-up after excision. J Bone Joint Surg 1995:77A:1357.

Wessel LM, Scholz S, Rusch M, Kopke J, Loff S, Duchene W, Waag KL. Hemarthrosis after trauma to the pediatric knee joint: what is the value of magnetic resonance imaging in the diagnostic algorithm? J Pediatr Orthop 2001 May-Jun;21(3): p338-42.

Wessel LM, Scholz S, Rusch M. Characteristic pattern and management of intra-articular knee lesions in different pediatric age groups. J Pediatr Orthop 2001 Jan-Feb;21(1): p14-9.

Yang KY, Lee EH. Isolated congenital pseudarthrosis of the fibula. J Pediatr Orthop B 2002 Oct;11(4): p298-301.

CHAPTER 11

Hip and Femur

Problems of the hip account for about 15% of the practice of orthopedists. Many hip problems in adults have their origin during growth.

General

Development

Ossification of the ischium, ilium, pubis, femoral shaft, and distal femoral epiphysis occurs before birth. The femoral head ossifies between the second and eighth postnatal months [A] and fuses with the neck between 15 and 21 years in boys and one year earlier in girls.

Growth of the upper femur occurs not only in the capital epiphysis and trochanteric apophysis but also along the neck of the femur [C]. Growth from the triradiate cartilage is a major contributor to acetabular development [B]. The deformities caused by trauma are site-specific [C].

Most growth of the acetabulum occurs from the triradiate cartilage. Closure will cause severe progressive dysplasia. Additional growth of the acetabulum occurs from the acetabular epiphysis. This growth is especially important late in childhood and during adolescence.

Damage to these growth centers, either from trauma or as a complication of treatment, is a common source of deformity and disability. The upper femur is very susceptible to vascular or epiphyseal injury.

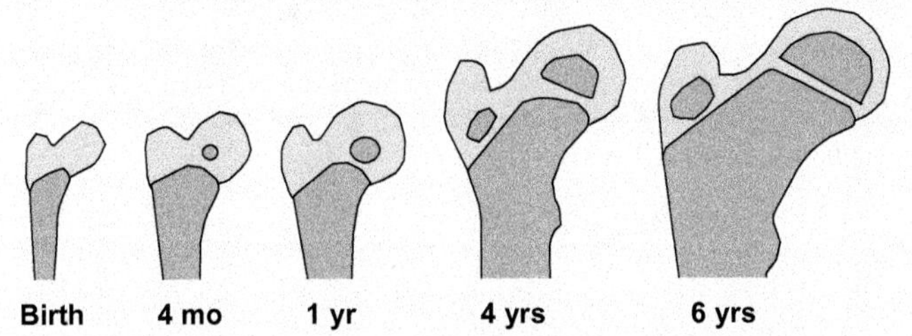

A Ossification of proximal femur This sequence shows ossification in the normal child. Redrawn from Tönnis (1984).

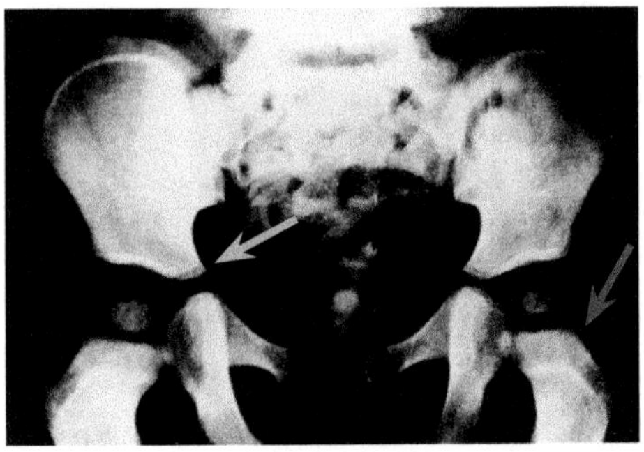

B Pelvic growth This child had a phosphorized oil dietary supplement as a child. Growth patterns are shown. Note the growth that occurs in the triradiate cartilage (orange arrow) and upper femur (red arrow). Courtesy I. Ponseti.

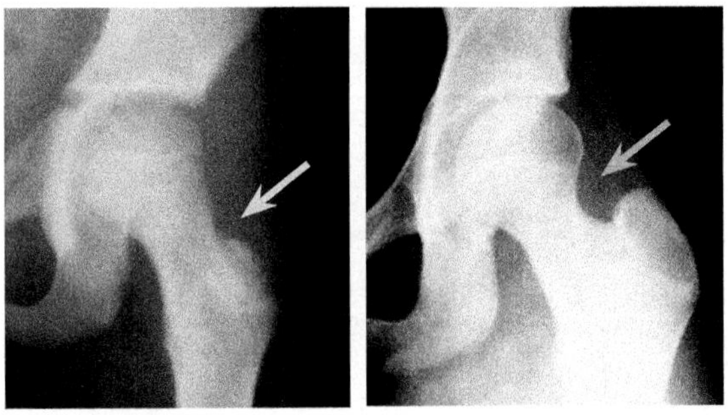

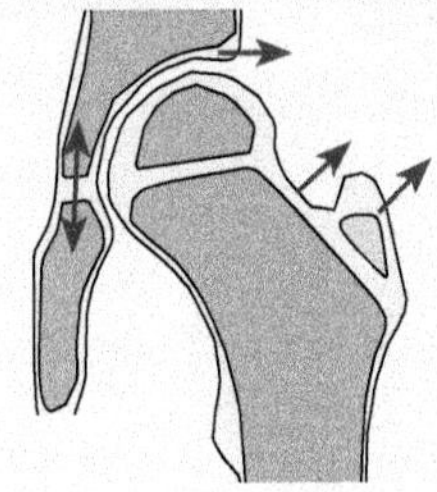

C Proximal femoral growth Note that growth (red arrows) occurs at many sites about the upper femur, including appositional growth of the femoral neck. Damage to the greater trochanteric apophysis from curettage for a bone cyst (yellow arrow) or from reaming to place an IM nail (orange arrow) causes a reduction in width and functional elongation of the femoral neck.

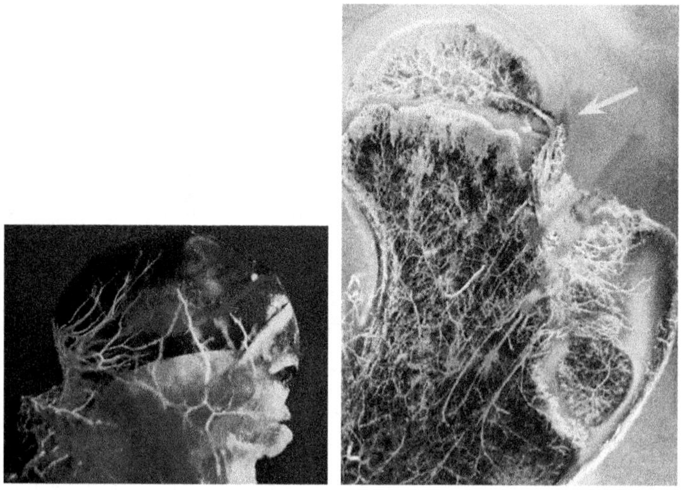

A Vascularity of the femoral head In infancy, transphyseal vessels are often present (red arrow). In childhood, the femoral head is supplied by the lateral retinacular vessels that must traverse the joint (yellow arrow). From Chung (1976).

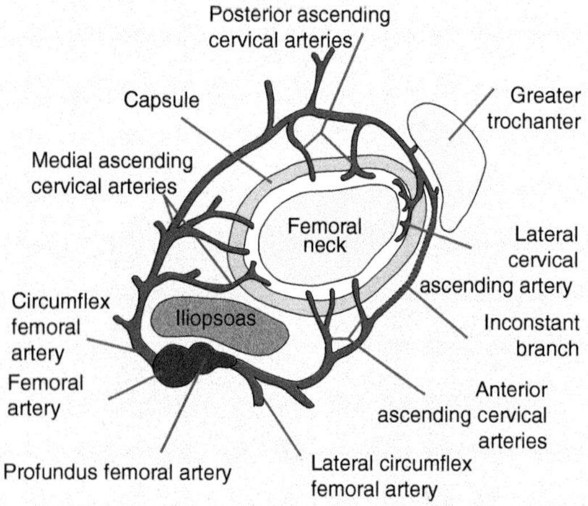

B Vascularity of the femoral head Note that the proximal femur is supplied by an arcade of vessels that arise from the profundus femoral artery.

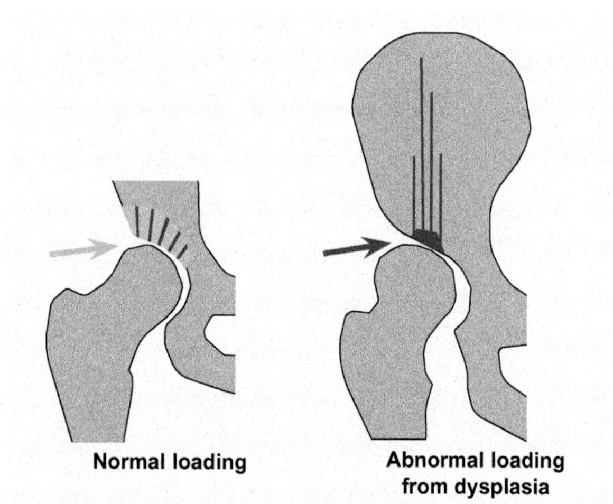

C Biomechanics of the hip In the normal hip, loading (green arrow) is low and well distributed. In dysplasia, loading is concentrated (red arrow), resulting in eventual cartilage degeneration.

Vascularity

Disturbances in blood supply to the upper femur are a common cause of many serious deformities and subsequent disability.

The femoral head may receive blood through the ligamentum teres, epiphyseal vessels, or metaphysis. The femoral head in the infant is supplied by epiphyseal vessels and vessels that traverse the epiphyseal plate [A]. These transphyseal vessels disappear as ossification develops in the femoral head. Circulation in the child is primarily through the metaphyseal vessels. Only in late childhood and adolescence do the ligamentum teres vessels make a significant contribution. After closure of the capital physeal plate, the metaphyseal vessels contribute to the circulation.

During most of childhood, this vascular supply is provided by two anastomotic rings formed by the medial and lateral circumflex vessels [B]. The pattern of distribution is variable, and deficiencies may contribute to the development of avascular necrosis.

Biomechanics

Loading within the joint is affected by the load-bearing area [C]. Increased loading is prominent when the hip is subluxated or shallow. Increased loading leads to osteoarthritis in adult life.

Operative procedures, especially osteotomies of the pelvis and femur, dramatically affect the biomechanics of the hip. The hip joint normally carries about four times its body weight. Hip joint loading is reduced by varus femoral osteotomy or by medializing the joint, as done in the Chiari osteotomy. When reconstructing a hip, try to achieve as normal an anatomy as possible.

Term	Definition
Coxa	**Refers to joint**
Vara	Reduced neck–shaft angle
Valga	Increased neck–shaft angle
Plana	Flattened femoral head
Magna	Enlarged femoral head
Breva	Shortened femoral neck
Hip dysplasia	**Abnormal features of the hip joint**
Acetabular	Dysplastic acetabulum
Femoral	Dysplastic femur
Joint status	**Acetabulofemoral relationship**
Congruous	Concentric reduction
Subluxated	Loss of concentricity
Dislocated	No joint elements in contact
Joint fit	**Joint surface relationship**
Spherical	Round femoral head
Congruous	Congruous fit
Incongruous	Incongruous
Aspherical	Femoral head nonspherical
Congruous	Congruous fit
Incongruous	Incongruous

D Nomenclature for deformity These terms are commonly used to describe various patterns of hip deformity.

Nomenclature

Hip terminology is reasonably straightforward [D, previous page]. The most significant recent change was the replacement of the term *congenital* with *developmental* in hip dysplasia. Congenital hip disease (CDH) thus becomes developmental hip dysplasia (DDH). Hip disorders caused by muscle disorders secondary to neurologic disorders such as cerebral palsy are called *neurogenic* dysplasia of the hip (NDH). The term *dysplasia* is a broad term covering disorders that may involve the acetabulum, upper femur, or both elements.

Evaluation

A thorough evaluation of the hip is important due to the vulnerability of the hip joint to damage, especially from impaired blood supply. Delays in diagnosis of DDH, septic arthritis, and slipped epiphysis are relatively common and sometimes result in joint destruction. The deep position of the hip joint makes evaluation more difficult than most extremity joints such as the knee or ankle. This, together with its tenuous vascularity, places the hip at special risk.

History

Is there a family history of hip problems? DDH is familial. Has the child complained of pain? Night pain suggests a neoplastic origin. Remember that hip pain may be referred to the knee [A]. Has the child limped? Were there systemic signs? Has the problem been getting worse or has it plateaued? Be certain to rule out septic arthritis and slipped epiphysis as acute disorders and DDH as a long-term problem.

Physical Examination

Observation Does the child appear ill? Is there spontaneous movement of the limb? Pseudoparalysis is common in trauma and infections. Does the child limp? Limping from hip problems is usually antalgic or due to an abductor lurch.

Palpation Palpate for tenderness over the bony prominences. Tenderness is often found in the adolescent with bursitis, tendonitis, or overuse syndromes. By determining the point of maximum tenderness exactly, a presumptive diagnosis can often be made.

Range of Motion Hip disorders often result in loss of motion. Inflammatory disorders usually cause a reduction in internal hip rotation early on and eventually flexion and adduction contracture of the hip.

Hip rotation Assess with the child prone. Assessing the range of medial rotation is a valuable screening test [B]. The finding of asymmetric hip rotation is abnormal and indicates the need for a radiograph of the pelvis.

Flexion Detect the presence of a contracture using the Thomas or prone extension test [C]. The prone extension test is most accurate, especially in children with neuromuscular disorders.

Abduction–Adduction Assess while stabilizing the pelvis with one hand.

Trendelenburg Test

Assess an abductor lurch using the Trendelenburg test [D]. Ask the child to lift one leg at a time. The pelvis should rise on the elevated side. A drop of that side is a positive sign and suggests that the abductor mechanism is weak on the opposite side. This lurch may be due to weakness of the muscles, a change in shape of the upper femur, or inflammation of the joint.

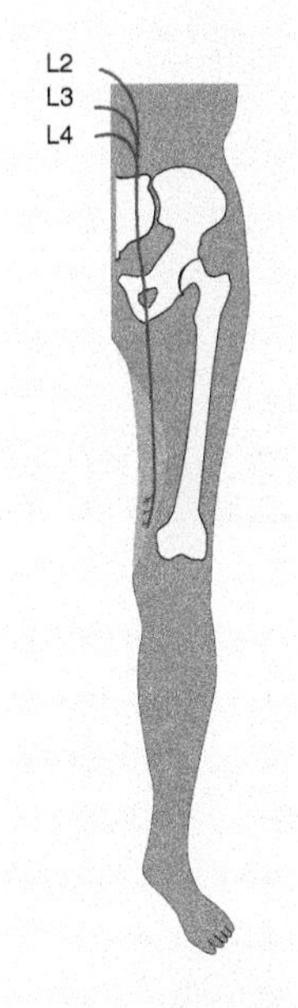

A Hip pain referred to knee The obturator nerve supplies articular branches to the hip and cutaneous coverage about the knee. Hip disorders may present with knee pain.

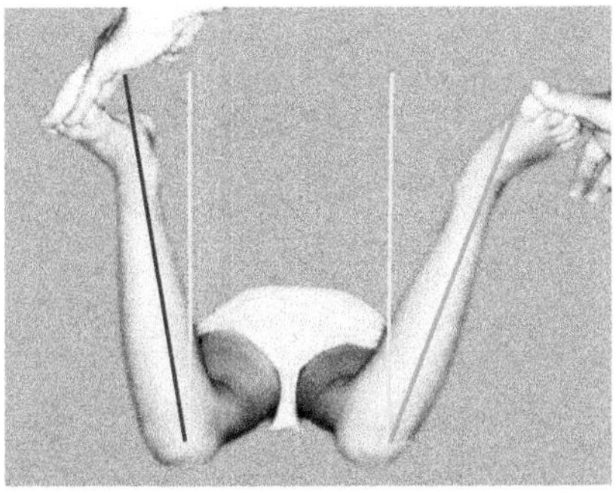

B Hip rotation test Position the child prone with the knees flexed to 90°. Rotate the hips internally and note any guarding and the extent of rotation. Asymmetry of rotation is usually abnormal. In this child with Legg-Calvé-Perthes disease on the left hip, rotation was limited compared to the normal right hip.

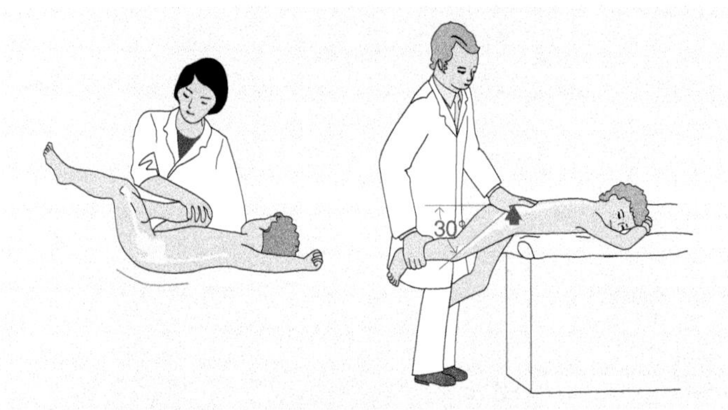

C Hip flexion contracture assessment The Thomas test (left) is performed with the contralateral hip flexed. Extend to measure the degree of contracture. The prone extension test (right) is performed with the child prone. Gradually extend the hip until the hand on the pelvis begins to rise. The horizontal–thigh angle indicates the degree of contracture.

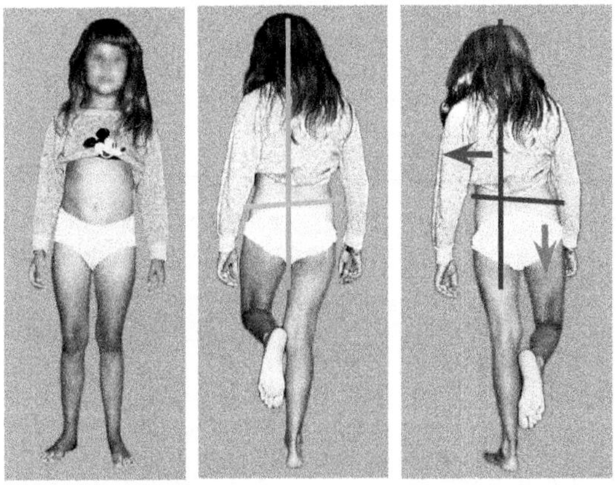

D Trendelenburg test This girl has DDH with weakness of the left hip abductors. When standing on her right leg, right hip abductors contract to elevate the left pelvis to maintain the head centered over the body (green lines). When standing on the weaker left leg, abductor weakness allows the right pelvis to fall (blue arrow). She must then shift her weight over the left leg (red lines).

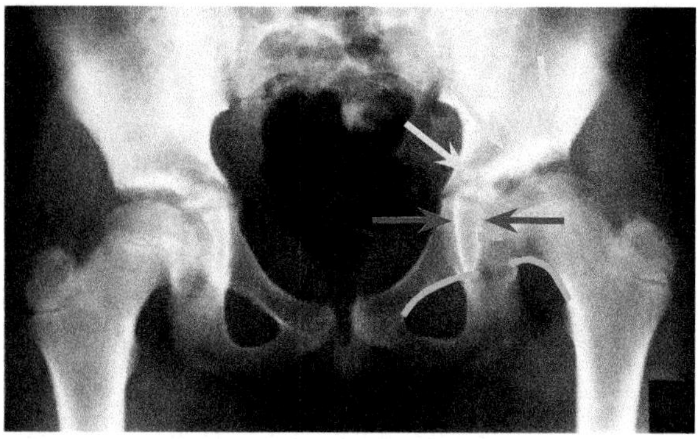

A AP x-ray of pelvis Much can be learned from this simple study. The right hip is normal. Acetabular dysplasia is present on the left. Note the triangular shape of the tear drop (red arrows). Note that the joint space (orange line) is widened. Shenton's line (green lines) is disrupted. The sourcil, or acetabular roof (yellow arrows), is sclerotic. The left hip joint is slightly higher and more laterally positioned than the normal side.

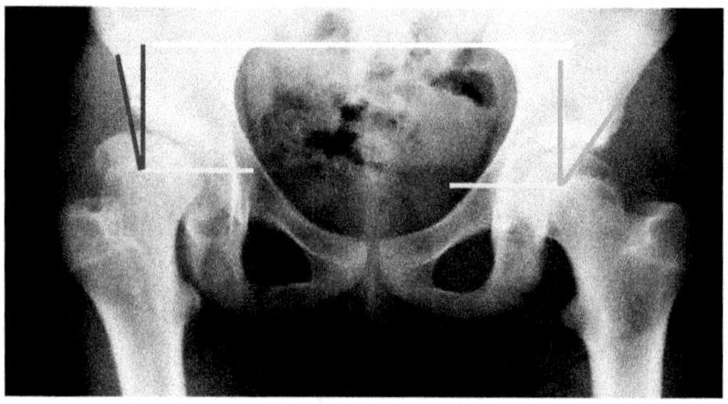

B Center–edge (CE) angle This child has a normal left hip with a CE angle of 30°. The right hip is aspherical and subluxated, and the CE angle is 10°. Note that measures are made with the pelvis level (white line).

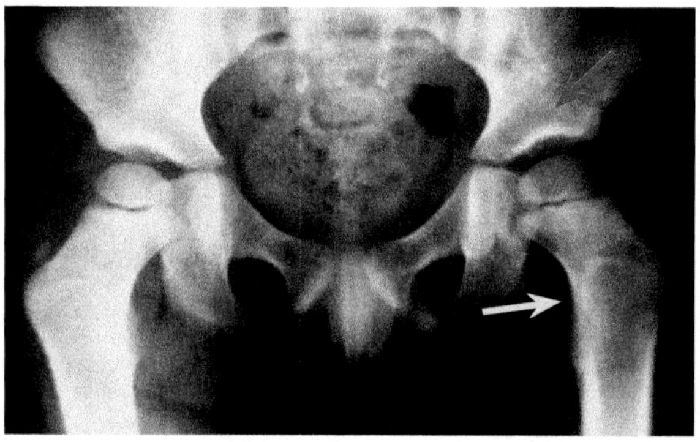

C Hemideossification Note the bone loss of the left hemipelvis (red arrow) due to an osteoid osteoma (yellow arrow) of the proximal femur.

Laboratory Studies

A CBC and an ESR and CRP are often helpful in evaluating hip disorders. The ESR and CRP are useful in differentiating septic arthritis from toxic synovitis. Infections usually elevate the ESR above 25–30 mm/hr. Toxic synovitis causes only a slight elevation in the ESR and CRP. Hematologic disorders such as leukemia and sickle cell disease may cause pelvic pain.

Hip Joint Aspiration

The aspiration of the hip is the most certain method of establishing the diagnosis of septic arthritis. Aspirate the joint promptly if the diagnosis of septic arthritis is seriously included in the differential. Although a negative aspirate (even when documented by an arthrogram) is not absolutely definitive, it is highly suggestive that the problem is not within the joint.

Delays in diagnosing septic arthritis may be catastrophic because it jeopardizes the vascularity to the femoral head and articular cartilage. Joint aspiration does not affect bone scans and should not be delayed by plans to perform imaging procedures.

Imaging

Imaging is required to evaluate hip disorders in children. Imaging is the only way to establish a prognosis. The vast majority of hip problems in children can still be managed adequately by careful examination and conventional radiographs.

Conventional radiography Evaluate most hip problems with conventional radiography. Except for the initial study, use a gonad shield. Obtain a single AP study [A]. Several useful measures may be made from this simple study [B, and A, next page]. Note any asymmetry in ossification of the pelvis. A painful condition such as an osteoid osteotomy results in hemideossification [C]. Be aware of the situations in which false negative studies are commonly misleading. A negative study does not rule out DDH in the neonate or an early septic arthritis. An AP radiograph may not show a mild slipped capital femoral epiphysis (SCFE).

Add other views as necessary. The frog-leg lateral allows comparison of both upper femora. The true lateral is useful in assessing the degree of slip in SCFE, the degree of involvement in Legg–Calvé–Perthes disease, or anterior coverage in DDH [D].

Useful special views include the abduction–internal rotation study for hip dysplasia [E], maximum abduction and adduction views for assessing hinge abduction problems, and anteversion studies. Femoral anteversion measurement is seldom necessary.

The load-bearing area of the hip significantly affects its longevity. A reduction in this area may be due to one or more of the following factors:

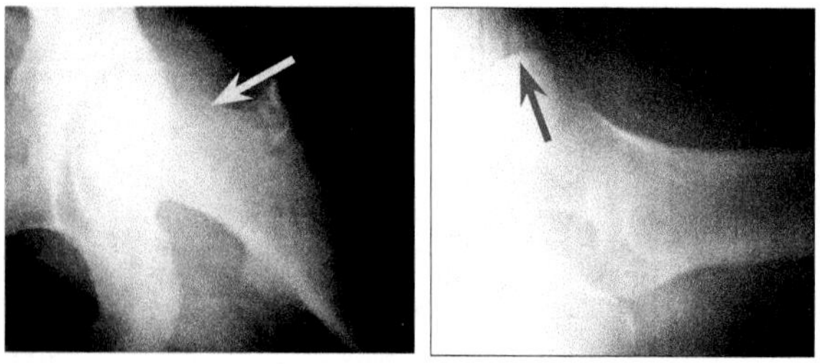

D Lateral x-rays of the proximal femur Frog-leg lateral (red arrow) is only an oblique view. A true lateral (yellow arrow) requires special positioning but provides more information, as it is made at right angles to the AP view. Note the lack of anterior coverage on lateral (red arrow).

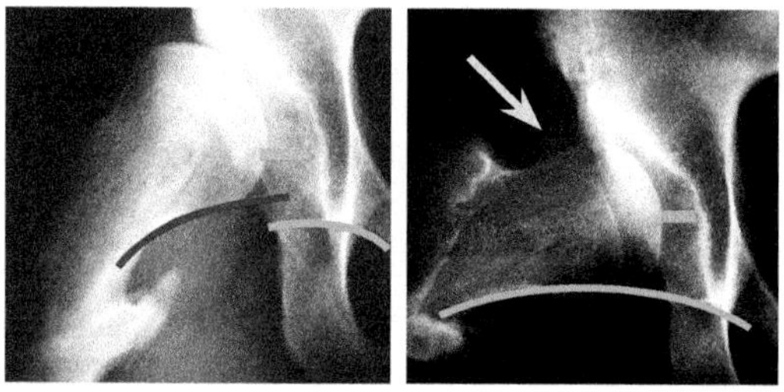

E Abduction internal rotation (AIR) view The resting position (red arc) shows the hip in a 14-year-old child with cerebral palsy. The hip is subluxated (orange lines), and Shenton's line (green arc) is disrupted (red arc). The AIR view (yellow arrow) shows improved congruity and less subluxation and restoration of Shenton's line.

Simple hip dysplasia The hip joint is either maldirected or shallow. Both reduce contact area. The depth of the acetabulum is often assessed by the CE angle. This angle increases during childhood as the joint ossifies. At the end of growth, values are like those of adults, with a normal range of 25°– 45°. Features of the normal hip are used as a basis for assessing deformity [A] and planning reconstruction.

Incongruity reduces contact area The femoral head is normally round and matches the shape of the acetabulum [B]. An aspherical femoral head is usually due to vascular problems. In the young child, the acetabulum usually remodels to become congruous, and the hip becomes aspherical and congruous [C]. If acetabular remodeling fails to occur, the hip may be aspherical and incongruous—a bad combination.

Displacement of the femoral head The relationship between the femoral head and acetabulum is normally congruous. If the head is displaced, it becomes subluxated. If all cartilage contact is lost, the joint is dislocated.

Ultrasonography (US) Ultrasound studies are of greatest value when readily available and performed by an orthopedist in conjunction with the overall evaluation. Cost, restricted access, and operator inexperience may limit value. Ultrasound's greatest potential usefulness is in assessing DDH in early infancy. Assessing joint effusion, localizing abscesses, and assessing the severity of SCFE, head size in LCP disease, and neck continuity in coxa vara are other applications. This imaging technique is underutilized in North America.

Scintigraphy Bone scans (BS) are useful in localizing inflammatory processes about the pelvis [D] and in assessing the circulation of the femoral head. Order high-resolution or pinhole-collimated AP and lateral scans of both proximal femora when assessing avascular necrosis (AVN). The bone scan is useful in confirming a preslip and assessing bone tumors.

Arthrography The usefulness of this procedure is limited, as it is invasive and requires sedation or anesthesia. Arthrography is appropriate to confirm joint penetration in negative taps for suspected joint sepsis and for special situations in managing DDH. The role in LCP disease is more controversial.

Magnetic resonance imaging (MRI) These studies are the most expensive and require sedation for infants and young children. MRI studies are most useful in assessing intraarticular disorders of the hip. Cartilaginous loose bodies or fracture fragments, deformity of the cartilaginous femoral head, status of the growth plate, and avascular necrosis are usually definable.

Computerized tomography (CT) Order CT studies to evaluate inflammatory conditions such as an iliopsoas abscess or the configuration of the upper femur and acetabulum. CT scans have replaced tomography in assessing AVN and physeal bridges.

Three-dimensional CT reconstructions are often helpful in visualizing complex deformities of the hip, which is necessary when planning surgery [E].

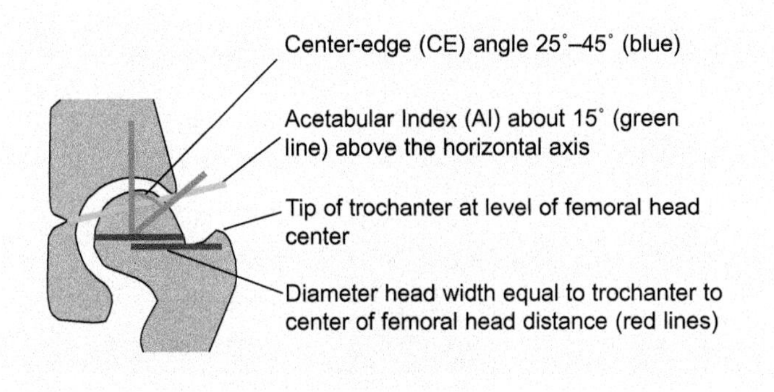

A Normal measurements These are measurements of the normal adolescent hip.

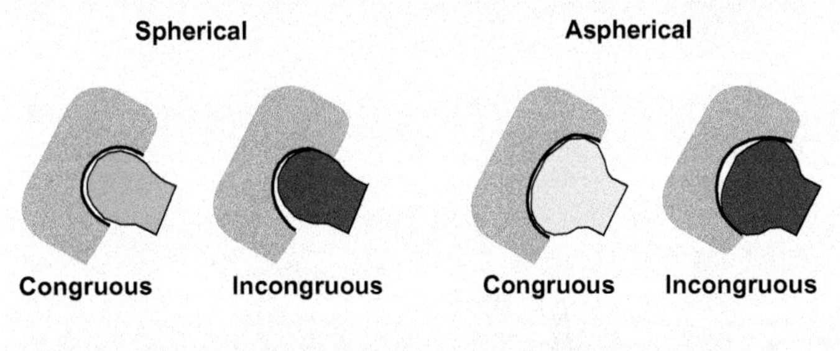

B Congruity Congruity of the hip may be either spherical or aspherical and congruous or incongruous. Incongruity (red) results in areas of excessive load, causing excessive cartilage wear and eventually osteoarthritis.

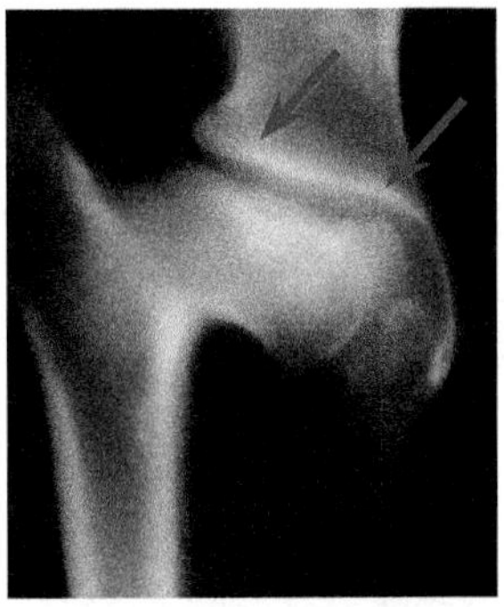

C Aspherical congruity This deformity resulted from Legg-Calvé-Perthes disease during middle childhood. The head became flattened and the acetabulum remodeled (red arrows) to become congruous.

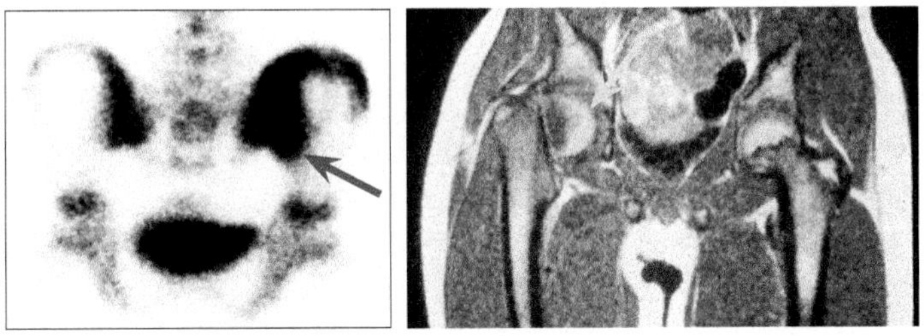

D Imaging options This bone scan shows inflammation of the sacroiliac joint (red arrow), and in a different patient, the MRI shows a slipped epiphysis (yellow arrow).

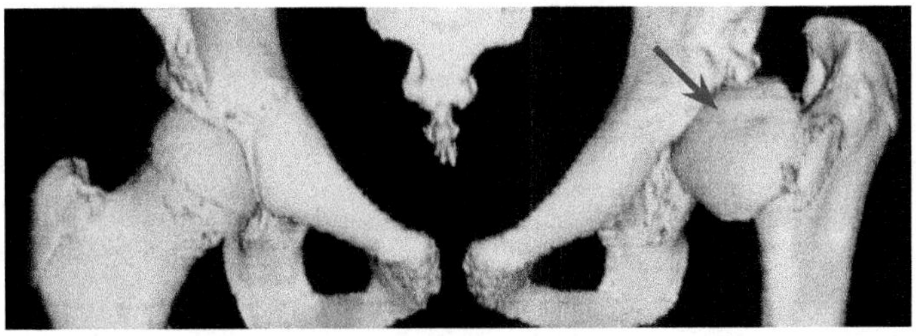

E Three-dimensional CT reconstructions Reconstructions are useful in assessing complex hip deformity prior to surgery. The deformity of the proximal femur (red arrow) is secondary to avascular necrosis associated with DDH management in infancy.

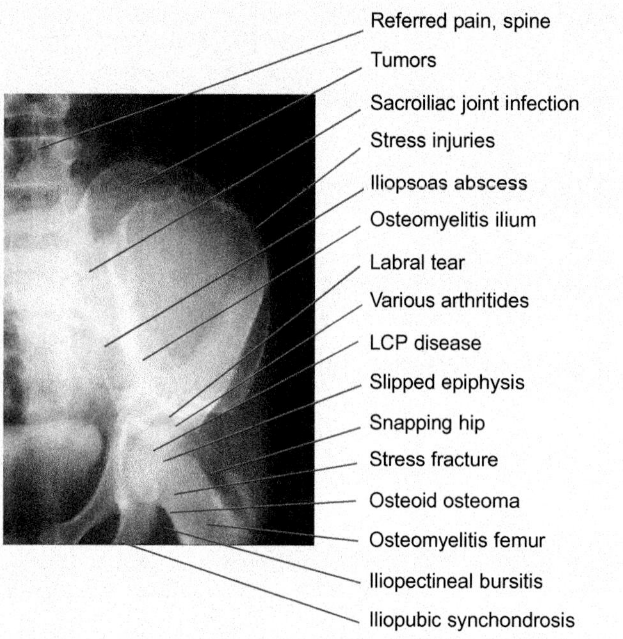

A Causes of hip pain in children The differential diagnosis is extensive.

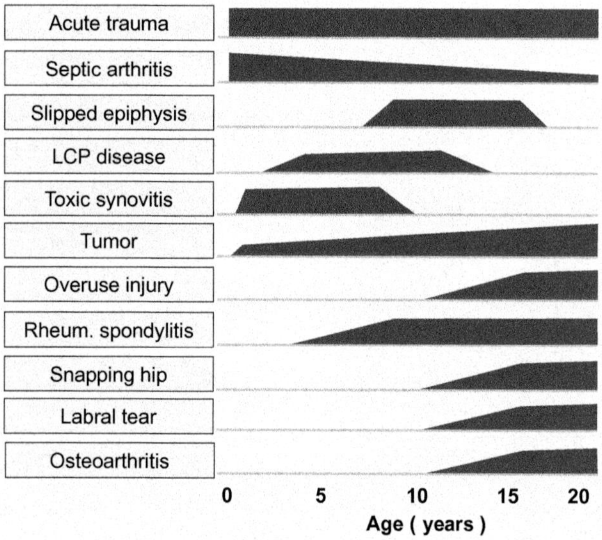

B Hip pain causes by usual age of onset These are ages when conditions are most common.

Hip and Pelvic Pain

The causes of hip and pelvic pain are numerous [A], sometimes making the diagnosis difficult.

Diagnosis

Detailing these features may help to establish the diagnosis.

Age Consider the age of the child with hip pain [B]. For example, LCP disease is most common in boys in middle childhood [B]. SCFE must be considered in the older child or adolescent. Overuse syndromes are most common in the adolescent.

Onset Acute onset is suggestive of injury or a rapid onset of infection. SCFE may be chronic or sudden. Acute slips are characterized by a mild injury and inability to walk. LCP disease onset is usually insidious. Overuse syndromes are most painful when active.

Spontaneous movement The most consistent physical finding for septic arthritis of the hip is a loss of spontaneous movement of the affected limb.

Systemic illness The child is ill with septic arthritis, and less sick with toxic synovitis, rheumatoid spondylitis, and tumors.

Resting position of the limb Intraarticular hip disorders usually result in the spontaneous positioning in slight flexion and lateral rotation [C]. This position reduces the intraarticular pressure.

Tenderness Palpate to determine the site of tenderness [D].

Hip rotation test Guarding and a loss of medial rotation suggest the problem is within the joint [E].

Night pain Nocturnal pain suggests the possibility of a malignant tumor.

Back stiffness Limitation of forward bending suggests that the disorder may be referred from the spine.

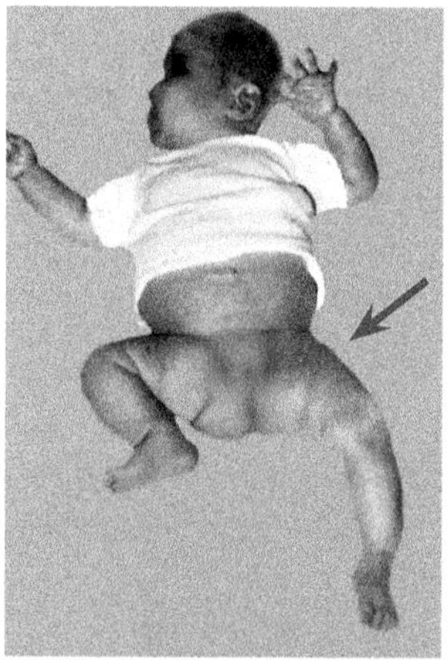

C Observation Observation revealed pseudoparalysis of the left leg, and the left hip is positioned in slight flexion and external rotation. These findings are typical for septic arthritis of the left hip.

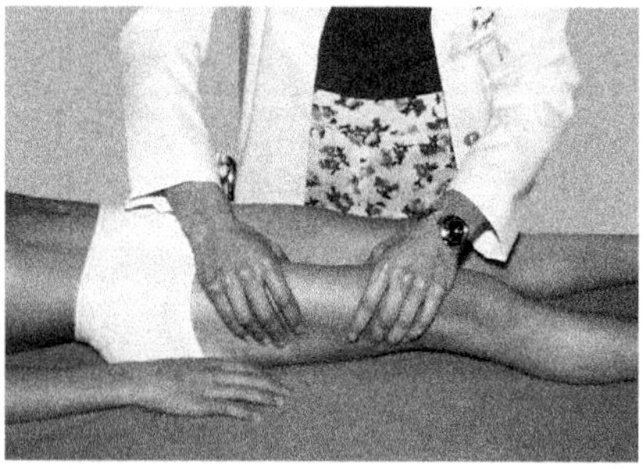

D Thigh tenderness Palpate for localized tenderness.

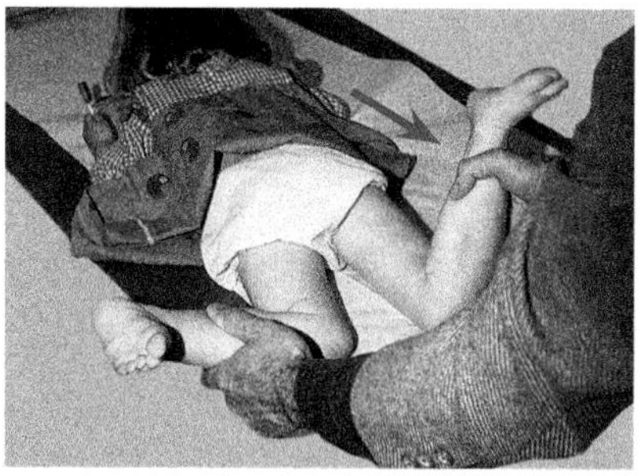

E Hip rotation test This child has reduced medial rotation of the right hip due to toxic synovitis.

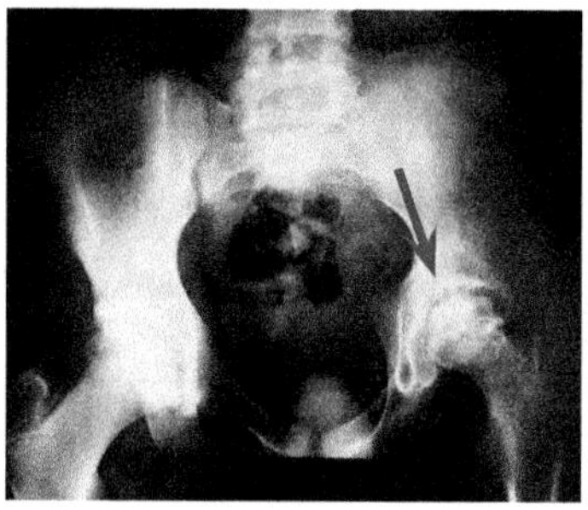

F Joint damage from septic arthritis Note the severe joint damage from septic arthritis treated two weeks after onset.

Causes

Establish the diagnosis by considering the features and the common causes of hip pain [A].

Infection is a common cause of pelvic pain. The early diagnosis of septic arthritis is critical because it may severely damage or destroy the hip joint [F, previous page]. Because of the tenuous vascularity of the hip, joint infections must be diagnosed and drained promptly. Soft tissue abscess, such as the psoas abscess, may be suspected by the finding of tenderness on rectal examination and soft tissue swelling on the AP radiograph of the pelvis. Confirm the diagnosis by CT or MRI studies. Sacroiliac infections are identified by bone scans.

Stress injuries or repetitive microtraumas may cause hip pain. Such pain is most common during the second decade and often follows vigorous activity. It may involve the upper femur, but more commonly it involves the origin of muscles such as the greater trochanter and iliac spines. The diagnosis is usually suggested by the history, physical findings of well-localized tenderness, and negative radiographs but a positive bone scan.

Tumors A variety of tumors occur about the hip and pelvis. Osteoid osteoma is common in the proximal femur and produces pain in a pattern that is nearly diagnostic. The pain is nocturnal and relieved by aspirin. The tumor produces reactive bone with a radiolucent nidus on conventional radiographs [B].

Toxic synovitis (or transient synovitis) is a idiopathic benign inflammation of the hip joint [C] that occurs in children. This condition is important, as it may be confused with septic arthritis and less commonly with LCP disease. The condition causes pain and irritability of the hip. It subsides spontaneously over several days.

Idiopathic chondrolysis This uncommon condition is seen in late childhood or adolescence. The hip becomes painful and stiff, and joint space narrowing is present [D]. See page 228.

Rheumatoid spondylitis Unlike juvenile rheumatoid arthritis, hip involvement may be the first sign of rheumatoid spondylitis. Establish the diagnosis with serologic tests.

	Night pain	Trauma history	Sick child	Pseudoparalysis	Hip rotation test +	Localized tenderness	Snapping hip	Radiographs	Bone scan	MRI	Ultrasound
Acute trauma		+		+		+		+			
Septic arthritis			+	+	+						+
Slipped epiphysis					+			+			
LCP disease					+			+			
Toxic synovitis					+						
Tumor	+							+			
Overuse injury		+				+			+		
Rheum. spondylitis					+						
Snapping hip							+			+	
Labral tear							+			+	
Chondrolysis					+			+			

A Hip pain and major diagnostic features These are some of the major clinical features that differentiate each cause of pain.

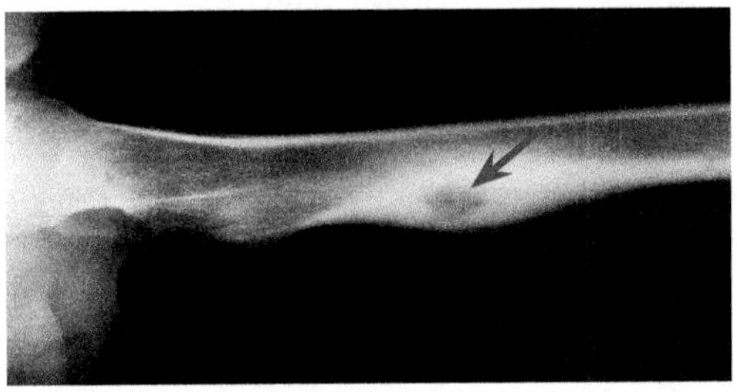

B Osteoid osteoma These lesions are common in the proximal femur and cause night pain.

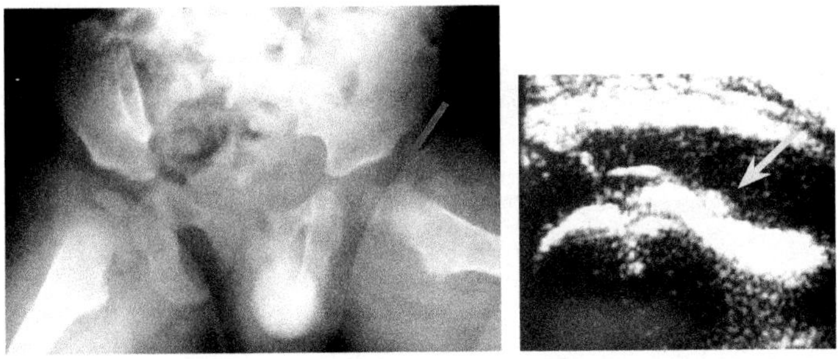

C Toxic synovitis The hip is often positioned in slight flexion and external rotation (red arrow). Ultrasound studies often show an effusion (yellow arrow).

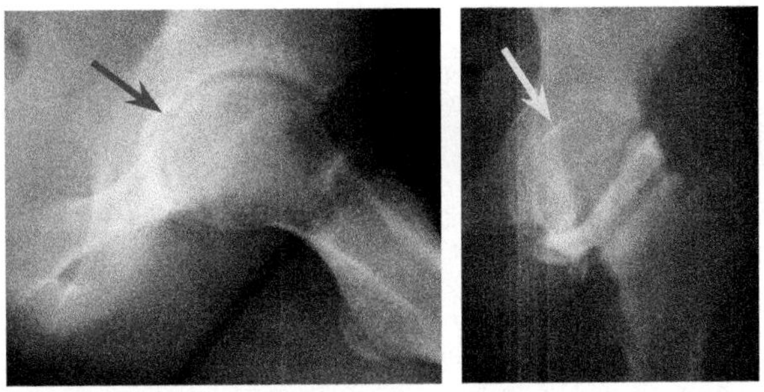

D Chondrolysis This hip shows narrowing of the joint space on conventional radiographs (red arrow), and the arthrogram (yellow arrow) shows thinning of the cartilage on the femoral head.

Developmental Hip Dysplasia

DDH is a generic term describing a spectrum of anatomic abnormalities of the hip that may be congenital or develop during infancy or childhood. The spectrum covers mild defects such as a shallow acetabulum to severe defects such as *teratologic* dislocations. Teratologic dislocations occur before birth and include severe deformity of both the acetabulum and proximal femur.

Incidence

DDH incidence depends on how much of the spectrum is included [A]. At birth, hip instability is noted in 0.5–1% of joints, but classic DDH occurs in about 0.1% of infants. The incidence of mild dysplasia contributing to adult degenerative arthritis is substantial. It is thought that half of the women who develop degenerative arthritis have preexisting acetabular dysplasia.

Etiology

DDH is considered to be inherited by a polygenic mode. DDH is more common in breech deliveries [B], in children with joint laxity [C], and in girls.

Pathology

The acetabulum is often shallow and maldirected. The proximal femur shows antetorsion and coxa valga. Structural interpositions between the displaced femoral head and acetabulum are common [D]. The iliopsoas tendon is insinuated between the femoral head and acetabulum, causing a depression in the joint capsule. This gives the capsule an hourglass configuration. The acetabular labrum is inverted into the joint, the ligamentum teres is enlarged, and the acetabulum may contain fat (pulvinar).

Natural History

Residual acetabular dysplasia is common in DDH. This may occur even following an apparently good early reduction [F]. The disability from dysplasia is related to the degree of displacement [E]. Greater displacement causes more function disability. Pain is most common with severe subluxation or articulation in a false acetabulum [G].

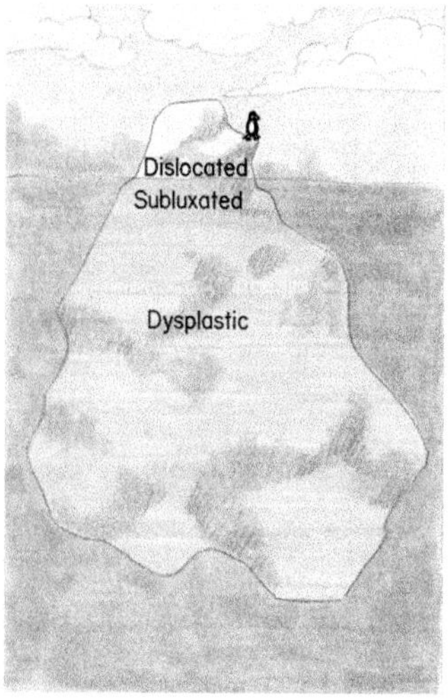

A Spectrum of hip dysplasia Dislocated hips are usually diagnosed during infancy, but hip dysplasia may not become evident until adult life and then present as degenerative arthritis.

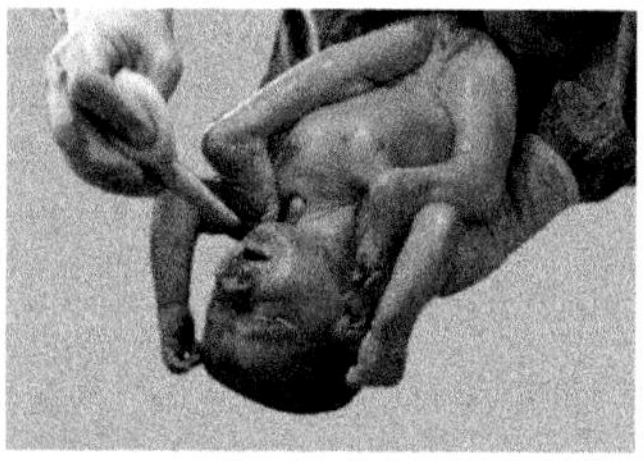

B Breech association DDH is often associated with breech presentation.

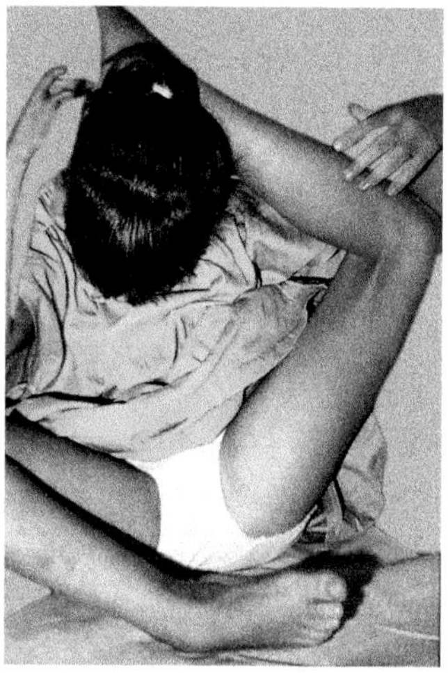

C DDH and joint laxity Children with DDH often show excessive joint laxity.

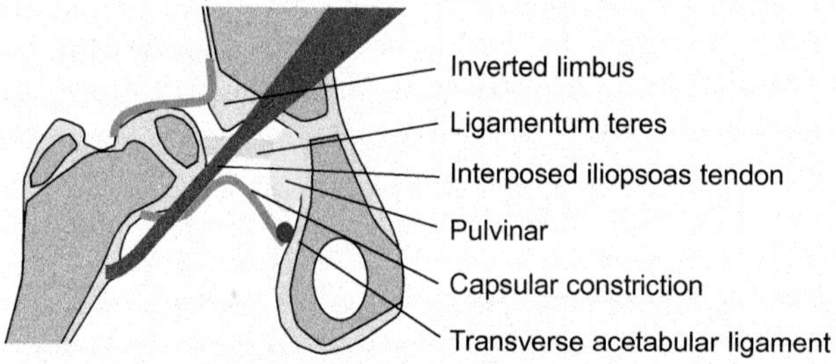

D Structures blocking reduction in DDH These interpositions may block reduction of the hip.

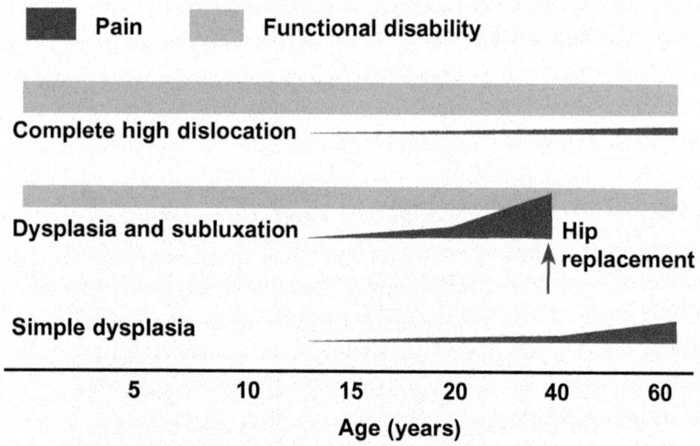

E Conceptual chart showing disability from DDH Pain, altered function, and cosmetic problems often result from persisting hip deformity due to DDH.

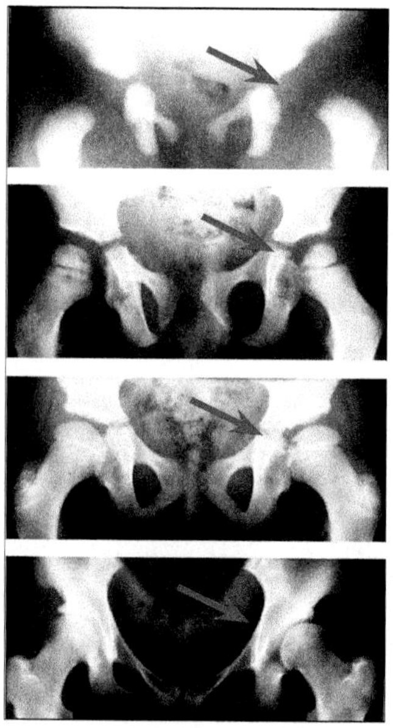

F DDH with residual acetabular dysplasia Radiographs at birth, 3, 10, and 19 years (top to bottom) show persisting dysplasia.

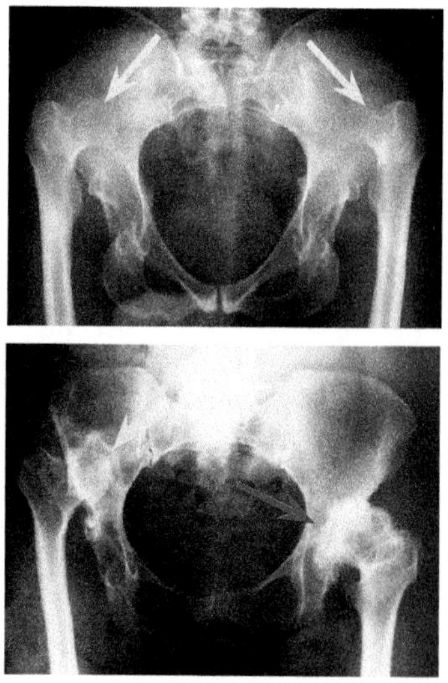

G Adult degenerative arthritis Note that arthritis is most severe in the subluxated (red arrow) hip as compared with the totally dislocated hips (yellow arrows).

Diagnosis

The early diagnosis of DDH is critical to a successful outcome. Acetabular development is abnormal if a hip is subluxated or dislocated. Delays in management result in residual abnormalities and eventual degenerative arthritis.

Neonatal examination Every newborn should be screened for signs of hip instability. The hip should be examined using both the Barlow and Ortolani techniques [A and B]. Examine one hip at a time. The infant should be quiet and comfortable so the muscles about the hip are relaxed. Use no force. Test for instability in several positions.

Changing manifestations of DDH The signs of DDH change with the infant's age [C]. For example, the incidence of hip instability declines rapidly, 50% within the first week. The classic findings of stiffness and shortening increase over the first few weeks of life. These signs become well established in the older infant [D].

Repeated examinations The hip should be examined during each "well baby" examination. In the neonatal period, DDH is detected by different signs, based on the infant's age. In early infancy, instability is the most reliable sign. Later, limitation of abduction and shortening are common. Beware of bilateral dislocations, as they are more difficult to identify [E]. If hip abduction is less than about 60° on both sides, order an imaging study.

Mother's intuition Although not proven, a common clinical experience is the accuracy of the mother's sense that something is wrong. Take the mother's intuition seriously [F].

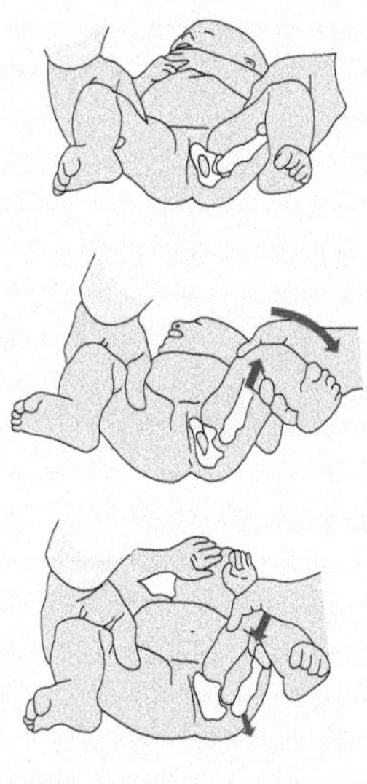

A Barlow's sign Hip instability is demonstrated by attempting to gently displace the hip out of the socket over the posterior acetabulum.

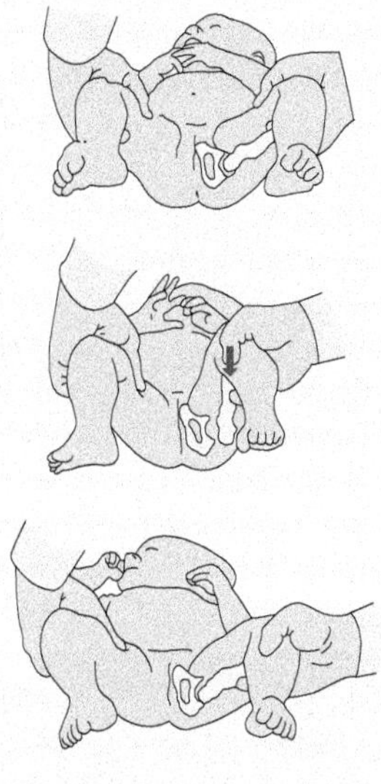

B Ortolani's sign The thigh is first adducted and depressed to subluxate the hip. The thigh is then abducted. The hip reduces with a palpable "clunk."

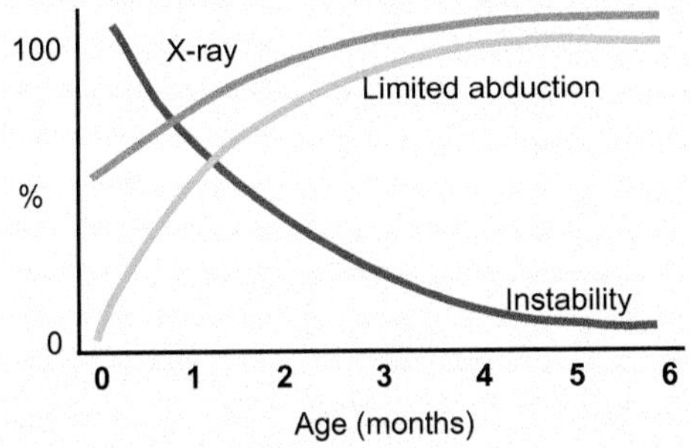

C Changing signs of DDH With increasing age, signs change.

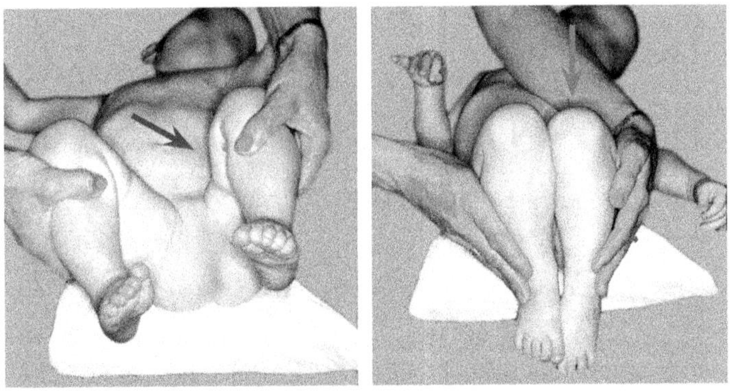

D DDH in older infant Note the limited abduction (red arrow) and shortening (blue arrow) on the affected left side.

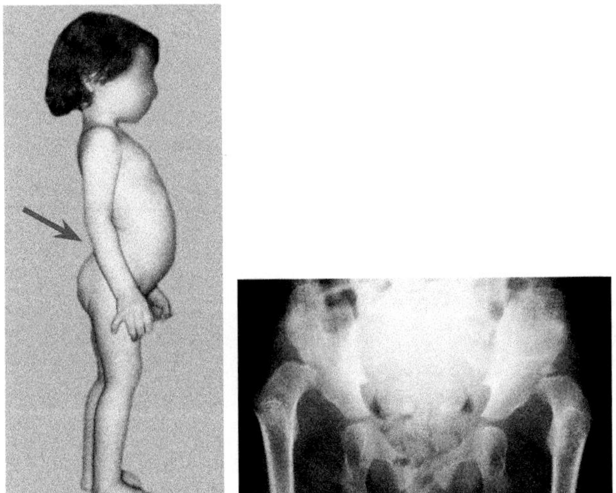

E Bilateral DDH This girl has symmetrical bilateral dislocations. The hip symmetry makes early diagnosis more difficult. Note the typical lumbar lordosis (arrow) that occurs with high dislocations.

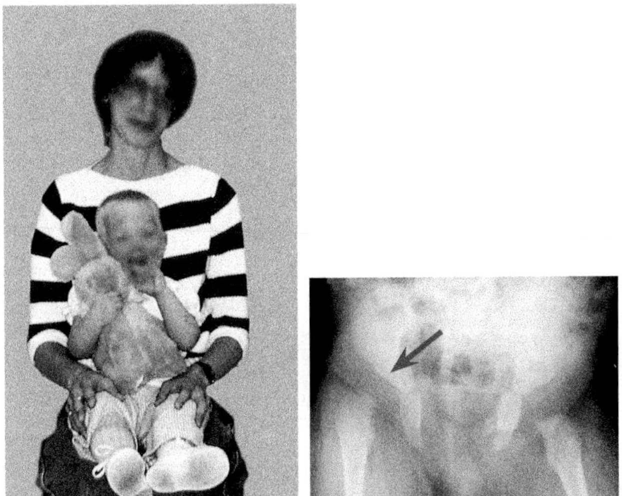

F Mother's intuition This mother had DDH as a child. She suspected that her son's hip was abnormal, but the primary care physician found nothing on examination. She insisted on a radiograph. This study demonstrated a dislocation (red arrow). This scenario is not uncommon.

Factor	Comment
Positive family history	Increases risk tenfold
Breech position	Increases risk five- to tenfold
Torticollis	Associated deformity
Foot deformities Calcaneovalgus Metatarsus adductus	Intrauterine constraint
Knee deformities Hyperextension Dislocation	Associated with teratogenic type dislocation

A Risk factors These factors increase the risk of DDH and signal the need for careful and repeated examinations and imaging studies.

Hip-at-risk factors The presence of several factors increase the risk of DDH [A and C]. When risk factors are present, the infant should be examined repeatedly and the hip imaged by ultrasound or radiography.

Hip "clicks" and asymmetrical thigh folds Hip clicks are fine, short-duration, high-pitched sounds that are common and benign. These are to be differentiated from "clunks," the sensation of the hip being displaced over the acetabular margin. Clicks and asymmetrical thigh folds are common in normal infants [B].

Radiography Radiographs become progressively more diagnostic with increasing age. By 2–3 months of age, radiography is reliable and this is the optimum age for screening by this method. A single AP radiograph is adequate. Draw the reference lines and measure the acetabular index. Normally, the AI in early infancy falls below 30°, is questionable in the 30°– 40° range, and abnormal if above 40°. Hip subluxation or dislocation may often be demonstrated by the metaphysis of the femur positioned lateral to the lateral acetabular marginal line [D].

Ultrasound imaging The effectiveness of ultrasound imaging depends upon the skill and experience of the examiner. A skillful ultrasound evaluation is an effective screening technique for DDH [E]. The major problem with this screening is in the interpretation of the findings. If the hip is unstable, imaging is unnecessary. Imaging is appropriate to evaluate a suspicious finding, when hip-at-risk factors are present, and to monitor the effectiveness of treatment.

Documentation Document your hip evaluation. The failure to diagnose DDH is a common cause of suits against physicians. If the diagnosis is delayed, a record showing that appropriate examinations of the hip were made provides the best defense. DDH may be missed by even the most skilled examiners. Failure to screen for DDH is not acceptable by current standards.

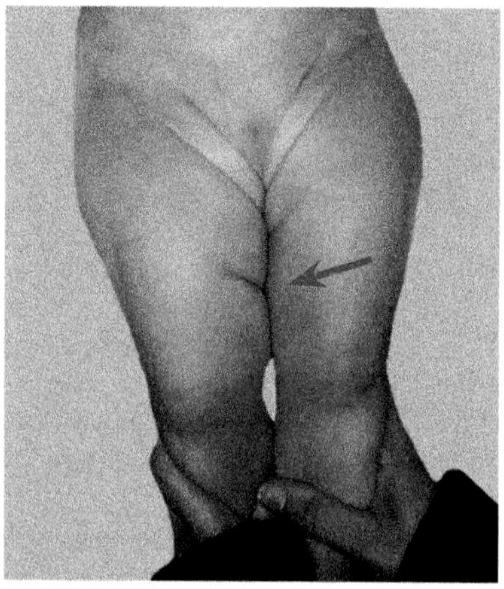

B Asymmetrical thigh folds These occur in up to 20% of normal infants.

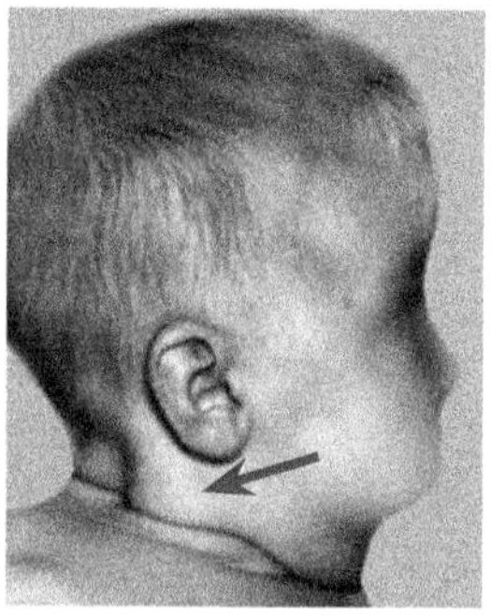

C DDH and torticollis This infant showed the typical features of muscular torticollis with a sternocleidomastoid tumor (red arrow). A radiograph of the pelvis demonstrated DDH.

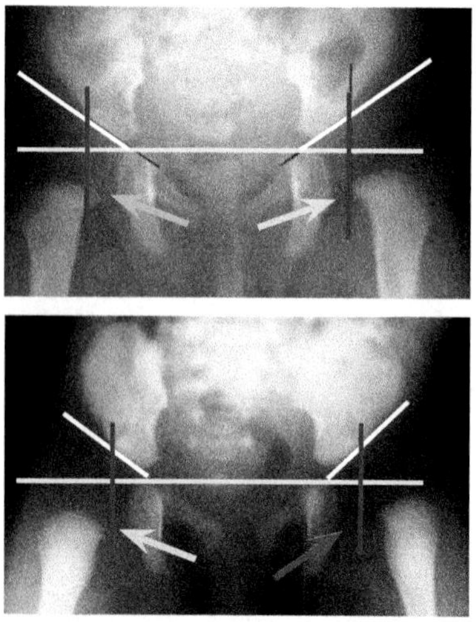

D Assessing radiographs in early infancy Note that in the normal hip (green arrow) the femoral metaphysis lies medial to the acetabular line. In the subluxated hip (yellow arrow) and dislocated hip (red arrow) the metaphysis falls progressively more lateral.

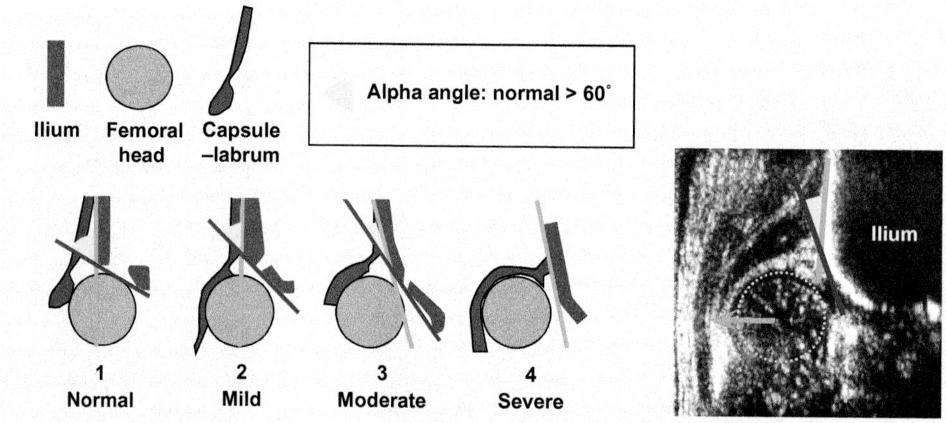

E Graf grading of DDH by ultrasound Drawing shows how the hips can be graded by measurements based on the ultrasound evaluation. The grades shown are divided by Graf into four types. Each is subdivided into subtypes (not shown). Reference lines are drawn to show the iliac margin (green), and the joint inclination (red). The alpha angle (yellow arc) can be constructed to show severity. The ultrasound image shows a severe displacement (orange arrow) of the femoral head (tan circle) in an infant with DDH.

Management

The management of DDH is challenging. Delays in diagnosis or problems in management often lead to residual anatomic defects and subsequent degenerative arthritis. The objectives of management include early diagnosis, reduction of the dislocation, avoidance of avascular necrosis, and correction of residual dysplasia.

Birth to 6 Months

This is the ideal age for management [A]. Treat DDH in this age group first with an abduction orthosis such as the Pavlik harness.

Pavlik harness This widely used orthosis allows motion in flexion and abduction. Be certain that it is fitted properly [B], both initially and as applied by the parents. Advise the family on ways of transporting the infant [C and E].

See the infant weekly in the brace. Make certain the brace is being fitted properly [D] and progress is being made. The hip should become progressively more stable.

If harness treatment is successful, continue full-time bracing for 6–8 weeks to allow the hip to become stable. Monitor with ultrasound imaging or by AP radiographs of the pelvis about every 2–4 weeks. Continue the brace at night until the radiographs are normal.

If a dislocated hip has not reduced by 3–4 weeks, abandon Pavlik treatment. Persisting with this treatment may cause head deformity and posterior fixation, making closed reduction difficult or impossible. Proceed with closed or open reduction. Manage as is described for infants over 6 months of age.

Night splinting After the hip is reduced and stable, continue with night splinting to facilitate acetabular development. Continue until the radiographs are normal. A simple abduction splint is inexpensive and is well accepted by the infant.

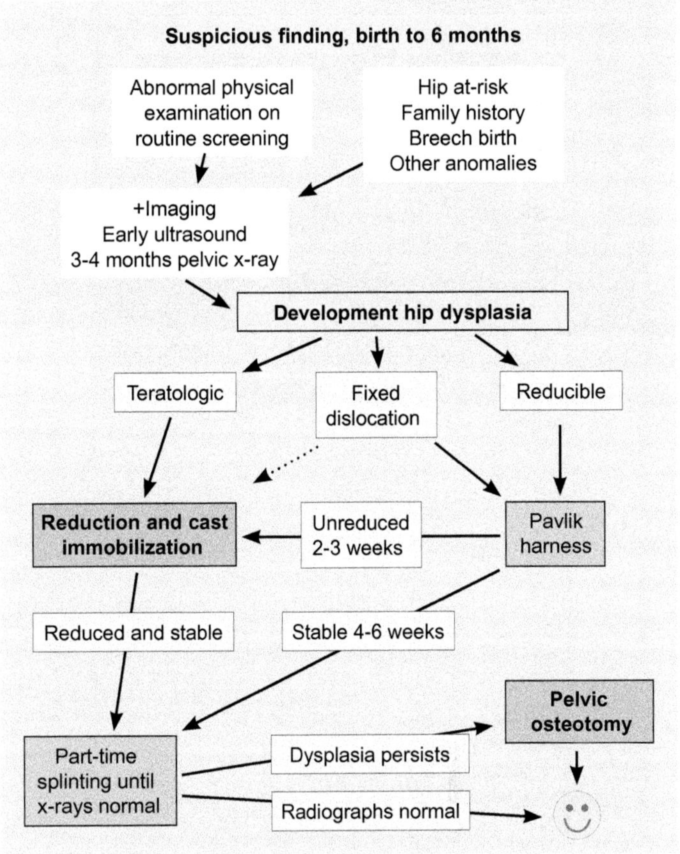

A DDH management flowchart, birth to 6 months

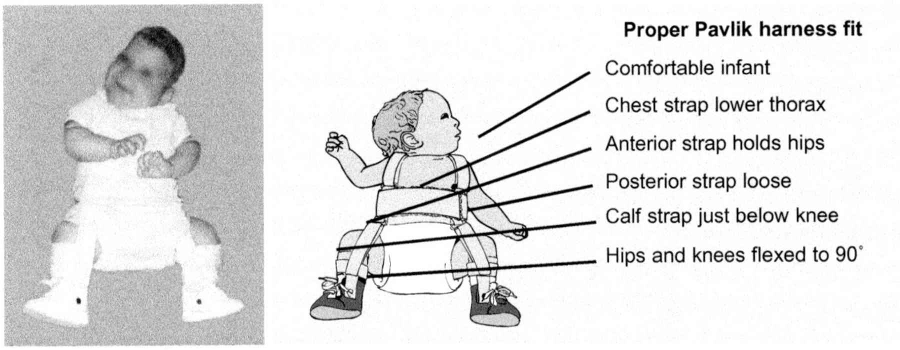

B Proper fit of Pavlik harness The harness should be carefully fitted. Make certain it is the proper size for the infant. The harness must be comfortable. Check the fit after the parent applies the harness to assess problems before the parent leaves the clinic.

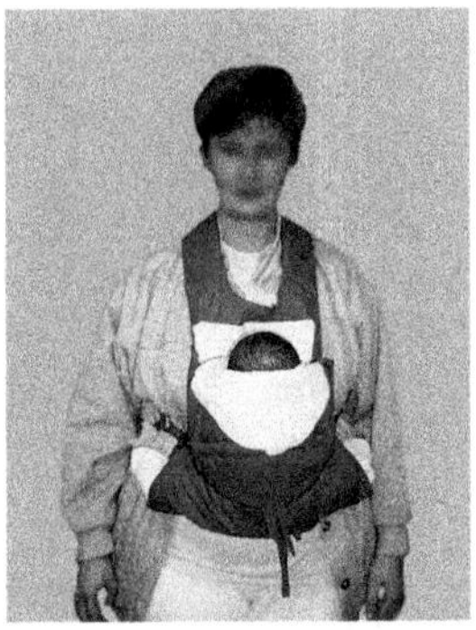

C DDH mobility These carriers are ideal, as they provide abduction, mobility, and comfort for the infant and parent.

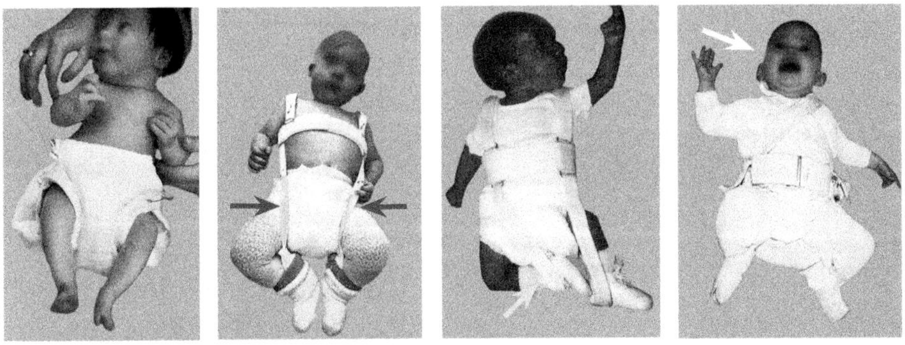

D Pitfalls in management Triple diaper management (orange arrow) is ineffective and gives a false sense that treatment has been initiated. Pavlik harness errors are common. Make certain that the straps are not too tight (red arrows), the calf strap is not too low (yellow arrow), and the infant is comfortable (white arrow).

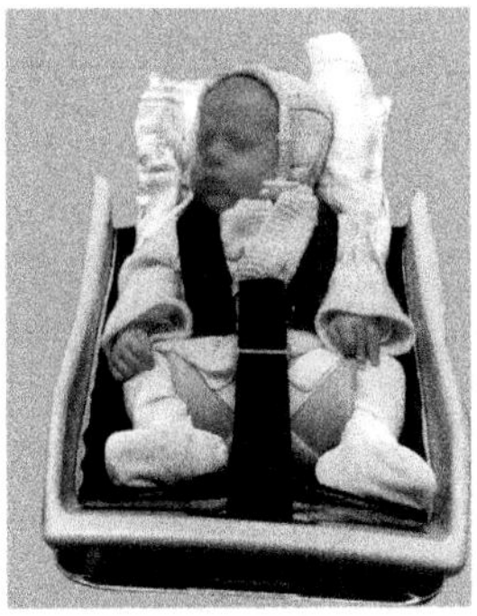

E DDH splints and car transportation These splints should fit into standard infant car seats.

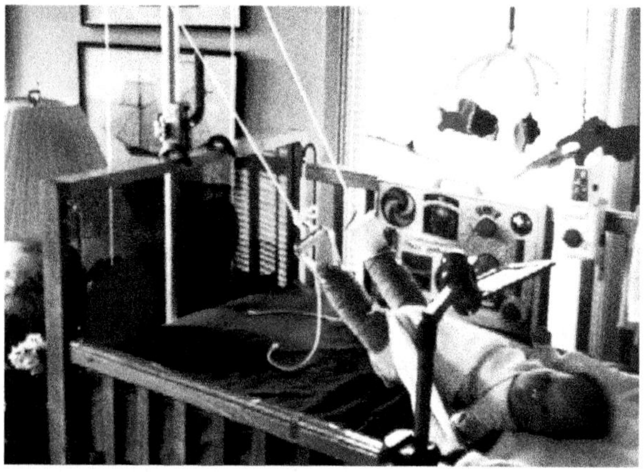

A Home traction Setup at home is less expensive, less stressful for the infant, and often more convenient for the family.

6 to 18 Months

In this age group, most cases of DDH can be managed by closed reduction and spica cast immobilization [A and C].

Traction The need for traction is controversial. The current practice is to omit traction in most cases. Traction may be useful if the hip is stiff and closed treatment is planned. Use home traction when possible. Maintain for about 3 weeks with the legs flexed and abducted about 45° with 2–3 pounds of traction applied to each limb [B].

Scheduling Schedule and obtain consent for a closed, or possibly open, reduction.

Reduction by closed means is first tried. If unsuccessful, open reduction is required.

Arthrography is useful when the quality of reduction is uncertain or the decision regarding management is difficult.

Follow-up After reduction, the infant should be followed carefully to assess the effect of time on growth, reduction, and acetabular development. Follow with AP radiographs made quarterly through infancy, yearly though early childhood, and then about every third year during middle and late childhood. The frequency of follow-up studies should be individualized based on the severity of any residual dysplasia.

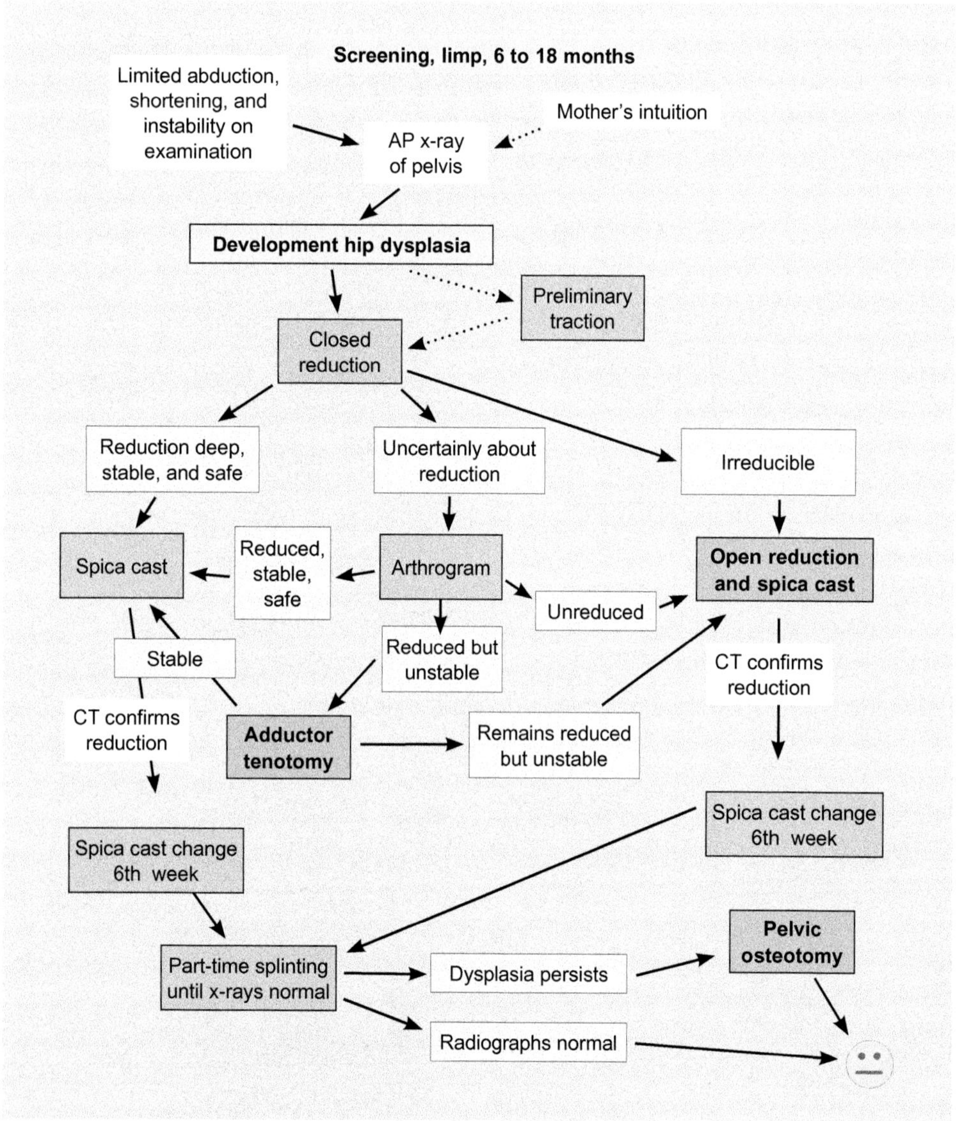

B DDH management flowchart, 6 to 18 months

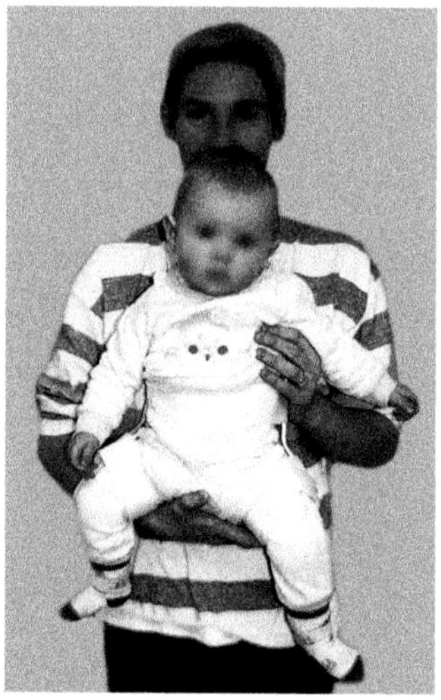

C Spica cast immobilization Infants require cast immobilization to retain the reduction of a dislocated hip.

18 to 30 Months

In this age group, operative management is usually required [A]. Occasionally, an infant with a "loose dislocation" can be managed as described in the flowchart for infants 6–18 months of age [B, previous page]. If the hip is unusually stiff, be prepared to add femoral shortening, as described for management of children over 30 months of age (next page).

Management Manage with an open reduction through an anterolateral approach and perform a concurrent Salter or Pemberton osteotomy. The open reduction is technically challenging. Add the pelvic osteotomy to improve results and save the child a second procedure.

Open reduction is the most difficult part of the procedure. The pelvic osteotomies are relatively simple, but the reduction can sometimes be difficult. The open reduction requires good exposure, careful dissection to minimize the risk of avascular necrosis, and a concentric reduction. The obstacles to reduction must be corrected [C].

Iliopsoas tendon This tendon is interposed between the femoral head and acetabulum and must be released.

Capsular constriction Open the capsule widely to ensure a complete release.

Transverse acetabular ligament This structure lies across the base of the acetabulum and will block a deep concentric reduction unless released.

Pulvinar is fatty fibrous tissue that often fills the depth of the acetabulum. Remove with a rongeur.

Ligamentum teres is elongated and sometimes hypertrophied. Removal is usually required. The vascular contribution through this ligament is minimal.

Limbus is often inverted and hypertrophied. Do not excise this structure. Once the hip is concentrically reduced, the limbus will remodel and form the labrum, an important structure for hip stability and longevity.

Concurrent osteotomy This choice may be based on the pathology and on the experience and preference of the surgeon.

Femoral osteotomy Proximal femoral varus osteotomy is becoming less commonly used because the acetabular dysplasia is the more significant deformity. Include only minimal rotational correction.

Salter innominate osteotomy is suitable for unilateral mild to moderate dysplasia. The procedure is simple, risks are few, and results good.

Pemberton pericapsular osteotomy [B] is more versatile because it can be performed bilaterally, does not destabilize the pelvis, provides greater correction, and requires no internal fixation. Avoid overcorrection. Stiffness is more common with this procedure, as the operation changes the shape of the acetabulum.

Postoperative care is determined by the treatment. If closed or open reduction is performed with an osteotomy, plan at least 12 weeks of spica cast immobilization. Usually, the cast is changed once or twice during this period. If a concurrent osteotomy is performed, stability is improved and only 6 weeks of immobilization are necessary.

Follow-up must be continued until the end of growth. Usually, a single AP radiograph of the pelvis is made every 6 months for 3 years, then yearly for 3 years, then every 3 years until maturity. At each visit, compare the current study with previous radiographs to determine the effect of time and growth on the development of the hip.

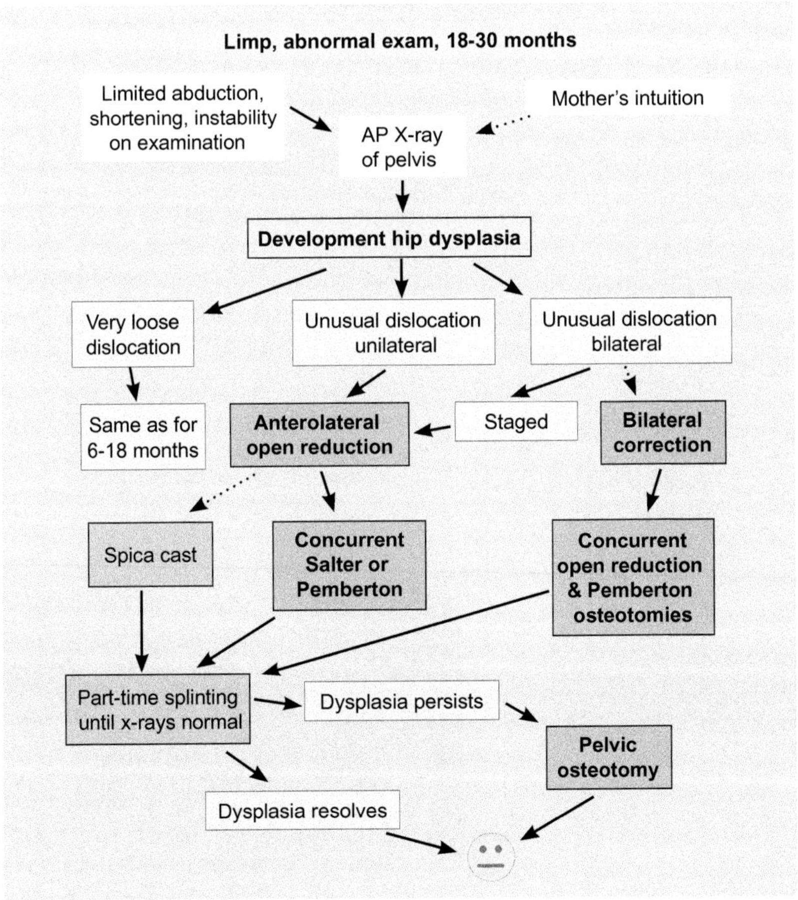

A DDH management flowchart, 18 to 30 months.

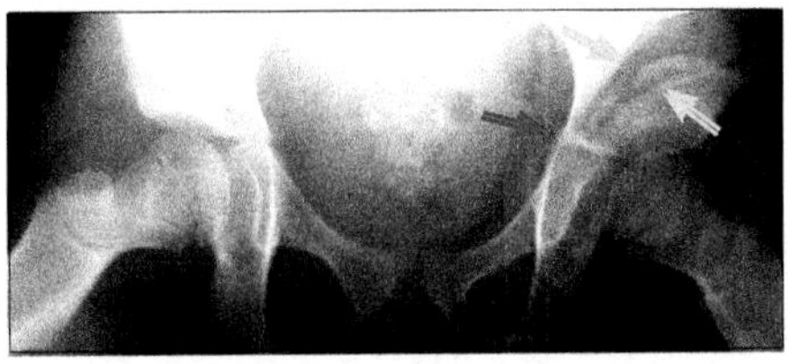

B Pemberton pericapsular osteotomy The osteotomy hinges at the triradiate cartilage (red arrow) and graft wedges open the osteotomy (yellow arrows).

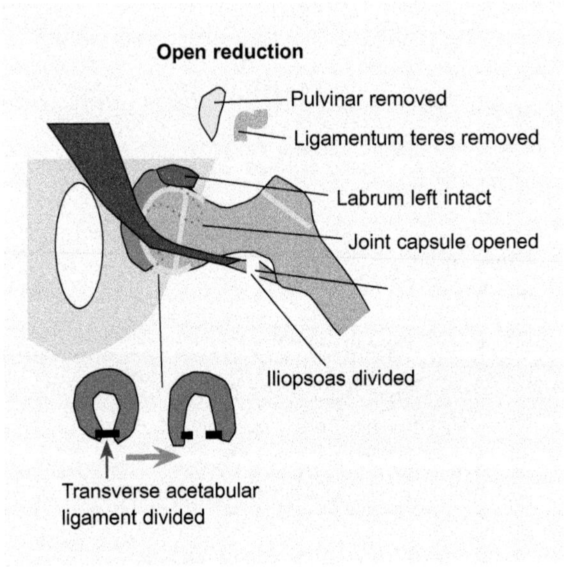

C Open reduction Open reduction is often difficult, and obstruction must be corrected.

30+ Months

In this older age group, the opportunity to achieve an early reduction has passed [C]. Avascular necrosis is still a threat and dysplasia is a certainty. Management is much more difficult and controversial, and a poor outcome with degenerative arthritis in early adult life is likely [B].

Indications for reduction Consider the child's age, bilaterality, the family's values, and the experience of the surgeon [C].

Early childhood In early childhood, reduction is usually appropriate. This requires a femoral shortening, open reduction, and a pelvic osteotomy [A]. If the dislocations are bilateral, correct one side at a time. Allow 6 months between procedures to allow the child to recover. Reduction improves function, reduces the limp, and may make performing some salvage procedure more effective.

Mid or late childhood In the older child, leaving the hip unreduced is a reasonable option, especially when the condition is bilateral [D]. The child will limp but is less likely to have pain. Hip arthroplasty may be elected after maturity.

Pelvic osteotomy Select the type of osteotomy based on the severity of the dysplasia and the age at the time of treatment. Select the Salter osteotomy for mild dysplasia. This procedure can be performed at any age and it does not change the shape of the acetabulum. Select the Pemberton osteotomy if dysplasia is moderate or severe. Avoid this osteotomy if the child is older than 6 years of age or if the acetabulum is hypoplastic.

Femoral osteotomy Femoral shortening osteotomy is nearly always necessary. If the deformity is severe, the femoral shortening is performed first, then the open reduction, followed by the pelvic osteotomy. The femoral fragments are then aligned, with gentle traction on the limb. The overlap is then determined and the overlapping distal femoral segment is resected. The procedure is primarily a shortening osteotomy with little or no varus or rotational components required.

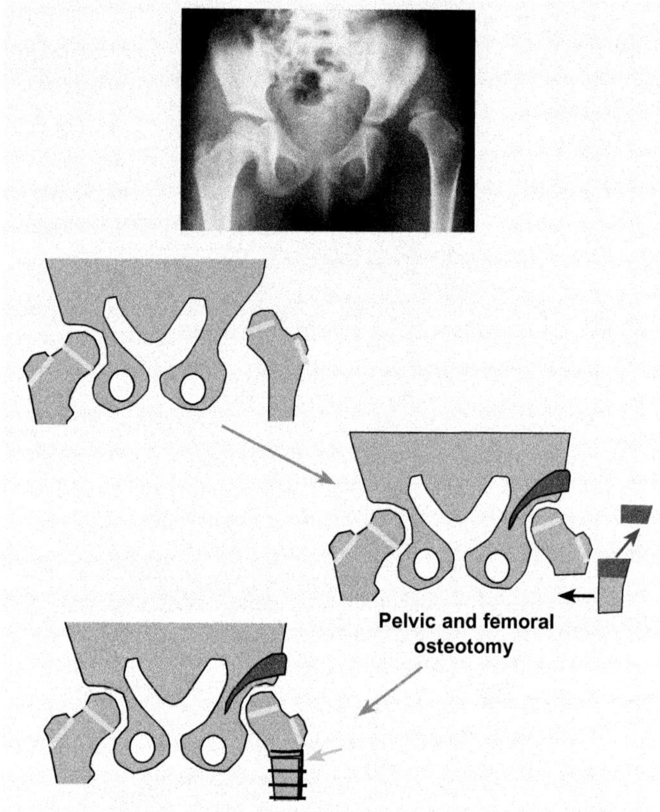

A Unilateral open reduction and pelvic and femoral osteotomy This combination of procedures is necessary in the child. Femoral shortening (red arrow) must be added to allow tension-free reduction. The distal fragment is aligned (black arrow) and fixed (green arrow).

DDH Management Objectives

Early concentric reduction
Avoid avascular necrosis
Overcome dysplasia

B DDH Management Avoiding avascular necrosis is often not appreciated as one of the primary objectives.

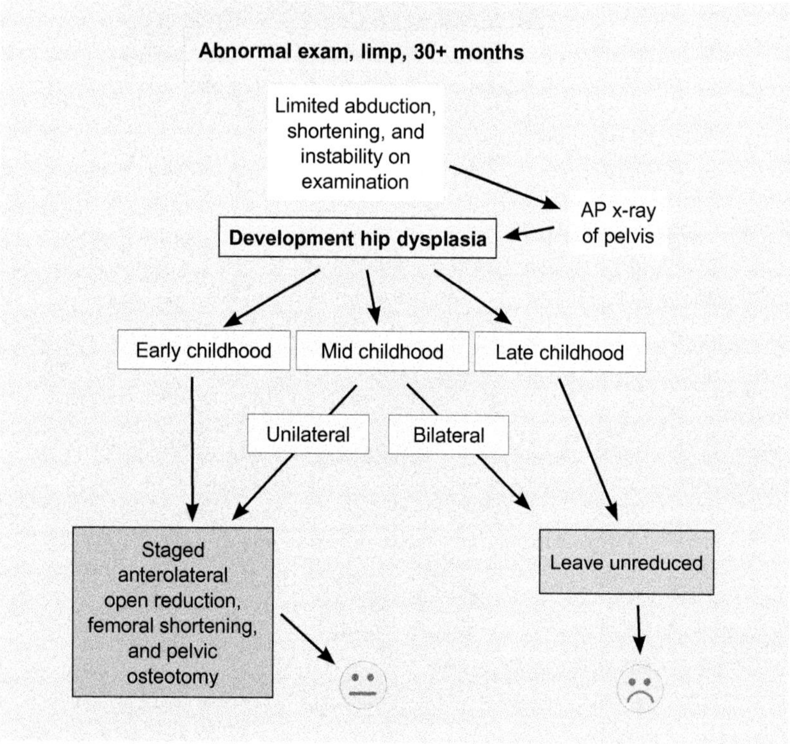

C DDH management flowchart, 30+ months Outcomes are seldom good or excellent in this age range.

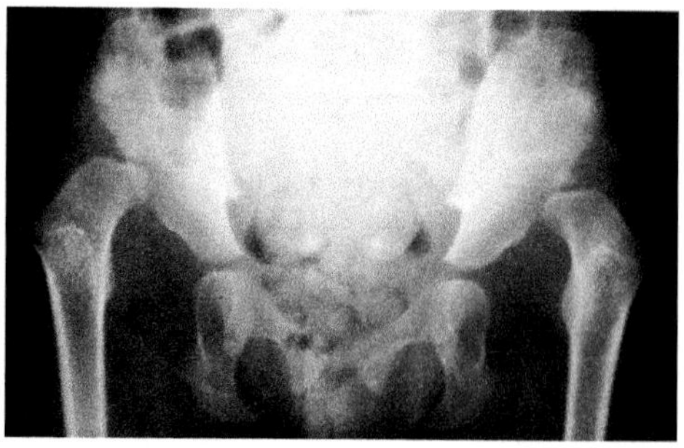

D Bilateral DDH in the child Staged corrections can be done in early childhood. In late childhood or adolescence, leaving the hips unreduced may be prudent.

Avascular Necrosis

Next to achieving a concentric reduction, preventing AVN is of utmost importance. Unless the necrosis is mild, this complication causes altered proximal femoral growth, creates deformity [A], and often leads to premature degenerative arthritis.

Types AVN includes severe necrosis, extensive physeal bridge formation [B], and shortening of the femoral neck, which leads to degenerative arthritis during adult life. At the other end of the AVN spectrum is the mild resolving form characterized by irregular ossification but without physeal bridge formation and subsequent deformity.

Type 1 This pattern is common and usually resolves spontaneously with no residual deformity.

Type 2 This type of bridge is common and may not be apparent in early childhood, becoming obvious toward the end of growth. These bridges cause a tethering of growth and, if eccentric, a tilting of the growth plate [E].

Type 3 This type of bridge is relatively uncommon and produces some shortening of the inferior aspect of the femoral neck and a more vertical orientation of the physis.

Type 4 Central bridges cause total arrest with shortening of the femoral neck, relative trochanteric overgrowth, and mild femoral shortening.

Management Manage the deformity based on its severity and the type of deformity [F].

Prevention Attempt to prevent AVN by using preliminary traction and open reduction in stiff hips with an obstructing limbus, percutaneous adductor tenotomy, femoral shortening in the child, and immobilization in the "safe" or human position. Despite all precautions, AVN may still occur [C].

Early signs The early signs of AVN [D] are often followed by evidence of a growth disturbance.

Deformity The type and severity of the deformity is related to the location and extent of the physeal bridge. The residual deformities of Type 4 AVN often require a combined distal and lateral transfer of the trochanter and a contralateral arrest of the distal femoral epiphysis. These procedures may be combined with the procedures performed at the age calculated to be appropriate for the epiphysiodesis to correct the leg length difference.

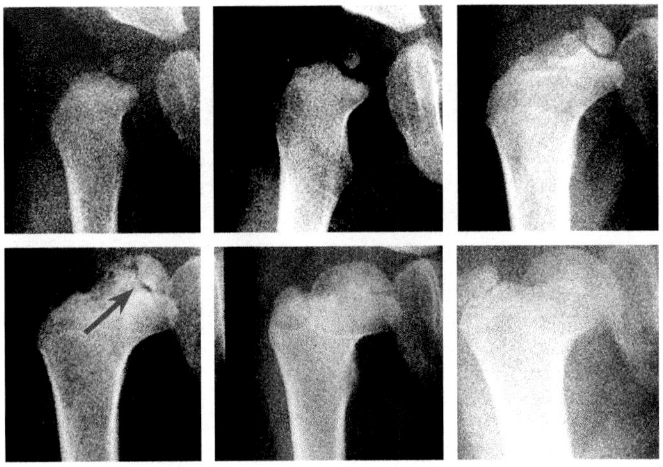

A Type 4 deformity Note the progressive changes throughout infancy and childhood from a central physeal bridge (red arrow) with shortening of the femoral neck and relative trochanteric overgrowth.

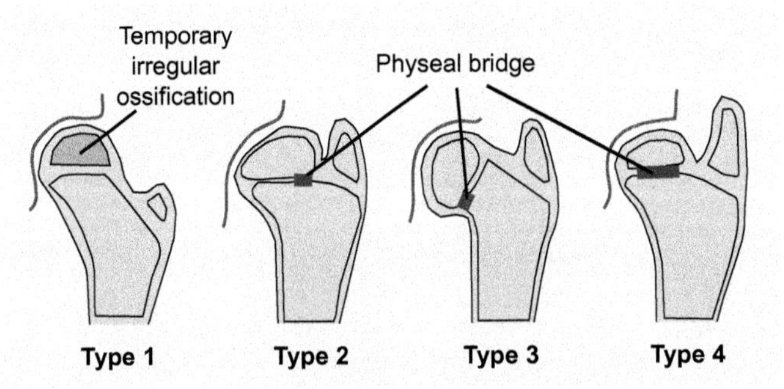

B Classification of AVN patterns These patterns depend upon the severity and location of the ischemic necrosis. Based on Kalamchi and MacEwen (1980) classification.

Reduction Pitfalls

Excessive abduction
Forced positions
Preliminary traction?
Reduction with inverted limbus?
Type of approach for open reduction?

C Reduction pitfalls Consider these factors. Some are controversial.

Early Signs of AVN

Failure of ossific nucleus to appear during the first year after reduction
Ossific nucleus fragments following reduction
Ossific nucleus fails to grow following reduction
Widening of the femoral neck

D Early signs of AVN These are signs that suggest AVN. From Salter.

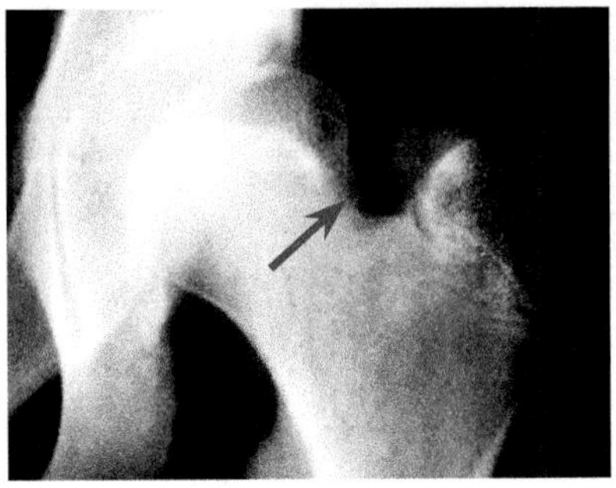

E Type 2 AVN Note the lateral bridge (arrow) with shortening of the superior portion of the femoral neck and tilting of the physis.

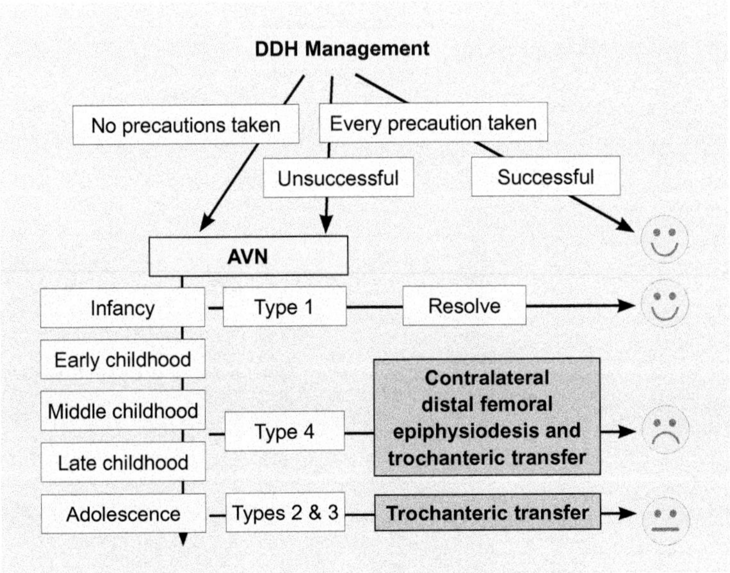

F Management of AVN occurring as a complication of DDH treatment

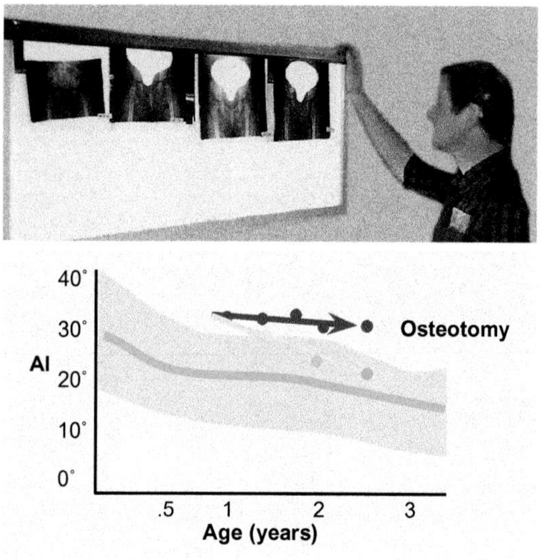

A Effect of growth on acetabular development Follow acetabular development by placing radiographs in chronologic order and assessing the effect of time. Measure the acetabular index (AI) for each study. Compare this sequence of measurements with the chart of normal AI measurements. If improvement occurs (yellow arrow) and the values become normal (green dots), treatment is not required. If AI values remain elevated (red dots and arrow), then pelvic osteotomy will be necessary.

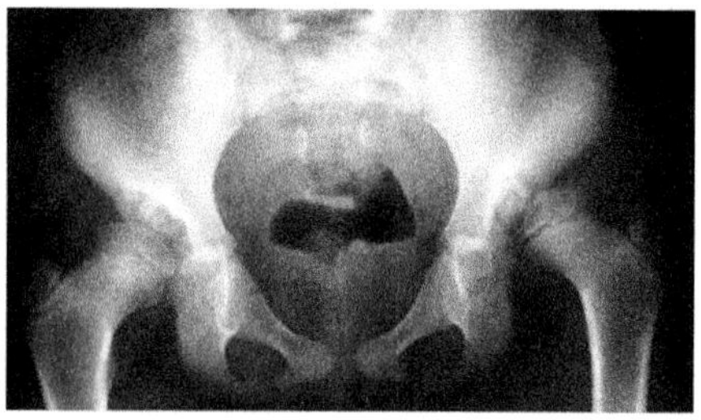

B Severe acetabular dysplasia Attempt to correct acetabular dysplasia before it becomes this severe.

Persisting dysplasia

The third objective in DDH management is the correction of persisting hip dysplasia [A]. Dysplasia should be corrected during growth to prevent osteoarthritis.

Dysplasia may involve the femur, the acetabulum [B], or both. The most pronounced deformity is in the acetabulum. The most severe dysplasia includes subluxation. Subluxation and dysplasia cause osteoarthritis, which may begin during the teen years. Disability occurs later with simple dysplasia.

Femoral dysplasia The proximal femur is anteverted and the head may not be spherical due to the dislocation. The deformity may be due to ischemic necrosis.

Acetabular dysplasia is the most pronounced deformity and includes shallowness and anterolateral orientation of the socket.

Acetabulofemoral relationship The femoral head is subluxated if not concentric with the acetabulum. The head may also be lateralized following growth with the head subluxated. The acetabulum often becomes saucer shaped, causing instability.

The femoral head may be spherical or aspherical as a result of ischemic necrosis. The fit with the acetabulum may be congruous or incongruous. Aspherical incongruity is common because, over years of growth, the acetabulum assumes a shape to match that of the femoral head.

Timing of correction Correct hip dysplasia as soon as it is evident that the rate of correction is unsatisfactory, preferably before age 5 years [C]. Establish a time line of a series of AP radiographs [A] of the pelvis taken at 4–6 month intervals during infancy and early childhood. Measure the acetabular index, note the smoothness of the acetabular roof (sourcil), and observe the development of the medial acetabulum (tear drop). Assess by studying the sequence of films. Perform a pelvic osteotomy if the AI remains abnormal and the other features remain dysplasic after 2 to 3 years of observation. Avoid delaying an obvious need for correction [B].

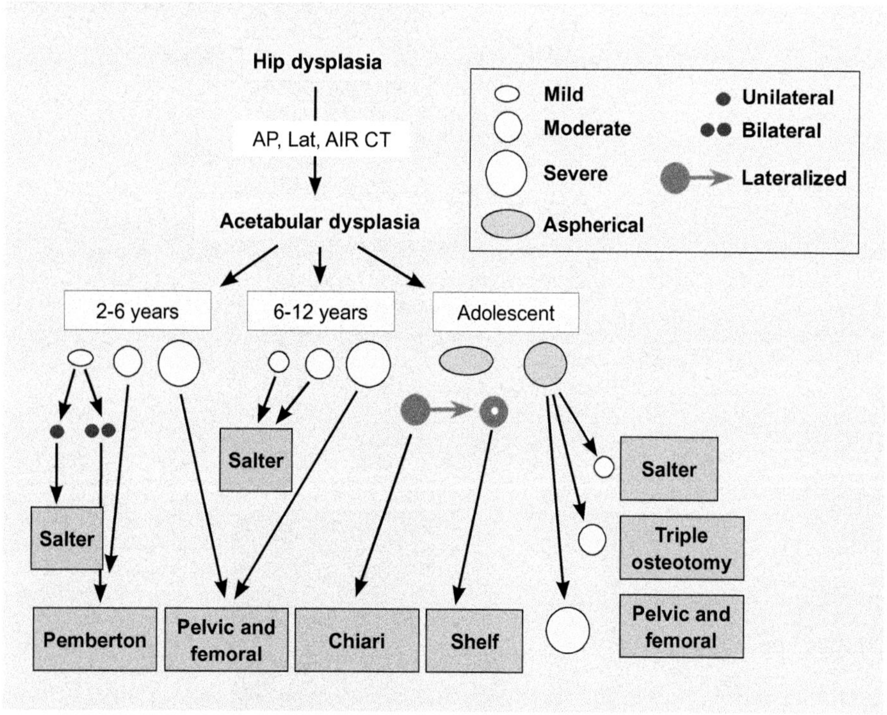

C Management of acetabular dysplasia Manage based on age, severity, congruity, and lateralization.

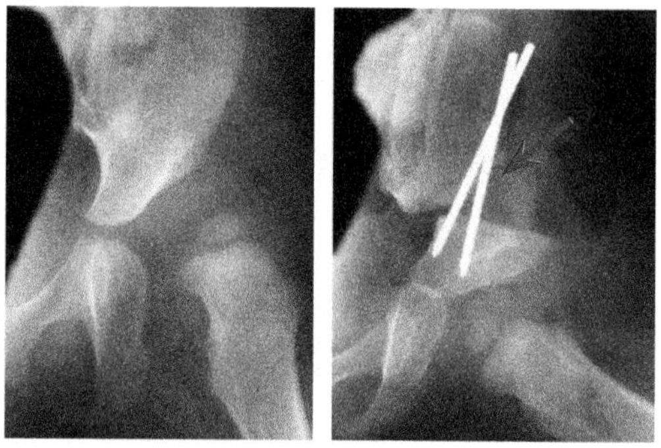

D Salter osteotomy This procedure is useful for mild to moderate dysplasia and may be performed at any age after about 18 months.

Principles of correction Proper correction of hip dysplasia in DDH follows these certain basic principles:

1. Correct the primary or most severe deformity. This is usually the acetabular deformity.
2. Correction should be adequate. If the deformity is severe, combine a pelvic and femoral osteotomy or perform a shelf operation.
3. Avoid creating incongruity. Avoid the Pemberton procedure in the older child. Consider the shelf or Chiari procedure if aspherical congruity is present.
4. Medialize the lateralized hip in the older child with a Chiari osteotomy.
5. Articular cartilage is more durable than fibrocartilage as develops in the shelf and Chiari procedures.

Reconstructive procedures These are procedures that provide articular cartilage for load bearing. Select the appropriate procedure based on the site of deformity, age, severity, and congruity [C, previous page]. The choices are numerous [A].

Femoral osteotomy Femoral shortening is essential in the older child with unreduced DDH. Remove just enough bone to allow reduction. Reduce the neck–shaft angle by about 20°. Limit rotational correction to about 20°.

Salter osteotomy This is the best choice for correcting mild deformities at any age [D, previous page]. The osteotomy will reduce the AI about 10°–15° and the CE angle by 10°.

Pemberton osteotomy This is the best choice for bilateral or moderate to severe dysplasia [B] in children under the age of 6 years.

Dega osteotomy The osteotomy is more posterior in the ilium, providing posterior and lateral coverage most suitable for neurodysplasia correction.

Triple osteotomies Several types are available. They provide the best choice for correcting moderate dysplasia in adolescence when spherical congruity is present [C]. These procedures are technically challenging.

Ganz osteotomy This periacetabular osteotomy allows major correction appropriate just before or after skeletal maturity [C]. The procedure is technically challenging.

Sutherland procedure This procedure is a double innominate osteotomy seldom performed because correction is limited.

Salvage procedures These procedures create an articular surface of fibrocartilage that is more prone to degeneration with time.

Chiari osteotomy This is appropriate when the hip is lateralized and severely dysplasic. It may be used with aspherical congruity. Avoid excessive medialization. Coverage is by fibrocartilage.

Shelf procedure This procedure enlarges the acetabulum with fibrocartilage. It is versatile and may be considered for severe dysplasia without lateralization when aspherical congruity exists. This is the least risky of the major procedures.

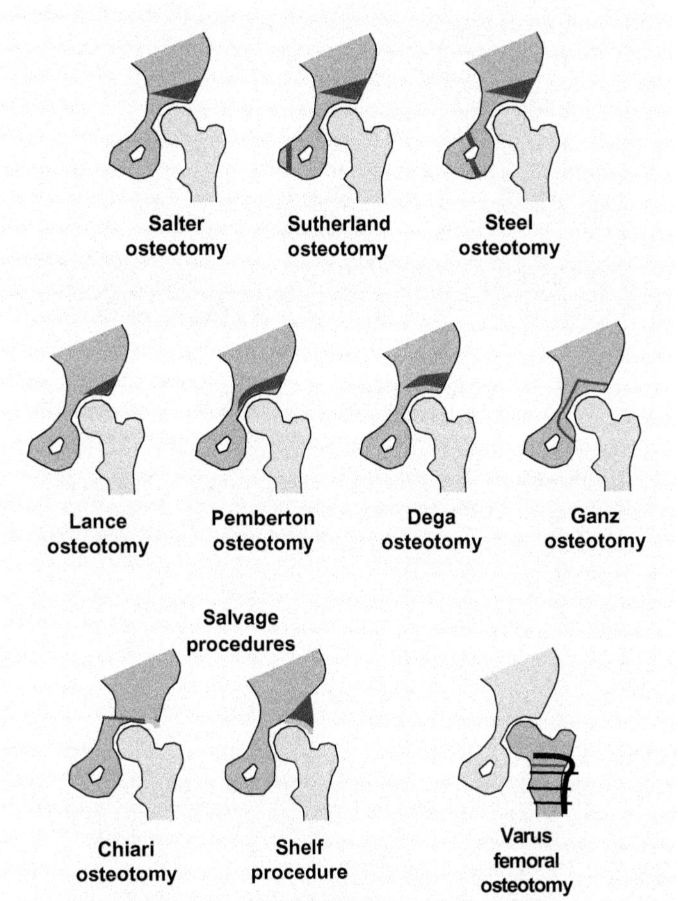

A Options for osteotomies of the hip Procedure is shown in red. Orange lines show fibrocartilage articulations.

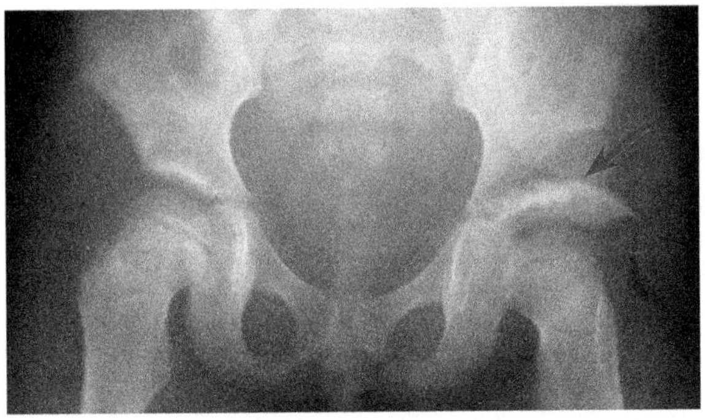

B Pemberton osteotomy This osteotomy extended into the triradiate cartilage and provided excellent correction (red arrow).

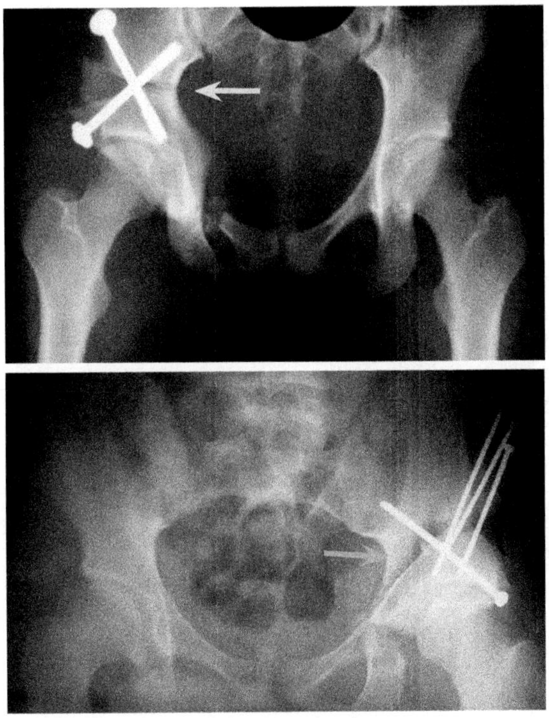

C Pelvic osteotomies These procedures are useful in dysplasia in the adolescent patient. The triple innominate osteotomy (yellow arrow) and the Ganz osteotomy (orange arrow) are shown.

Legg-Calvé-Perthes Disease

Legg-Calvé-Perthes Disease (LCP), or simply Perthes, disease is an idiopathic juvenile avascular necrosis of the femoral head. Synonyms include Waldenström's disease and coxa plana. It affects about 1 in 10,000 children. Males are affected four times more often than girls, and it is bilateral in 10–15% of subjects.

Etiology

The cause of LCP disease is unknown. Affected children are small and delayed in maturation, suggesting a constitutional disorder. Vascularity is tenuous in early childhood, and developmental variations in vascular pattern [A] are more common in boys, predisposing some individuals. In addition, trauma, alterations in the coagulability of blood, and endocrine and metabolic disorders may be contributing factors [C]. Possibly several factors combine to cause the disease.

Pathology

The pathology is consistent with repeated bouts of infarction and subsequent pathologic fractures. Synovitis and effusion, cartilaginous hypertrophy, bony necrosis, and collapse are present. Widening and flattening of the femoral head follow. Most deformity occurs in the "fragmentation phase." If necrosis is extensive and the support of the lateral pillar is lost, the head collapses, mild subluxation occurs, and pressure from the lateral acetabular margin creates a depression, or "furrow" in the femoral head.

Healing requires replacement of dead bone with living bone. Over time in young children, the deformity remodels and the acetabulum becomes congruous. At maturation, the head is reasonably round and the prognosis fair to good. If growth arrest occurs, or the child is older, remodeling is limited. Thus, the capacity of the acetabulum to remodel to congruity is reduced and osteoarthritis is likely in adult life.

Natural History

The prognosis for LCP disease is fair. The most important prognostic factor is the sphericity of the femoral head at skeletal maturation. This sphericity is related to the age of onset [A and B, next page]. The younger the age, the more likely the head will be spherical [B]. Physeal bridges may occur at any age but are more likely in the older patient and those with more severe disease [D].

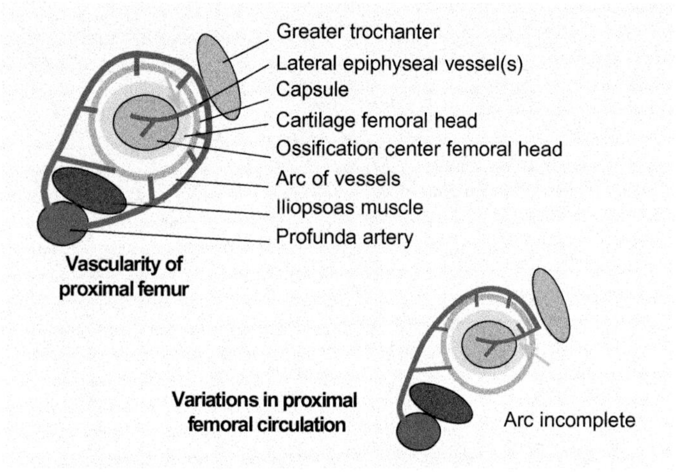

A Circulation to the proximal femoral epiphysis This conceptual drawing illustrates the redundant vascular arcade of the proximal femur in the normal child (upper). Congenital or developmental alterations may make the circulation to the femoral head vulnerable to vascular compromise. Note that the circulation is redundant for the proximal femur except for the epiphysis, which is supplied by the lateral retinacular vessels (green arrow).

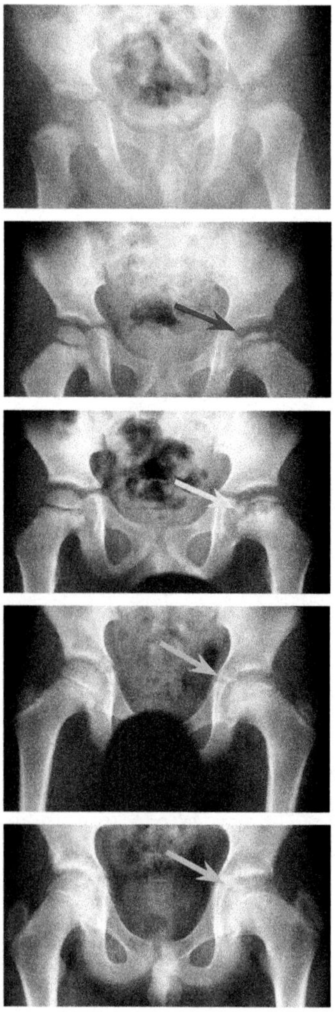

B Natural history of early onset LCP disease These radiographs were taken at ages 2, 3, 5, 8, and 15 years. Note at age 3 years (red arrow) how total head avascular necrosis is evident. Without treatment, healing (yellow arrow) and remodeling (green arrows) occur.

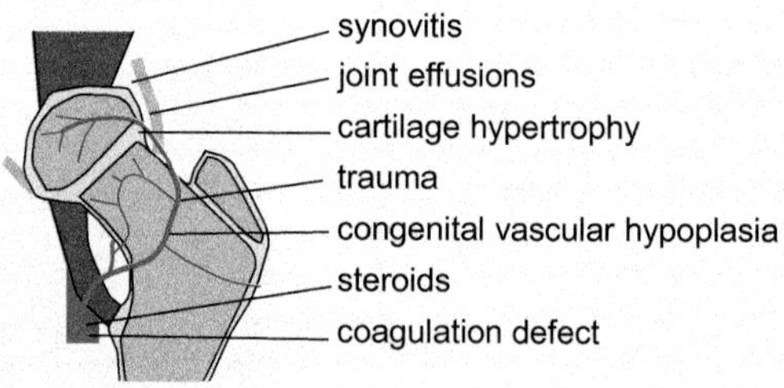

C Causes of LCP disease These are some of the causes of LCP disease. They may act alone or in combination to cause ischemia of the femoral head.

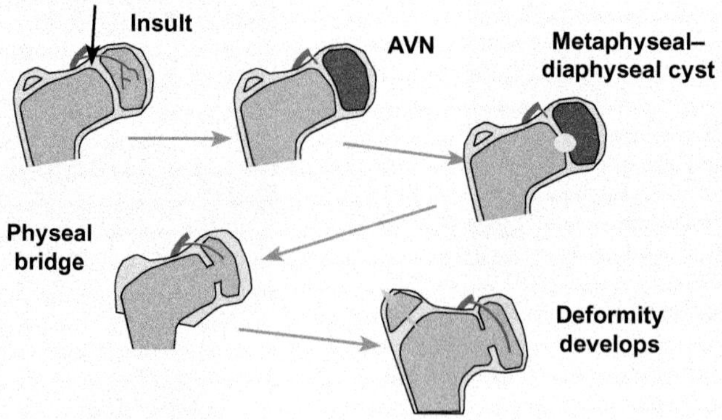

D Physeal bridge formation Cysts may fill in with bone across the growth plate. This creates a bony bridge that tethers growth and causes progressive deformity. The deformity includes shortness of the femoral neck, relative overgrowth of the greater trochanter, and persistence of flattening of the femoral head.

The longer the period between the completion of healing and skeletal maturity, the longer the period of remodeling. This remodeling cannot occur if a physeal bridge develops. Physeal bridging may occur in young patients and accounts for the occasional poor result seen in these young children. Physeal bridging is more likely in the older child.

Factors affecting prognosis are many, complicating assessment of treatment methods. During late childhood and adolescence, children may experience episodes of pain with vigorous activity. These episodes are transient, often lasting a day or two. More persistent disability may develop during middle to late adult life due to osteoarthritis. The need for joint replacement increases with advancing age and is most likely when the onset of LCP disease occurs after the age of 8 or 9 years [C].

Diagnosis

LCP occurs between 2 and 18 years of age, but most commonly develops in boys between ages 4 and 8 years. Bilateral involvement occurs with usually more than a year interval between onsets. The disease rarely follows toxic synovitis. An antalgic limp is usually the first sign. Pain may be present but is usually mild. Frequently, the child has recurring pain and a limp for several months before being seen by a physician.

Physical examination The child is comfortable, and the screening examination is normal except for the involved leg. The limp is antalgic, a Trendelenburg sign may be present, and mild atrophy is often present. The most prominent find is stiffness [D]. The loss of hip internal rotation is the earliest sign. The hip rotation test is positive. Abduction is nearly always limited. Flexion is least affected.

Imaging studies The stage of the disease determines the findings on imaging. Early in the disease, radiographs may be normal, show slight widening of the cartilage space, or often a pathognomonic radiolucent cleft in the femoral head viewed from a lateral position. Radiographic features are largely determined by the stage of the disease at the first visit. Ultrasound will show a joint effusion. The bone scan often shows reduced uptake on the affected side early in the disease [E]. The MRI shows evidence of marrow necrosis, irregularity of the femoral head, and a loss of the signal on the affected side [F]. In the majority of cases, only conventional radiographs are necessary to establish the diagnosis and provide management.

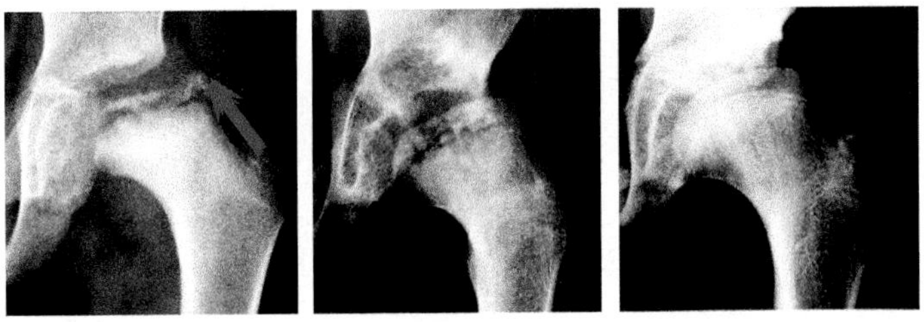

A Extrusion with residual coxa plana Note the extrusion in this 7-year-old child. Remodeling improves but does not resolve flattening.

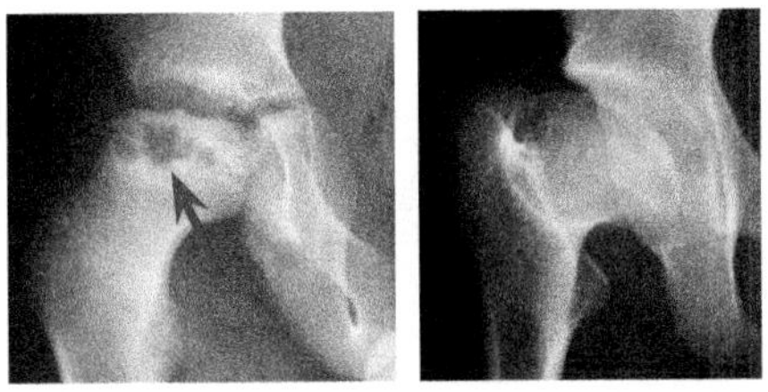

B Late onset LCP Note the metaphyseal–epiphyseal cyst at age 11 years (arrow). The head is aspherical and flat at age 18 years (right).

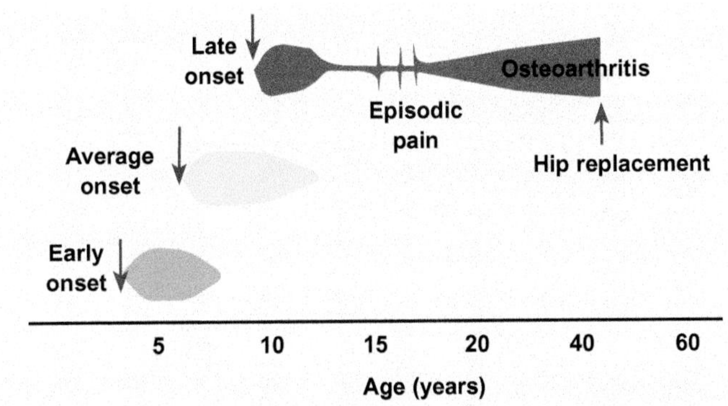

C Pain and age of onset of LCP disease Pain occurs during the acute disease. This lasts for 2–3 years. Pain occurs when deformity persists as episodic incongruity pain during activity and later persistent pain due to osteoarthritis (red).

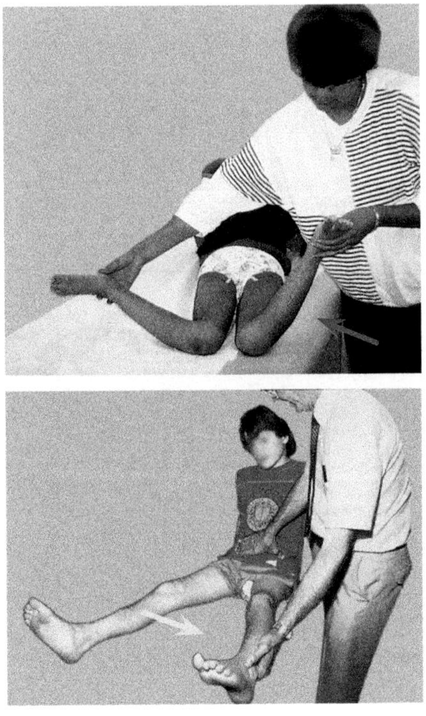

D Limited range of motion Note the reduction of medial rotation on the affected right side (red arrow) consistent with a positive hip rotation test. Examine with one hand spanning the iliac spines as a basis to estimate hip abduction that is reduced in LCP disease (yellow arrow).

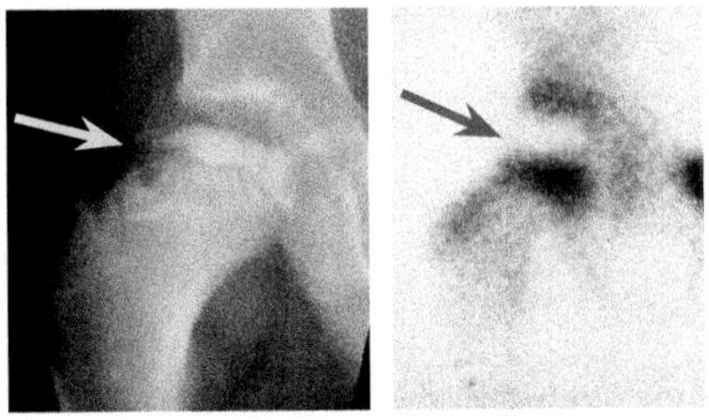

E Imaging Various features are shown based on the stage of the disease in the AP radiograph (yellow arrow). The bone scan often shows decreased uptake over the femoral head (red arrow).

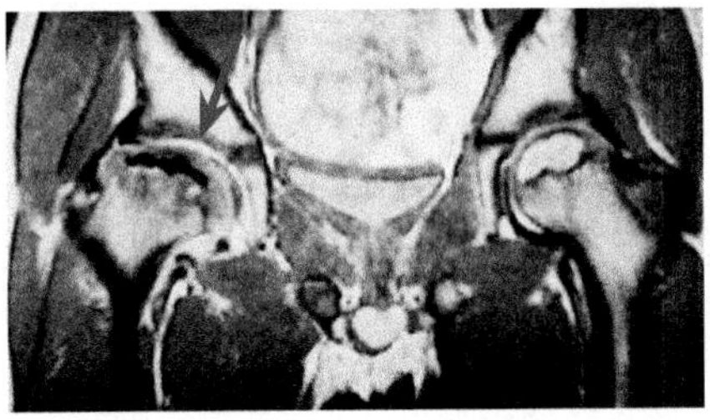

F MRI Marrow necrosis corresponding to the extent of the necrosis (arrow) is evident.

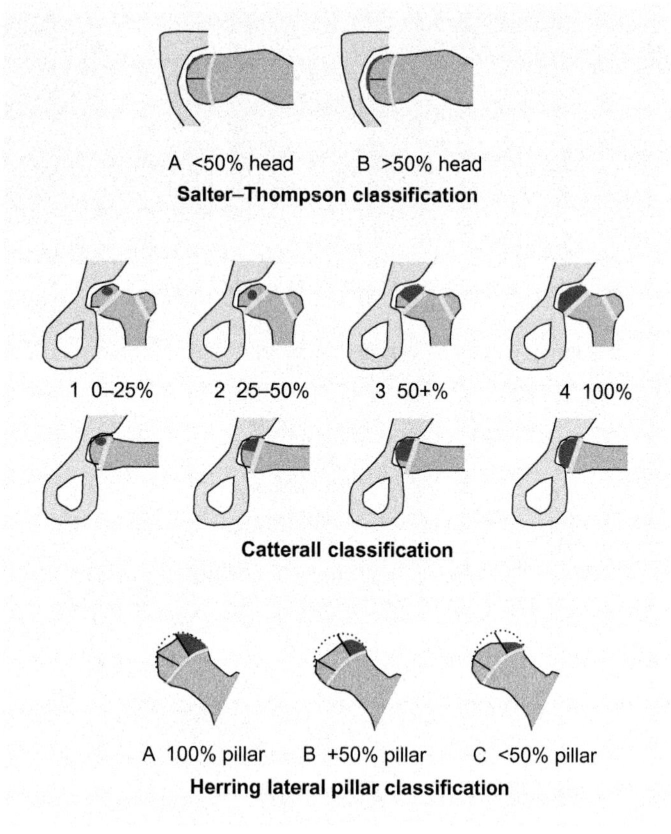

A Classifications of LCP disease severity

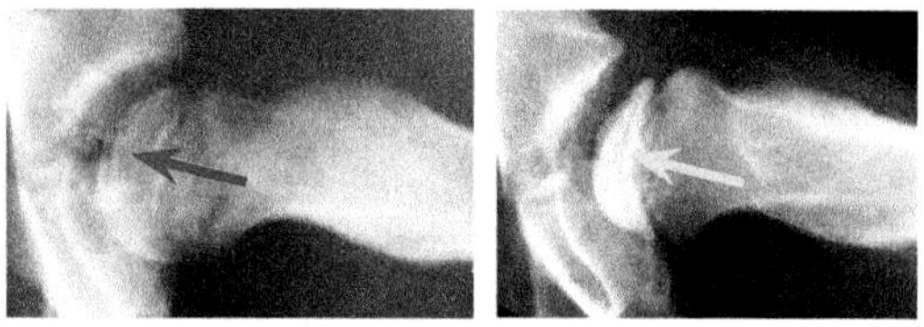

B Salter–Thompson classification Note the extent of the crescent sign (red arrow), which shows the extent of the area of necrosis (yellow arrow), as evident in the radiograph taken one year later.

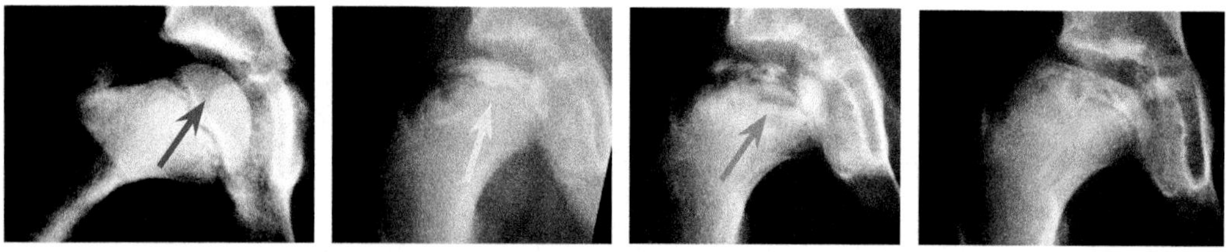

C Stages of LCP disease The disease progresses through the stage of synovitis (red arrow), necrosis (yellow arrow), fragmentation (blue arrow), and reconstitution (green arrow).

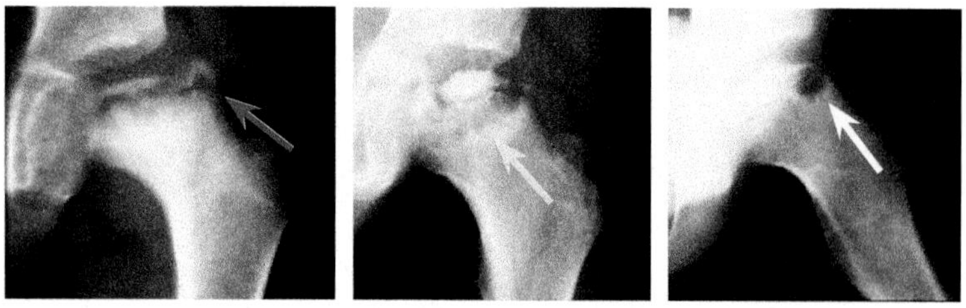

D Head-at-risk signs Extrusion (red arrow), metaphyseal reaction (yellow arrow), and lateral rarefaction or Gage's sign (white arrow) are shown.

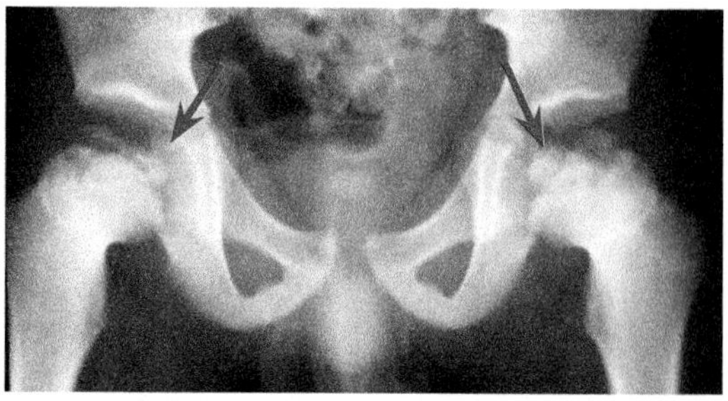

E Symmetrical involvement suggests another diagnosis This child has epiphyseal dysplasia.

Classification

LCP disease is classified by the extent of head involvement and by the stage of the disease.

Extent of involvement Several classification systems are in use for assessing the severity of involvement [A]. Salter–Thompson and Catterall grade the extent of involvement of the epiphysis, and Herring grades on the "lateral pillar." The Salter–Thompson classification is based on showing a cleft (crescent sign) in the lateral radiograph [B]. This cleft is a fracture line between the living and dead bone and shows the minimum extent of necrosis. This can be observed early in the disease. The other signs may show changes with time as grades progressively increase well into the fragmentation phase of the disease.

Stage of disease The disease is divided into four stages: synovitis, necrosis or collapse, fragmentation, and reconstitution [C]. The disease progresses through each stage and each part of the healing process. In some classifications, the first stage is omitted.

1. Synovitis This stage is of short duration (weeks) and shows the effect of ischemia. Synovitis produces stiffness and pain. Radiographs may show a slight lateralization of the epiphysis (cartilage hyperplasia), bone scans show reduced uptake, and the MRI shows a reduced signal.

2. Necrosis or collapse The necrotic portions of the femoral head undergo collapse, and radiographs show a reduction in size and an increased density of the head. This stage lasts 6–12 months.

3. Fragmentation In this healing stage, avascular bone is resorbed, producing the patchy deossification seen on conventional radiographs. Deformation of the femoral head often occurs during this stage. This stage persists for 1–2 years.

4. Reconstitution New bone is formed. Overgrowth often produces coxa magna and a widening of the neck.

Head-at-risk signs [D] include extrusion or ossification lateral to the femoral head, metaphyseal changes of rarefaction or cyst formation, and a radiolucency on the lateral aspect of the physis (Gage's sign).

Differential Diagnosis

Disorders that cause clinical and radiographic changes, such as LCP disease, are numerous [D]. Although these other causes are relatively rare, they should at least be considered before establishing the diagnosis. The most likely diagnoses to miss are hypothyroidism and epiphyseal dysplasia. Dysplasias usually affect both hips with symmetrical degrees of involvement [E, previous page]. Bilateral symmetrical involvement is very rare in LCP disease.

Management

The objective of management of LCP is to preserve the sphericity of the femoral head to reduce the risk of stiffness and degenerative arthritis while preserving the emotional well-being of the child.

The management of LCP is very controversial. In the past, treatment regimens have varied from operating on every case to no treatment at all. Children have been subjected to years of hospitalization in recumbency and various types of ineffective bracing [A] and operative treatments.

Management Principles The following is a list of currently accepted principles of managing LCP:

1. Avoid treatment of patients who will do well without treatment. The young child and children of any age with minimal involvement do not require treatment.

2. Consider the psychosocial situation [B]. The emotionally dysfunctional child should not be subjected to orthotic management. Due to the long duration of the disease, treatment often imposes severe emotional stress for the child. Be sensitive to the child's overall well-being.

3. Provide "containment" to maintain or improve the sphericity of the femoral head [C]. The acetabulum is used as a mold to contain the plastic femoral head. This requires positioning the hip in abduction in a brace or a surgical procedure that increases acetabular coverage of the femoral head.

4. Attempt to maintain or gain a satisfactory range of motion [E]. Motion is nearly always reduced. The degree of stiffness is related to the severity of the disease and the activity level of the child. Gaining motion by curtailing activity has its limits. What constitutes a satisfactory range of motion is seldom defined. A minimum is about 20° of abduction.

5. Control the cost of management. Inpatient traction, MRI studies, arthrography, and operative procedures are most expensive. Conventional radiographs, rest at home, and the selective use of imaging and procedures provides optimum care at least cost.

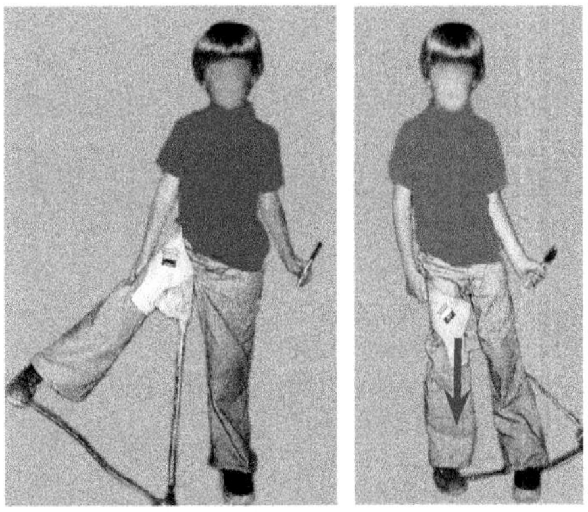

A Adaptive boy The boy circumvented treatment by dropping the brace (arrow) so he could walk on both feet.

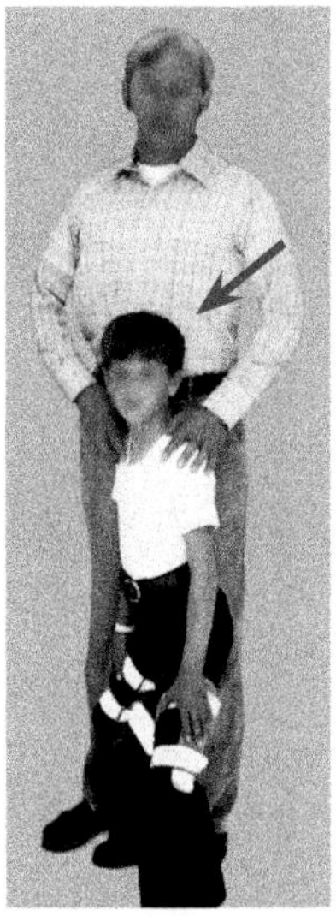

B Head at risk This is a difficult disease for children.

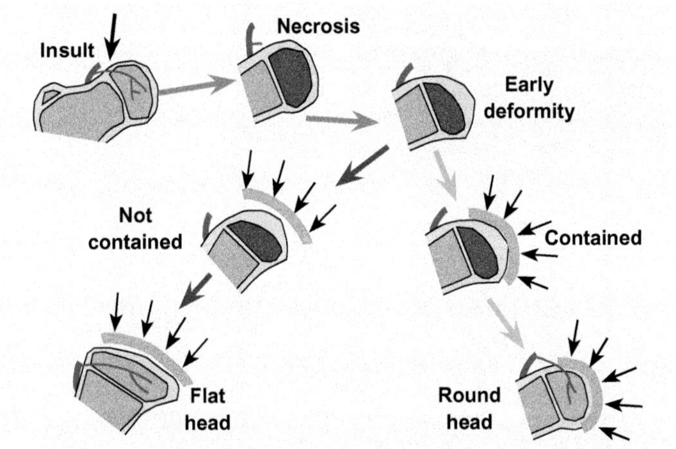

C Concept of containment treatment Containment is provided by positioning the leg or the acetabulum to encompass the femoral head. Without containment (red arrows), the head becomes flattened. The contained head (green arrows) becomes round. Both heads become revascularized.

Category	Disease	Comment
Syndromes	Gaucher's disease Mucopolysaccharidosis Multiple epiphyseal dysplasia Spondyloepiphyseal dysplasia	Often produce bilateral AVN, which is symmetrical in severity and stage
Hematologic	Sickle cell disease Hemophilia Lupus erythematosis	May be related to steroid treatment
Infection	Septic arthritis Femoral osteomyelitis	Complication in delayed drainage of an infected hip
Metabolic	Hypothyroidism	
Trauma	Femoral neck fractures Hip dislocation Slipped epiphysis	Common causes of AVN
Inflammation	Toxic synovitis	Occurs in 1-3% of cases
Tumors	Lymphoma	

D Differential diagnosis of LCP Several disorders may be confused with LCP. Often, the primary disease makes the cause of the avascular necrosis clear.

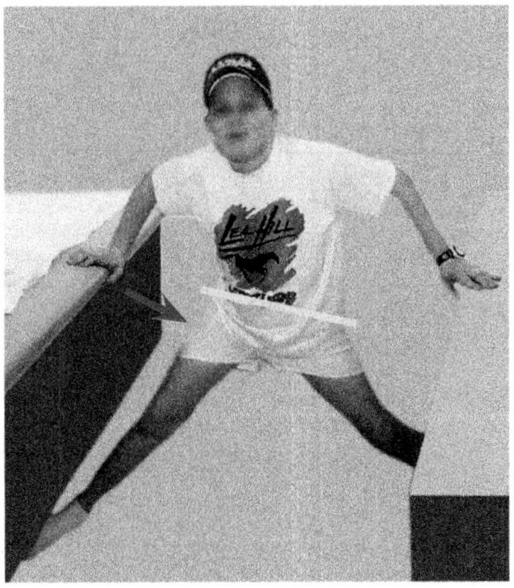

E Tight abductors The pelvis tilts (yellow line) and abduction is limited on the right side (red arrow).

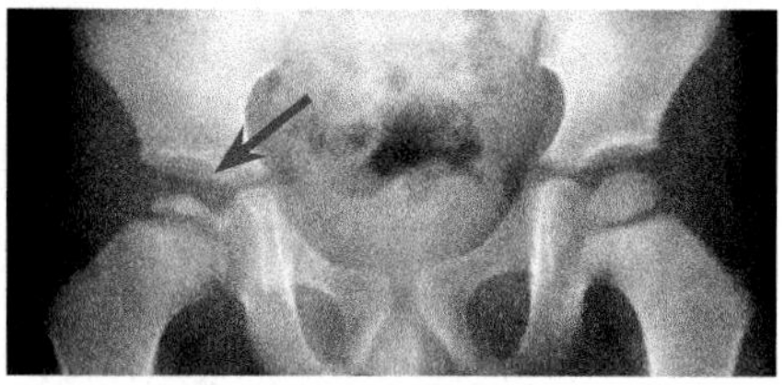

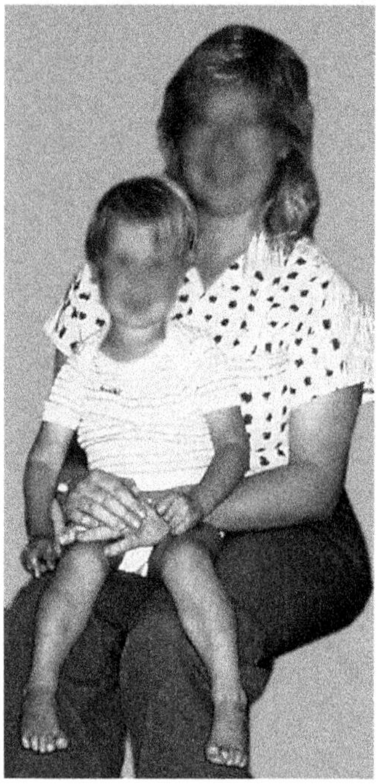

A LCP disease in a young child This 3-year-old girl was managed without treatment. The outcome was good.

Management Algorithm

The flowchart based on the Herring A, B, and C categories [C] is one of many approaches to management. The management of LCP disease is one of the most controversial in orthopedics. Consider each of the following variables in planning management.

Age is the most important variable and the first consideration. Prognosis is mostly dependent on the age of onset. Divide ages into the young child group (0–5 years), the middle age group (5–8 years), and the older child group (8+ years). This older group has a much poorer prognosis.

Early childhood The prognosis is usually excellent in early childhood [A] unless a physeal bridge develops. The development of bridging is not preventable. In this age group, treatment is not necessary or helpful. Asking the parents to limit the child's activity is asking the parents to do the near impossible. It is neither fair nor helpful. Simply ask the parents to redirect the child's activity when feasible into some activity that is less physical. If metaphyseal cysts develop, follow the child with an AP radiography every two years to assess growth, as physeal bridging may occur. If this complication develops, it may be necessary to transfer the trochanter in late childhood or adolescence.

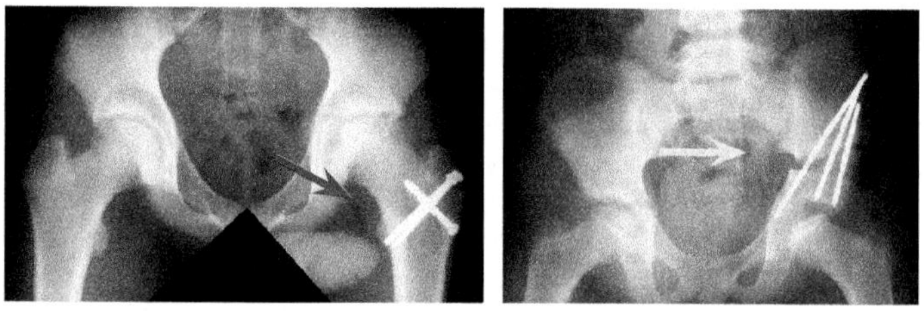

B Moderate containment Containment is provided by a varus osteotomy (red arrow) or a single innominate osteotomy (yellow arrow).

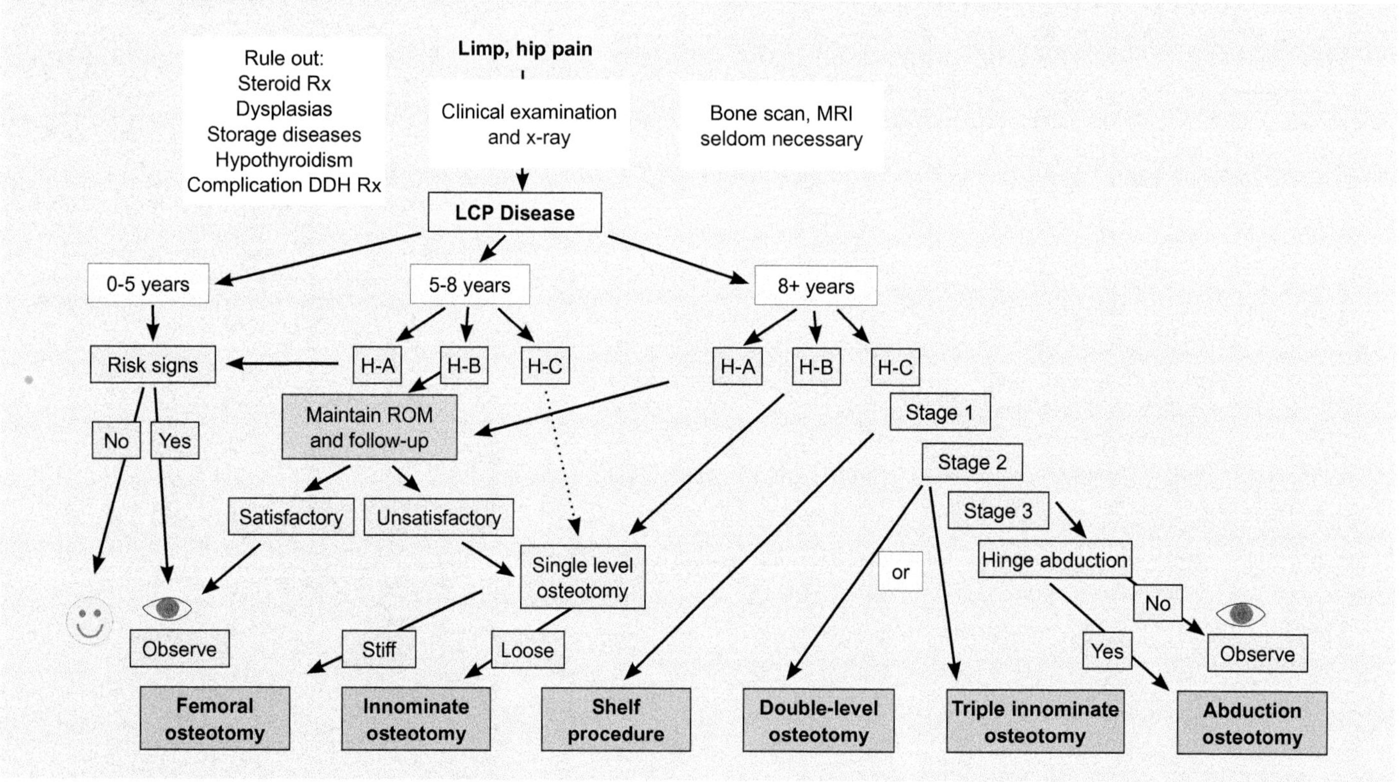

C Management of LCP disease This flowchart considers age, severity, range of motion (ROM), and stage of disease in determining appropriate management.

Middle childhood Avoid treatments that are either ineffective or present special hardships for the child [A]. Manage Herring A and B without containment. Encourage abduction exercises. Provide follow-up. Consider treating Herring C by containment [B, previous page]. Such treatment is controversial.

Late childhood Consider operative containment in Herring B and C hips if seen during stage 1 or 2. An option is abduction casts or braces, but most children find this treatment very difficult. In stage 1, the shelf procedure [C] is effective and least invasive. In stage 2, the double-level osteotomy [B] is often necessary. The head is still plastic and will remodel when well contained. In stage 3, the deformity is permanent. If hinge abduction is present, an abduction osteotomy may improve motion and reduce discomfort [D]. If motion is satisfactory and not painful, accept the deformity [E].

Severity Be aware that the Salter–Thompson cleft sign, when visible, will predict severity earlier than either the Herring or Catterall methods. The Herring method does not become fully clear until the stage of late necrosis or early fragmentation.

Operative choices These choices [C, previous page] demonstrate the many options in management. The choices do not include brace management. This option is still viable but poorly accepted by most children and families due to the long duration required.

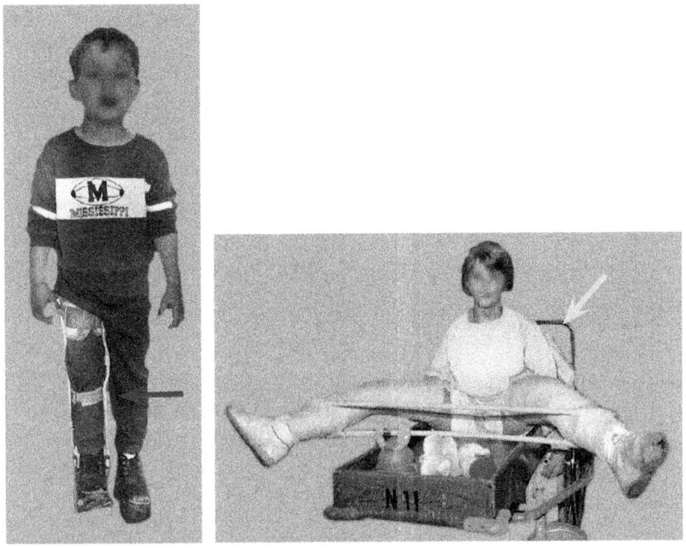

A Extremes in management The pattern bottom brace (red arrow) has been shown to increase hip loading and provides no containment. Wide abduction casts (yellow arrow) are effective but very difficult for the child.

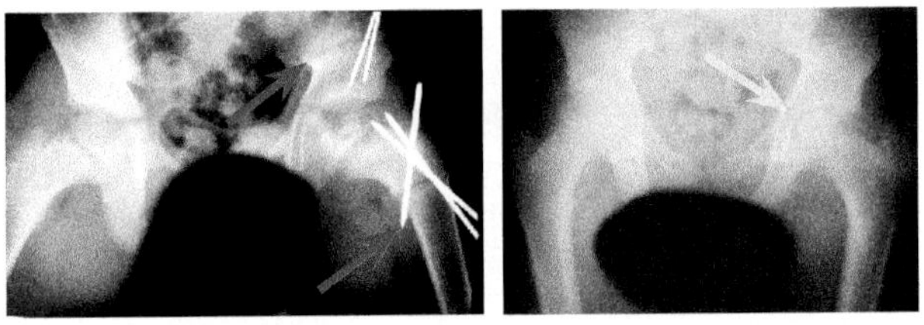

B Double-level osteotomy for LCD disease Containment in this 10-year-old child with H–C was provided by an innominate and femoral osteotomy (red arrows). A round head is shown at age 15 years (yellow arrow).

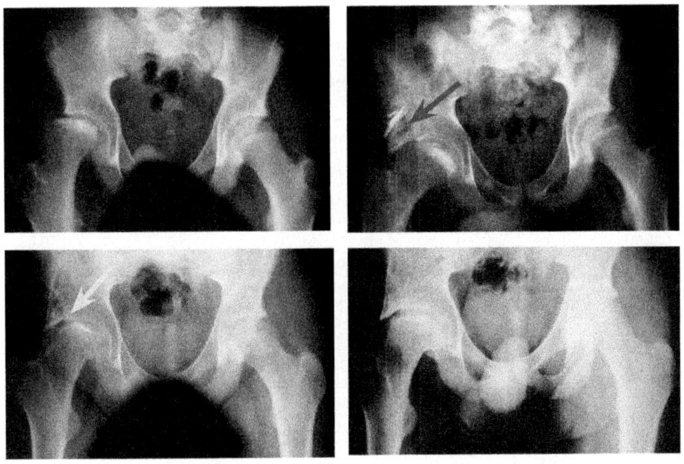

C Shelf containment in LCP disease This 10-year-old girl is H–C and in stage 1. A shelf procedure was performed. Radiographs are shown at age 10 years (red arrow), 11 years (yellow arrow), and 12 years (orange arrow).

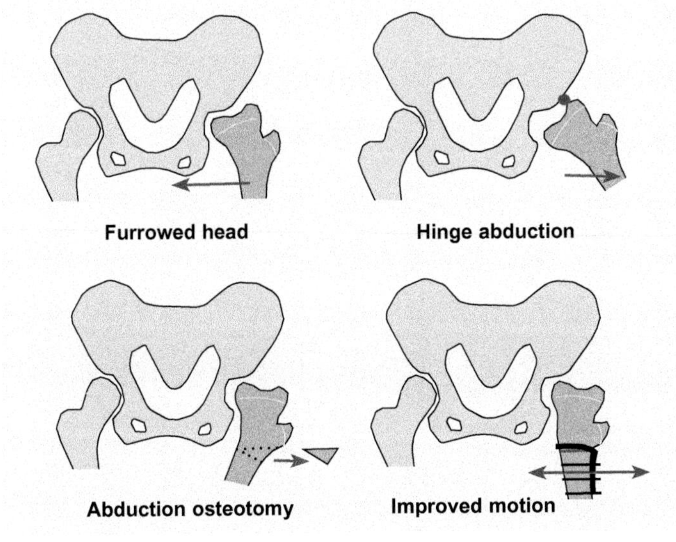

D Hinge abduction With flattening or furrowing of the femoral head, adduction is full, but abduction causes the lateral margin of the femoral head to hinge on the pelvis, in turn causing widening of the medial joint space and pain. Pain and motion may be improved by an abduction osteotomy.

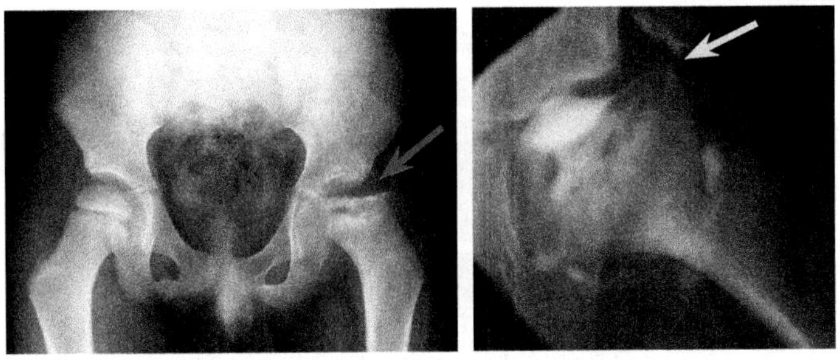

E Severe deformity Severe deformity on AP radiograph (red arrow) and by arthrogram (yellow arrow) in an 11-year-old boy in stage 3. The deformity was established and no treatment was recommended.

Slipped Capital Femoral Epiphysis

Slipped capital femoral epiphysis (SCFE) is a displacement of the upper femoral epiphysis on the metaphysis [A]. SCFE is the most common adolescent hip disorder. It occurs in about 1 in 50,000, most commonly in obese boys. The peak age is 13 years for boys and 11 years for girls, with a range from middle childhood to maturity. SCFE is bilateral in about one-fourth of cases, with possibly slight silent slippage in even more.

Etiology

The cause of SCFE is complex. In early adolescence, the growth plate is relatively weaker, as evident from the incidence of physeal injuries at other sites at this age. The hip is vulnerable, as it carries about four times its body weight. Retroversion or a reduced neck shaft angle may increase the verticality of the plate, making it mechanically less stable. The risk is further increased by any constitutional disorder that adds to this physeal weakness. Endocrine disorders, such as hypothyroidism, hypopituitarism, or hypogonadism, and metabolic disorders, such as rickets or treatment with radiation or chemotherapy, may contribute. If obesity [A] or trauma is added to this, the plate may fail—gradually, acutely, or as a combination of gradual and acute components.

Natural History

Failure of physis and slipping may occur from age 6 years until the plate is fused. Most slips are gradual over a period of many months [B]. Often the progress on the slip is variable; acute episodes are superimposed on gradual slipping. Closure of the plate as the result of treatment or as it occurs naturally at the end of growth halts the process. Following slipping, remodeling may reduce the deformity. The risk of osteoarthritis is increased when the slip is more severe, the child is older, and especially if avascular necrosis or chondrolysis complicate management.

Patients with SCFE have a normal acetabulum, and the articular cartilage is often preserved. Thus, despite the presence of significant deformity, many do well for many decades. Chondrolysis and avascular necrosis cause early degeneration.

An enigma is the significance of the so-called pistol grip deformity. This deformity is often seen in males who develop osteoarthritis. Speculation is that this deformity is secondary to unappreciated SCFE. Why such mild deformity should cause early degeneration is unclear, however.

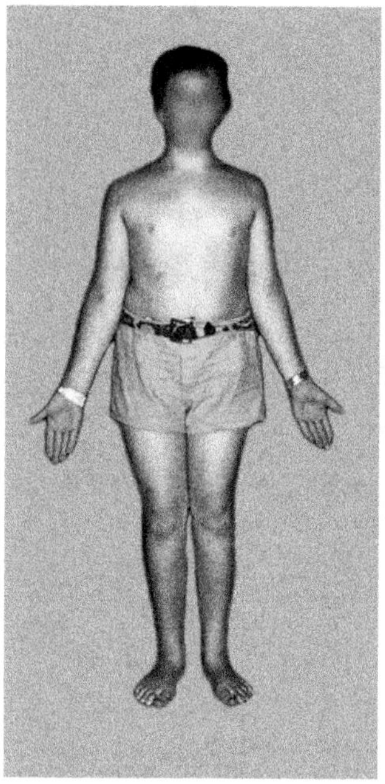
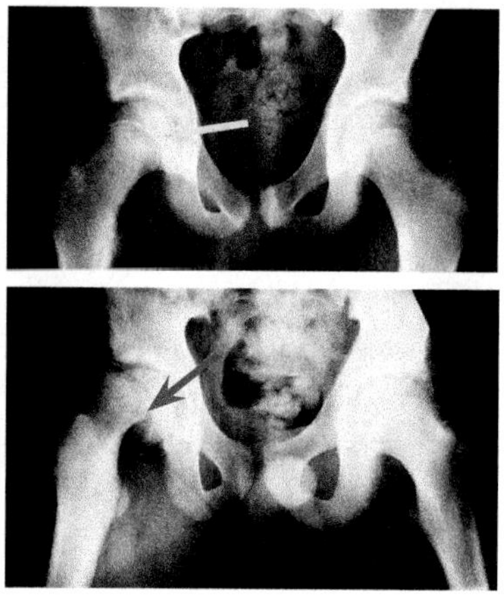

A Slipped capital femoral epiphysis Typical habitus is shown (left). The upper radiograph was made in an orthopedist's office where diagnosis of SCFE (yellow arrow) was made. An acute slip (red arrow) occurred in the parking lot on the way to the hospital.

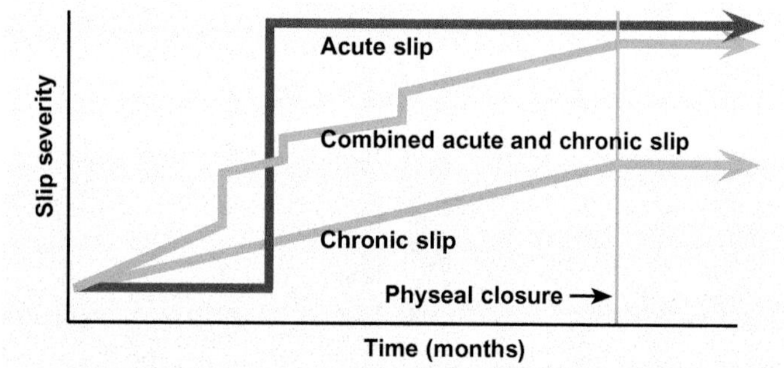

B Patterns of slippage Slipping occurs over a period of months. At physeal closure, progression ceases.

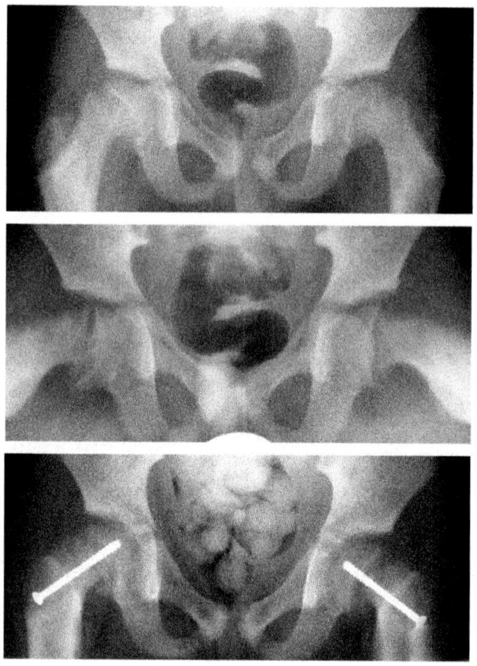

C Bilateral SCFE Bilateral involvement suggests the possibility of some underlying disorder. This patient had renal osteodystrophy.

Atypical SCFE

- Renal osteodystrophy
- Radiotherapy
- Chemotherapy
- Endocrine disorders

D Atypical SCFE Underlying disease or treatment increases the risk for SCFE.

Diagnosis

The diagnosis of SCFE is made more difficult because the onset of the common chronic slip is insidious and the pain is often referred to the knee. Knee pain occurring between the ages of 6 years and maturity should promote an evaluation of the hip. Long-standing slips will produce an out-toeing gait, an abductor lurch, and limb atrophy.

Screening is done with a hip rotation test (see page 28). The loss of medial hip rotation is due to inflammation of the joint and to the posterior inferior slippage of the femoral head, causing a deformity similar to femoral retroversion. A positive finding requires further evaluation with a "frog-leg" lateral radiograph of the pelvis.

Radiography The diagnosis of SCFE can nearly always be made on conventional radiographs of the pelvis. The frog-leg lateral best shows the posterior slippage of the epiphysis. The AP radiograph usually shows widening of the growth plate and rarefaction of the adjacent metaphysis [A]. Sometimes these are the only findings, and the condition is called a "preslip." Subtle displacement is identified by a loss of the normal relationship at the epiphysis–neck interface. On the AP radiograph, the head lies above and lateral to a line drawn along the superior margin of the neck. On the lateral radiograph, any slipping will disrupt this alignment [B]. On the AP radiograph, assess severity by the percentage of contact between the head and neck. For a more accurate assessment, obtain a true lateral view and measure the slip angle [E].

Other imaging Pinhole (high-resolution) lateral bone scans of both femoral heads will show increased uptake in preslips [C]. Ultrasound imaging will demonstrate the "step off" at the site of displacement. The MRI shows AVN or altered head position [D].

Atypical slips Underlying disorders that weaken the physeal plate or increase the loading may increase the risk of involvement. Bilateral involvement increases the possibility of some problems [C, previous page]. Often a history of some endocrine or renal or special treatment is given [D, previous page].

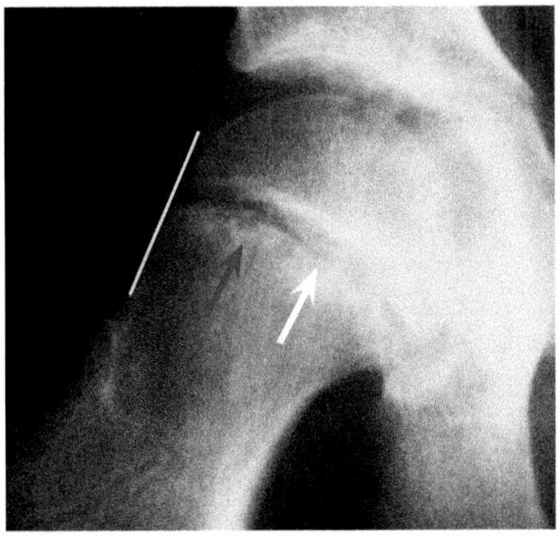

A Classic AP radiographic features Note that the head is displaced inferior to a line (yellow) drawn along the superior margin of the neck. Metaphyseal rarefaction (red arrow) and slight widening of the growth plate (white arrow) are seen.

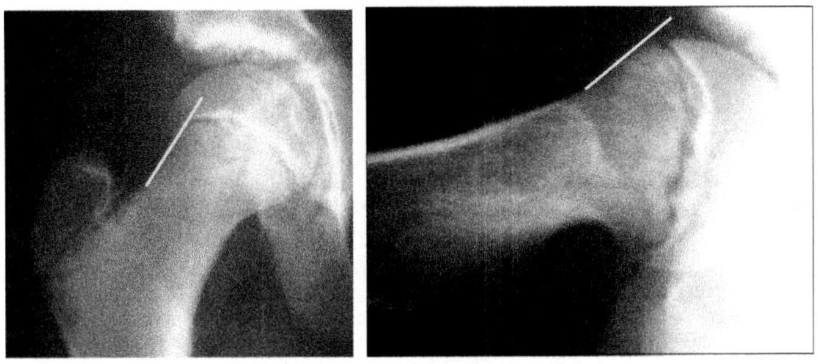

B Very early slip Note that on the AP view, no change is seen in the head–neck relationship. The slight slip is clearly evident on the lateral view, though.

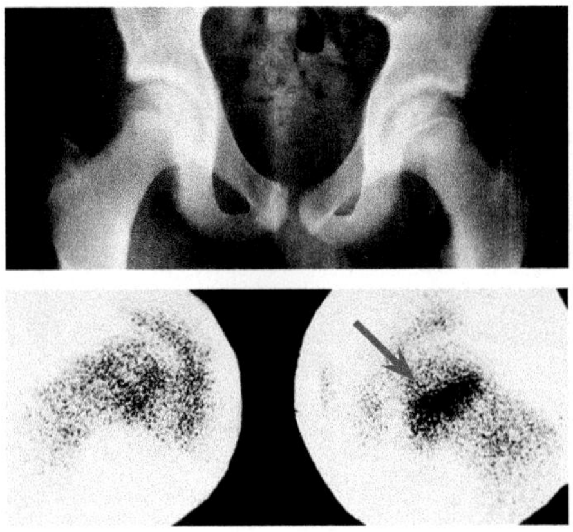

C Bone scan in preslip The diagnosis of a preslip can be confirmed by a high-resolution bone scan. Increased uptake of the physis (red arrow) is noted, as compared to the opposite uninvolved side.

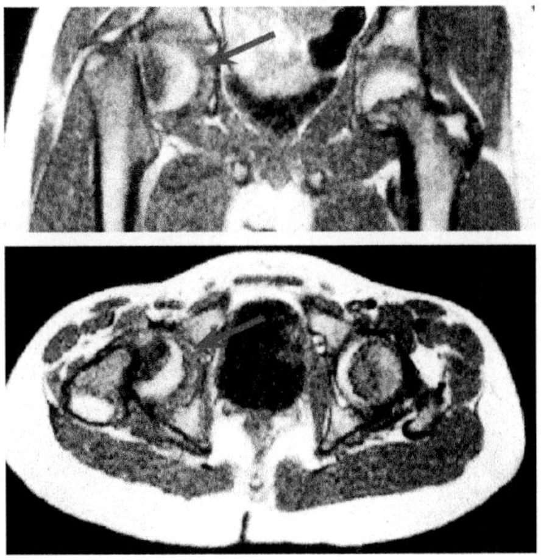

D MRI view of SCFE This study shows a severe slip (red arrows).

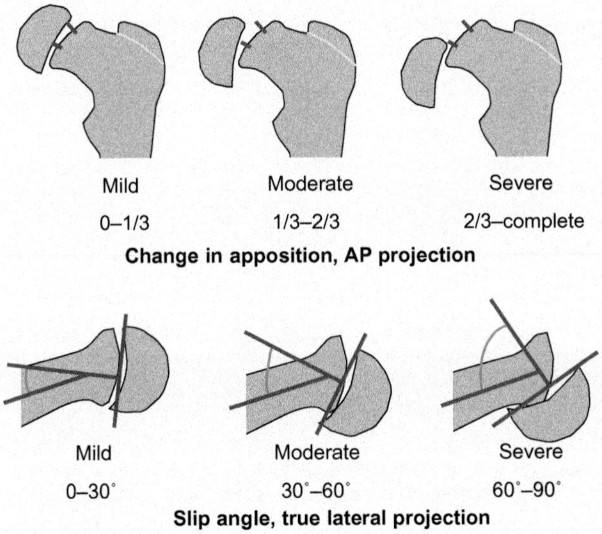

E Grading severity of SCFE Severity can be expressed as a grade based on the displacement seen in the AP projection. A more accurate measurement is the slip angle measured from a true lateral radiograph.

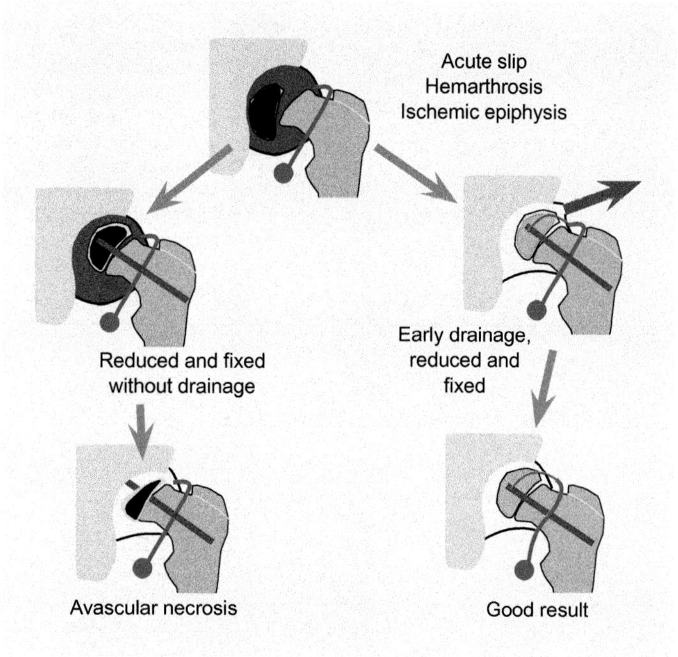

A Prevention of AVN by early drainage Some surgeons recommend early emergency decompression, reduction, and fixation to prevent AVN in acute SCFE.

Management

The objective of management is to stabilize the growth plate to prevent further slippage and to avoid complications [B]. Achieve this by a screw, pins, epiphysiodesis, or immobilization with a spica cast.

Unstable slips Five to ten percent of all slips cause instability and increase the risks of avascular necrosis (AVN). They occur suddenly, causing an inability to walk. Because the slip is unstable, any movement of the leg causes pain.

Unstable slips are often more severe than gradual slips. Management is difficult and controversial, and the outcome is sometimes poor. Acute management choices include traction, manipulation, cast immobilization, acute decompression, reduction, and fixation. Mounting evidence suggests that early decompression and fixation reduces the risk of AVN [A].

Admit the patient. Arrange for screw fixation. If the procedure is delayed, consider applying skin traction with the limb supported on a pillow. Reduction may occur from traction or when the limb is in position in the operating room for fixation. Fix as with a stable slip. Supplement the fixation with a second screw if the first pin is not optimal or if the patient is obese or even more unreliable about self-care than most adolescents. Encourage bedrest for 3 weeks and then nonweight-bearing activity until early callus is seen. Follow up to observe for AVN (see next page).

Stable SCFE Fix mild and moderate stable slips in situ with a single screw. This prevents further slippage and leads to fusion of the growth plate (see next page). In the child under age 8 years, fix with smooth pins to allow growth.

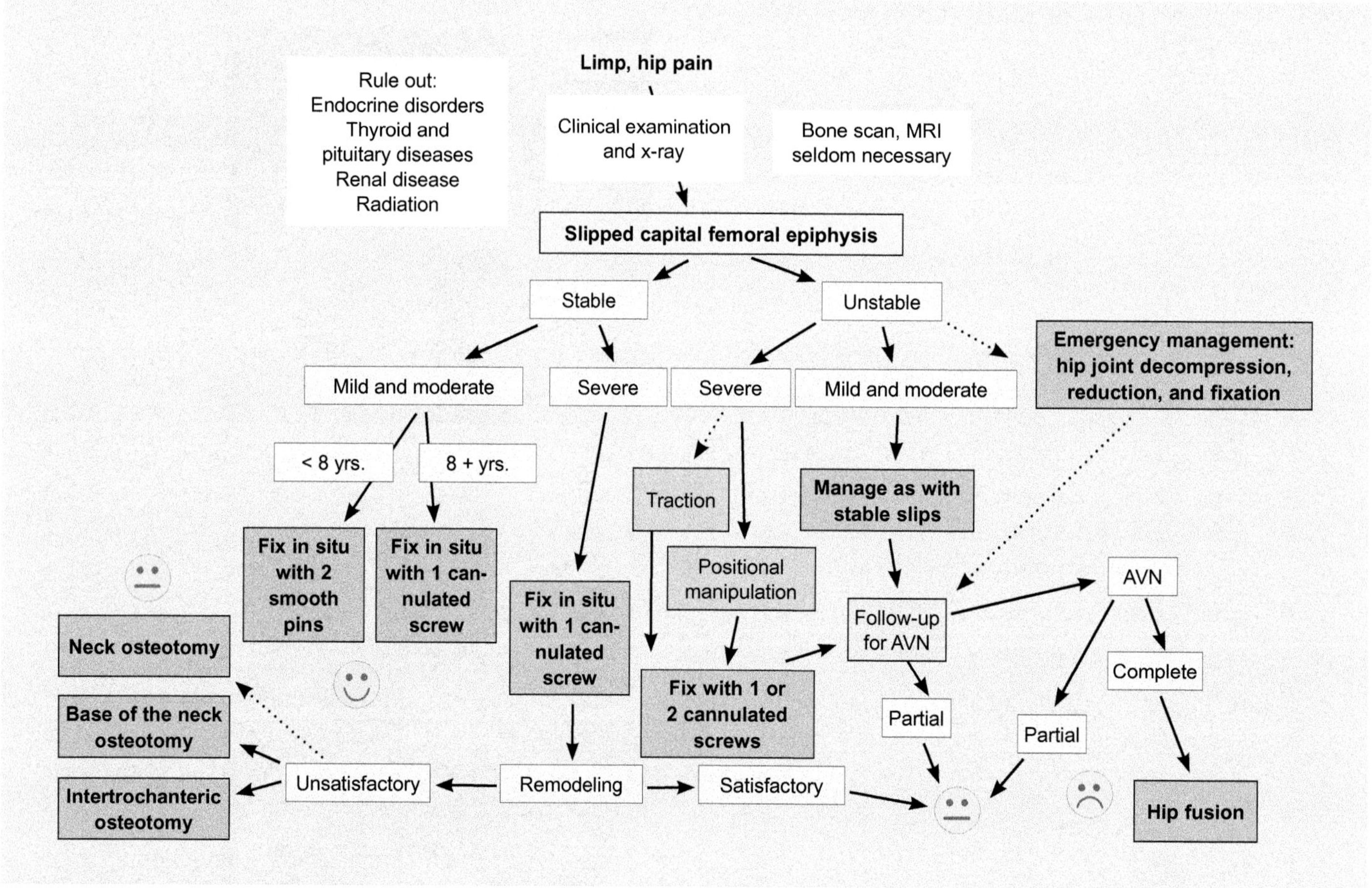

B Management flowchart for SCFE

Osteotomy The procedure can occur at several different levels [A]. In general, osteotomies closest to the site of deformity provide the most anatomic correction but the greatest risk of avascular necrosis. The following are the operative choices.

Cervical osteotomy This shortening valgus osteotomy is made at the site of deformity, providing excellent correction. Due to the risk of causing avascular necrosis, this procedure is usually performed only by surgeons with considerable experience with the technique. Fixation is simple.

Base of the neck osteotomy This provides safety with good correction, as the procedure is extracapsular and relatively close to the deformity. An anterolaterally based wedge of bone is removed at the base of the neck. Any prominences are shaved off. Fixation is simple.

Intertrochanteric osteotomy This is extracapsular, and contact surfaces are large, providing stability and rapid healing. Fixation is more complicated, and the osteotomy is distant from the site of deformity.

Subtrochanteric osteotomy Because the osteotomy is most distal and fixation more difficult, this procedure is not commonly performed. The base of the neck or the intertrochanteric osteotomy levels are preferred because correction is good and risks are minimal.

Osteoplasty Residual prominence of the anterior portion of the femoral neck impinges on the acetabulum in flexion and internal rotation. Removal improves motion. The procedure is simple and safe but does not position articular cartilage in a load-bearing configuration, as is achieved by osteotomy procedures. This procedure is underappreciated and underutilized.

Prophylactic pinning Bilateral slips occur in about one-fourth of patients. Always carefully evaluate the apparently uninvolved side. Pin the other side if an early slip is suspected or if some underlying metabolic disorder, such as renal osteodystrophy, is present. Other factors that increase the risk for the other hip to slip are an age under 10 years and severe obesity.

Severe slips Severe slips complicate management.

In situ fixation Plan fixation, allow remodeling to correct deformity and follow with an osteotomy to improve motion should that be necessary. Marked displacement makes in situ fixation difficult. Make the point of entry for the screw on the anterior aspect of the femoral neck. This allows central placement of the pin in the displaced femoral epiphysis.

Initial osteotomy The more difficult approach is to perform an osteotomy that includes correction of the deformity and stabilization of the slip. Stabilization may be achieved by placing fixation across the physis or positioning the physis in a horizontal position.

Complications

Complications are common in SCFE.

Avascular necrosis AVN is a serious complication that often follows management of unstable slips. Do everything possible to prevent this disastrous outcome. Avoid manipulative reductions [C]. AVN is a serious complication that often follows management of unstable slips. Follow the patient's progress clinically. Be suspicious if hip rotation becomes guarded or progressively more restricted. Necrosis is usually clear radiographically in 6–12 months, or earlier on MRI studies.

Chondrolysis may occur with or without treatment [B]. Joint penetration by guide pins or screws is a doubtful cause. The joint space narrows, hip motion decreases, and an abduction contracture often develops. Relieve weight bearing and encourage motion. The value of aspirin, hospital traction, and capsulotomy is uncertain. Most improve with time. Rarely, the disease progresses to joint destruction and arthrodesis. The combination of chondrolysis and AVN is devastating and usually ends in hip fusion.

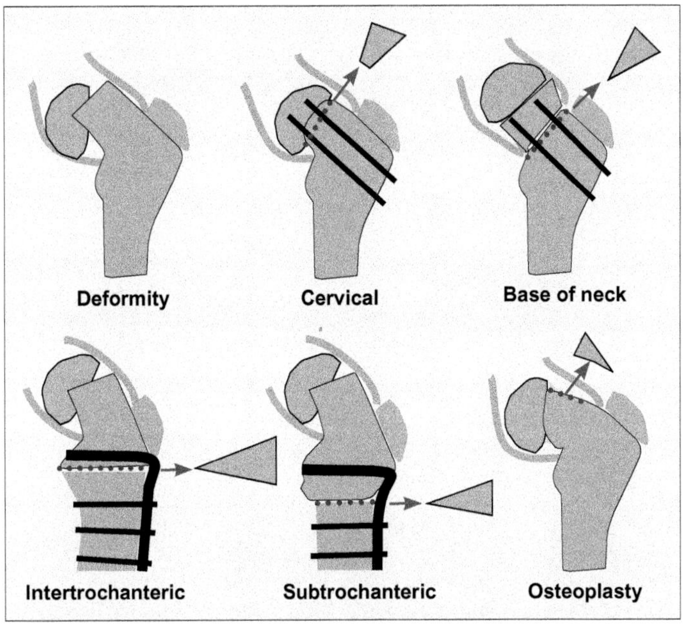

A Osteotomies for correction of deformity These are the choices for the site of an osteotomy to correct the deformity of a severe slip.

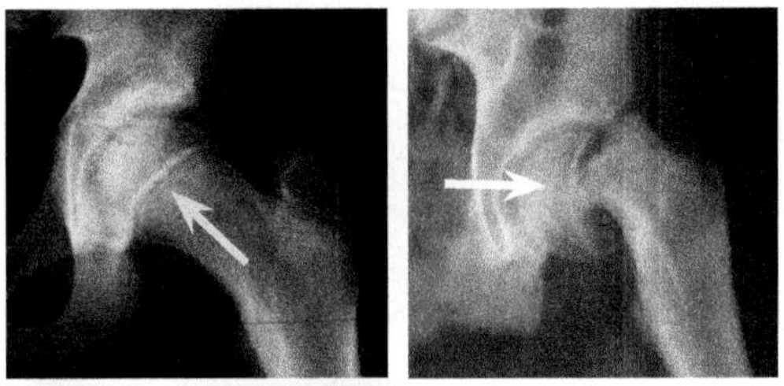

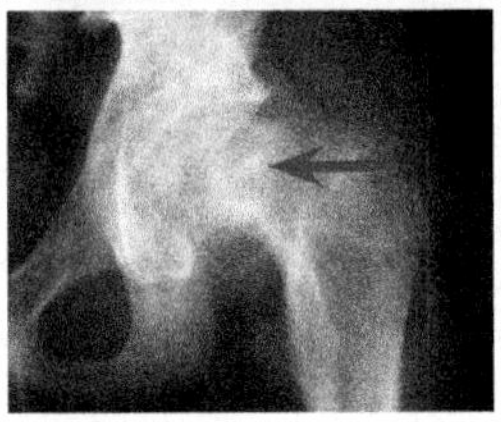

B Acute slip and avascular necrosis and chondrolysis These preslip metaphyseal changes were not appreciated (yellow arrow), and an unstable slip occurred (white arrow), complicated by avascular necrosis and chondrolysis (red arrow).

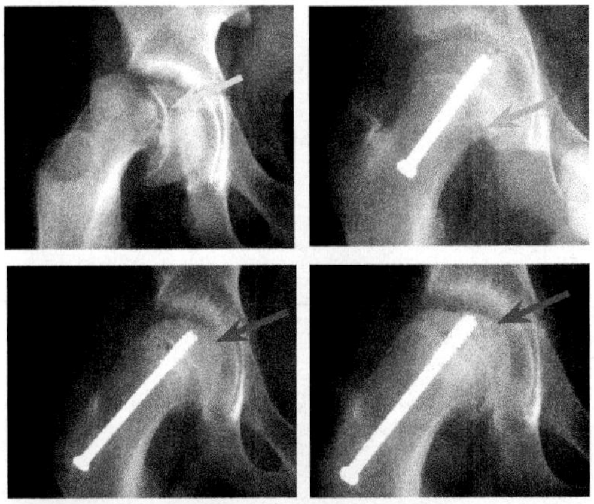

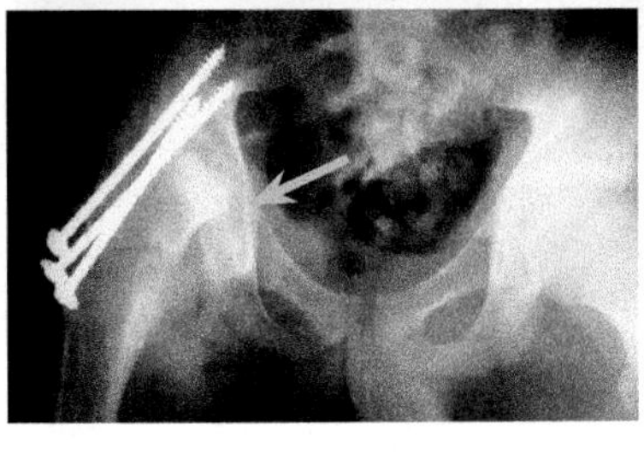

C Unstable slip with avascular necrosis This acute slip (yellow arrow) was reduced and pinned (orange arrow) without drainage. The hip underwent AVN (red arrows) and eventually required a hip fusion (green arrow).

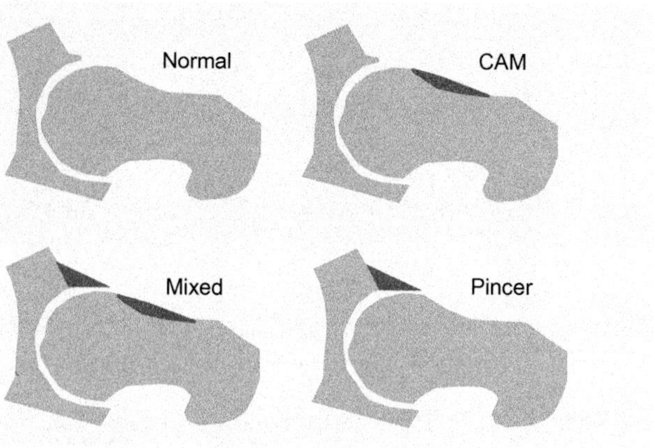

A Types of femoral acetabular impingement The lateral view of normal hip, and deformity with *CAM*, mixed, and *Pincer* type deformity. Impingement occurs with flexion of the hip.

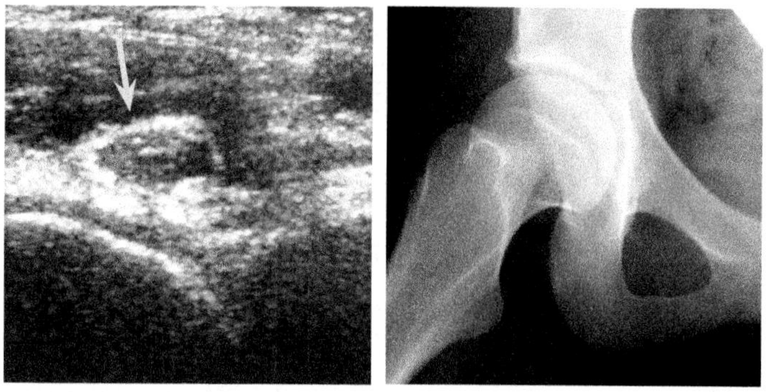

B Snapping hip The ultrasound shows movement of the iliopsoas tendon (arrow). The radiograph is normal.

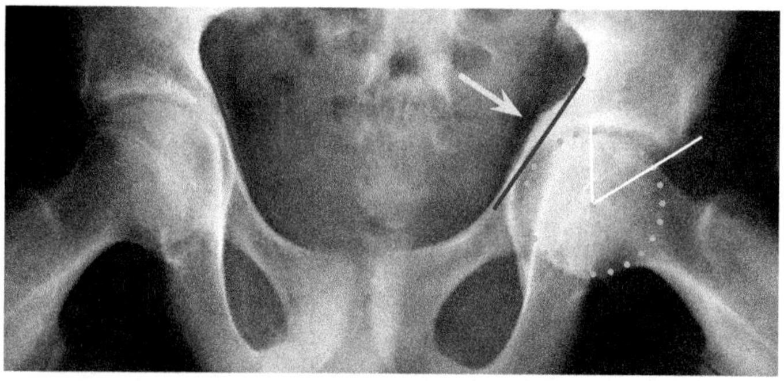

C Acetabular protrusion Note the deepening of the acetabulum and displacement medial to the ilioischial line (red lines) and a CE angle of 60°.

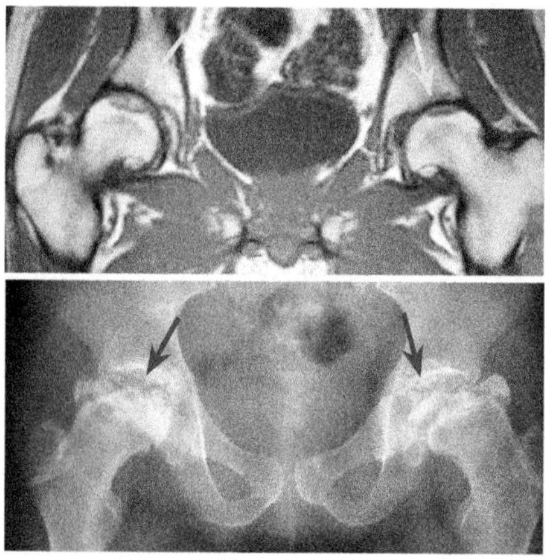

D Steroid induced AVN The early MRI shows early bilateral AVN (yellow arrows). Note the extensive necrosis 2 years later (red arrows).

Miscellaneous Hip Disorders

Femoral Acetabular Impingement (FAI)

Impingement [A] is of two types. *Pincer impingement* is due to excessive anterior acetabular coverage that cause impingement on the femoral head and neck during hip flexion. It is often secondary to acetabular retroversion. The second type is *CAM impingement* due to an anterior prominence of the femoral neck due to residual of slipped capital femoral epiphysis, LCP disease, or avascular necrosis complicating DDH management. Both types cause limitation of motion of the hip, increased risk of damage to the labrum, and premature osteoarthritis. Refer FAI to a specialist as management is technically difficult. Generally, correction is accomplished by excision of the source of impingement. Resection may be performed by exposure using arthroscopy, minimally invasive exposure, or open hip dislocation. Labral repair is performed during the same procedure.

Labral Tears

Labral tears can occur spontaneously in adolescents following trauma or associated with acetabular dysplasia and deformities from LCP disease or SCFE. The symptoms include snapping and catching, but they seldom cause pain with normal activity. Internal rotation and extension may elicit discomfort. Pain relief follows injection of a local anesthetic into the joint. The diagnosis can be confirmed by MRI or arthroscopy.

When possible, first correct any underlying problem such as acetabular dysplasia. Prescribe NSAIDs. Limited arthroscopic debridement may be helpful. Labral tears increase the risk of the hip undergoing degenerative changes.

Idiopathic Chondrolysis

This idiopathic disorder is characterized by chondrolysis with a spontaneous onset resulting in pain, stiffness, and narrowing of the joint and cartilage space [A]. Its natural history is variable. Restoration of the joint space often occurs over several years. In others, the hip becomes ankylosed, and fusion is required.

Manage by weight release with crutches while encouraging active motion through activities such as swimming.

Snapping Hip

Snapping hip may occur in the adolescent. The iliopsoas tendon subluxates, creating a snap and causing pain. The subluxation can be demonstrated by ultrasound [B]. Manage with rest, injection, or rarely with tendon lengthening.

Protrusio Acetabuli

Protrusio is rare in children. It occurs in Marfan syndrome, seronegative spondyloarthropathy, and conditions that weaken bone. Pain, stiffness, medial displacement of the acetabulum, and an increased CE angle are typical features [C]. Manage the underlying disease. Consider early fusion of the triradiate cartilage in Marfan syndrome or in severe deformity. An osteotomy of the pelvis to shift the loading more laterally (reverse triple innominate osteotomy) may be required.

Steroid-Induced AVN

This catastrophic complication of steroid management causes severe involvement that is often bilateral [D]. The mechanism by which steroids reduce femoral head blood flow is uncertain. High doses of steroid are more causative than the cumulative dose or duration of therapy. AVN may follow the completion of therapy of up to 3 years and is the most severe form of AVN. Management includes early core decompression and total joint arthroplasty.

Coxa Vara

Coxa vara (CV) describes a deformity in which the neck–shaft angle is reduced below 110° [A]. CV has many causes [B] and can be a primary isolated deformity or associated with other disorders.

Measurements Measurements of the shape of the upper femur in addition to the neck–shaft angle include the epiphyseal angle and the articular trochanteric distance (ATD). The ATD is an important measurement in assessing abductor muscle deficiencies. Normally, the center of the femoral head lies at the level of the tip of the trochanter. The ATD is positive. A reduction in the ATD may be due to coxa vara or relative trochanteric overgrowth from loss of growth of the capital femoral epiphysis.

Disability Coxa vara causes limb shortening and abductor muscle weakness. Because the deformity increases the epiphyseal angle, the deformity is sometimes progressive.

Congenital coxa vara is often associated with a short femur [C], or it can be associated with a skeletal dysplasia such as spondyloepiphyseal dysplasia.

Acquired coxa vara may be associated with other problems, as is common in fibrous dysplasia, or it may be iatrogenic, as may occur after a varus osteotomy treatment of LCP disease [D].

Developmental coxa vara may develop over time.

Management is based on the category of deformity.

Progressive coxa vara may be congenital or developmental. Perform a valgus osteotomy that reduces the epiphyseal angle to less than about 40°. This more horizontal position provides stability and reduces the risk of recurrence.

Valgus osteotomy Residual deformity is most common when the procedure is performed late in childhood, when the time for remodeling is limited. The effect of this osteotomy is sometimes minimized by a concurrent greater trochanteric arrest.

Trochanteric transfer This procedure is simple and effective and often the best way to manage residual coxa vara in the older child or adolescent. Note that the transfer is both distal and lateral. The lateral component is most important to improve abductor strength and reduce the child's limp.

Coxa Valga

An increased neck–shaft angle is seldom a problem. This increase in the neck–shaft angle as seen on an AP radiograph of the pelvis may be due to true coxa valga, femoral antetorsion, or a combination of the two.

True coxa valga This deformity may occur following arrest of the greater trochanteric apophysis or neck cartilage that may follow surgical procedures. On the AP radiographs, the neck appears elongated.

Apparent coxa valga from femoral antetorsion may be seen in children with this syndrome.

Combinations In neuromuscular disorders such as cerebral palsy, the deformity is usually a combination femoral antetorsion and a true coxa valga. The neck is elongated, the true lateral radiography shows an increase in anterior inclination of the femoral neck, and CT scans show increased anteversion.

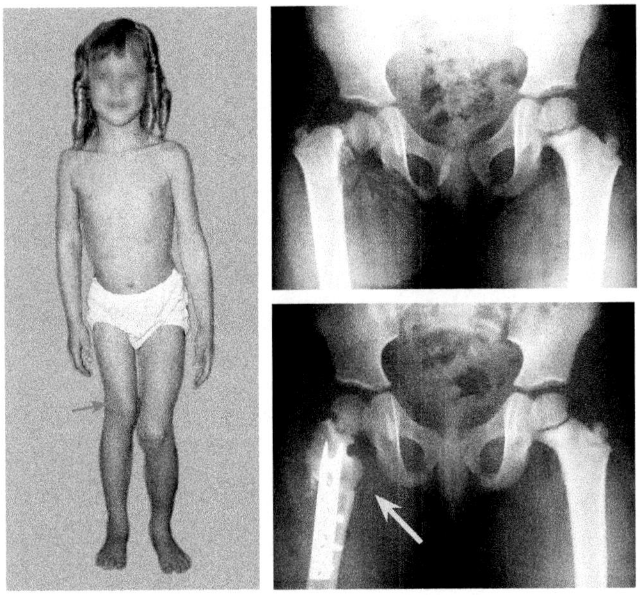

A Valgus osteotomy Note the shortening of the right leg (blue arrow). The varus deformity (red arrow) was corrected with a valgus osteotomy (yellow arrow).

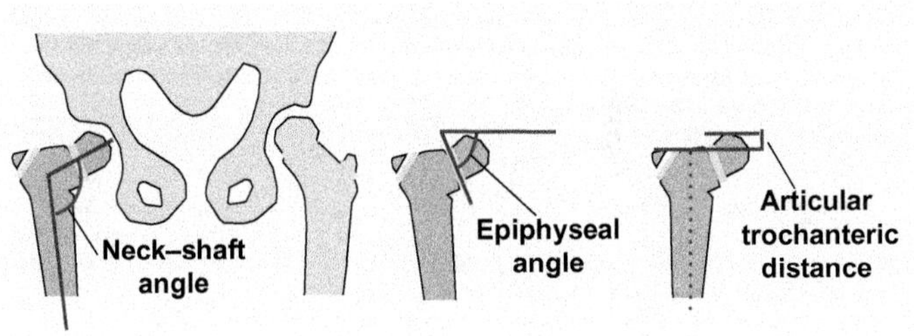

B Measurements of the proximal femur These measurements are often used in discussion of changes in the neck-shaft angle.

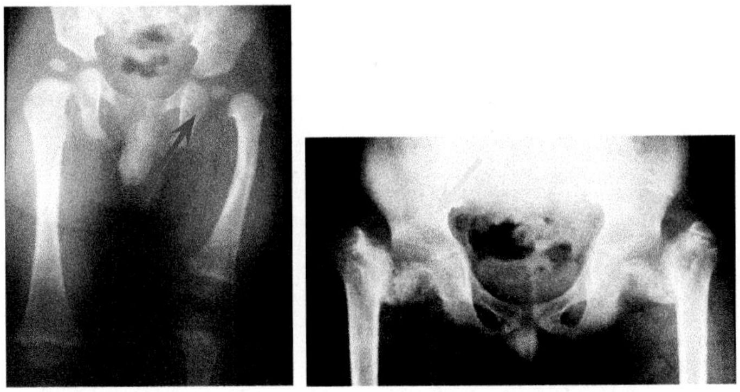

C Congenital coxa vara This deformity is often associated with congenital short femur (red arrow) or may occur as a feature of a bone dysplasia (yellow arrows).

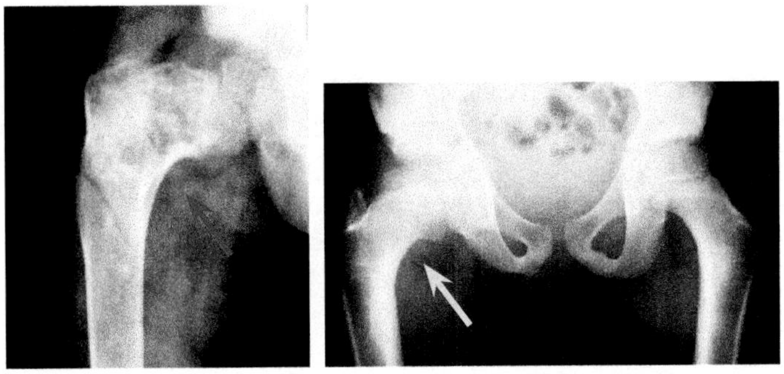

D Acquired coxa vara Varus deformity as seen in fibrous dysplasia (red arrow) and following varus osteotomy in Perthes disease (yellow arrow).

GENERAL

Chung, SMK The arterial supply of the developing proximal end of the femur. J. Bone Joint Surg. 58-B:961, 1976.

Hilton, J On the Influence of Mechanical and Physiological Rest in the Treatment of Accidents and Surgical Diseases, and the Diagnostic Value of Pain. London, 1863.

Pauwels, F Biomechanics of the Normal and Diseased Hip. New York, Springer-Verlag, 1976.

Trueta, J The normal vascular anatomy of the human femoral head during growth. J. Bone Joint Surg. 39-B:358, 1957.

DDH

Barlow, T.G. Early diagnosis and treatment of congenital dislocation of the hip. J. Bone Joint Surg. 44-B:292, 1962.

Chiari, K. Medial displacement osteotomy of the pelvis. Clin. Orthop. 98:55, 1974.

Dunn P.M. Clicking hips should be ignored. Lancet 1:846, 1984.

Ferguson, A.B. Jr. Primary open reduction of congenital dislocation using a median adductor approach. J. Bone Joint Surg. 55-A:671, 1973.

Galeazzi, R. Il Pio Istituto Rachitici di Milano. Milan, 1874-1913.

Ganz R., Klaue K., Vinh T.S., Mast J.W. New periacetabular osteotomy for treatment of hip dysplasias. Technique and preliminary results. Clin. Orthop. 232:26, 1988.

Graf, R. Classification of hip joint dysplasia by means of sonography. Arch. Orthop. Trauma Surg. 102:248, 1984.

Harcke H.T., Kumar, S.J. The role of ultrasound in the diagnosis and management of congenital dislocation and dysplasia of the hip. J. Bone Joint Surg. 73-A:622, 1991.

Harris, W.H. Etiology of osteoarthritis of the hip. Clin. Orthop. 213:20, 1986.

Hilgenreiner, H. Zur frühdiagnose und frühbehandlung der angeborenen huftgelenkuerrenkung. Med. Klin. 21:1385, 1925.

Le Damany, P. La Luxation Congénitale de la Hanche; Études d'Anatomie Comparée, d'Anthropogénie Normale et Pathologique, Déductions Thérapeutiques. Paris, 1912.

Lequesne, M., de Séze, S. Le faux profil du bassin. Nouvelle incidence radiographique pour l'étude de la hanche. Son utilité dans les dysplasies et les différentes coxopathies. Rev. Rhum. Mal. Oetoartic. 28:643, 1961.

Lorenz, A. The operative treatment of congenital dislocation of the hip. Trans. Am. Orthop. Assoc., 7:99, 1895.

Ludloff, K. Open reduction of congenital hip dislocation by anterior incision. Am. J. Orthop. Surg. 10:438, 1913.

Ortolani, M. Congenital hip dysplasia in the light of early and very early diagnosis. Clin. Orthop. 119:6, 1976.

Pavlik, A. Stirrups as an aid in the treatment of congenital dysplasias of the hip in children. J. Pediat. Orthop. 9:157, 1989. Translated by V. Bialik & N.D. Reis from Lékarské Listy, 5:81, 1950.

Pemberton, P.A. Pericapsular osteotomy of the ilium for treatment of congenital subluxation and dislocation of the hip. J. Bone Joint Surg. 87-A:65, 1965.

Perkins, G. Signs by which to diagnose congenital dislocation of the hip. (1928) Clin. Orthop. 274:3, 1992.

Rosen, S. von. Early diagnosis and treatment of congenital dislocation of the hip joint. Acta Orthop. Scand. 26:136, 1956.

Salter, R.B. Innominate osteotomy in the treatment of congenital dislocation of the hip. J. Bone Joint Surg. 43:72, 1961.

Sharp, I.K. Acetabular dysplasia. The actebular angle. J. Bone Joint Surg. 43-B:268, 1961.

Shenton, E.W.H. Disease in Bones and its Detection by X-Rays. London, 1911.

Smith-Petersen, M.N. A new supra-articular subperiosteal approach to the hip joint. Am. J. Orthop. Surg. 15:592, 1917.

Staheli, L.T. Slotted acetabular augmentation. J. Pediat. Orthop. 1:321, 1981.

Steel, H.H. Triple osteotomy of the innominate bone. J. Bone Joint Surg. 55-A:343, 1973.

Sutherland, D.H., Greeknfield, R. Double innominate osteotomy. J. Bone Joint Surg. 59-A:1082, 1977.

Tönnis D. Normal values of the hip joint for the evaluation of X-rays in children and adults. Clin. Orthop. 119:39, 1976.

Tönnis D., Behrens K., Tscharani F. A modified technique of the triple pelvic osteotomy: early results. J. Pediat. Orthop. 1:241, 1981.

Trendelenburg, F. Dtsch. Med. Wschr. 21:21, 1895.

Wagner, H. Osteotomies for congenital hip dislocation. In, Proceeding of the Fourth Open Scientific Meeting of the Hip Society. St. Louis, 1976.

Wagner, H. The Hip. Proceedings of the Fourth Open Scientific Meeting of the Hip Society. St. Louis, 1976.

Wedge J.H., Wasylenko M.J. Natural history of congenital disease of the hip. J. Bone Joint Surg. 61-B:334, 1979.

Wiberg, G. Studies on dysplastic acetabula and congenital subluxation of the hip joint. Acta Orthop. Scand. Suppl. 58:1, 1939.

LCP

Calvé, J Sur une forme particulière de pseudo-coxalgie greffée sur des déformations caractéristiques de l'extrémité supérieure du fémur. Rev. Chir. 42:54, 1910.

Catterall, A The natural history of Perthes' disease. J. Bone Joint Surg. 53-B:37, 1971.

Gage, HC A possible early sign of Perthes' disease. Brit. J. Radiol. 6:295, 1933.

Herring, JA, Neustadt, JB, Williams, JJ The lateral pillar classification of Legg Calvé Perthes disease. J. Pediatr. Orthop. 12:143, 1992.

Köhler, A Die Normale und Pathologische Anatomie des Hüftgelenkes und Oberschenkels in Röntgenographischer Darstellung. Hamburg, 1905.

Legg, AT An obscure affection of the hip-joint. Boston Med. Surg. J. 162:202, 1910.

Little, DG, Kim, HKW. Potential for bisphosphonate treatment in Legg-Calvé-Perthes disease. J. Pediatr. Orthop. 31(2 Suppl):S182-8, 2011.

Meyer, J Dysplasia epiphysealis capitis femoris. A clinical-radiological syndrome and its relationship to Legg-Calvé-Perthes disease. Acta Orthop. Scand. 34:183, 1964.

Miyamoto, Y., Matsuda, T., Kitoh, H., Haga, N., Ohashi, H., Nishimura, G., Ikegawa, S. A recurrent mutation in type II collagen gene causes Legg-Calve-Perthes disease in a Japanese family. Hum. Genet. 121: 625-629, 2007.

Mose, K Legg-Calvé-Perthes disease. A comparison among three methods of conservative treatment. Thesis at Universitesforlaget, Arthus, Denmark, 1964.

Perthes, GC Über arthritis deformans juvenilis. Deutsch. Ztschr. Chir. 107:111, 1910.

Petrie, JG, Bitenc, I The abduction weight bearing treatment in Legg-Perthes disease. J. Bone Joint Surg. 53-B:54, 1971.

Rowe, SM, Kim, HS, Yoon, TR Osteochondritis dissecans in Perthes' disease. Report of seven cases. ActaOrthop. Scand. 60:545, 1989.

Salter, RB, Thompson, GH Legg-Calvé-Perthes disease. The prognostic significance of the subchondral fracture and a two group classification of the femoral head involvement. J. Bone Joint Surg. 66-A:479, 1984.

Stulberg, SD, Cooperman, DR, Wallensten, R The natural history of Legg Calvé Perthes disease. J. Bone Joint Surg. 63-A:1095, 1981.

Waldenström, H Der obere tuberkulöse collumherd. Ztschr. Orthop. Chir. 24:487, 1909.

Waldenström, H The first stages of coxa plana. Acta Orthop. Scand. 5:1, 1934.

Wynne-Davies, R, Gormley, J. The ætiology of Perthes' disease. J. Bone Joint Surg. 60-B:6, 1978.

SCFE

Boyer, DW, Mickelson, MR, Ponseti, IV Slipped capital femoral epiphysis. Long-term follow-up of 121 patients. J. Bone Joint Surg. 63-A:85, 1981.

Carney, BT, Weinstein, SL, Noble, J Long-term followup of slipped capital femoral epiphysis. J. Bone Joint Surg. 73-A:667, 1991.

Dunn, DM Treatment of adolescent slipping of the upper femoral epiphysis. J. Bone Joint Surg. 46-B:621, 1964.

Fahey, J, O'Brien, E Acute slipped capital femoral epiphysis. J. Bone Joint Surg. 47 A:1105, 1965.

Fröhlich, A Ein fall von tumor der hypophysis cerebri ohne akromegalie. Wein. Klin. Rdsch. 15:883-906, 1901.

Ganz, R, Gill, TJ, Müller, ME, Gautier, E, Ganz, K, Krügel, N, Berlemann, U. Surgical dislocation of the adult hip. A technique with full access to the femoral head and acetabulum without the risk of avascular necrosis. J Bone Joint Surg. 83-B:1119-1124, 2001.

Hall, JE The results of treatment of slipped femoral epiphysis. J. Bone Joint Surg. 39 B:659, 1957.

Harris, WR The endocrine basis for slipping of the femoral epiphysis. J. Bone Joint Surg. 32-B:5, 1950.

Heyman, CH, Herndon, CH, Strong, JM Slipped femoral epiphysis with severe displacement. A conservative operative treatment. J. Bone Joint Surg. 39-A:293, 1957.

Imhäuser, G Spätergebnisse der sog. Imhäuser-osteotomie bei der epiphysenlösung. Zugleich ein beitrag zum problem der hüftarthrose. Z. Orthop. 115:716, 1977.

Ingram, AJ, Clarke, MS, Clarke, CS, Marshall, RW Chondrolysis complicating slipped capital femoral epiphysis. Clin. Orthop. 165:99, 1982.

Ippolito, E, Mickelson, M, Ponseti, I A histochemical study of slipped capital femoral epiphysis. J. Bone Joint Surg. 63-A:1109, 1981.

Jerre, T A study of slipped capital femoral epiphysis with special reference to late functional and roentgenological results and the value of closed reduction. Acta Orthop. Scand. 6:1, 1950.

Key, J Epiphyseal coxa vara or displacement of the capital epiphysis of the femur in adolescence. J. Bone Joint Surg. 8:53, 1926.

Klein, A, Joplin, RJ, Reidy, JA Treatment in cases of slipped capital femoral epiphysis at Massachusetts General Hospital. Arch. Surg. 46:681, 1943.

Lacroix, P, Verbrugge, J Slipping of the upper femoral epiphysis. A pathological study. J. Bone Joint Surg. 33-A:371, 1951.

Lehman, WB, Grant, A, Rose, D, Pugh, J, Norman, A A method of evaluating possible pin penetration in slipped capital femoral epiphysis using a cannulated internal fixation device. Clin. Orthop. 186:65, 1984.

Loder, RT, Richards, BS, Shapiro, PS, Reznick, LR, Aronson, DD Acute slipped capital femoral epiphysis. The importance of physeal stability. J. Bone Joint Surg. 75 A:1134, 1993.

Moseley, C The "approach-withdraw phenomenon" in the pinning of slipped capital femoral epiphysis. Orthop. Trans. 9:497, 1985.

Murray, RO The etiology of primary osteoarthritis of the hip. Brit. J. Radiol. 38:810, 1965.

Resnick, D The "tilt deformity" of the femoral head in osteoarthritis of the hip, a poor indicator of previous epiphysiolysis. Clin. Radiol. 27:355, 1976.

Waldenström, H On necrosis of the joint cartilage by epiphyseolysis capitis femoris. Acta Chir. Scand. 67:936, 1930.

Weiner, DS, Weiner, S, Melby, A, Hoyt, WA A 30-year experience with bone graft epiphysiodesis in the treatment of slipped capital femoral epiphysis. J. Pediatr. Orthop. 4:145, 1984.

Wilson, P, Jacobs, R, Schector, L Slipped upper femoral epiphysis. An end result study. J. Bone Joint Surg. 47-A:1128, 1965.

Zionts, LE, Simonian, PT, Harvey, JP Transient penetration of the hip joint during in situ cannulated-screw fixation of slipped capital femoral epiphysis. J. Bone Joint Surg. 73 A:1054, 1991.

OTHER

Khan, M, Adamich, J, Simunovic, N, Philippon, MJ, Bhandari, M, Ayeni, O. Surgical management of internal snapping hip syndrome: a systematic review evaluating open and arthroscopic approaches. J. Arthroscop. 29(5): 942-948, 2013.

Klaue K., Durnin, C.W., Ganz, R. The acetabular rim syndrome. A clinical presentation of dysplasia of the hip. J. Bone Joint Surg. 73-B:423, 1991.

Wild, AT, Sponseller, PD, Stec, AA, Gearhart, JP. The role of osteotomy in surgical repair of bladder exstrophy. Sem. Pediatr. Surg. 20(2):71-78, 2011.

CHAPTER 12
Spine and Pelvis

Spine problems in children have the potential to cause considerable disability and must be taken seriously. Whereas the majority of adults have back pain at times, back pain in children is less common and often due to some specific organic disease that requires treatment. Deformity is of greater concern in the child because of the potential for progression with growth. Conversely, minor truncal asymmetry [A] is common in children and may cause undue concern, leading to unnecessary apprehension and treatment.

Normal Development

The axial system develops during the embryonic period.

Embryo

During the fourth week, mesenchymal cells from the sclerotome grow around the notochord to become the vertebral body and around the neural tube to form the vertebral arches [B]. Cells from adjacent sclerotomes join to form the precursor of the vertebral body, an intersegmental structure. Between these bodies, the notochord develops into the intervertebral disc. Cells surround the neural tube to become the vertebral arches.

During the sixth fetal week, chondrification centers appear at three sites on each side of the mesenchymal vertebrae. The centrum is formed by the coalition of the two most anterior centers. Chondrification is complete before the ossification centers appear [C]. The centrum, together with an ossification center of each arch, make a total of three primary ossification centers for each vertebra.

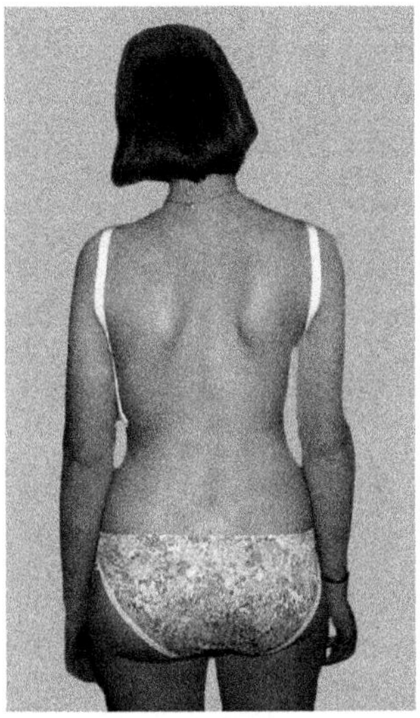

A Mild truncal asymmetry These mild asymmetries are variations of normal, do not require treatment, and cause no disability.

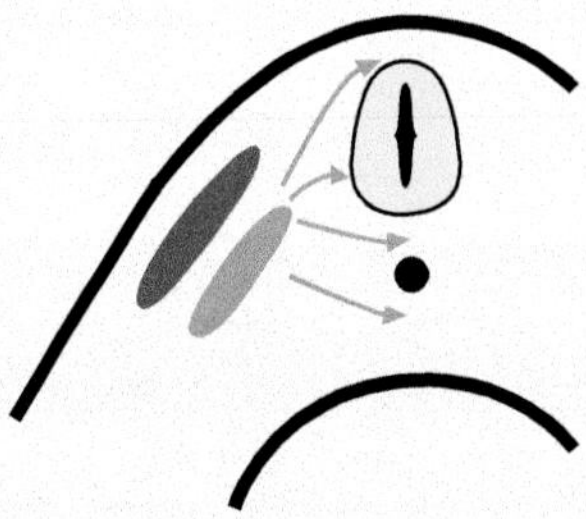

B Sclerotome growth Cells from the sclerotome grow around the notochord and neural tube.

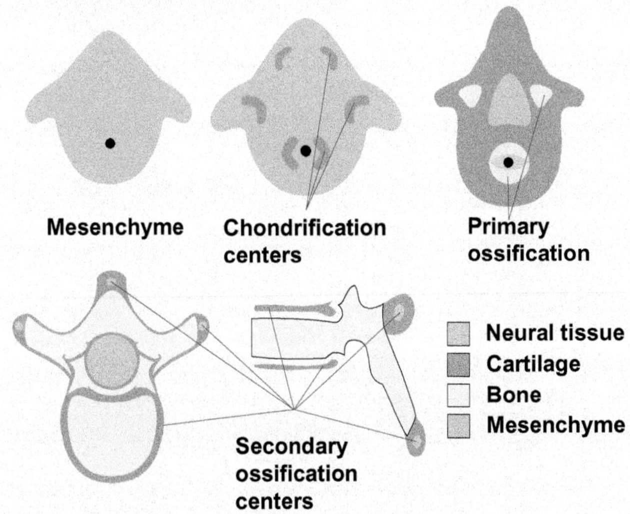

C Vertebral development Vertebrae develop first as mesenchyme, then cartilage, and finally bone. Secondary ossification centers develop during childhood and fuse during adolescence or early adult life. From Moore (1988).

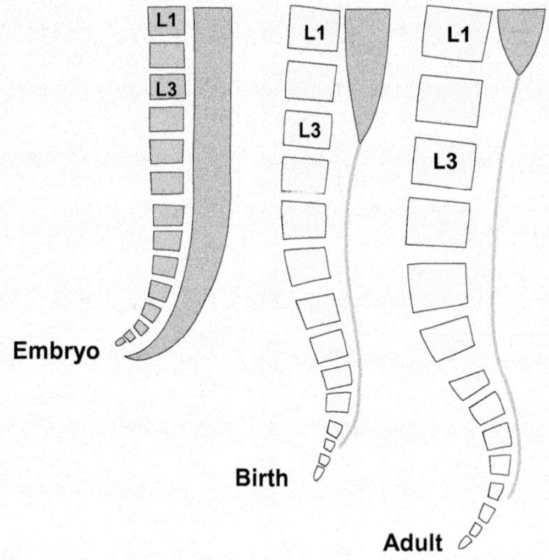

A Spinal cord vertebral column relationship During the fetal period, the spinal cord fills the vertebral canal. With growth, the cord ends at a progressively higher level.

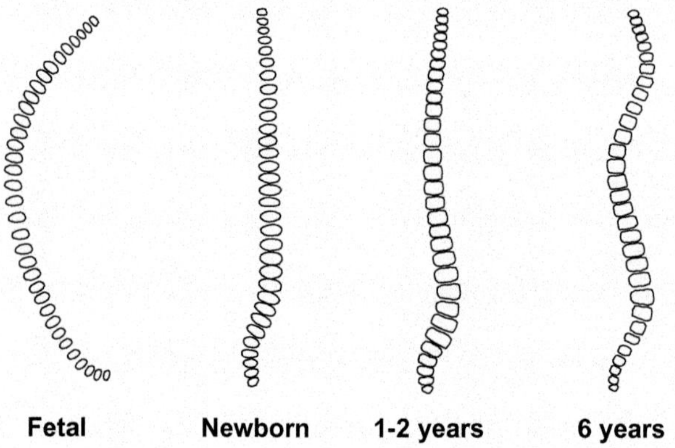

B Normal spine development (sagittal plane) The spine changes from a single curve at birth to a triple curve during childhood.

Childhood

During early childhood, the centers of each vertebral arch fuse and are joined to the vertebral body by a cartilaginous *neurocentral junction.* This junction allows growth to accommodate the enlarging spinal cord. Fusion of the neurocentral junction usually occurs between the third and sixth years. Anterior notching of the vertebrae is sometimes seen in the infant's or child's vertebrae and shows the site of somite fusion [C].

Secondary ossification centers develop at the ends of the transverse and spinous processes and around the vertebral end plates at puberty. These fuse by age 25 years. Congenital defects are common in the axial system. Variations in the lumbar spine occur in about one-third of individuals. Spina bifida occulta is common. Hemivertebrae result from a failure of formation or segmentation. Such lesions are frequently associated with genitourinary abnormalities and less frequently with cardiac, anal, and limb defects; tracheoesophageal fistula; and conductive hearing defects if the cervical spine is involved.

Cord level Initially, the neural and bony elements of corresponding somites lie opposite each other. Thus, the caudal end of the spinal cord fills the spinal canal, and the spinal nerves pass through the corresponding intervertebral foramina. By the 24th fetal week, the cord ends at S1; at birth, at L3; and in the adult, at L1 [A]. This differential growth rate results in the formation of the caudal equina: the accumulation of the nerves traversing the subarachnoid space to the intervertebral foramina. The end of the cord is attached to the periosteum opposite the first coccygeal vertebra by the filum terminale. The filum is the residual of the embryonic spinal cord.

Sagittal configuration In the frontal projection, the spine is relatively straight throughout growth. In the lateral projection, the spine evolves from a single curve at birth to a triple curve pattern in the child [B]. Although this triple curve pattern is necessary to assume an upright posture, the obliquity imposes an added load on the lumbar spine. This load contributes to development of spondylolysis in the child, intervertebral disc herniation in the adolescent, and degenerative arthritis in the adult.

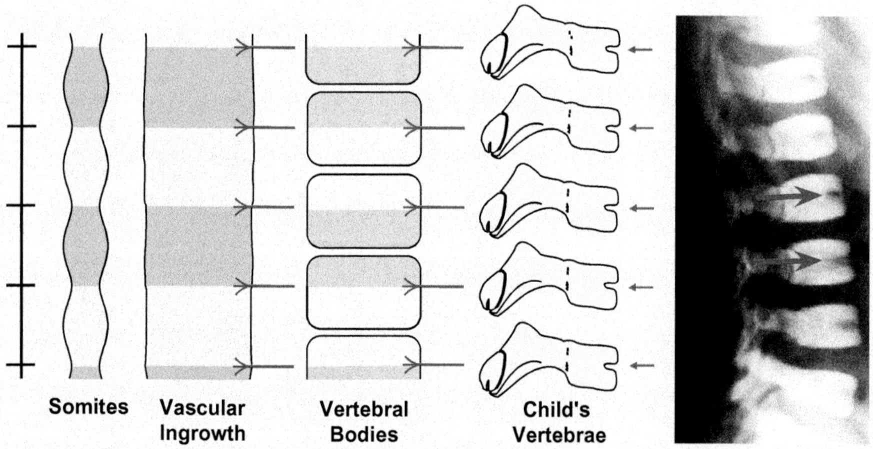

C Vertebral intersegmental development The vertebral bodies form as intersegmental structures. As blood vessels grow between somites, their final position is midvertebral. The site of blood vessel entry and somite fusion is sometimes seen radiographically as an anterior notch in the vertebral body of the child (red arrows).

Evaluation

The spine is evaluated as part of a screening examination or to assess pain or deformity.

History and Physical Examination

Screening examination Is there some underlying disorder? Marfan syndrome, neurofibromatosis, osteochondrodystrophies, or mucopolysaccharidoses are readily obvious in the older child but may not be so apparent in the infant.

History Inquire about the onset, progression, disability, and duration. Family history is of great importance because scoliosis and hyperkyphosis are often familial. Back pain is also familial.

Posture Note asymmetry of shoulder height, scapular prominence, flank crease, or asymmetry of the pelvis. Note any skin lesions, especially those in the midline. The presence of midline skin lesions, such as dimples, hemangioma or hair patches, cavus feet, or leg atrophy, are often associated with underlying spinal lesions. Café au lait spots are associated with neurofibromatosis, a cause of scoliosis.

Be aware that minor truncal asymmetries occur in about 10% of children. These are benign, cause no disability, and require no treatment. Avoid calling attention to such normal asymmetries because it only worries the patient and family.

Forward bending Perform the forward bending test [A]. This is best done with the examiner seated in front or behind the child. Control the child's forward bend by holding the hands together. Slowly guide the child's forward bending while observing the symmetry of each level of the spine. Any significant scoliosis will be readily apparent.

For children unable to stand, examine the child sitting with forward bending. If unable to sit, examine the child prone and look for truncal asymmetry.

Assess asymmetry with a scoliometer [B], which measures inclination. Minor degrees of asymmetry are usually only a variation of normal, but require follow-up examination. If any abnormalities are found, a detailed physical and screening neurological examination is essential to avoid diagnostic errors. Hesitation, a list to one side, or restricted motion is abnormal. Lesions such as spinal cord tumors, spondylolisthesis, disc herniations, or discitis limit the mobility or symmetry on forward bending.

Side view As viewed from the side, the back should curve evenly without any sharp angulation. A sharp angular segment of the spine is seen in Scheuermann kyphosis.

Neurological examination should be part of the examination. In addition to the routine assessment, assess abdominal reflexes. Abdominal reflexes are assessed by gently stroking each quadrant of the abdominal wall [C]. Absence or marked asymmetry suggests a subtle neurological abnormality that may indicate the need for more intensive neurological investigation, such as MRI.

Imaging Studies

Radiographs and other imaging studies are indicated to measure the vertebral curves and to further assess specific problems identified by the physical examination [D].

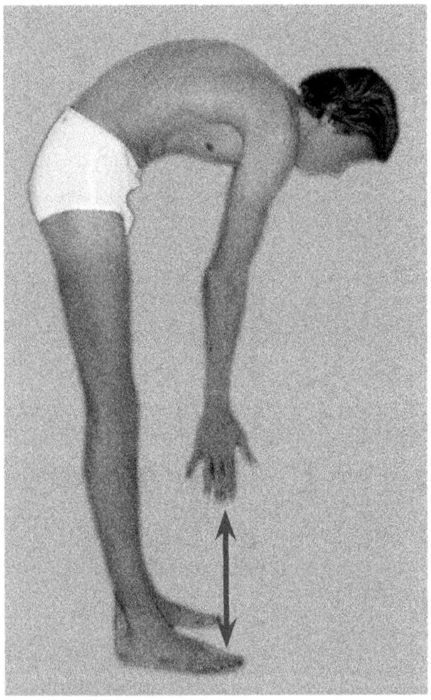

A Limited forward bending Limited forward bending (red arrow) is seen in a variety of diseases. It is an important sign that suggests the need for additional studies.

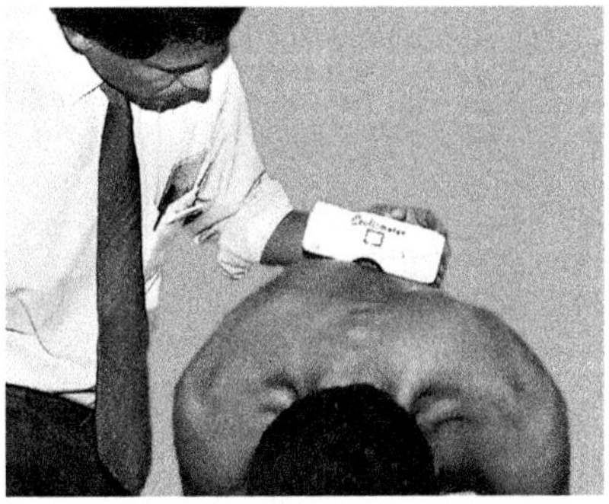

B Truncal inclination Asymmetry may be assessed with an inclinometer or scoliometer. Measures above 5°-7° are an indication for radiographic studies.

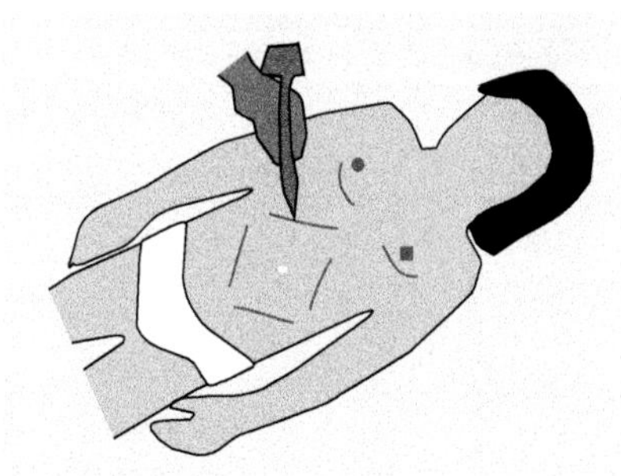

C Abdominal reflexes Stroke each quadrant of the abdomen with the base of a reflex hammer to assess the symmetry of the reflex.

Imaging Method	Condition
Radiography	Initial study
PA radiograph	36-inch standing for scoliosis
Lateral radiograph	36-inch standing for kyphosis or lordosis
Lumbar oblique	Spot L-S spine for spondylolysis
CT Scan	Fractures, spondylolysis
Bone scan	Back pain, infections, or tumors
MRI	Spinal dysraphism, cord lesions, tumors, abscess or disc herniation
SPECT scans	Spondylolysis

D Uses of imaging methods for spinal disorders Avoid ordering a battery of studies, as this is expensive and often exposes the child to unnecessary radiation.

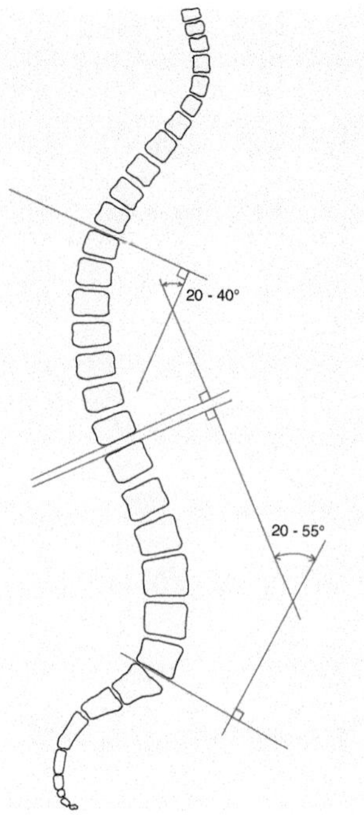

A Method of measuring spinal alignment Select the endplate of the upper and lower vertebrae with greatest deviation from the horizontal plane. Construct an endplate and right angle line (red). The enclosed angle is the degree of kyphosis or lordosis.

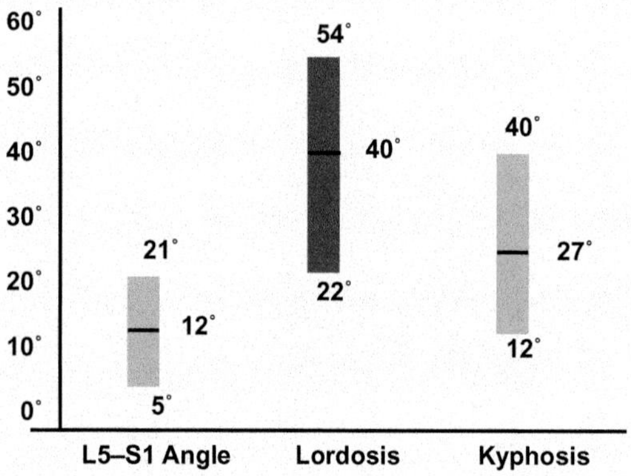

B Normal values of sagittal measures of the spine in children The range includes values from the 10th to the 90th percentiles. The L5-S1 angle includes measures between the inferior surface of L5 and the superior surface of S1 (green). Lordosis is measured using the Cobb method between L1 and L5 (red). Kyphosis is measured using the Cobb method between T5 and T12 (blue). From Propst-Proctor & Bleck. JPO 3:344, 1983.

Radiographs Make PA and lateral spine films in the upright position on 36-inch film using shielding and techniques that avoid excessive radiation exposure. Order oblique lumbosacral views to assess the pars if spondylolysis is suspected and not seen on lateral view.

SPECT Single-photon emission computed tomography (SPECT) imaging is useful to assess subtle pars reactions.

CT studies are useful to detail bony deformities or lesions.

MR imaging is used to study patients with neurological findings, those with unexplained progression of deformity, and certain types of deformity, as well as preoperatively for children with neurological impairment. These studies are helpful in evaluating tumors, congenital abnormalities such as Chiari malformation [C], various cysts, tethered cords, and filum terminale anomalies.

Multiple studies Order only those imaging studies that are definitely necessary during the initial evaluation [D].

Normal variability Measurements of deformity are made from standing radiographs [A]. Be aware of the normal range in the sagittal plane [B].

Sagittal plane The normal range for dorsal kyphosis falls between about 20° and 45°. Kyphosis between 45° and 55° is marginal. Kyphosis below 20° is referred to as hypokyphosis, and above 55° as hyperkyphosis. Hyperkyphosis is sometimes referred to as a "round back" deformity. Normal levels for lumbar lordosis fall between 20° and 55°. Likewise, reduced lordosis is termed hypolordosis, and increased lordosis is termed hyperlordosis. Hypolordosis is called a "flat back" and hyperlordosis either a "lordotic deformity" or a "swayback."

Frontal plane Mild curves that cause truncal asymmetry are usually normal variants. These variations are <10° by Cobb and <5° by scoliometer measure. These asymmetries have not been shown to cause any disability in childhood or adult life. Bone scans are usual in assessing back pain when radiographs are negative or equivocal.

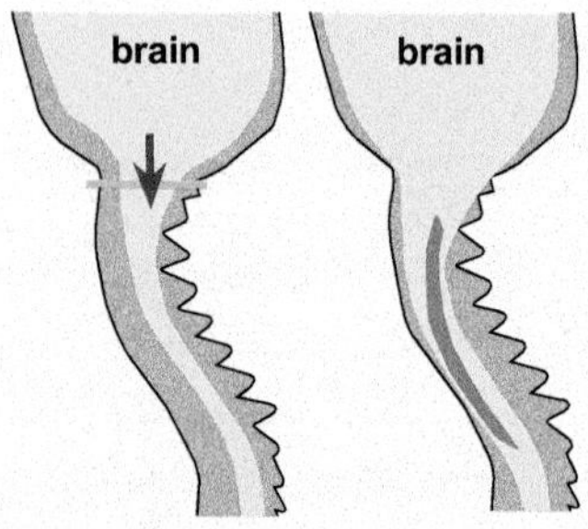

C Chiari malformation and syrinx This malformation is a displacement of the cerebellum into the spinal canal (red arrow). These lesions may be associated with a syrinx (blue).

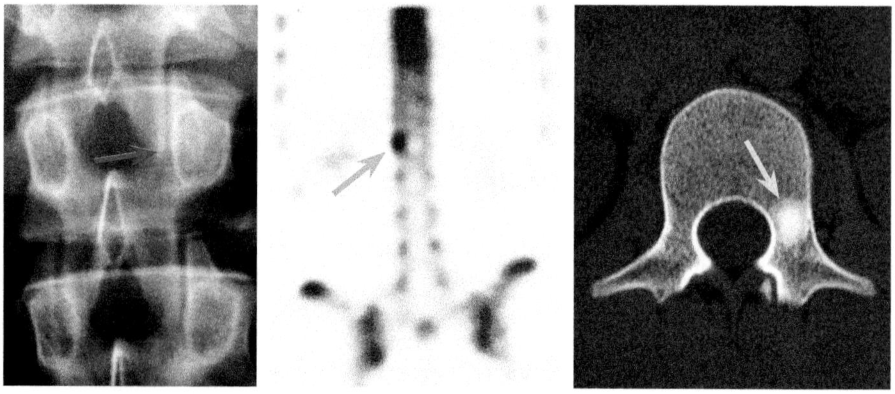

D Osteoid osteoma spine This lesion caused severe night pain. Enlargement of pedicle is seen on radiographs (red arrow). The bone scan showed a focal hot spot (orange arrow) and the CT scan shows the sclerotic lesion (yellow arrow). Excision was curative.

Congenital Deformities

Diastematomyelia

This is a congenital defect with a central cartilaginous–bony projection that divides the spinal cord [A].

Diagnosis Cutaneous lesions occur in most patients with a hairy patch, dimple, hemangioma, subcutaneous mass, or teratoma at or near the level of the diastematomyelia. Other deformities are common. Nearly all have some associated anomaly, such as spinal dysraphism, asymmetry of the lower extremities, clubfoot, or a cavus foot. Two-thirds have congenital scoliosis. Two-thirds are located in the lumbar spine. Half have neurological abnormalities.

Management Resect the spur in a patient with progressive neurological findings. Follow the others and consider resection should neurological findings develop or if correction of spinal deformity is planned.

Sacral Agenesis

Caudal regression or sacral agenesis includes a spectrum of abnormalities [B] with hypoplasia or aplasia [C] of the sacrum, which is most common in offspring of diabetic mothers.

Clinical features include knee-flexion contractures with popliteal webbing, dislocations and flexion contractures of the hips, scoliosis, equinovarus deformities of the foot, and instability at the spinal–pelvic junction. These deformities vary in severity with the level of the agenesis and the resulting loss of motor power. Neurological features may be most predictive of progression, and MR imaging is helpful in assessment.

Management is often difficult and depends upon the deformity, motor, and sensory status. Knee flexion deformities are difficult to correct, and recurrence is common. The combination of limited operative procedures and orthotic or mobility aids are tailored to the child. Spine–pelvic instability and hip dislocations are often better tolerated than the stiffness caused by surgical stabilization or reduction.

Exstrophy Bladder

A failure of anterior closure of the pelvis results in pelvic diastasis and an open bladder [D]. In the more severe form, cloacal exstrophy, an omphalocele containing intestinal contents, is also present.

Clinical features include pelvis diastasis, acetabular retroversion, and lateral rotation of limbs with out-toeing gait. This out-toeing tends to improve with age.

Management Orthopedic disabilities are insufficient to require correction. A pelvic osteotomy may be required during bladder reconstruction to facilitate closure. Perform bilateral supra-acetabular osteotomies and stabilize with a spica cast following urological repair.

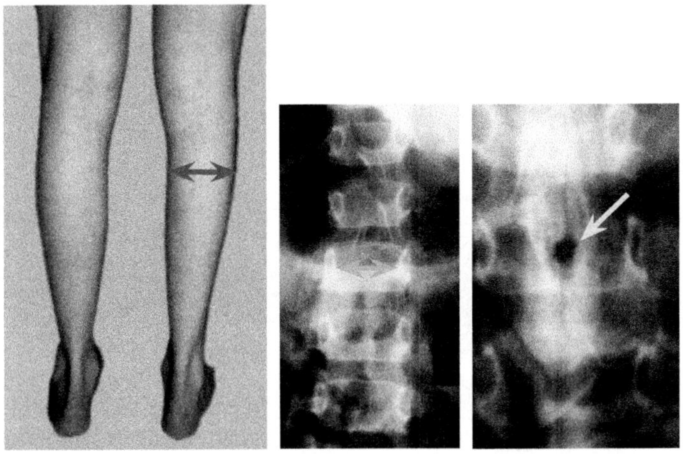

A Spinal dysraphism Diastematomyelia and other congenital spine defects should be considered in children with cavus feet or limb hypoplasia (red arrow). The interpedicular distance is widened (orange arrow) and a midline bony bar bisects the spinal cord, as shown on myelography (yellow arrow).

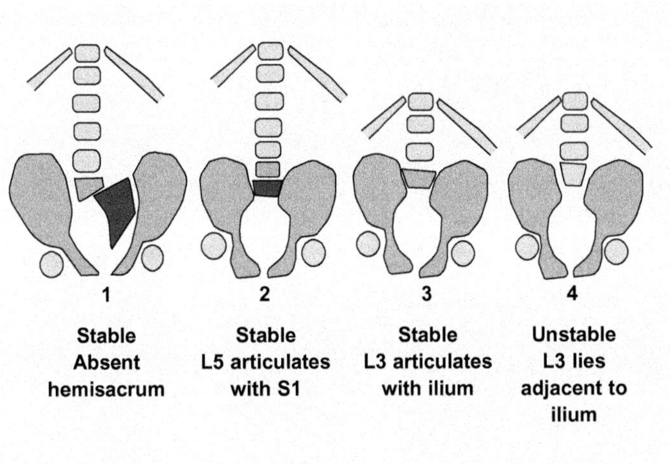

B Sacral agenesis classification by Renshaw. The sacrum may be hypoplastic or completely absent (red). The spine-pelvic relationship may be stable or unstable. Based on Renshaw (1978).

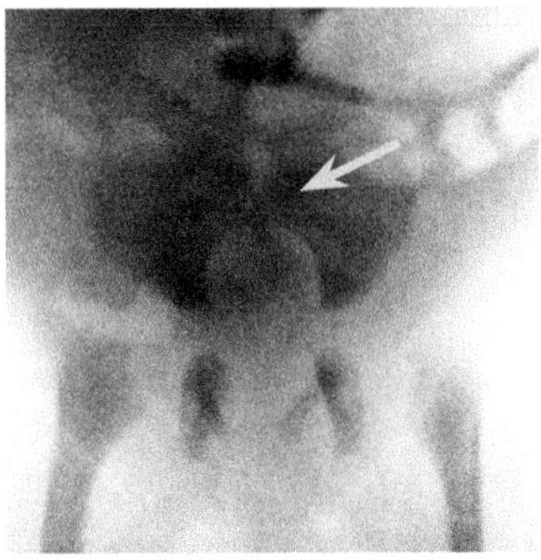

C Sacral agenesis Radiographs show a type 3 deficiency (yellow arrow).

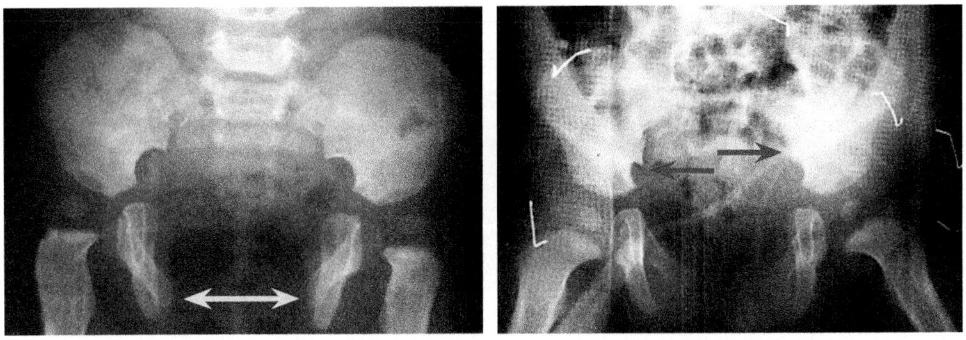

D Bladder exstrophy This is associated with separation of the pubic bones (yellow arrow) and retroversion of the acetabula. Bilateral iliac osteotomies (red arrows) were performed to facilitate bladder reconstruction.

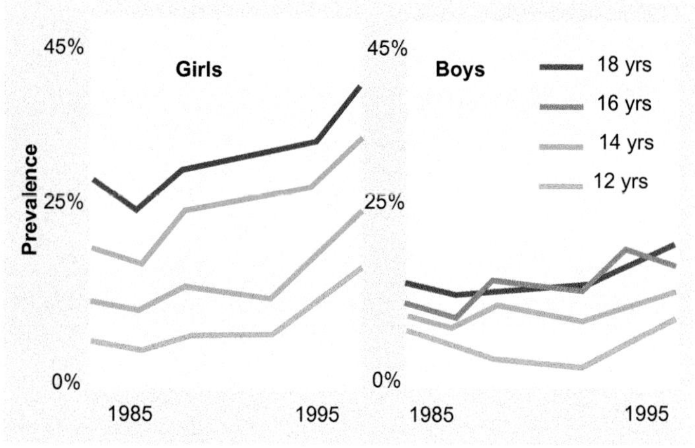

A Back Pain Children Prevalence by date, age, and gender. From Hakala et al, BMJ 325:737, 2002.

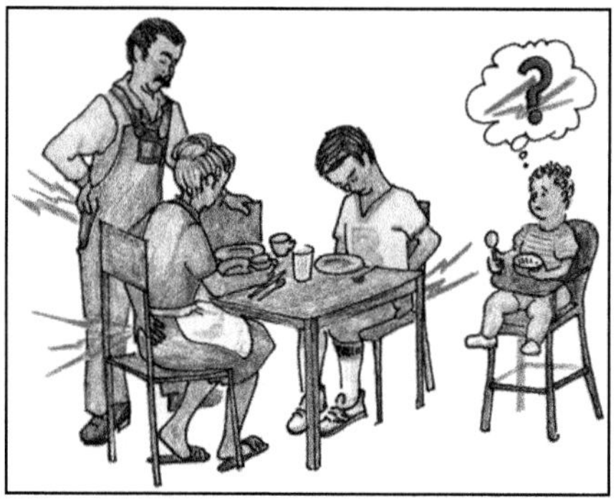

B Familial back pain The child may learn about back pain from siblings and parents.

Causes of back pain

- Trauma
- Spondylolisthesis and spondylolysis
- Scheuermann disease
- Schmorl nodes
- Spine tumors
- Discitis
- Rheumatoid spondylitis
- Functional disorders
- Overuse syndromes

C Causes of back pain in children These are the major causes of back pain in children and adolescents.

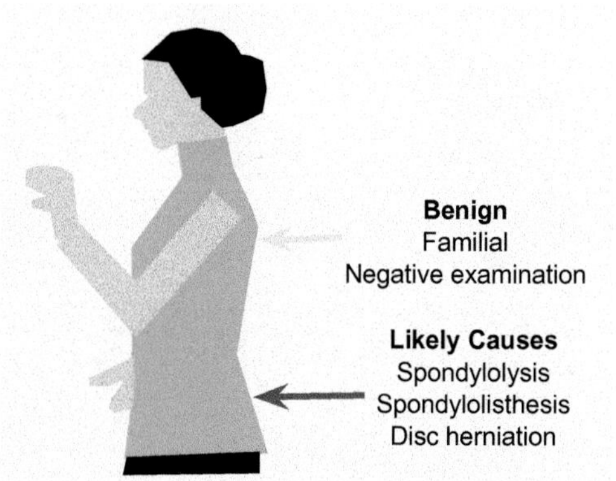

D Location and seriousness Lower back plain (red arrow) is much more likely to require treatment than upper and mid back pain (yellow arrow).

Back Pain

During the past several decades, back pain in children has become increasingly common [A]. This is especially true in adolescents and late teens. This increase is associated with increasing stress, complexities in family relationships [B], diminished physical activity, and increasing time with television and electronics. Because of the prevalence and social/cultural factors, the role of the primary care provider has increased significantly.

Prevalence

Back pain has becomes increasingly common especially among girls in late teens [A].

Evaluation

Be aware of the causes of back pain [C]. Worrisome features include onset before age 4 years, symptoms persisting beyond 4 weeks, interference with function, systemic features, increasing discomfort, night pain, neurological findings, and recent onset of scoliosis.

The location is significant [D]. Thoracic back pain is more common in girls, more common in late teens, and much less likely to be serious and require treatment.

Perform a careful physical examination. On bending, look for symmetry, mobility, and evenness of the curvature. Note the location of any tenderness. Perform a neurological examination and check for tight hamstrings.

Generally, image by radiographs – anteroposterior and lateral studies – are sufficient. Be aware that oblique views and CT scans expose the child to significant amounts of radiation. Avoid ordering MRI and other expensive studies. The spine doctor will prefer to order exactly what is needed.

When to refer

Upper thoracic pain Can often be managed in primary care.

Low back pain Especially if associated with localized tenderness, limited spine mobility, limited straight leg raising, uneven curvature of the back when bending, or asymmetry.

Management

Adolescent benign back pain Some suggest limiting backpacks to less than 20% of body weight (not evidence based). Encourage activity, a healthy lifestyle, and weight control. Provide reassurance. Consider this as a common backache, requiring no treatment, and best ignored.

Prognosis If back pain is present in adolescence together with a positive family history of back pain, nearly 90% of these adolescents will have back pain in adult life. Psychosocial problems are more significant than structural abnormalities in determining the likelihood that back pain will become chronic [C].

Tumors

Tumors may be metastatic or primary. Primary tumors may arise from the cord or bone [A].

Metastatic Tumors

These tumors are most common in the thoracic, then lumbar, and least common in the cervical spine [B]. Manage with chemotherapy and radiation. Mortality is high. Those who survive are likely to have deformity. Early stabilization may prevent progression of the deformity.

Primary Tumors

Primary tumors may occur in the vertebrae or cord. Most vertebral tumors are benign, and most cord tumors are malignant. Either type may cause spinal cord compression [C].

Spinal cord tumors cause diagnostic difficulties. They may present to the orthopedist with torticollis, scoliosis, gait disturbances, foot deformities, or back pain. Often forward bending is limited and asymmetrical. Perform a careful neurological examination. Study with plain radiographs first. Look for changes in intrapedicular distance. MRI studies are usually diagnostic.

Vertebral tumors are more common. Most are benign. Most present with pain. Duration of symptoms from benign tumors is usually longer than those from malignant tumors. Most may be diagnosed by conventional radiographs.

Osteoid osteoma and osteoblastoma cause classic night pain, usually secondary scoliosis, limited spinal mobility [D], often tenderness, and sometimes classic radiographic features. Bone scans are often diagnostic. Excision is often necessary. Exactly localize with preoperative imaging. Percutaneous ablation is an option [E].

Eosinophilic granuloma causes pain, tenderness, limited mobility, and usually a focal lesion. The classic vertebrae plana [F] is often absent. For solitary, uncomplicated lesions, observational management is appropriate. If lesions are multiple or if neurological involvement is present, operative resection may be necessary.

Aneurysmal bone cysts cause pain, rarely cord or root compression, sometimes deformity, and limited mobility. Radiographs are often diagnostic with expansion and ballooning of the cortex [G]. Management is often difficult. Manage with preoperative selective arterial embolization, intralesional excision curettage, bone grafting, and fusion of the affected area if instability is present.

Vertebral Tumors

Benign
- Eosinophilic granuloma
- Osteoid osteoma
- Aneurysmal bone cyst
- Osteoblastoma
- Neurofibromatosis
- Osteochondroma

Malignant
- Ewing sarcoma
- Lymphoma of bone
- Leukemia

Spinal Cord Tumors

Benign
- Neurofibroma
- Lipoma
- Spinal cysts

Malignant
- Astrocytoma
- Ependymoma
- Mixed glioma
- Ganglioglioma

A Vertebral (bone) and spinal cord tumors

Metastatic Tumors
- Ewing sarcoma
- Rhabdomyosarcoma
- Adenocarcinoma
- Neuroblastoma
- Miscellaneous other tumors

B Metastatic tumors to spine From Freiberg (1993).

Cord Compression
- Neuroblastoma
- Sarcoma
- Astrocytoma
- Lymphoma

C Tumors causing cord compression in children From Conrad (1992).

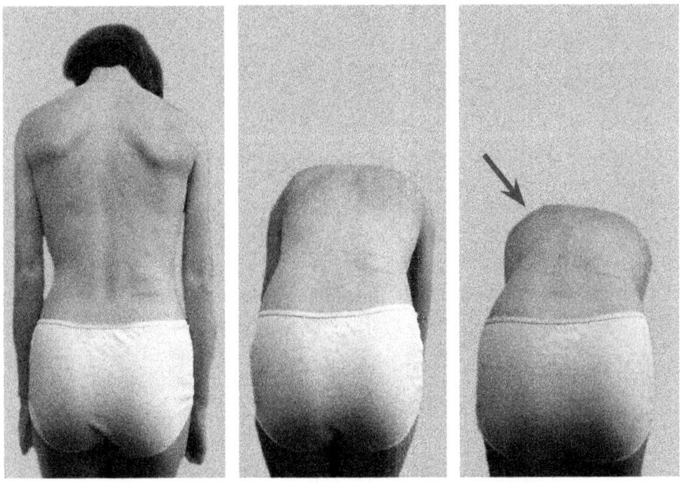

D List on forward bending This boy with an osteoid osteoma shows asymmetrical forward bending. Bending is restricted on the left side (arrow).

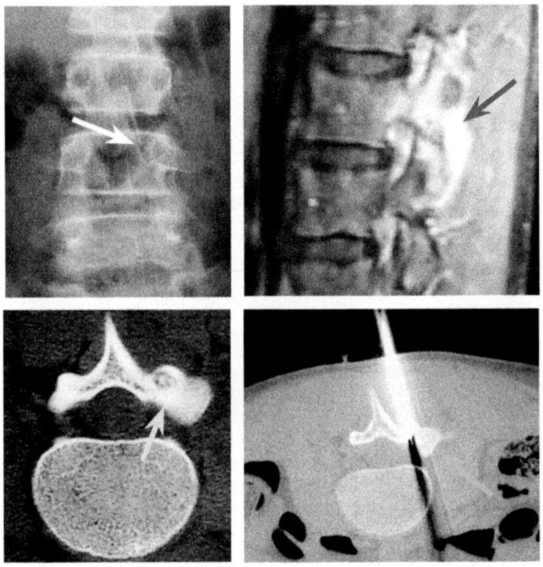

E Percutaneous ablation of osteoid osteoma The lesion is difficult to image on the radiograph (white arrow), but inflammation is readily apparent on MRI (red arrow), well defined on CT (yellow arrow), and ablated percutaneously, as shown by intraoperative imaging (green arrow).

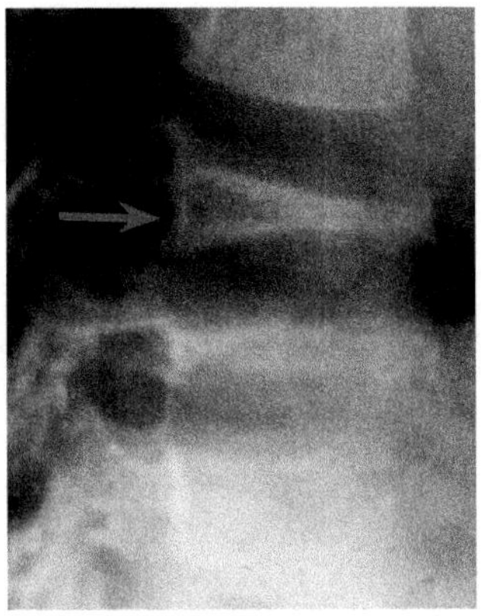

F Disc collapse from eosinophilic granuloma Note the vertebral collapse. The appearance is classic.

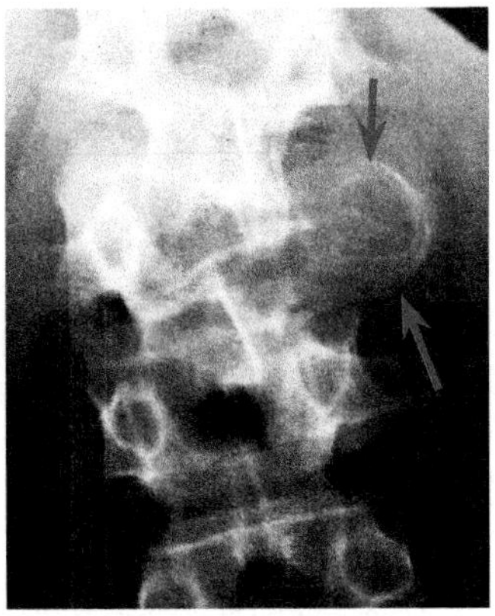

G Aneurysmal bone cyst in 15-year-old boy Note the expansile cystic lesion (arrows).

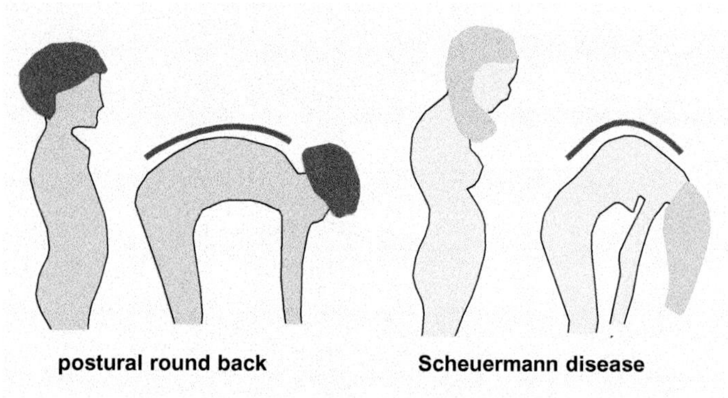

A Differentiating postural round back and Scheuermann disease Note the smooth contour of the back on forward bending in the child with round back as compared with the angular pattern in the child with Scheuermann disease.

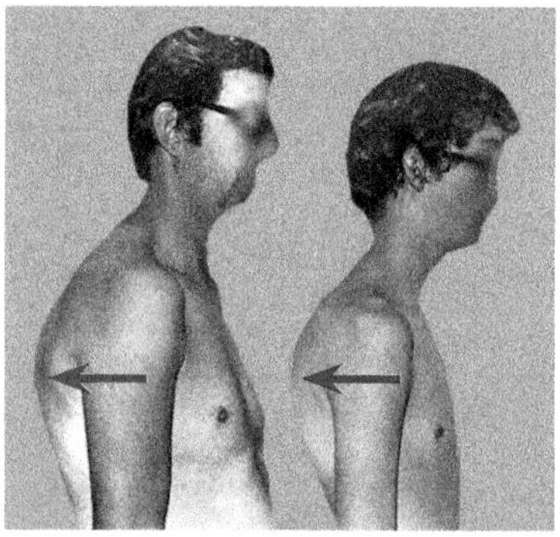

B Familial Scheuermann This father and son have the same fixed deformity.

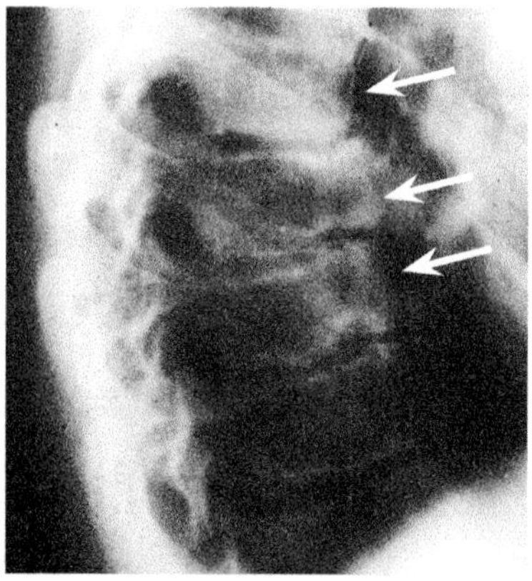

C Painful kyphosis This 16-year-old male has pain and tenderness over the lower thoracic spine. Note the narrow disc spaces, as well as erosion and deformity of the vertebral bodies (arrows).

Scheuermann Disease

Scheuermann disease is a familial disorder of the thoracic spine producing vertebral wedging and kyphosis greater than about 45° [A] and often causing back pain.

Clinical Features

A history of heavy physical loading from athletics or work is common. Often the deformity is familial [B]. Patients often complain of deformity, fatigue, and sometimes pain. The normal even contour of the spine is lost with an abrupt kyphotic segment at or above the thoracolumbar level. Tenderness over the apex may be present. Radiographs show anterior body wedging. Mild scoliosis is common. The strict definition requires a wedging of at least 5° involving three vertebrae [C].

Management

Treat the pain by NSAIDs, rest, and stress reduction. Sometimes a thoracolumbar sacral orthosis (TLSO) will be helpful in controlling the pain. Management of the deformity is discussed on page 253.

Schmorl Nodes

These nodes are vertical herniations of the intervertebral disc through the vertebral endplate, causing narrowing of the disc space [D]. Sometimes the condition is referred to as *lumbar Scheuermann disease*. This herniation is most common in adolescents, is often associated with trauma, and may be the cause of back pain. The lesions may be seen on plain radiographs, although MR imaging is most sensitive and may be indicated when the diagnosis is uncertain. Manage by rest, NSAIDs, and sometimes a TLSO.

Disc Herniation

Disc herniations occur rarely in adolescents. Predisposing features include positive family history, recent trauma, facet asymmetry, spinal stenosis, transitional vertebrae, and spondylolisthesis.

Clinical Features

Herniations usually occur at the L4–L5 or L5–S1 levels, often producing radicular pain and secondary spinal deformity. The patient may be seen because of scoliosis or a list. Straight leg raising is limited, and neurological changes are variable. Radiographs are usually normal. Occult spina bifida is more common in these patients. MRI studies or myelography shows the lesion [E]. Disability is increased if the herniation is associated with spinal stenosis. Be aware that fracture of the lumbar vertebral ring apophysis may be confused with disc herniations.

Management

Manage first with NSAIDs, rest, limited activities, and a TLSO. Persisting or increasing disability are indications for MRI and operative disc excision. Endoscopic or open discectomies are successful in 90% of cases.

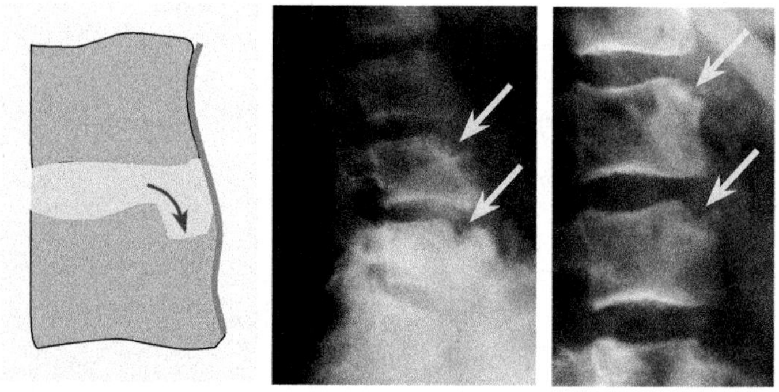

D Schmorl nodes With vertical loading, the nucleus may herniate into the vertebral body (red arrow) producing pain and atypical radiographic defects (yellow arrows).

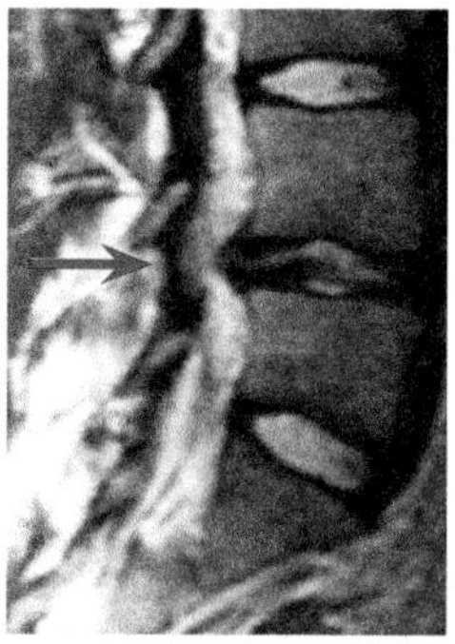

E MRI in disc herniation The posterior bulging disc at L4-L5 is clearly demonstrated on MRI.

Discitis

Discitis is an inflammation (probably an infection) that involves the lower thoracic or upper lumbar disc spaces in infants and children. Unlike other musculoskeletal infections, discitis usually resolves spontaneously.

Clinical Features

The clinical features of discitis are age related. Discitis in the infant is characterized by fever, irritability, and an unwillingness to walk. The child may show constitutional illness with nausea and vomiting. The adolescent may complain of back pain. Because the symptoms are vague and poorly localized, the diagnosis is often delayed. The findings of fever and malaise, a stiff back, unwillingness to walk, and an elevated ESR and CRP are suggestive of discitis.

Imaging Early in the disease, a bone scan may show increased uptake over several vertebral levels [A]. After 2–3 weeks, narrowing of the disc space is seen on a lateral radiograph of the spine. MRI often shows worrisome features and may lead to overtreatment [B].

Aspiration or biopsy Disc space aspiration is not necessary unless the disease is atypical.

Management

Manage based on the stage and severity of the disease. If the child is systemically ill, antistaphylococcal antibiotic treatment is appropriate. If the child is acutely ill, an intravenous route is appropriate. Otherwise, oral medication is adequate. Discitis is more severe in the older child [C]. Continue antibiotics until the ESR returns to normal. For comfort, consider immobilization in a "panty spica" or brace [D] for a period of several weeks.

Prognosis

Long-term studies show a variety of abnormalities that include residual narrowing [A, right], block vertebrae, and limited extension, but the likelihood of back pain is not increased.

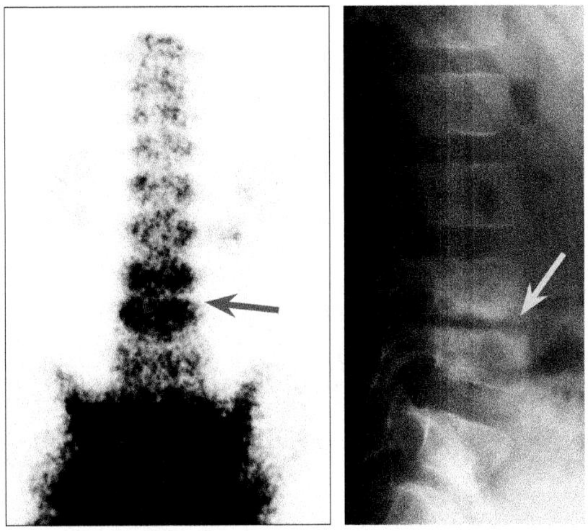

A Discitis L4-L5 The typical features of discitis are shown on different imaging studies. The bone scan shows increased uptake (red arrow), and later the lateral radiograph shows narrowing (yellow arrow) of the disc space.

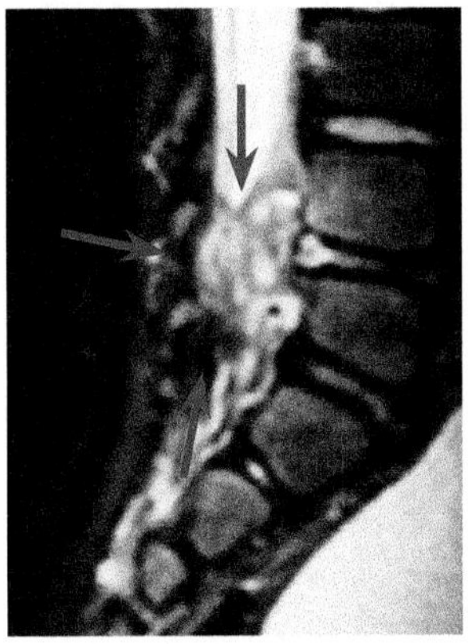

B MRI of discitis The typical intense inflammatory reaction seen on MRI may lead to concern about abscess formation and lead to unnecessary operative draining.

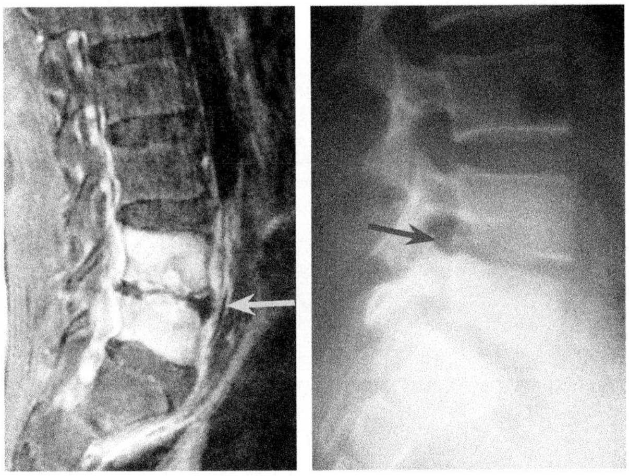

C Discitis in an older child Discitis is more severe in the older child. Note the extensive inflammation of adjacent vertebrae in the MRI (yellow arrow) and the residual narrowing (red arrow).

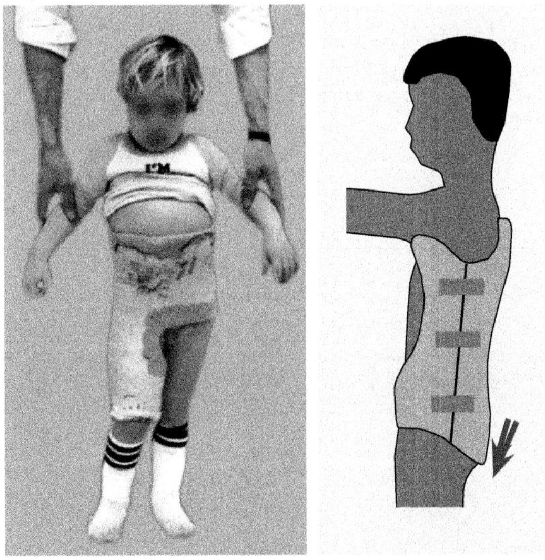

D Immobilization of the back reduces discomfort Most complete immobilization includes the back and one limb to immobilize the lumbosacral spine (left). Adequate immobilization is often achieved with a custom TLSO that extends well down over the pelvis (arrow).

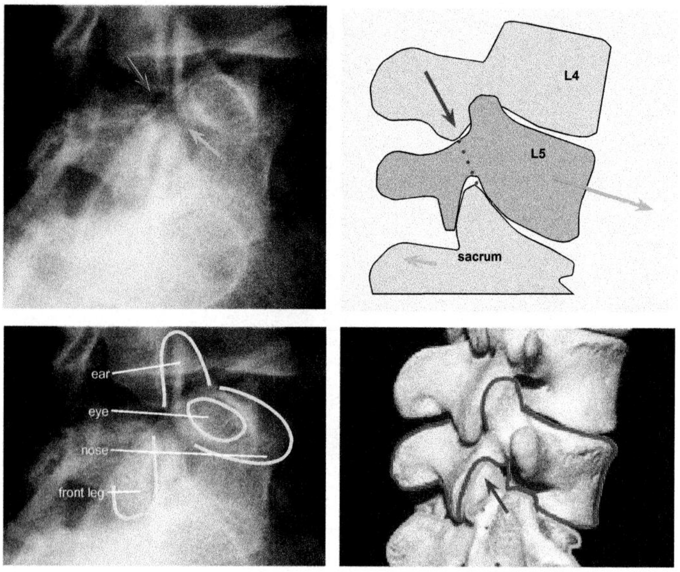

A Spondylolysis The fracture through the pars is shown by red arrows. Note the fracture through the pars as shown on the oblique radiograph (upper left) and diagram (upper right). The scotty dog analogy is often used (lower left) to describe the vertebral elements (yellow lines). The neck is the site of fracture. The superior facet of the sacrum (green arrow) normally prevents forward displacement of L5. This restraint is lost when the pars fractures. The model (lower right) shows the site of the fracture.

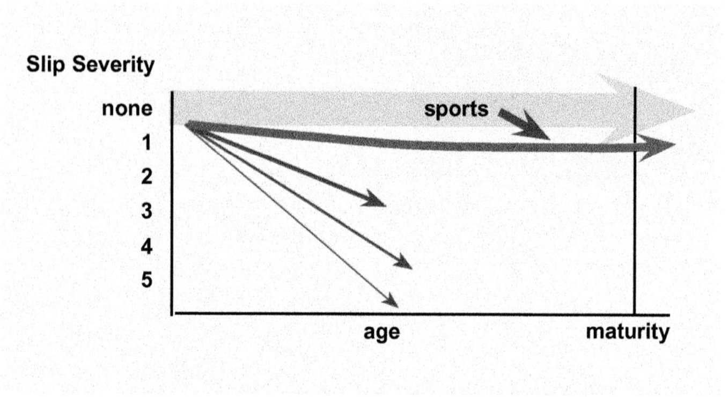

B The natural history of pars defects Most defects develop during early childhood and remain mild. Others develop in late childhood, usually due to repetitive trauma from certain sports or less commonly due to acute trauma.

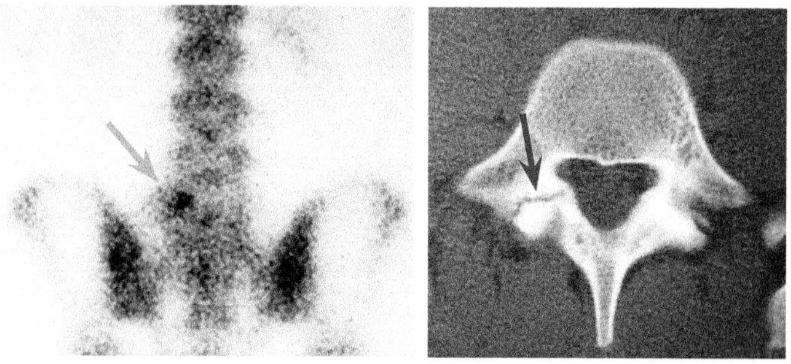

C Unilateral spondylolysis These studies were performed in a 15-year-old girl with a history of back pain for one month. This bone scan shows an active unilateral defect (orange arrow), and the CT scan shows the defect clearly (red arrow).

Spondylolysis and Spondylolisthesis

Bilateral or unilateral defects of the pars interarticularis cause spondylolysis [A]. This defect may allow displacement of the vertebrae, which is called spondylolisthesis. These lesions are the most common cause of structural back pain in children and adolescents.

Pathogenesis

In children, these conditions are usually due to a stress fracture through a congenitally dysplastic pars interarticularis. This inherent weakness occurs more commonly in certain races (such as Inuit peoples), families, or individuals. The defects often are associated with spina bifida occulta. Spondylolisthesis occurs in about 4% of 4-year-old children and increases to about 6% by maturity. Spondylolisthesis occurs in about a third of those with pars defects, especially in those with mechanical instability. These lesions occur more commonly in children with abnormal bone or connective tissue, as occurs in conditions such as Marfan syndrome and osteopetrosis. Lesions are common in children who participate in certain sports that cause hyperextension of the lumbar spine with rotation, such as gymnastics, wrestling, diving, and weightlifting [B]. Progression after adolescence is unusual.

Clinical Features

History and physical examination The child usually complains of back pain. Tenderness may be present at the L5-S1 level. If the displacement is severe, a prominence is palpable over the defect. Straight leg raising and forward bending may be limited. The neurological examination is usually normal. If the condition is acute, secondary scoliosis may be present.

Imaging First, order a standing lateral radiograph of the lumbosacral spine. A forward displacement of the body of L5 or L4 establishes the diagnosis. If no displacement is present, order oblique radiographs of the lower lumbar spine to assess the status of the pars. Spina bifida occulta is common in children with the defect. A bone scan may show reaction [C] before radiographs show a defect and may be used to determine the activity and healing potential of the lesion. Even more sensitive is SPECT imaging in demonstrating the stress reaction of spondylolysis.

Classification Wiltse classifies spondylolisthesis into two types:

Dysplastic is a congenital facet deficiency allowing slippage.

Isthmic allows slippage due to a defect in the pars interarticularis. These lesions may be due to a fatigue fracture, a stress fracture, or elongation without fracture.

Grade the degree of slip in severity and activity (duration).

Severity Grade on the basis of slip angle [A, next page] and displacement [C, next page]. Slip angle changes usually occur with slips greater than 50%.

Activity Grade on the duration or activity. Recent fractures are active and show increased uptake on bone scan. Cold lesions are chronic, inactive, and less likely to heal.

Progression Pain is most pronounced at the time of onset or fracture. Most isthmic lesions become stable and painless with time. Pain is aggravated by activity, especially competitive sports. Lesions often are symptomatic in adolescence but become painless in adult life when activity levels are reduced. The incidence of back pain is comparable to normal population levels.

Management

Management is based on the patient's age, degree of deformity, type of lesion, activity, and physical activity level.

Spondylolysis management depends upon the activity of the lesion.

Acute lesions from an acute injury or recent overuse experience are managed by reduction of activity and usually an under-arm brace [B]. Often these lesions will heal.

Established lesions Manage symptoms with NSAIDS and activity modification. Operative stabilization is seldom necessary.

Spondylolisthesis is managed based on the severity of the slip, considering the displacement and slip angle. If fusion is required, it is often performed without reduction.

Grade 1–2 slips Manage with NSAIDS, activity modification, and TLSO as necessary to control symptoms. Follow with standing lateral radiographs.

Grade 3 slips Most require operative stabilization in children. Fuse L4–S1 level with posterolateral autogenous grafting.

Grade 4 slips These slips may require fusion of L4-S1, as the displacement may be significant, making identification of the transverse process of L5 difficult. If slip angle is severe, reduction is sometimes performed.

Grade 5 (spondyloptosis) management is controversial. In situ fusion provides pain relief and safety, but the deformity remains. Reduction incurs greater risk but improves appearance and posture.

Special situations require tailoring of management.

L4 spondylolisthesis is less common, more mechanical in etiology, often causes more symptoms, and is more likely to require operative stabilization.

Spondylolysis with persisting symptoms may be managed by repair of the pars defect with grafting and fixation.

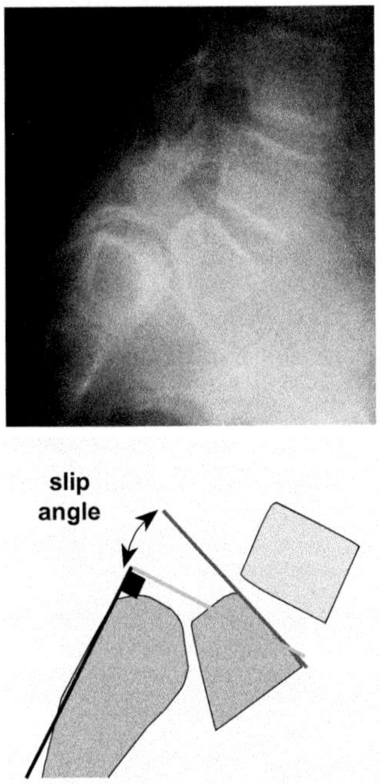

A Slip angle Draw the sacral line (black) along the posterior margin of the sacrum. Construct a right angle line to sacral line (green). Draw the L5 body line along the superior margin of the body of L5 (red line). The slip angle is the angle between the green and red lines.

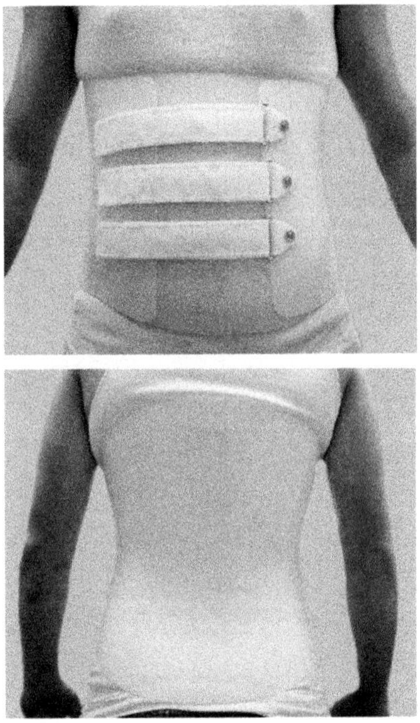

B Brace for spondylolysis The brace from the front and back shows the anterior closure and posterior extension to provide optimal immobilization for an under-arm brace.

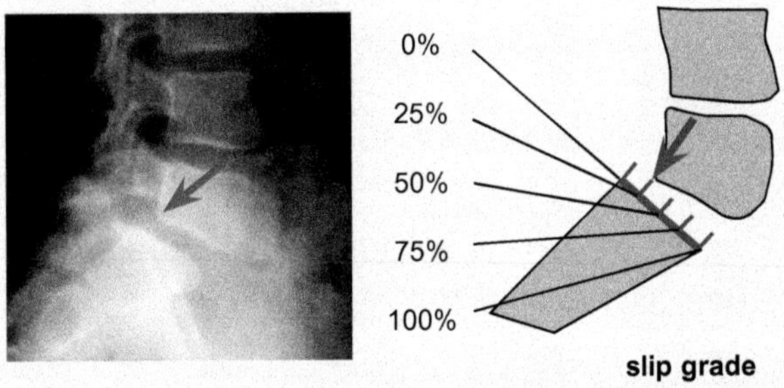

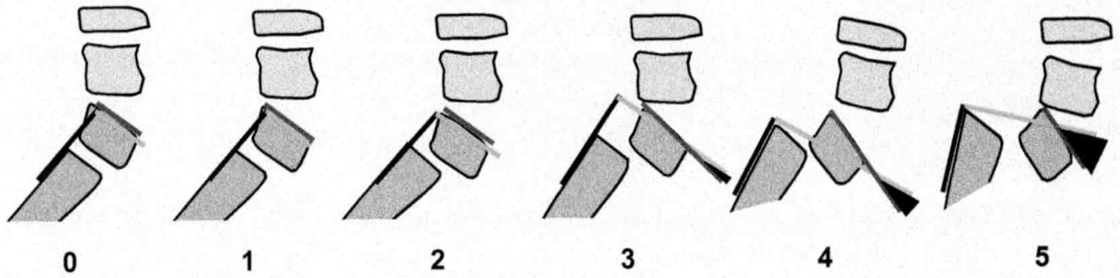

C Slip displacement The severity of the slip is assessed by the degree of displacement of L5 relative to the sacrum (red arrows) and the slip angle (black triangles). Slips are graded into five categories based on degree of displacement. Note that the slip angle increases progressively through grades 3 to 5.

Category	Disease
Secondary	Muscle spasm Leg length inequality Functional disorders
Congenital	Failure of formation or segmentation Neurotissue disorders
Neuromuscular	Upper neuron lesions – cerebral palsy Lower neuron lesions – poliomyelitis Myopathies – muscular dystrophy
Constitutional	Certain syndromes Metabolic disorders Arthritis
Idiopathic	Infantile Juvenile Adolescent
Miscellaneous	Traumatic Neoplastic Contractures Iatrogenic – radiation, thoracoplasty

A Classification of scoliosis Scoliosis is classified into general categories.

Condition	Comment
Spondylolisthesis	Only with severe displacement
Herniated disc	Often causes scoliosis
Osteoid osteoma	Focal painful lesion
Intraspinal tumor	Most serious cause
Discitis	Older child

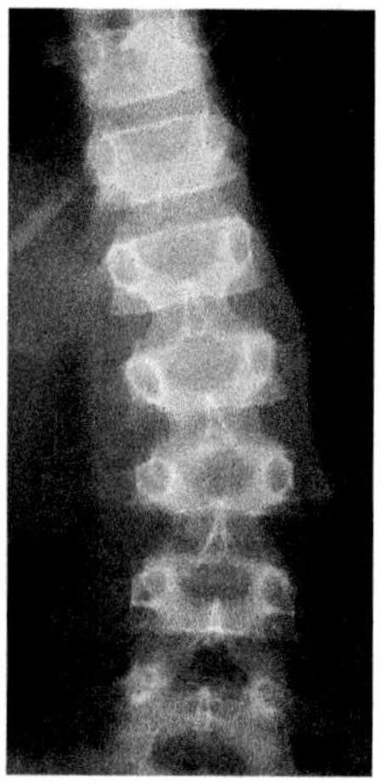

B Underlying causes of scoliosis due to muscle spasm These conditions should be ruled out if the scoliosis is atypical, associated with pain, list, stiffness, tenderness, or obvious muscle spasm.

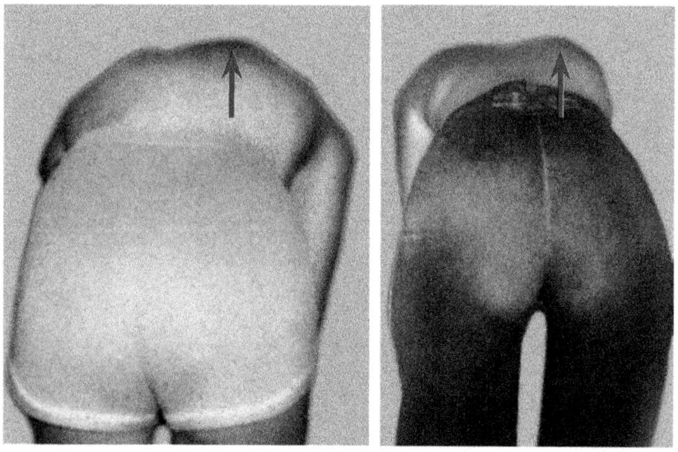

C Familial scoliosis Scoliosis runs in families. Perform a forward bending test on the parents and siblings. This mother (right) was unaware of her scoliosis.

Scoliosis

Scoliosis is often defined as simply a frontal plane deformity of the spine >10°. The deformity is much more complex, however, and includes significant transverse and sagittal plane components. The causes of scoliosis are numerous [A]. Mild truncal asymmetry occurs in as much as 10% of the population and may be considered as a variation of normal. Curves greater than 10° are abnormal, and in the growing child may progress to cause a significant problem. Scoliosis is the most common back deformity.

Secondary or Functional Scoliosis

This type of scoliosis can also be described as "functional" because it is secondary to some other problem [B]. The scoliosis usually resolves when the underlying problem is corrected. The scoliosis is usually flexible and nonstructural. There are no bony changes, and the rotational elements are minimal. The common causes of functional scoliosis are leg length inequality and muscle spasm.

Leg length discrepancy Differences in limb length produce a transient functional scoliosis. This type of scoliosis seldom becomes rigid or structural, presumably because the scoliosis is present only when the child is standing on both feet. Thus with lying, sitting, and walking, the spine is straight. The fear of causing a structural scoliosis or other back problems is not a valid reason for ordering a shoe lift or for performing limb length equalization procedures.

Muscle spasm Scoliosis may be the presenting sign for several inflammatory or neoplastic disorders. The spinal curvature often functions to relieve discomfort. For example, the back is curved to reduce pressure on a nerve root from a herniated disc. Management is directed at the underlying disorder. Scoliosis will disappear once the underlying problem is corrected.

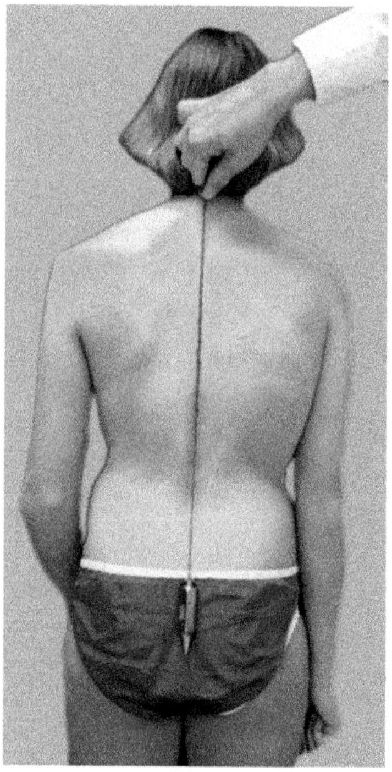

D Balance Assess alignment with a plumb line.

Evaluation

The evaluation should establish the diagnosis, determine the severity, and allow an estimation of the potential for progression of the scoliosis.

History Inquire about the age of onset, progression, and previous management. A family history of deformity [C, previous page] or pain is important as both run in families. Painful scoliosis in the child suggests an inflammatory or neoplastic basis for the scoliosis.

Screening examination Start with a screening examination. Look for conditions such as Marfan syndrome or the café au lait spots of neurofibromatosis. Assess the child's limb lengths and gait, and perform a neurological examination.

School screening The value of school screening is controversial. The advantage is the earlier detection of deformity. The disadvantage is the large numbers of children with "scoliosis," those with minimal truncal asymmetry that are referred to physicians, often studied radiographically, and subjected to the anguish of having *scoliosis.* Proposals to be more efficient have included establishing a threshold of 7° scoliometer reading and biannual screening.

Back examination Note truncal symmetry [A]. Note differences in shoulder height, scapular prominence, flank crease, and pelvic symmetry. Ask the patient to bend forward. Be concerned about stiffness or a list, as these suggest an underlying neoplastic or inflammatory process.

Perform the forward bending test Visually scan each level of the spine to assess symmetry. If a "rib hump" is present, measure it with a scoliometer. This simple device measures the tilt of the rib hump. Assess the balance of the spine using a plumb line [D, previous page]. Record the displacement of the weight from the buttock crease.

Radiographs Radiographs are indicated if the scoliometer reading is greater than 7° or if progression is likely. Progression is more likely if the child is under 12 years of age, when others in the family have significant curves, or if any findings suggest that the curve may not be simply idiopathic. Radiographs should be made on 36-inch film and taken standing with shielding. A single PA radiograph is satisfactory for screening or a baseline study.

Cobb angle This method [B] measures the level with the greatest tilt. Note the "apical vertebra," as this defines the level of the curve. Curves greater than 10° are considered significant.

Flexibility Left and right bending studies show the rigidity of the curves [D]. The value of these studies is controversial.

Level A general classification of the level of the curve is used for general description without regard for management considerations [C, next page].

Maturity is assessed by clinical evaluation (Chapter 1) or by the status of the triradiate cartilage or the Risser sign [C].

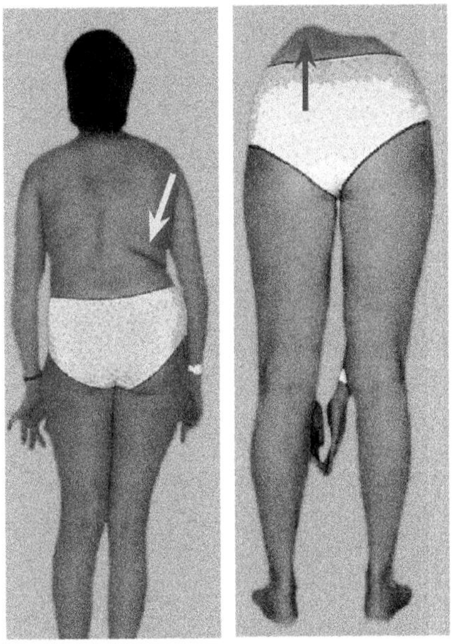

A Adolescent idiopathic right thoracic left lumbar scoliosis The flank crease (yellow arrow) and thoracic prominence (red arrow) are shown.

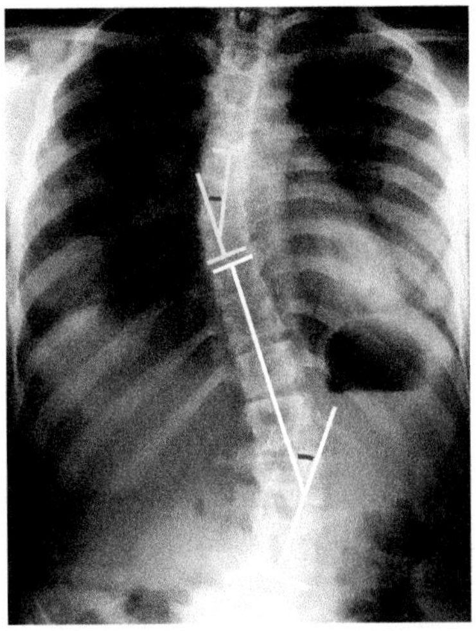

B Cobb measure of curve The degree of scoliosis (red arcs) is the angular difference between right angle lines drawn to the most tilted vertebral bodies. Note the double curve with the thoracic apex at T8 and the lumbar curve at L4.

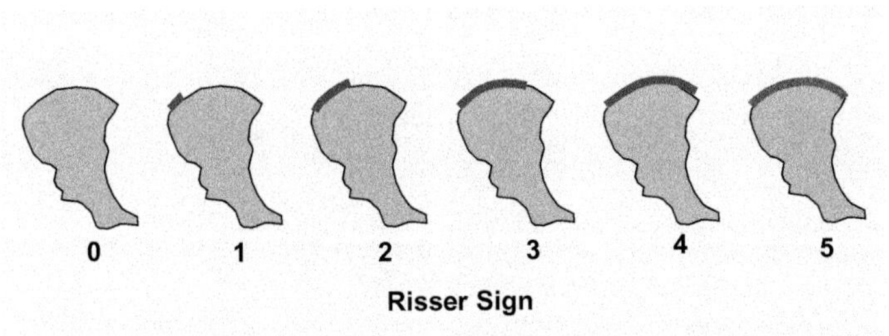

C Risser sign The status of the iliac apophysis is a traditional method of assessing maturity. The apophysis may be unossified (0), partially ossified (1–4) or fused to the ilium (5).

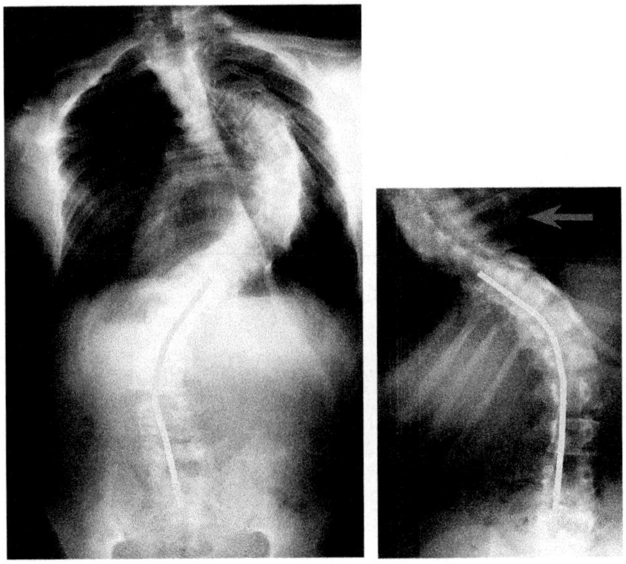

D Flexibility study The left bending study (arrow) shows full correction of the lumbar curve.

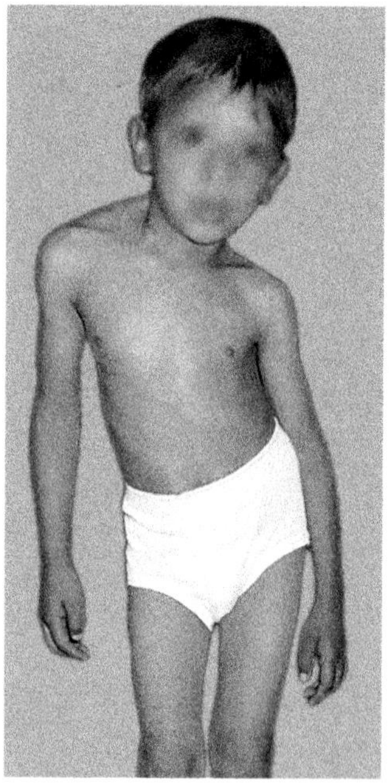

A Congenital scoliosis This child has upper thoracic congenital scoliosis with severe deformity. This type of deformity should be prevented by early surgery.

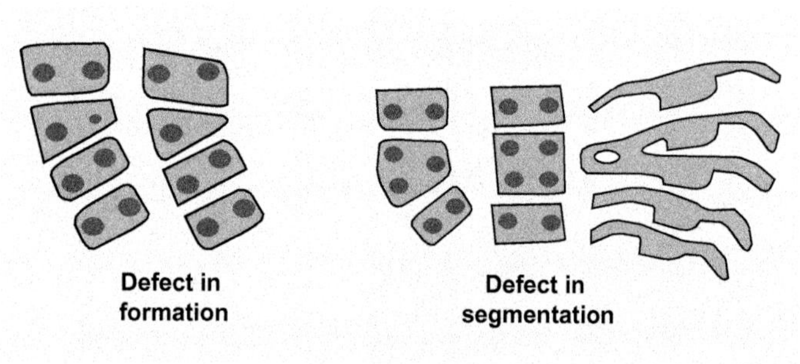

B Types of congenital scoliosis. The common defects are a failure in formation or segmentation. Complex deformities may show mixed patterns.

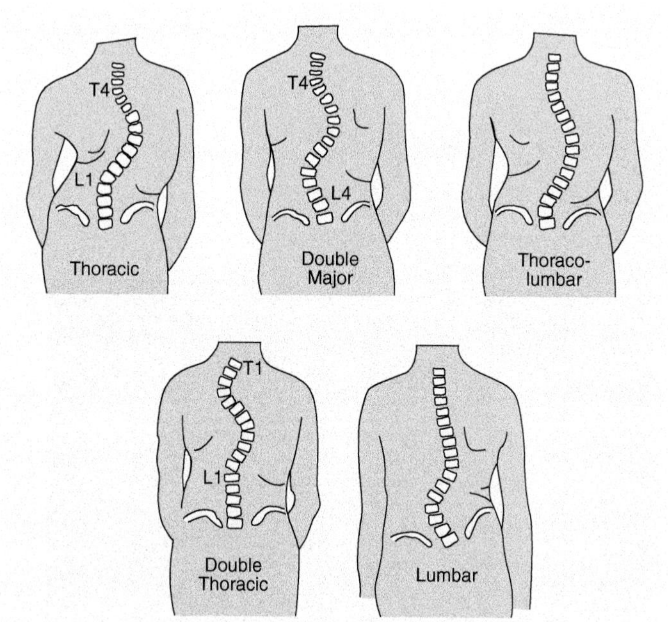

C Classification of scoliosis Scoliosis is classified into general categories by level.

Congenital Scoliosis

Congenital structural defects may cause a variety of spinal curves [A]. Such curves are often complex and may require special imaging techniques for assessment. Because these malformations are due to an abnormality of the fetal somite formation, associated lesions in the same somite are common. Thus, the finding of congenital scoliosis, especially one involving the thoracolumbar region, should prompt an ultrasound evaluation of the urinary system and consideration about syndromes such as the VACTERL association.

Pathogenesis

Congenital scoliosis is usually caused by a failure of formation or segmentation [B]. The progression of the curve is related to the type of bony defect. Curves that are most likely to progress are those with unilateral unsegmented bars that restrict growth on one side while the opposite side grows normally.

Evaluation

Note the severity, symmetry, and flexibility of the curve. Screen the child for additional disorders of the urinary and cardiovascular systems. Murmurs should be evaluated by a pediatric cardiologist. Order a renal ultrasound, as 10–20% will have congenital urinary abnormalities, some of which are life-threatening.

Imaging Study the pattern of the curve on AP and lateral radiographs of the entire spine and additional imaging methods for special situations [A, next page]. Categorize the curve pattern to assess the likelihood of progression. If the curve pattern is ambiguous, CT scans of the apical region are sometimes necessary. MR studies are indicated if neurological abnormalities are found. Plan follow-up and repeat the radiographs in 3–6 months.

Management

The management of congenital scoliosis depends upon the pattern and severity of the curve [D] and rate of progression.

Observation is appropriate when the potential for progression is uncertain. Evaluate every 3 months during the first 3 years and again during puberty when spinal growth is greatest.

Orthotic treatment of congenital scoliosis is controversial and less effective than for idiopathic curves. Congenital curves that are long and flexible are most likely to respond to brace treatment.

Operative treatment The goal is to obtain a balanced trunk and spine and to prevent any neurological defects with the least disturbance in normal growth. Operative treatment is required in about half of children with congenital scoliosis. Several options are available.

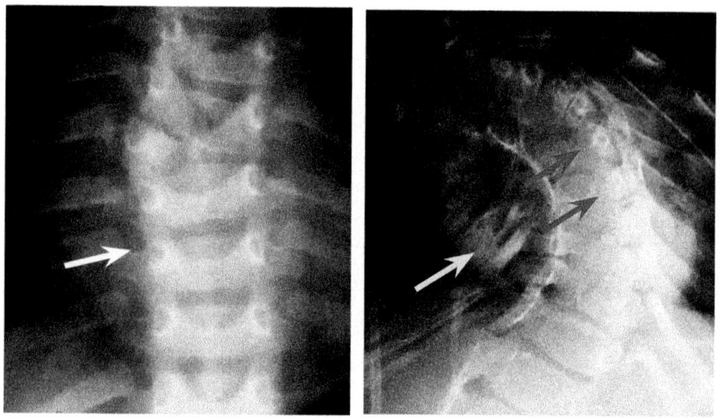

D Grades of severity The hemivertebrae (white arrow) often produce little deformity. On the other extreme, unilateral fusions of the vertebrae (red arrows) and ribs (yellow arrow) cause progressive severe deformity. This curve was fused in infancy to prevent further progression.

In situ fusion is indicated for curves due to unilateral bars or mild to moderate curves demonstrating progression. In children under 10 years of age, both anterior and posterior fusions are necessary to prevent a crankshaft phenomenon.

Hemivertebra resection This procedure may be indicated for severe curves with spinal imbalance at or below the thoracolumbar junction in young children.

Instrumentation and fusion Moderate curves in the older child may be managed by limited correction. Limited correction and careful monitoring are necessary to prevent neurological complications.

Osteotomy or resection and instrumentation These aggressive measures may be necessary for severe deformity and imbalance. Preoperative halo traction and staged correction are techniques that may reduce the risk of neurological complications.

Hemifusion on the convex side may be considered for lumbar curves in infants or young children to provide some correction with growth.

Thoracic Insufficiency Syndrome

This syndrome may accompany congenital scoliosis. This syndrome includes rib fusions and the inability of the thorax to support normal respiration or lung growth.

Management

Campbell and associates have developed a technique for correction that includes an opening wedge thoracostomy with use of a chest-wall distractor known as a vertical expandable prosthetic titanium rib [C]. This lengthens and expands the constricted hemithorax, allowing growth of the thoracic spine and the rib cage. The procedure is usually performed in early childhood with repeat lengthenings of the prosthesis performed at 4–6 month intervals. The procedure may also be used for bilateral insufficiency [B].

Results

The procedure corrects most components of chest-wall deformity and indirectly corrects congenital scoliosis without the need for spine fusion. Scoliosis is reduced and vital capacity is increased.

Complications

The most common complication is asymptomatic proximal migration of the rib fixation devices through the ribs.

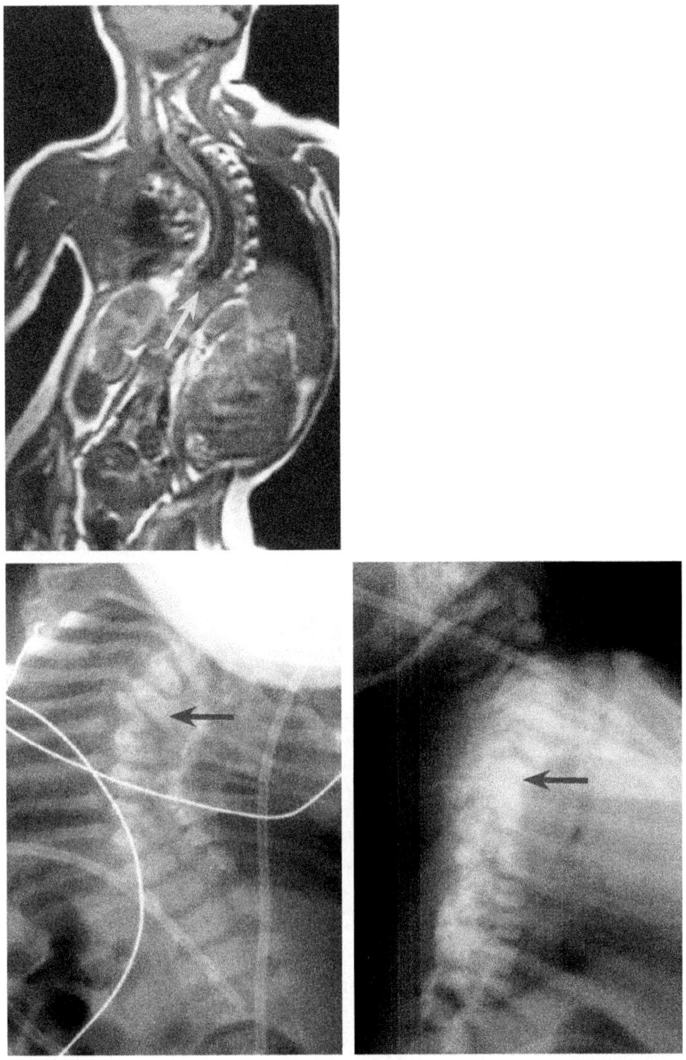

A Special imaging in congenital scoliosis. This congenital scoliosis (red arrows) in a newborn was imaged with MRI because of a neurological deficit. Note the hydromyelia (yellow arrow).

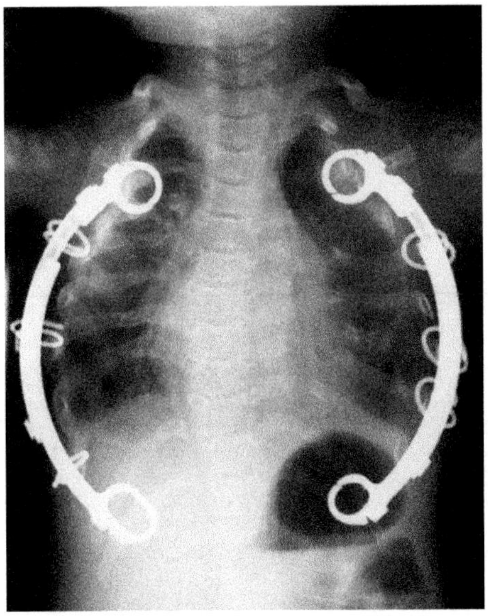

B Bilateral expansion Titanium ribs were used for bilateral chest wall expansion to improve pulmonary function.

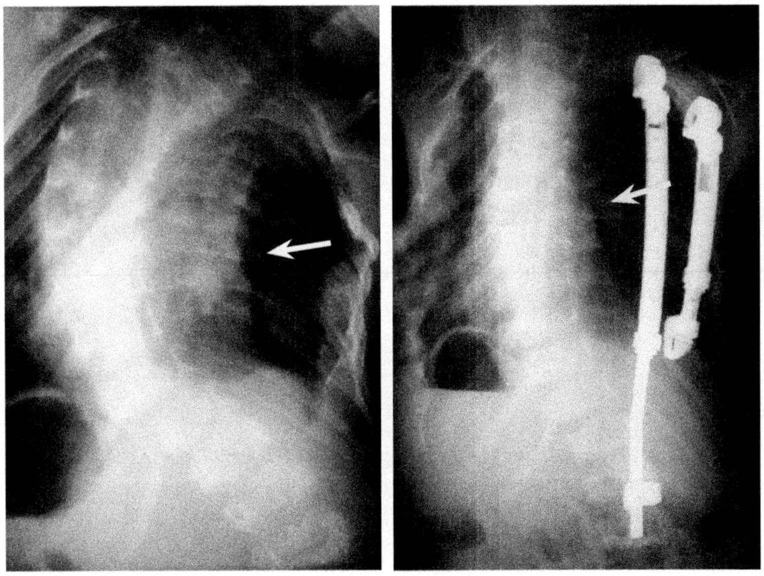

C Hemithorax expansion Vertical expandable prosthetic titanium ribs were used to reduce scoliosis and expand a constricted hemithorax. The preoperative appearance (white arrow) and the result following distraction (yellow arrow) are shown.

Etiology	Comment
Hormonal factors	Melatonin deficiency? Growth hormonal role?
Spinal growth	Asymmetrical growth? Thoracic lordosis causing rotation deformity
Collagen defect	Marfan syndrome example
Muscle imbalance	Muscular dystrophy example
Genetic factors	Multifactorial pattern likely
Brain or cord defect	Syringomyelia or Chiari malformation examples

A Possible causes of idiopathic scoliosis These are suggested possibilities.

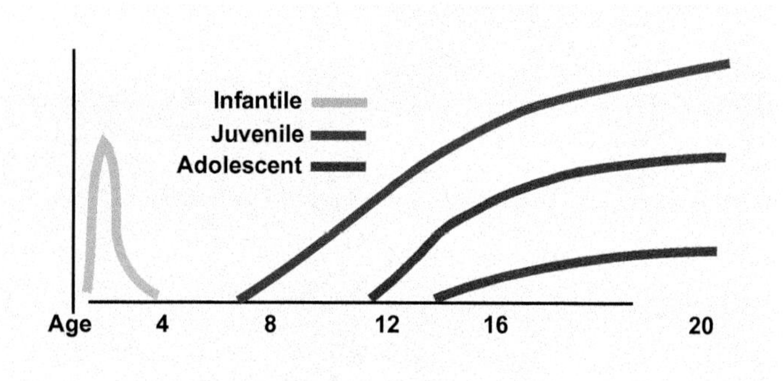

B Natural history of idiopathic scoliosis Progression of severity is related to the age of onset of the scoliosis.

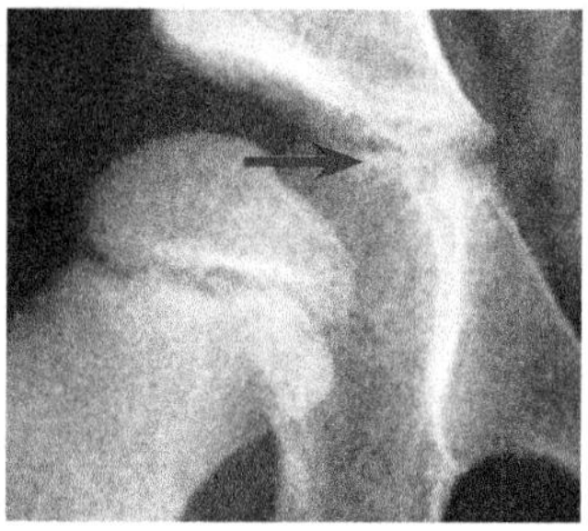

C Triradiate cartilage An open triradiate cartilage (arrow) indicates skeletal immaturity and an increased risk of curve progression.

Idiopathic Scoliosis

Prevalence

Mild truncal asymmetry occurs in about 10% of the population and is a normal variant. The diagnosis of scoliosis is reserved for curves >10°, and this occurs in 2–3% of children, with boys and girls equally affected. Progressive curves are more common in girls by 4–7:1, with a prevalence of 0.2% with >30° and 0.1% with >40°. About 10% of children identified with scoliosis require treatment.

Etiology

The cause of idiopathic scoliosis is uncertain. The deformity has a genetic component, as the concurrence among twins is greater than 50% and about a quarter of the daughters of mothers with significant scoliosis also have the deformity. Several theories have been proposed [A].

Natural History

Progression The potential for progression depends upon the age of onset [B], curve severity [D] and level of skeletal maturity, Risser sign [E], and status of the triradiate cartilage [C]. Progression is greatest during the adolescent growth spurt, which occurs just prior to menarche.

In adults, curves <30° progress little, and curves 30–50° progress about 10–15° over a lifetime. Curves 50–76° progress about 1° a year. Curves above T12 are more likely to progress.

Morbidity Patients with untreated adolescent idiopathic scoliosis of the lumbar and thoracolumbar spine have been shown to have radiographic degenerative changes of the spine at 50-year follow-up, but have not been shown to have an increased level of disability compared to the general population.

Pulmonary function Restrictive lung disease can be detected in patients with Cobb angles >100 degrees. Increased early mortality has been demonstrated only for severe early onset scoliosis. Ventilation perfusion scans show that the concave lung is the most affected in the majority of cases. Correction of adolescent idiopathic scoliosis has been demonstrated to increase vital capacity an average of 15% in short-term follow-up studies. Individuals with scoliosis have normal mortality rates.

Pain Back pain occurs in about 80% of the cases, which is comparable to the general population. Curves at the lumbar and thoracolumbar regions are most likely to be painful.

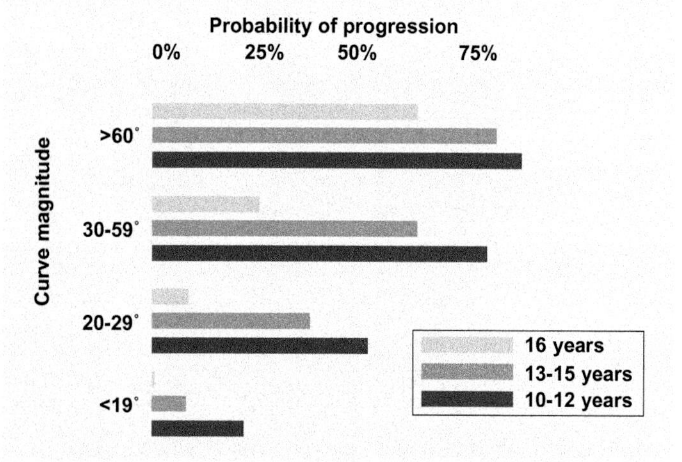

D Probability of progression Progression of >5° is based on the magnitude of the curve at the age of initial detection. From data of Nachemson, Lonstein, and Weinstein (1982).

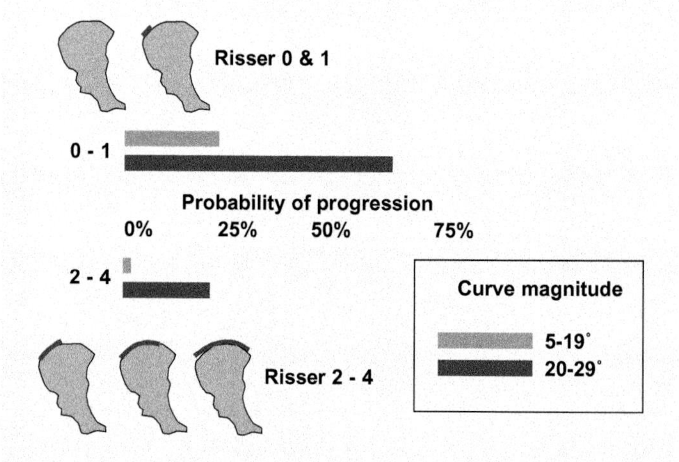

E Risser sign Likelihood of progression is based on the Risser sign and curve magnitude. From data of Lonstein and Carlson (1984).

Classification

Idiopathic scoliosis is the most common spinal deformity. Idiopathic scoliosis is often divided into categories based on age of onset and curve pattern.

Age of onset Onset may be described simply as *early* or *late*. Traditionally, three categories have been used.

Infantile Onset occurs in the first 3 years

Juvenile Onset at age 3 to 10 years.

Adolescent Onset at age 10 years to maturity.

Curve pattern The patterns may be described simply by location. This classification is useful for all types, independent of cause. For idiopathic scoliosis, curves are classified to facilitate management and communication.

Lenke This classification includes six curve types [A], a lumbar spine modified (A, B, or C) and a sagittal thoracic modified (–, N, or +), creating a total of 42 different curve types. The lumbar modified more precisely defines the position of the lumbar curve. The thoracic modified defines the sagittal alignment as being hypokyphotic, normal (curve 10°–40°), or hyperkyphotic. This classification system has been shown to be quite reliable, and its use is increasing.

Management Principles

Manage scoliosis by observation, bracing, or surgery. Exercises, electrical stimulation techniques, and manipulation are ineffective and should be avoided. Ninety percent of curves are mild and require only observation. The objectives of management are to avoid unnecessary treatment, to minimize the morbidity of required treatment, and to successfully arrest progressive curves or correct curves that cause or will likely cause disability.

Reassurance is an important part of management. Avoid the term *scoliosis* for mild curves, and simply refer to the deformity as a "mild truncal asymmetry." This reduces the apprehension that is associated with the diagnosis of *scoliosis*. This diagnosis often causes apprehension, as scoliosis is usually equated with treatment either by bracing or surgery.

Indications for treatment should be individualized; however, some generalizations can be made [B].

Observation only is indicated for patients with curves of less than 25°. Mature patients may be discharged or advised only if they become symptomatic. Follow immature adolescents with a radiograph every 6 months until maturity.

Brace treatment is indicated for immature patients (Risser 0 or 1) with curves of 25°–40°. Boys may be treated with Risser 2–3 if the curve exceeds 30° and is progressive. Observe smaller curves for progression. Progression is defined as a documented increase of 5 or more degrees.

Operative treatment is usually indicated for immature patients with curves >40° and mature patients with curves >50°.

Importance of Duration of Use in Brace Management

The BrAIST study of 2013 helped to resolve fundamental questions about the role of brace treatment of adolescent scoliosis. The findings included:

Effectiveness Bracing for mild to moderate curves was found to be effective in preventing progress and the need for operative correction.

Hours worn per day important The duration of wear was related to the effectiveness [C].

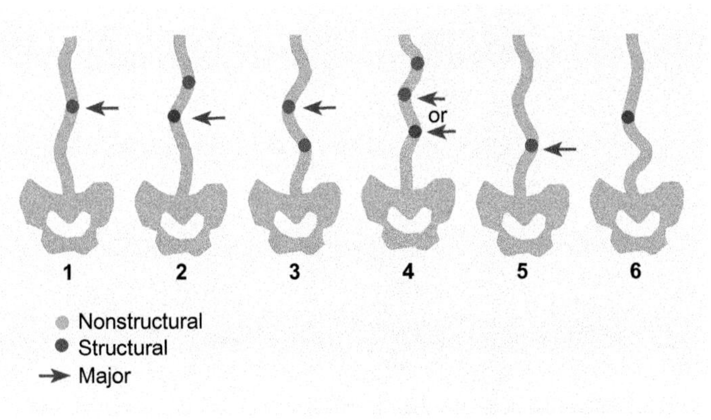

A Lenke classification Curves are described as proximal thoracic, main thoracic, and thoracolumbar/lumbar in location. Structural curves (red dots) and nonstructural curves (green dots) are differentiated by flexibility. The major curve has the largest Cobb measurement (red arrow).

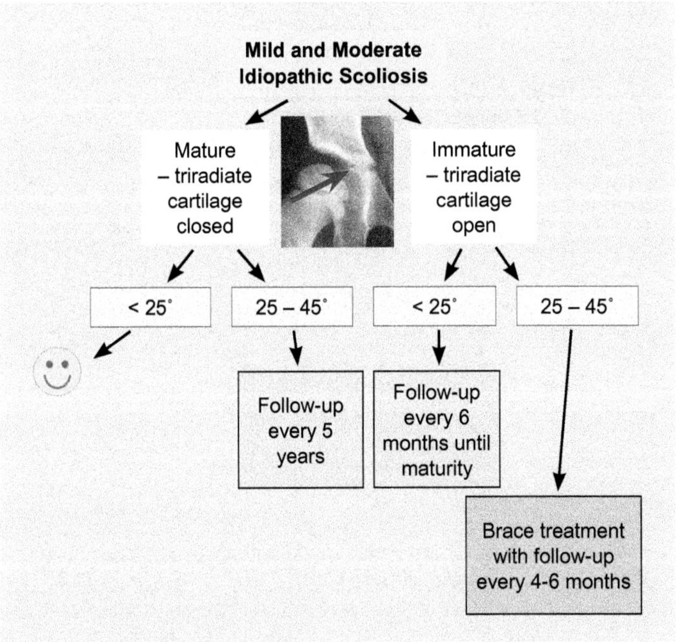

B Mild to moderate curve management Curves less than about 45° are managed based on curve severity (Cobb angle) and maturation.

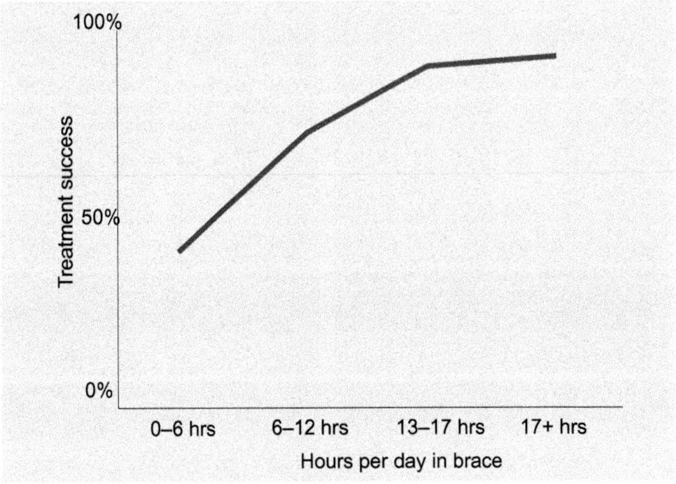

C Mild to moderate curve management Curves less than about 45° are managed based on curve severity (Cobb angle) and maturation. See Weinstein et al, NEJM 2013 369:1512.

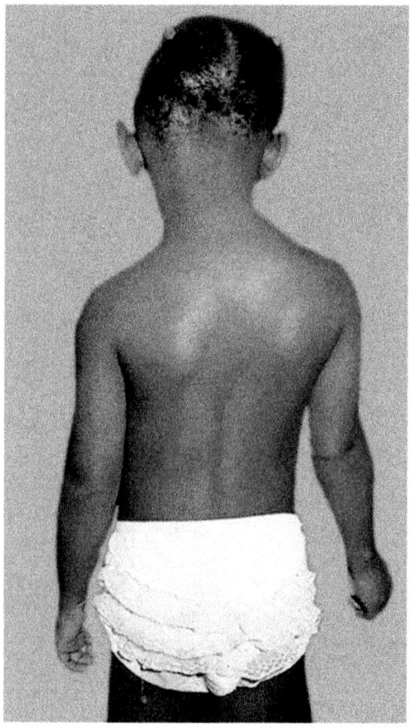

A **Juvenile scoliosis** This girl shows an elevated right shoulder and thoracic asymmetry.

Infantile Scoliosis

Infantile idiopathic scoliosis occurs in infants and children under 3 years of age. Because the deformity often is associated with plagiocephaly and hip dysplasia, it is thought to be a positional deformity. Like other position deformities, spontaneous resolution usually occurs. In some cases, the scoliosis is secondary to an underlying spinal abnormality. These cases progress to become severe. Infantile scoliosis is rare in North America.

Evaluation

Boys with left thoracic curves are the most common group to have infantile scoliosis. Study by radiographs and measure the apical-rib-vertebral angle difference, or RVAD [B]. If the RVAD exceeds 20°, study with an MRI, as about a quarter will show a significant neuroanatomical abnormality such as Chiari-1 malformations.

Management

Curves with angles of <20° resolve and require only observation. Follow closely curves >20°. If curves progress and exceed 30°, manage with a brace. Curves uncontrolled by bracing that exceed 40° may require operative correction. Several operative options are available.

Rib distractors Titanium rib distraction with lumbar laminar fixation may be serially expanded for gradual reduction in curve severity [C].

Spinal instrumentation Instrumentation without fusion preserves growth [D].

Fusion Consider anterior and posterior fusion to arrest progression and prevent crankshaft deformity. Be aware that, following fusion, trunk height will be lost at about 0.07 cm per level fused times the years of remaining growth.

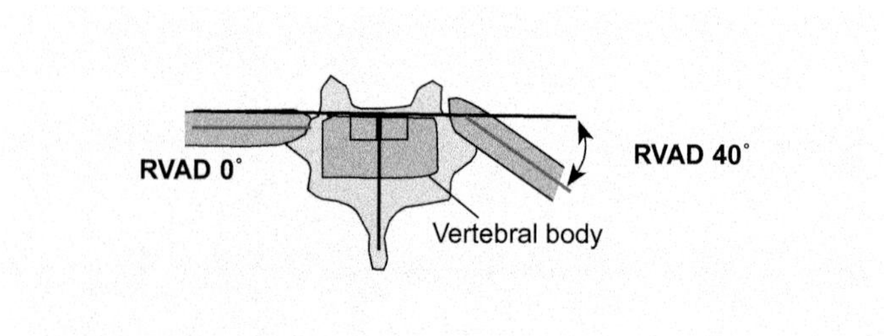

B **Rib-vertebral angle difference** This is the angle between the axis of the ribs (red lines) and a right angle to the body of the vertebrae (black line). Note on the left side here that the lines are parallel, giving a RVAD of 0°.

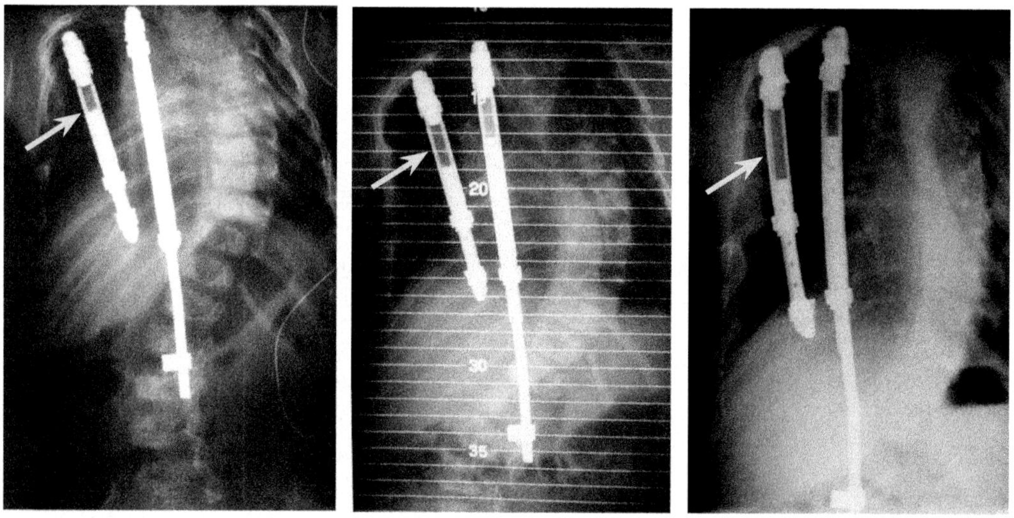

C **Progressive correction by rib expanders** This young child with scoliosis was managed by expandable fixation (yellow arrows), utilizing rib fixation at three sites and a single lumbar hook. Note the progressive reduction in curve magnitude.

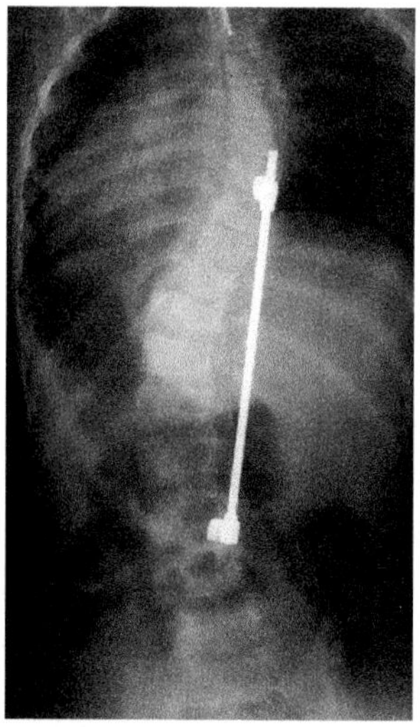

D **Instrumentation without fusion** This distraction rod was placed to prevent progression while allowing the spine to continue to grow.

Juvenile Scoliosis

This form of scoliosis is identified between 3 and 10 years of age [A, previous page]. Gender ratios are about equal for the younger patients, but girls become predominant toward puberty. About two-thirds of the curves are progressive. Most require bracing.

Evaluation

Measure the Cobb angles. For children with a Cobb angle >20°, study with a full spine MRI, as 20–25% will show a significant spinal abnormality such as Chiari I malformations or tumor. Hypokyphosis with values <20° suggests a poorer prognosis and complicates orthotic management.

Management

Follow for progression. A few curves resolve spontaneously. Institute orthotic management for progressive curves that exceed 20° [A].

Bracing Manage curves with an apex below T7 with a TLSO. A Milwaukee brace is necessary for more proximal curves. Considering the long duration of bracing necessary, balance brace time with tolerance. Avoid bracing for too many years, as the child must endure many years of brace treatment as well as the final surgical correction.

Operative correction is indicated for curves exceeding 40°–50°. Anterior and posterior fusions are necessary for young children to prevent the crankshaft deformity. Be certain to correct or maintain normal sagittal alignment. Instrumentation without fusion may be considered in young children, as described for the infantile form.

Adolescent Scoliosis

Idiopathic scoliosis with an onset after age 10 years is the most common and classic form.

Brace Principles

Bracing usually slows or arrests progression of most spinal curvatures in immature patients with progressive curves between 25° and 40°. Brace curves with documented progression above 25° or curves above 30° when first seen.

Bracing options Select the orthosis based on the type and level of curve and the anticipated tolerance of the patient [A]. The most effective bracing types and protocols are also the most restrictive and cause the greatest psychosocial disability. Select a balance that is best for the patient.

Nighttime braces are best tolerated, but effectiveness is controversial. The Charleston bending brace is most widely used. The brace is worn only at night, allowing the child freedom during the day.

TLSO brace This is the most commonly used orthosis. It is appropriate for curves with an apex in the midthorax and below. The Boston brace [B] is prefabricated with custom pads applied by the orthotist. Most include a 15° lordosis correction. The brace may be worn on a 16- to 23-hour-per-day protocol.

Milwaukee brace For upper thoracic curves, the Milwaukee brace may be necessary. This brace is the most restrictive and is compatible with limited activity.

Introduce the brace over a period of several weeks. Encourage acceptance as quickly as possible. Discomfort in the brace should be corrected by making necessary modifications early. Continued discomfort reduces compliance, increasing the risk of bracing treatment failure. Modifications in the brace will correct this problem. Encourage normal activities while being braced.

Improving acceptance Several methods can be used to reduce the adverse effects of brace treatment of scoliosis [C]. The bracing schedule may be tailored to the patient. Some patients are already at or beyond their tolerance limits. It may be best to maintain a relationship with the patient and family and to follow the patient without treatment. If the curve is advanced, it may be best to elect an operative option earlier than is normally appropriate. Make certain the patient and family are aware that the time in the brace and the control of the curve are proportional.

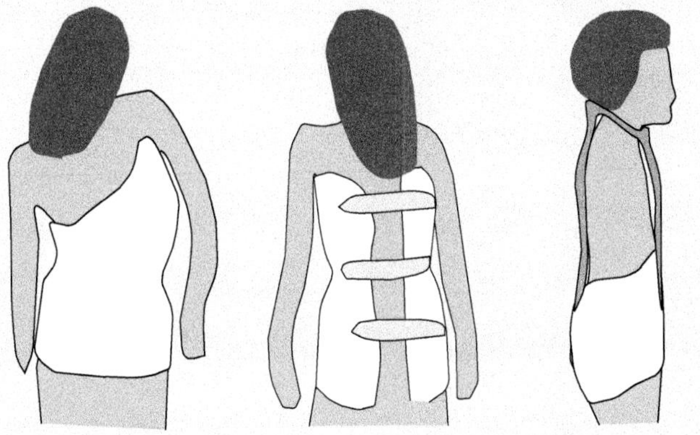

Charleston	TLSO	Milwaukee
Least obtrusive	Moderate	Most difficult to accept
Nighttime only	16–22/24 hours	16–22/24 hours
Most curves	Most curves	High curves

A Types of braces These are common braces and generalizations about their use.

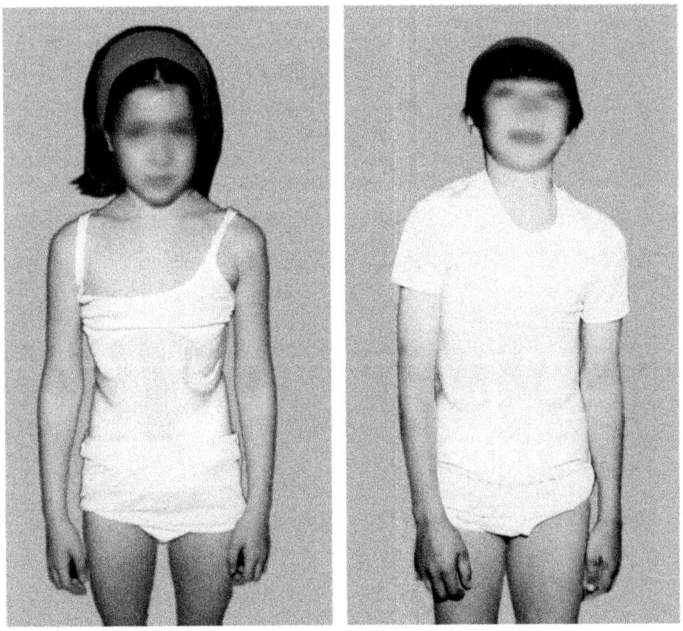

B Boston brace These underarm braces are useful for low thoracic and lumbar curves. They can be hidden by clothing for both genders.

Technique	Comment
Education	Reassurance
Support groups	Organize or arrange with other patients wearing braces
Type of brace	Tailor to situation
Activities	Encourage to remain active
Day vs night use	Most will find nighttime least obtrusive
Out of brace activities	Plan physical activity in time out of brace

C Improving acceptance of brace treatment These are techniques that may be used to keep the management within the tolerance limit of the patient.

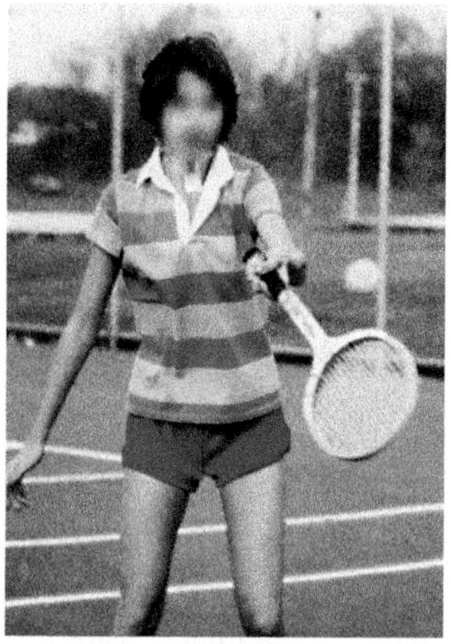

A Physical activity This girl remains physically active even while wearing a Milwaukee brace.

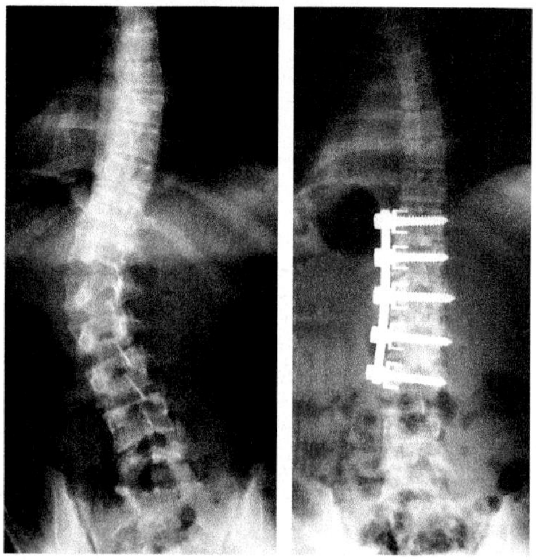

B Anterior fixation This lumbar curve was instrumented and fused, involving only five vertebrae.

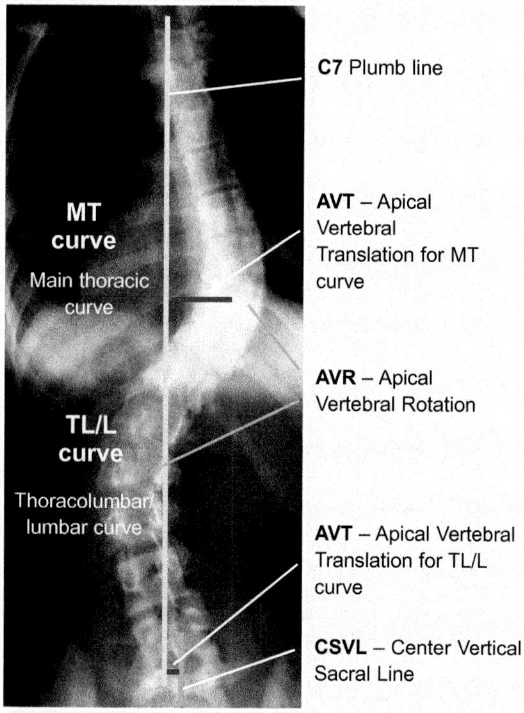

C Curve definitions These are definitions by Lenke and associates for assessing and defining curve configuration in planning instrumentation and fusion.

Initial response should show a reduction of the curve by >50%.

Follow-up Schedule follow-up visits every 4 to 6 months to assess fit, size, compliance, and curve progression. Obtain a standing PA radiograph out of the brace to assess progress.

Dealing with compliance Bracing is uncomfortable, often adversely affects self-image, and imposes some difficulties with social and athletic activities. The patient should participate in most prebracing activities [A]. All of these problems further complicate an already difficult time in life. The physician must not exceed the "tolerance limit" of psychological stress on the patient. If this tolerance limit is exceeded, the patient will become noncompliant and may not return for follow-up. He or she may simply ignore the problem or seek nonconventional methods of treatment that are less demanding. Make the patient and family aware that control or correction of the curve is related to the time in the brace.

Discontinue bracing about 2 years post-menarcheal or Risser 4 for girls and Risser 5 for boys. Progression while bracing may indicate the need for operative stabilization.

Operative Treatment Principles

Indications Operative management is the most definitive and effective method of management of scoliosis. It is appropriate for curves that exceed 40°–50°.

Approaches Select the approach based on the curve characteristics and the experience of the surgeon.

Posterior fusion This standard approach allows correction and instrumentation of the majority of curves and levels.

Anterior fusion The advantages of anterior fusion include a reduction in the number of vertebra requiring fusion [B], less dissection, and correction of hypokyphosis. Anterior fixation provides excellent stability when extended to or just beyond the neutral vertebrae.

Fusion levels It is important to establish fusion levels thoughtfully. Too short a fusion may result in progression; fusion too long increases the risk of pain and degenerative changes. Inappropriate fusion levels may cause spinal malalignment, changes in posture, and postfusion back pain. Definitions are useful in planning instrumentation and fusions [C]. Note the rotation of the apical vertebra [D].

Curves Fuse the major curve or largest curve, regardless of its flexibility, and minor or structural curves.

Upper and lower end vertebrae may extend to the neutral vertebra, which is defined as the lowest vertebra bisected by the CSVL.

Combined anterior and posterior fusion This procedure is indicated to prevent crankshaft phenomenon in children, for correction of severe curves, or to reduce the risk of recurrence in patients with constitutional disorders such as Marfan syndrome.

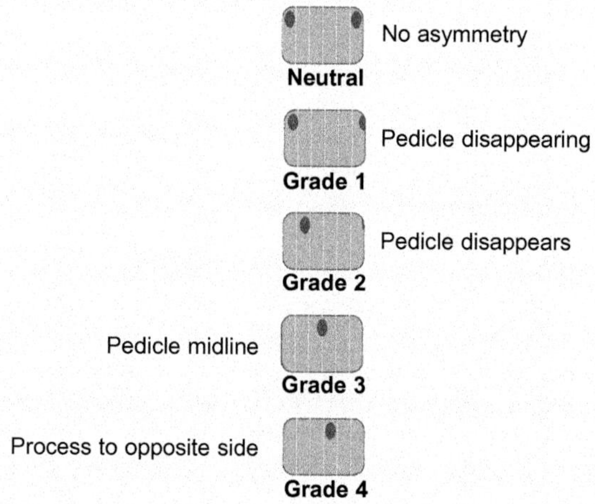

D Apical vertebral rotation The degree of rotation is graded based on the relationship of the pedicles to the vertebral body. Based on Nash (1969).

Operative Technique

Instrument to reduce the scoliosis and maintain or improve sagittal alignment. Avoid excessive distraction, and incorporate solid fixation. Decorticate carefully, excise facet joints when feasible, and add supplemental bone. This supplemental bone may be autogenous, bank bone, or agents that induce osteogenesis.

Harrington instrumentation was the initial standard that incorporated distraction and compression of the ends of the curves. This technique provided little control of sagittal alignment and has been largely replaced.

Luque fixation utilizes sublaminar wires fixed to posterior rods.

Drummond fixation employs spinous processes to posterior rod fixation.

Cotrel and Dubousset introduced a universal system that provides translation and rotation in addition to distraction, which permits a solid three-dimensional correction. Many modifications of this form, such as the Isola and TRSH systems, have been developed.

Hybrid fixation utilizes options such as dual rods, laminar wires, pedicle screws, and cross links to achieve maximum stability [A].

Video-assisted thoracoscopy These procedures allow closed anterior releases, rib resection and harvesting, and insertion of correctional implants to reduce operative morbidity [B]. Such procedures require special skills and instrumentation and carry a steep learning curve. Due to the increased complication rate, the procedure is controversial.

Spinal Monitoring

Monitoring is utilized to reduce risk of neurological injury during spinal exposure and instrumentation.

Wake-up test Intraoperative wake-up neurological testing is effective and inexpensive but difficult to use, and has largely been replaced by continuous monitoring methods.

Intraoperative neurophysiological monitoring includes transcranial motor-evoked potentials (TcMEP) and neurogenic motor-evoked potentials (NMEP).

Complications

Operative complications are not uncommon because of the magnitude of the procedure and also the vulnerability of the cord and nerve routes [C]. These complications are described as early, such as neurological injuries, and late, such as pseudarthrosis.

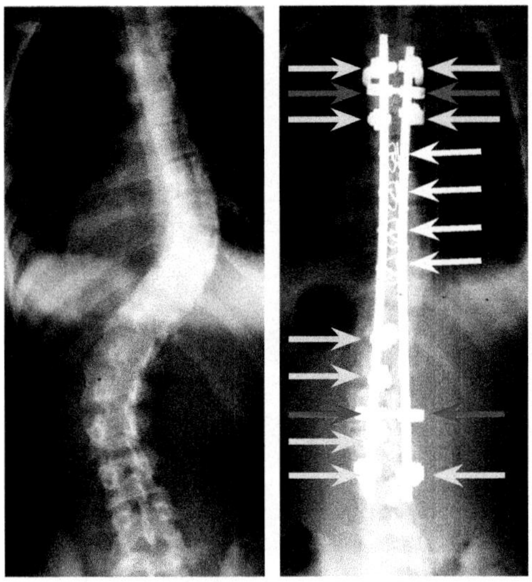

A Hybrid instrumentation Correction and fixation of this curve utilized dual rods, pedicle screws (yellow arrows), laminar wires (white arrows), and cross links (red arrows).

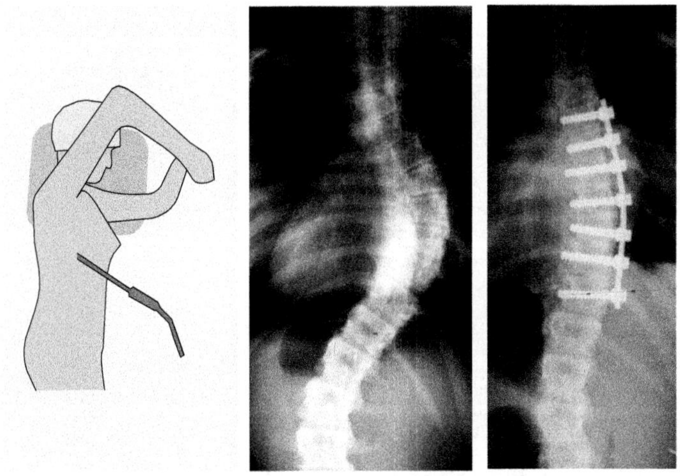

B Thoroscopic instrumentation This curve was instrumented percutaneously with video assistance.

Complication	Comment
Pseudarthrosis	Less common with rigid fixation
Back pain	May occur from a variety of problems including sagittal malalignment, pseudarthrosis, infection, etc.
Flat back syndrome	Pain secondary to abnormal posture
Crankshaft deformity	Secondary to relative anterior overgrowth
Infection	May be delayed in onset
Spinal cord injury	May be reduced with monitoring
Hardware problems	May be due to prominence or breakage
Dural tears	Require intraoperative repair
Superior mesenteric artery syndrome	Most common with correction of sagittal plane deformity

C Complications following scoliosis surgery These complications may follow surgical correction of idiopathic scoliosis.

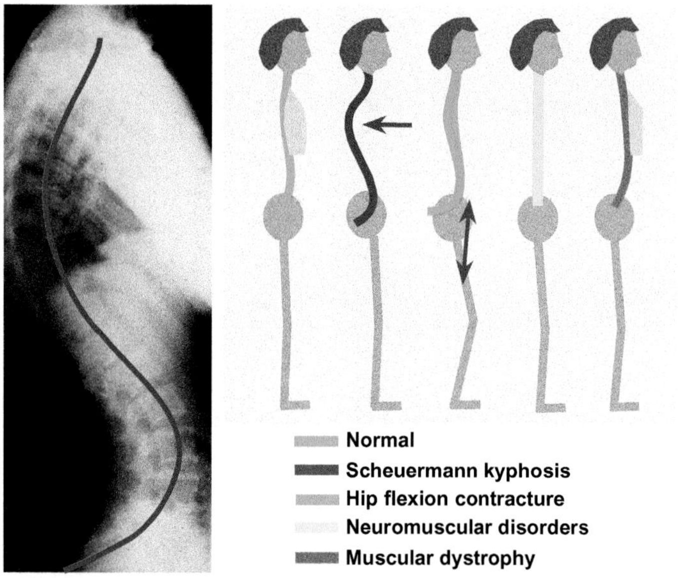

A Patterns of sagittal deformity Normal (green), Scheuermann kyphosis (red); hyperlordosis secondary to hip flexion contracture (blue); flat back (yellow) and associated neuromuscular disorders; and thoracic lordosis (brown) with pulmonary compromise, as seen in muscular dystrophy.

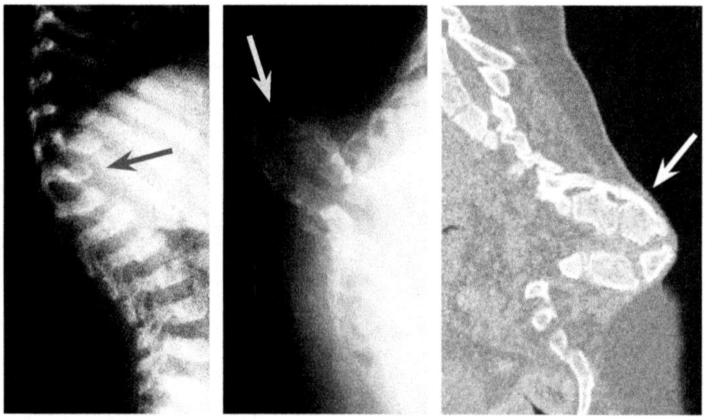

B Congenital kyphosis Vertebral hypoplasia may lead to paraplegia (red arrow). Kyphosis in spina bifida (yellow arrow) often shown best by CT scans (white arrow). This severe kyphosis may cause skin breakdown over the apex and difficulty in positioning.

Sagittal Deformity

Sagittal alignment [A] is affected by our upright posture and significantly affects appearance, cardiopulmonary function, and potential for degenerative arthritis of the spine. Because the spine has greater mobility in flexion and extension than side bending, sagittal deformities are not complicated by a rotational component, as occurs with scoliosis. The spine has three curves: cervical lordosis, thoracic kyphosis, and lumbar lordosis. Upright posture requires that these curves be balanced; they are interrelated. Furthermore, lower extremity alignment affects the spine. For example, excessive lumbar lordosis is usually compensated by hip flexion.

Kyphosis

Kyphosis is a posterior convex angulation of the spine. Kyphosis is normal for the thoracic spine with normal range from about 20° to 50°.

Postural round-back This is a normal variation. The major problem is cosmetic. It is flexible, as the posture can be improved by asking the child to straighten up, and it does not cause a permanent deformity.

Congenital kyphosis Congenital kyphosis may be due to a failure of formation, segmentation, or mixed types [B] and [C]. The apex of the curve is most common between T10 and L1. Deformities secondary to a failure of formation are usually progressive and may lead to paraplegia. Assess the apex with high-quality radiographs and a CT study if necessary. Classify the type of deformity. For progressive deformities under about 55°–60°, fuse posteriorly. More severe deformities may require anterior and posterior fusions.

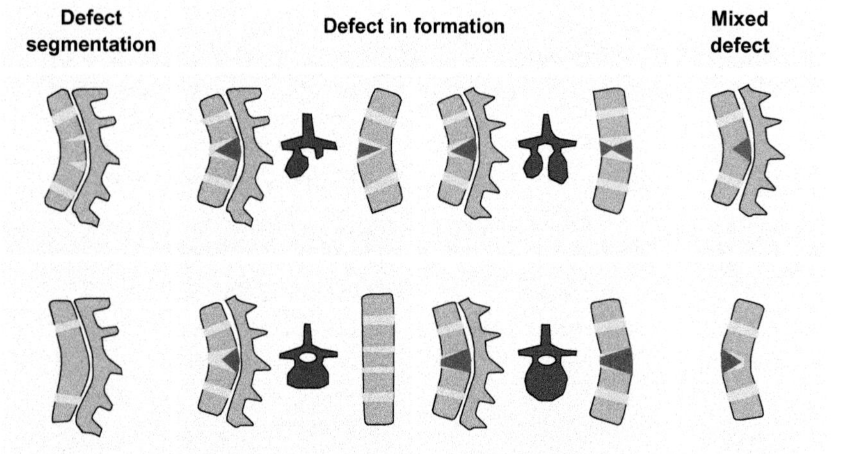

C Classification of congenital kyphosis and kyphoscoliosis Based on McMaster and Singh (1999).

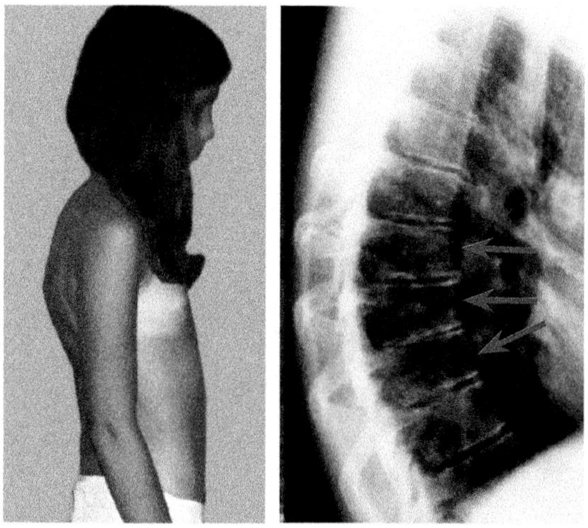

D Scheuermann kyphosis Note the round back deformity and anterior wedging of vertebrae (red arrows).

Scheuermann Kyphosis

This disease often causes both pain and deformity [D, previous page]. The deformity may present with back pain, as discussed on page 238, or as a deformity.

Deformity Management of the deformity is controversial, as long-term disability is mild and effective treatment is difficult.

Moderate curves <60° Manage with observation and encourage physical activity. Curves >60° in skeletally immature children (Risser sign <3) may be improved by brace treatment. Consider applying a preliminary hyperextension plaster cast to improve flexibility. For curves above T7, use a Milwaukee brace [A]. For lower curves, use an underarm brace. Brace initially for 20 hours daily. Once the curve is controlled, taper the brace to nighttime use.

Curves >80° uncontrolled by bracing may require operative correction with posterior instrumentation and fusion.

Natural history of this condition is usually benign, except in individuals with kyphosis that was upper thoracic and >100° who were likely to have restrictive lung disease.

Lordosis

Lordosis is the anterior convex angulation of the lumbar spine. The normal range of lordosis is from about 30° to 50°.

Developmental lordosis This developmental variation is common in the prepubescent child [B]. Parents are concerned. The deformity is flexible, and the screening examination is normal. Radiographs are not necessary. Resolution occurs with growth.

Functional hyperlordosis This deformity is functional, a compensation for a fixed deformity above or below the lumbosacral level.

Hyperkyphosis is the primary deformity, and the hyperlordosis is compensatory. This compensatory deformity remains flexible, and this flexibility is demonstrated by correction of the lordosis on forward bending.

Hip flexion contracture causes a functional increase in lordosis, usually >60°. This deformity is very common in cerebral palsy. Assess with the prone extension test [C]. Lordosis is also common in children with bilateral developmental hip dislocations or coxa vara.

Structural Hyperlordosis or Hypolordosis

Hyperlordosis may follow laminectomy in children for conditions such as tumors or trauma. This deformity is best prevented by decompression or exposures that save posterior elements or early posterior fusion in wide excisions in growing children. Operative procedures that arrest growth of the posterior lumbar vertebrae, such as shunting or rhizotomy, may result in increasing lordosis with growth.

Spondyloptosis causes a secondary hypolordosis with flattening of the buttocks.

Neuromuscular disorders such as muscular dystrophy may cause hypolordosis.

Fractures with malunion may cause an increase or decrease in lordosis.

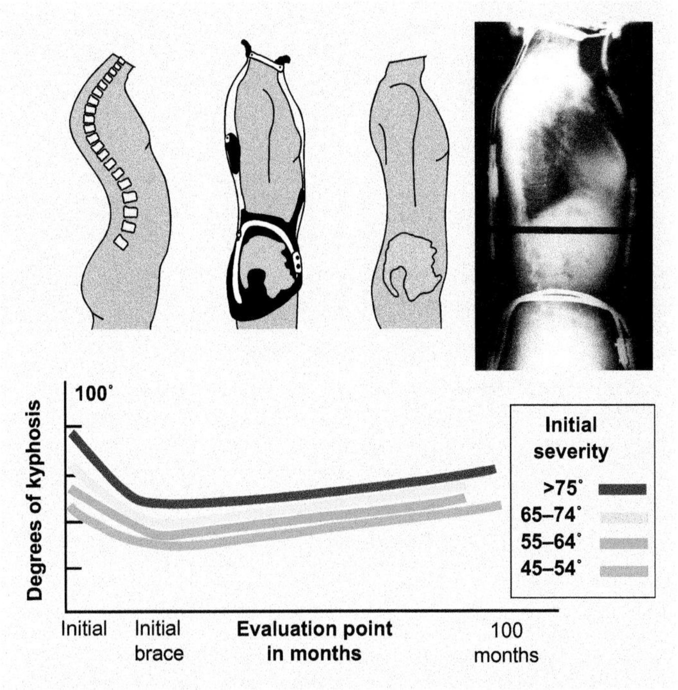

A Milwaukee brace management of juvenile kyphosis The Milwaukee brace is effective in managing kyphosis. The outcome is related to the severity of the curve at the beginning of treatment. Based on Sachs et al. (1987).

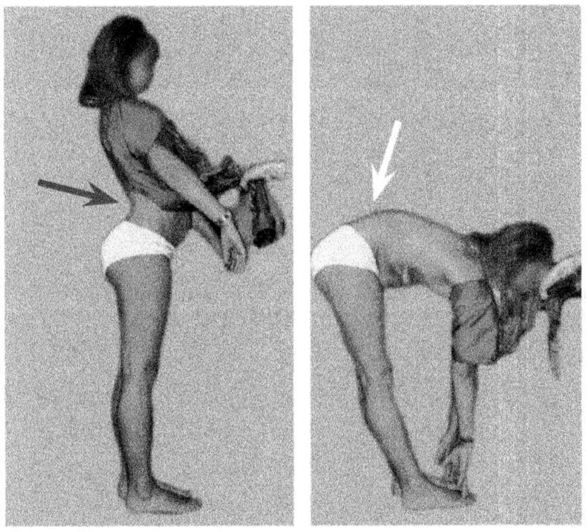

B Physiologic lordosis of puberty This form of lordosis (red arrow) is seen during late childhood just prior to puberty. The spine is flexible and the lordosis disappears on forward bending (white arrow).

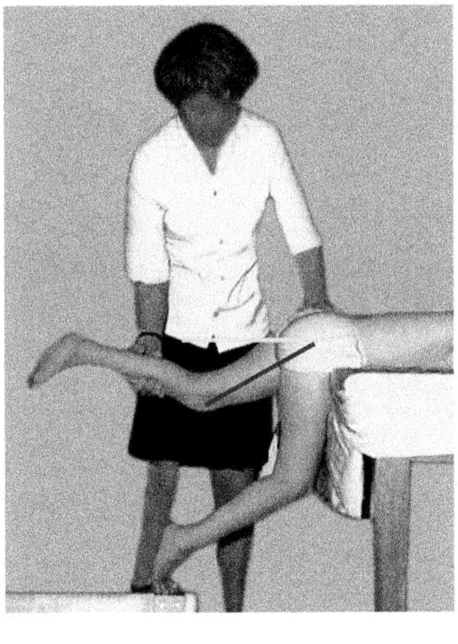

C Prone extension test for assessing hip flexion contracture The thigh is gradually lifted until the pelvis starts to extend. This indicates the limit of hip extension. The contracture is the angle between the thigh (red line) and the horizontal (yellow line).

Cervical Spine

Cervical spine problems that often present with neck complaints are covered in Chapter 9.

Radiographs

Conventional radiographs remain the most valuable method of imaging the neck and shoulder.

Pseudosubluxation at C2–C3 and less commonly at C3–C4 is common in children under the age of 9 years [A].

ADI The atlanto-dens interval (ADI) is the distance between the odontoid and anterior arch of axis [B]. This measure is most important in children. This distance is <4–5 mm in children. When the ADI >10–12 mm, all ligaments have failed. Flexion-extension lateral radiographs [C] demonstrate instability most graphically.

SAC The space available for the cord (SAC) is between the odontoid and the posterior arch of the axis.

Occiput–C1 relationship is often assessed by McRae and McGregor lines [B].

Special Studies

Additional imaging studies may be appropriate, depending upon the evaluation. Look for associated defects. For example, order a renal ultrasound evaluation if the diagnosis of Klippel-Feil syndrome is made. In children with disproportionate dwarfism, prior to any surgical procedure requiring anesthesia, order a screening flexion–extension lateral radiograph of the cervical spine. If instability is demonstrated, special intubation techniques will prevent injury to the cervical spinal cord.

Basilar Impression

Basilar impression is a congenital or acquired deformity in which the cervical spine extends into the foramen magnum. The deformity may be congenital or secondary to osteopenia due to conditions such as rickets or osteogenesis imperfecta. This deformity may cause symptoms during adolescence.

Occipital-Atlantal Instability

Instability at the occiput-C1 level is rare and usually due to a congenital bony defect or marked ligamentous laxity, as seen in Down syndrome. Seldom is operative stabilization by fusion necessary.

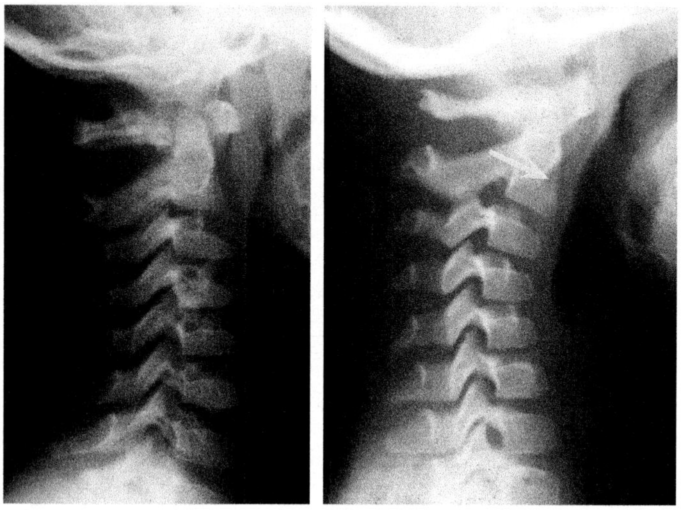

A Pseudosubluxation The normal alignment of the cervical spine is usually well demonstrated by a lateral radiograph. Pseudosubluxation is common in younger children with C2 displaced forward on C3 (yellow arrow).

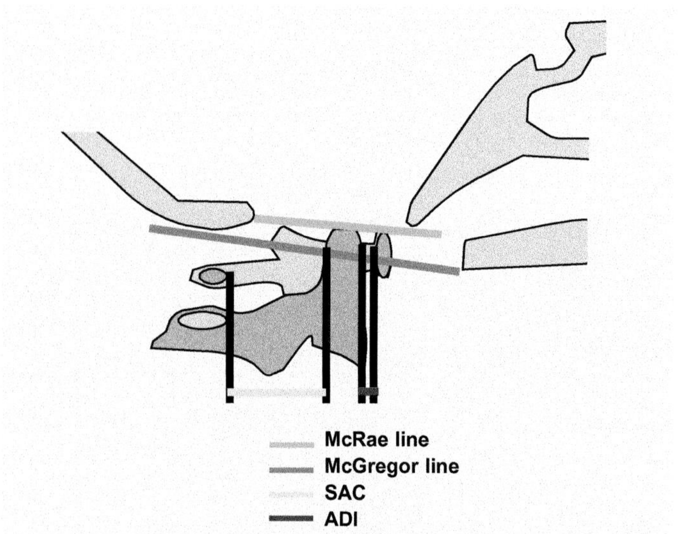

B Cervical measures These lines and measures are commonly used. The SAC, or space available for the cord (yellow line), and ADI, or atlanto-dens interval (red line), are expressed in mm.

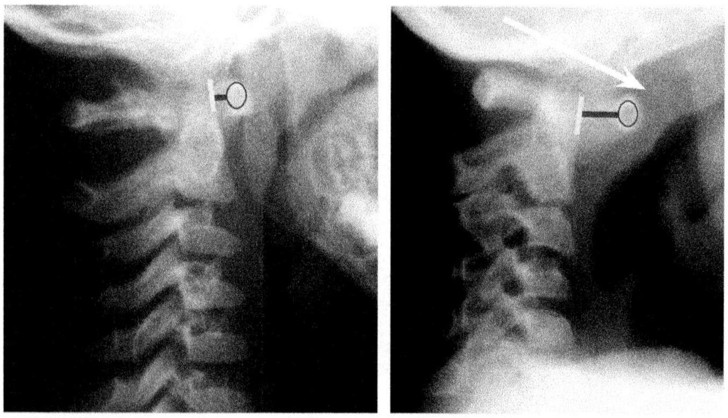

C Neutral and flexion views of cervical spine These studies show the relationship between arch of atlas (red ring) and the front of the odontoid (yellow line). The distance between is the ADI (red line). This relationship changes with neck flexion (right), demonstrating C1-C2 instability, with the ADI increasing from 2 to 10 mm due to rupture of the transverse atlantal ligament.

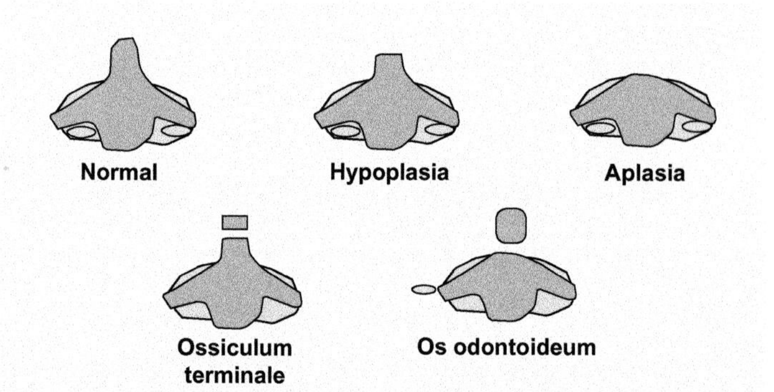

D Odontoid types These varied types contribute to varying degrees of instability. Based on Copley and Dormans (1998).

Atlantoaxial Instability

Instability at the C1–C2 level is relatively common [C, previous page]. Instability is due to abnormalities of the odontoid [D, previous page, and A] or to ligamentous laxity. Instability results from rupture or attenuation of the transverse atlantal or alar ligaments [B]. Such ligamentous deficiencies are common in Down syndrome and in rheumatoid arthritis. Instability is also common in disproportionate dwarfism. Children with these problems should avoid activities that cause cervical spine stress and should have an evaluation prior to being administered a general anesthetic.

Polyarticular Juvenile Rheumatoid Arthritis

Clinical stiffness and radiographic changes in the cervical spine occur commonly in polyarticular-onset and systemic-onset disease. Neck problems are rare in pauciarticular-onset disease. Although stiffness and radiographic changes are common, children seldom complain of neck pain.

Klippel–Feil Syndrome

The Klippel-Feil syndrome includes clinical [C] and radiographic [D] features. The syndrome is now known to be much more generalized.

Clinical features About half have the classic findings of fusions, low hairline, and stiffness. Classify the condition by the levels of fusions. Other clinical associations include congenital scoliosis, renal anomalies, Sprengel deformity, synkinesis, congenital heart disease, and impaired hearing [E]. Other deformities include odontoid abnormalities, occipitocervical fusion, and basilar impression.

Evaluate carefully with full spine examination, neurological, cardiac, renal, and hearing screening. Make radiographs of the entire spine. Order a renal ultrasound. If neurological findings are present, study with MR imaging.

Management includes advising the family of the risks and avoiding activities such as diving, football, and gymnastics, which place excessive loads on the cervical spine. Arthrodesis of unstable segments may be required if excessive instability and neurological abnormalities are present.

Natural history Affected individuals have instability problems above and degenerative problems below the levels of fusion. Adults have disability from this syndrome.

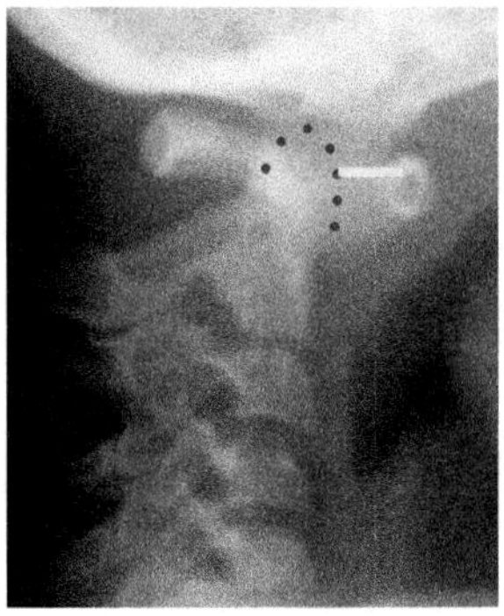

A Odontoid hypoplasia Note the hypoplastic odontoid and the instability, as demonstrated by an ADI of 8 mm.

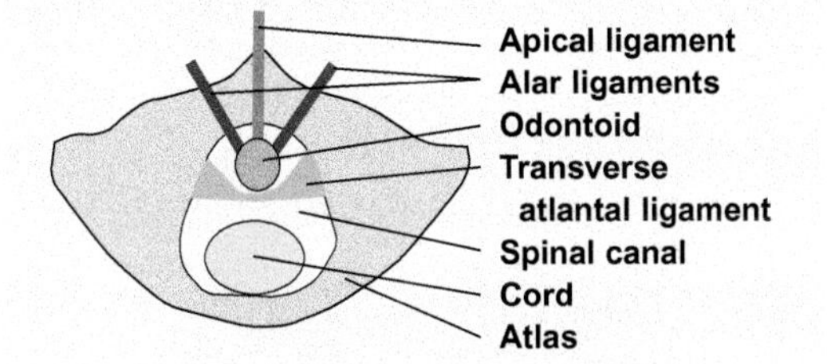

B Constraining ligaments These multiple ligaments usually prevent the odontoid from compressing the cord.

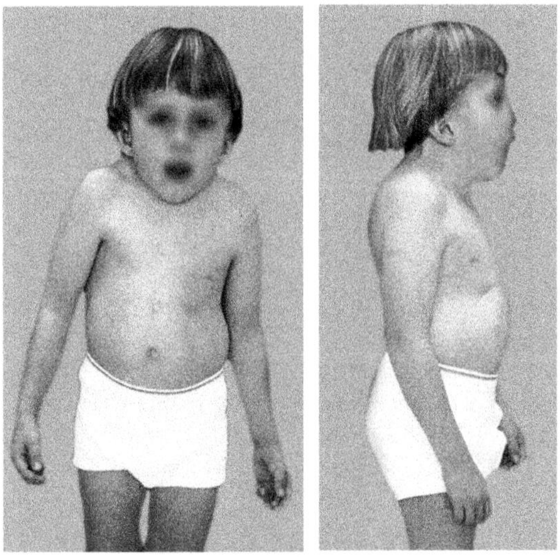

C Clinical features of Klippel-Feil syndrome This syndrome includes shortening of the neck, a low hairline and neck stiffness.

Disease	Associated Disorders
Klippel-Feil Syndrome	Scoliosis Renal abnormalities Sprengel deformity Deafness Synkinesis Congenital heart disease
Disproportionate Dwarfism	C1-C2 disorders causing instability

E Associations Disorders about the neck are often associated with other congenital defects. Renal and cervical instability problems may not be diagnosed unless special studies are ordered.

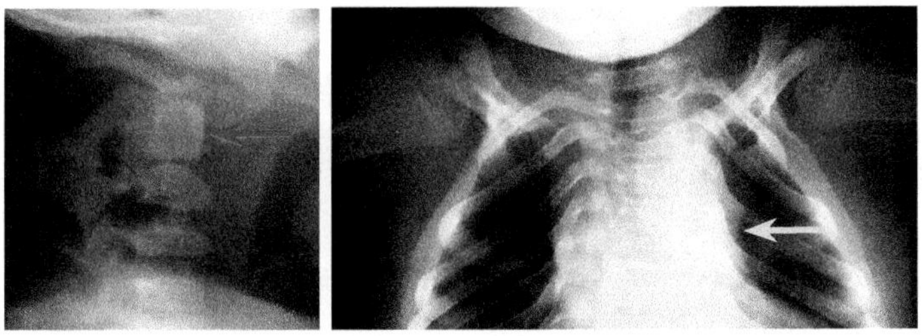

D Radiographic features of Klippel-Feil syndrome This syndrome includes shortening of the neck, cervical fusions (red arrow), and various other abnormalities, such as scoliosis (yellow arrow).

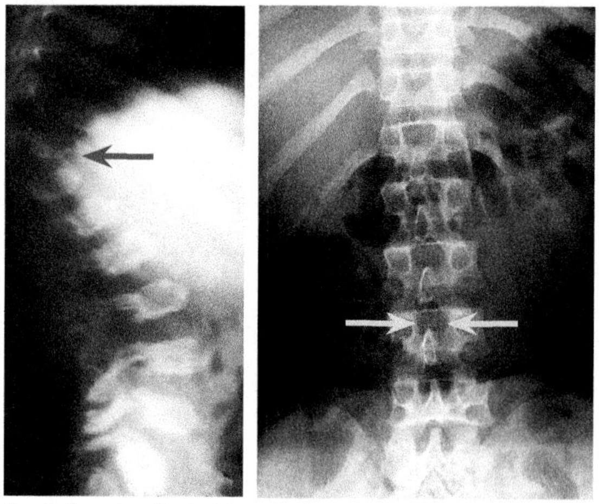

A Achondroplasia Note the kyphosis in the infant (red arrow) and the narrow lumbar canals in the adolescent (yellow arrows).

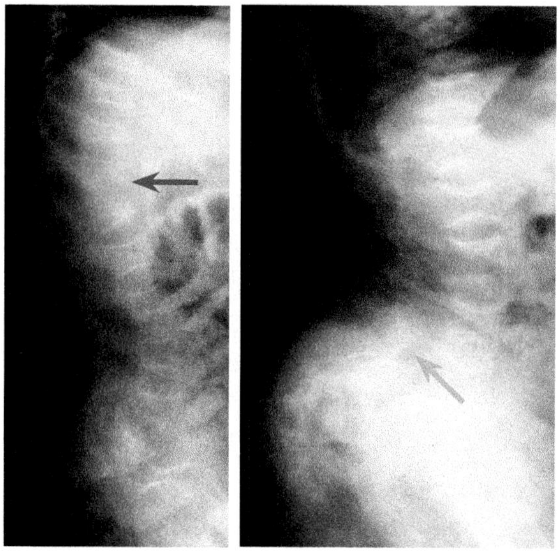

B Osteogenesis imperfecta Note the vertebral deformity (red arrow) and accentuated lumbar lordosis (orange arrow).

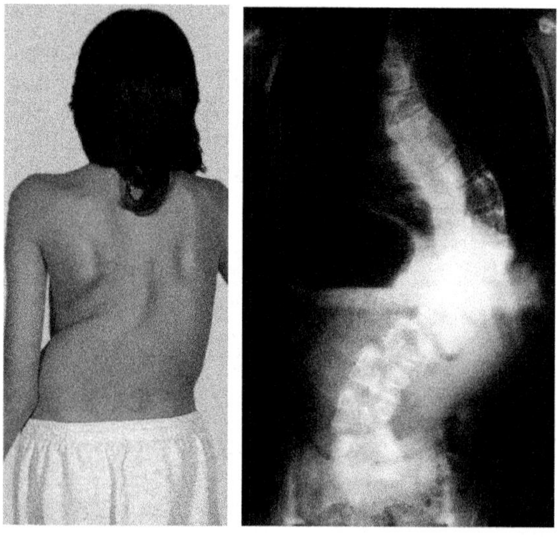

C Marfan syndrome Note the severe right thoracolumbar curve. This curve is not improved by bracing, making instrumentation and fusion necessary.

Spine in Generalized Disorders

Many constitutional disorders, such as the osteochondrodystrophies and metabolic and chromosomal abnormalities, are associated with scoliosis. In these children, during each clinic visit, screen for spinal deformity.

Achondroplasia

This is a rhizomelic short-limb dwarfism, which is usually readily recognized at birth. Major and disabling spine deformities occur often in these children [A].

Stenosis of the foramen magnum causes increased hypotonia, sleep apnea, and sudden infant death syndrome. Foramen magnum decompression, duroplasty, and cervical laminectomy may be necessary if symptoms are severe.

Thoracolumbar kyphosis is common in most infants. The deformity is usually flexible. Treat rigid curves >30° with an orthosis. If deformity exceeds 40° after age 5, anterior and posterior fusion may be required.

Spinal stenosis is common and often becomes symptomatic in early adult life. The stenosis may be aggravated by thoracolumbar kyphosis. This deformity is usually treated in adulthood.

Pseudoachondroplasia

This autosomal dominant short-limb dwarfism causes several spinal problems.

Atlantoaxial instability from odontoid deficiencies and generalized laxity is demonstrated by flexion–extension radiographs and MRI if unstable. Decompression and fusion may be required.

Thoracolumbar deformities include kyphosis and scoliosis.

Hyperlordosis may result from hip flexion contracture.

Osteogenesis Imperfecta

Deformity is due to osteopenia [B], and scoliosis and basilar invagination are serious problems. Bracing is inappropriate, as it may cause chest and rib deformity and is unlikely to arrest progression of the curve. Operative stabilization and fusion are indicated for curves exceeding 35°–45°. Instrument with posterior sublaminar segmental fixation and fusion. Add anterior fusion if the deformity is severe and/or associated with kyphosis.

Spondyloepiphyseal Dysplasia

This is a group of short-trunk dwarfism with dysplasia of the spine and long bones.

Atlantoaxial instability occurs in about 40% from odontoid deficiencies, and generalized laxity is demonstrated by flexion–extension radiographs and MRI if unstable. Decompression and fusion may be required.

Thoracolumbar scoliosis and kyphosis are common and may cause back pain in adults. Manage as with idiopathic scoliosis.

Diastrophic Dysplasia

This is an autosomal recessive disorder with short-limb dwarfism. Spine deformities include generalized cervical spina bifida, cervical spine kyphosis, and thoracolumbar kyphoscoliosis. These deformities may be severe and require instrumentation and fusion.

Marfan Syndrome

This is an autosomal dominant disorder of connective tissue.

Scoliosis develops in most patients [C, previous page]. Curve patterns are often double, major structural, right thoracic, left lumbar. Some curves are triple. Curves usually start earlier and are more progressive, refractory, and rigid.

Brace management is less effective than for idiopathic scoliosis but is used with similar indications and protocols.

Operative management is indicated for curves >50° with segmental fixation using sublaminar wires. Be certain to balance the spine and restore normal sagittal alignment.

Spinal deformities have included atlantoaxial instability and spondyloptosis, among others.

Morquio Syndrome

This mucopolysaccharidosis type IV is one of a spectrum of lysosomal storage diseases. The spine is normal at birth, but deformities develop with growth [A]. Odontoid dysplasia is common and life-threatening. Odontoid aplasia, hypoplasia, or os odontoideum may cause instability. This instability, combined with accumulation of mucopolysaccharides within the spinal canal, may compromise the cord, causing sudden death or quadriplegia. Manage instability with neurological compromise first with evaluation by dynamic MRI studies. Fuse occiput to C3 or more proximal if posterior elements are adequate. Consider prophylactic stabilization if instability is severe.

Neurofibromatosis

Spine involvement in neurofibromatosis is common [B]. Look for bony dysplasia associated with the scoliosis. If dysplastic features are present, consider MRI or CT studies. Follow carefully, as rapid progression may occur with growth.

Nondystrophic scoliosis Manage like idiopathic scoliosis.

Dystrophic scoliosis is often characterized by short angular progressive curves. Brace treatment is ineffective. Correct by combined anterior and posterior spinal fusion. Include the entire structural levels in both the fusion masses.

Rett Syndrome

Rett syndrome is a progressive encephalopathy observed only in girls, who are apparently normal until 6 to 12 months of age. It is characterized by autism, dementia, ataxia, stereotypic hand movements, hyperreflexia, spasticity, seizures, and scoliosis [C]. Scoliosis is usually progressive and seldom responds to brace management. Most require posterior fusion with segmental instrumentation.

Down Syndrome

Trisomy-21 syndrome includes characteristic faces, congenital heart disease, mental retardation, and excessive joint laxity. Upper cervical instability involving the occipito-cervical and the atlantoaxial levels develop in many children. This instability results from joint and ligamentous laxity.

Clinical manifestations of cord compromise from instability include disturbances in gait, exercise intolerance, and neck pain. Mild weakness and hyperreflexia may be found. Screen with flexion-extension radiographs by ages 5–6 years.

Management Be concerned if ADI >5 mm. Follow yearly with examination and every several years with radiographs. Some recommend fusion with ADI >10 mm.

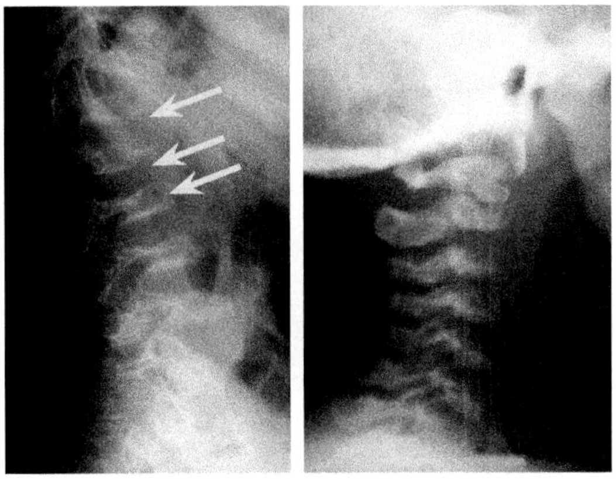

A Morquio syndrome Vertebral body changes (yellow arrows) are useful in evaluation. Odontoid hypoplasia (red arrow) is a serious defect.

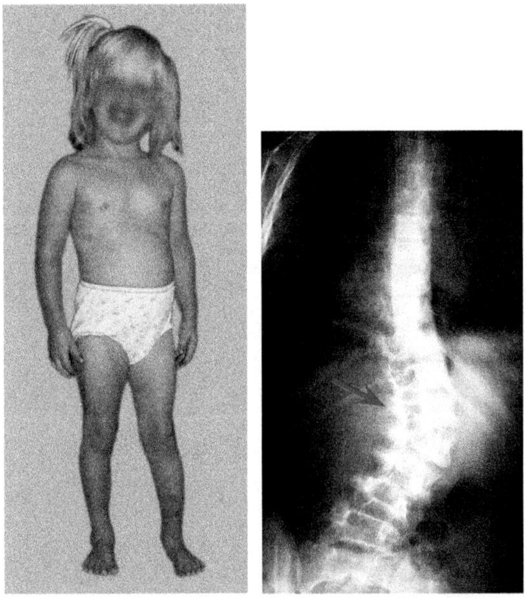

B Neurofibromatosis Curves tend to be sharp and progressive (red arrow).

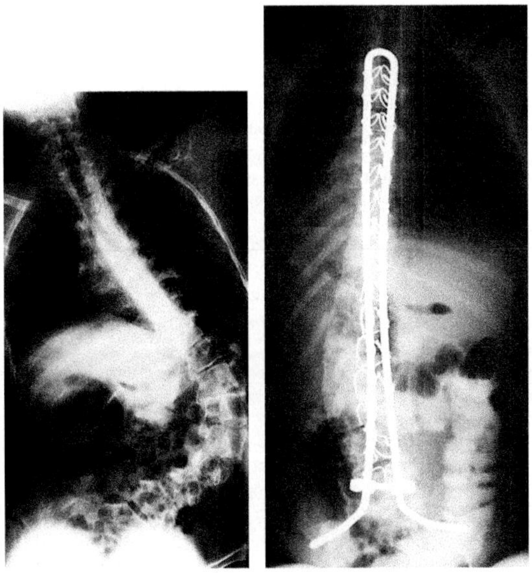

C Rett syndrome Deformity is severe and progressive, often requiring long fusion.

BACK PAIN

Feldman DS, Straight JJ, Badra MI, Mohaideen A, Madan SS. Evaluation of an algorithmic approach to pediatric back pain. J Pediatr Orthop. 2006;26:353-7.

Landman Z, Oswald T, Sanders J, Diab M, Spinal Deformity Study Group. Prevalence and predictors of pain in surgical treatment of adolescent idiopathic scoliosis. Spine. 2011 May 1;36(10):825-9.

IDIOPATHIC SCOLIOSIS - ADOLESCENT

Cotrel Y, Dubousset J, Guillaumat M. New universal instrumentation in spinal surgery. Clin Orthop Relat Res. 1988 Feb;227:10-23.

Diab M, Landman Z, Lubicky J, et al. Use and outcome of MRI in the surgical treatment of adolescent idiopathic scoliosis. Spine. 2011 Apr 15;36(8):667-71.

Dolan LA, Weinstein SL. Surgical rates after observation and bracing for adolescent idiopathic scoliosis: an evidence-based review. Spine. 2007 Sep 1;32(19 Suppl):S91-S100.

Hamill CL, Lenke LG, Bridwell KH, Chapman MP, Blanke K, Baldus C. The use of pedicle screw fixation to improve correction in the lumbar spine of patients with idiopathic scoliosis. Is it warranted? Spine. 1996 May 15;21(10):1241-9.

Harrington PR. Treatment of scoliosis: correction and internal fixation by spine instrumentation. J Bone Joint Surg Am.1962 Jun 01;44(4):591-634.

Luque ER. Segmental spinal instrumentation for correction of scoliosis. Clin Orthop Relat Res. 1982 Mar;(163):192-8.

Negrini S, Minozzi S, Bettany-Saltikov J, Zaina F, Chockalingam N, Grivas TB, Kotwicki T, Maruyama T, Romano M, Vasiliadis ES. Braces for idiopathic scoliosis in adolescents. Cochrane Database Syst Rev. 2010 Jan 20;(1).

Sanders JO. Maturity indicators in spinal deformity. J Bone Joint Surg Am. 2007 Feb;89 Suppl 1:14-20.

Weinstein SL, Dolan LA, Spratt KF, Peterson KK, Spoonamore MJ, Ponseti IV. Health and function of patients with untreated idiopathic Scoliosis. A 50-Year natural history study. JAMA. 2003;289(5):559-567.

Weinstein SL, Dolan LA, Wright JG, Dobbs MB. Effects of bracing in adolescents with idiopathic scoliosis. N Engl J Med. 2013 Oct;369:1512-1521.

IDIOPATHIC SCOLIOSIS - INFANTILE and JUVENILE

Akbarnia BA, Breakwell LM, Marks DS, McCarthy RE, Thompson AG, Canale SK, Kostial PN, Tambe A, Asher MA. Dual growing rod technique followed for three to eleven years until final fusion: the effect of frequency of lengthening. Spine (Phila Pa 1976). 2008 Apr 20;33(9):984-90.

Betz RR, Ranade A, Samdani AF, et al. Vertebral body stapling: a fusionless treatment option for a growing child with moderate idiopathic scoliosis. Spine. 2010 Jan 15;35(2):169-76.

Crawford CH, Lenke LG. Growth modulation by means of anterior tethering resulting in progressive correction of juvenile idiopathic scoliosis: a case report. J Bone Joint Surg Am. 2010 Jan;92(1):202-9.

Gupta P, Lenke LG, Bridwell KH. Incidence of neural axis abnormalities in infantile and juvenile patients with spinal deformity. Is a magnetic resonance image screening necessary? Spine 1998 Jan 15;23(2):206-10.

James JIP. Idiopathic scoliosis; the prognosis, diagnosis, and operative indications related to curve patterns and the age at onset. J Bone Joint Surg Br. 1954;36: 36-49.3636 1954.

Klemme WR, Denis F, Winter RB, Lonstein JW, Koop SE. Spinal instrumentation without fusion for progressive scoliosis in young children. J Pediatr Orthop. 1997 Nov-Dec;17(6):734-42.

Mehta MH. The rib-vertebra angle in the early diagnosis between resolving and progressive infantile scoliosis. J Bone Joint Surg Br. 1972 May;54(2):230-43.

Mehta MH. Growth as a corrective force in the early treatment of progressive infantile scoliosis. J Bone Joint Surg Br 2005;87(9):1237-1247.

Wynne-Davies R. Infantile idiopathic scoliosis. Causative factors, particularly in the first six months of life. J Bone Joint Surg Br. 1975 May;57(2):138-41.

CONGENITAL SCOLIOSIS

Basu PS, Elsebaie H, Noordeen MH. Congenital spinal deformity: a comprehensive assessment at presentation. Spine. 2002 Oct 15;27(20):2255-9.

Hedden D. Management themes in congenital scoliosis. J Bone Joint Surg Am. 2007 Feb; 89 Suppl 1:72-8.

Hedequist DJ, Emans J. Congenital scoliosis: a review and update. J Pediatr Orthop. 2007 Jan-Feb;27(1):106-16.

Kawakami N, Tsuji T, Imagama S, Lenke LG, Puno RM, Kuklo TR; Spinal Deformity Study Group. Classification of congenital scoliosis and kyphosis: a new approach to the three-dimensional classification for progressive vertebral anomalies requiring operative treatment. Spine. 2009 Aug 1;34(17):1756-65.

Lenke LG, Newton PO, Sucato DJ, et al. Complications after 147 consecutive vertebral column resections for severe pediatric spinal deformity: a multicenter analysis. Spine. 2013; 38(2): 119-132.

Marks DS, Qaimkhani SA. The natural history of congenital scoliosis and kyphosis. Spine. 2009 Aug 1;34(17):1751-5.

McMaster MJ. Spinal growth and congenital deformity of the spine. Spine (Phila Pa 1976). 2006 Sep 15;31(20):2284-7.

Ruf M, Jensen R, Letko L, Harms J. Hemivertebra resection and osteotomies in congenital spine deformity. Spine. 2009 Aug 1;34(17):1791-9.

Yazici M, Emans J. Fusionless instrumentation systems for congenital scoliosis: expandable spinal rods and vertical expandable prosthetic titanium rib in the management of congenital spine deformities in the growing child. Spine. 2009 Aug 1;34(17):1800-7.

KYPHOSIS - CONGENITAL

Kawakami N, Tsuji T, Imagama S, Lenke LG, Puno RM, Kuklo TR; Spinal Deformity Study Group. Classification of congenital scoliosis and kyphosis: a new approach to the three-dimensional classification for progressive vertebral anomalies requiring operative treatment. Spine. 2009 Aug 1;34(17):1756-65.

McMaster MJ, Singh H. Natural history of congenital kyphosis and kyphoscoliosis. A study of one hundred and twelve patients. J Bone Joint Surg Am. 1999 Oct;81(10):1367-83.

Noordeen MH, Garrido E, Tucker SK, Elsebaie HB. The surgical treatment of congenital kyphosis. Spine. 2009 Aug 1;34(17):1808-14.

KYPHOSIS - of SCHEUERMANN

Coe JD, Smith JS, Berven S, et al: Complications of spinal fusion for Scheuermann kyphosis: a report of the Scoliosis Research Society Morbidity and Mortality Committee, Spine 35:99, 2009.

Lowe TG, Line BG. Evidence based medicine: analysis of Scheuermann kyphosis. Spine. 2007 Sep 1;32(19 Suppl):S115-9.

Montgomery SP, Erwin WE. Scheuermann's kyphosis: long-term results of Milwaukee brace treatment. Spine 1981;6:5–8.

Murray PM, Weinstein SL, Spratt KF. The natural history and long-term follow-up of Scheuermann kyphosis. J Bone Joint Surg 1993:75A:236.

Riddle EC, Bowen JR, Shah SA, et al. The DuPont kyphosis brace for the treatment of adolescent Scheuermann kyphosis. J South Orthop Assoc 2003;12:135–40. http://www.ncbi.nlm.nih.gov/pubmed/14577720 (27).

Sachs B, Bradford D, Winter R, et al. Scheuermann kyphosis: follow-up of Milwaukee-brace treatment. J Bone Joint Surg [Am] 1987;69-A:50-7.

SPONDYLOLYSIS – SPONDYLOLISTHESIS

Agabegi SS, Fischgrund JS. Contemporary management of isthmic spondylolisthesis: pediatric and adult. Spine J. 2010 Jun;10(6):530-43.

Beutler WJ, Fredrickson BE, Murtland A, Sweeney CA, Grant WD, Baker D: The natural history of spondylolysis and spondylolisthesis: 45-year follow-up evaluation. Spine. 2003 ;28(10):1027-1035, discussion 1035.

Bradford DS, Iza J. Repair of the defect in spondylolysis or minimal degrees of spondylolisthesis by segmental wire fixation and bone grafting. Spine. 1985 Sep;10(7):673-9.

Buck JE. Direct repair of the defect in spondylolisthesis. Preliminary report. J Bone Joint Surg Br. 1970 Aug;52(3):432-7.

Hu SS, Tribus CB, Diab M, Ghanayem AJ. Spondylolisthesis and spondylolysis. Instr Course Lect. 2008;57:431-45.

Klein G, Mehlman CT, McCarty M: Nonoperative treatment of spondylolysis and grade I spondylolisthesis in children and young adults: A meta-analysis of observational studies. J Pediatr Orthop 2009;29(2):146-156.

Meyerding HW. Low backache and sciatic pain associated with spondylolisthesis and protruded intervertebral disc: incidence, significance, and treatment. J Bone Joint Surg 1941;23(2):461-70.

Steiner ME, Micheli LJ. Treatment of symptomatic spondylolysis and spondylolisthesis with the modified Boston brace. Spine. 1985;10:937-43.

Taillard WF. Etiology of spondylolisthesis. Clin Orthop Relat Res. 1976 Jun;(117):30-9.

DISCITIS

Wenger DR, Bobechko WP, Gilday DL. The spectrum of intervertebral disk-space infection in children. J Bone Joint Surg 1978;60A:100.

TUMORS

Beer SJ, Menezes AH. Primary tumors of the spine in children. Natural history, management, and long-term follow-up. Spine 1997:22:649.

OTHER

Kim HW, Weinstein SL. Spine update. The management of scoliosis in neurofibromatosis. Spine 1997:22:2770.

Lipton GE, Guille JT, Kumar SJ. Surgical treatment of scoliosis in Marfan syndrome: guidelines for a successful outcome. J Pediatr Orthop 2002 May-Jun;22(3): p302-7.

Papaioannou T, Stokes I, Kenwright J. Scoliosis associated with limb-length inequality. J Bone Joint Surg Am. 1982 Jan;64(1):59-62.

Vercauteren M,Van Beneden M,Verplaetse R,et al. Trunk asymmetries in a Belgian school population. Spine. 1982Nov-Dec;7(6):555-62.

UPPER LIMB

CHAPTER 13

The purpose of the upper limb is to position the hand for bimanual function within the field of vision. Management should preserve or enhance a range of joint motion that allows, at a minimum, hand access to the face and perineum. This requires mobility, sensibility, strength, and fine motor function.

Upper Limb Development

Growth

The upper limb bud appears along Wolf's crest during the third post-fertilization week. The leading edge of this bud is a thickened ridge called the *apical ectodermal ridge,* or AER. This AER contains the design plan for the limb for its developmental and three-dimensional orientation. This development is controlled by genes that include the Hox and WNT7 groups. Mutations of these genes have been linked to malformations. Most congenital upper limb defects have their origin during this period [A]. Vascular ingrowth occurs concurrent with limb bud development. Disruptions of this ingrowth may lead to transverse limb deficiencies. At about 56 days, a gene initiates the process of apoptosis, or dissolution of the interdigital webbing, to create separate digits. A failure of this process results in syndactyly.

The hand forms by about the 8th week [B] and reaches about a third of its adult size at birth [C]. Upper limb growth occurs most rapidly in the proximal humeral and distal forearm epiphyses [D].

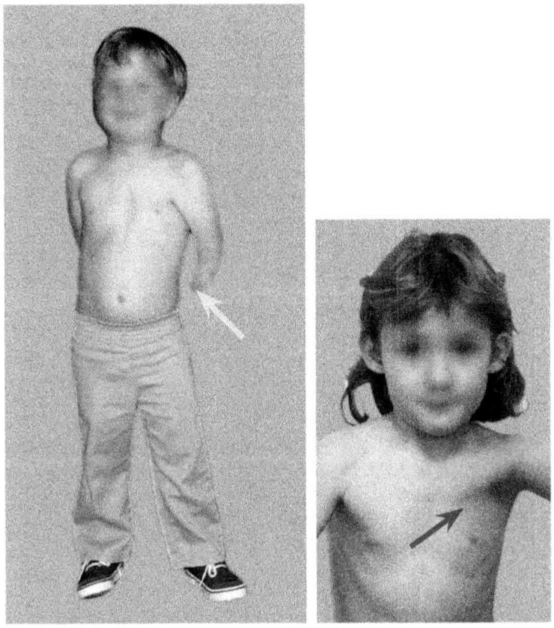

A Congenital anomalies Limb deficiencies (yellow arrow) and Poland anomaly (absence of the sternal head of the pectoralis – red arrow) are caused by a failure of vascular ingrowth during early development.

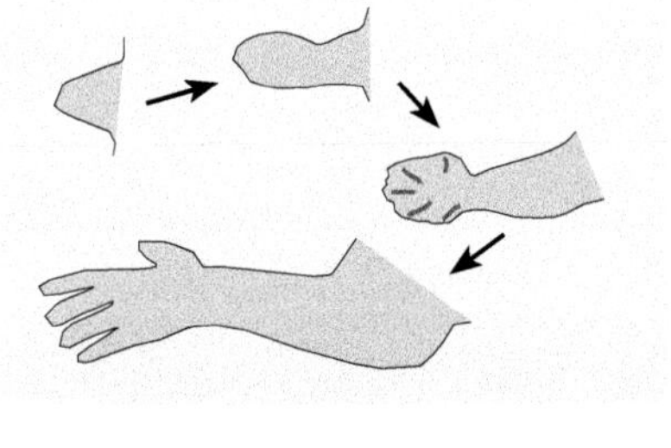

B Hand development The hand first as a bud at 3 weeks with progressive development and finally *apoptosis* or a dissolution of the interdigital webs to form fingers by about the 8th week. Redrawn from Arey (1980).

Age	Size
Fetal age 8 weeks	5 mm
Birth	60 mm
3 Years	120 mm
Adult	200 mm

C Hand growth The hand is about 5 mm when completely formed at the 8th fetal week, and about a third of its adult size at birth.

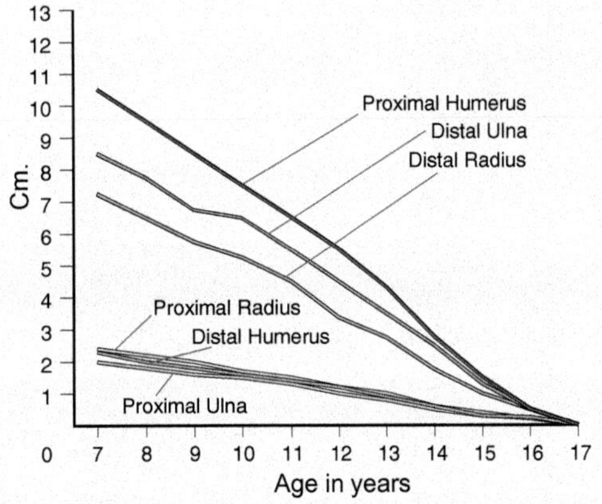

D Growth rates for upper limb The majority of growth of the upper limbs occurs from physes about the wrist and shoulder compared to the elbow. From Pritchett (1988).

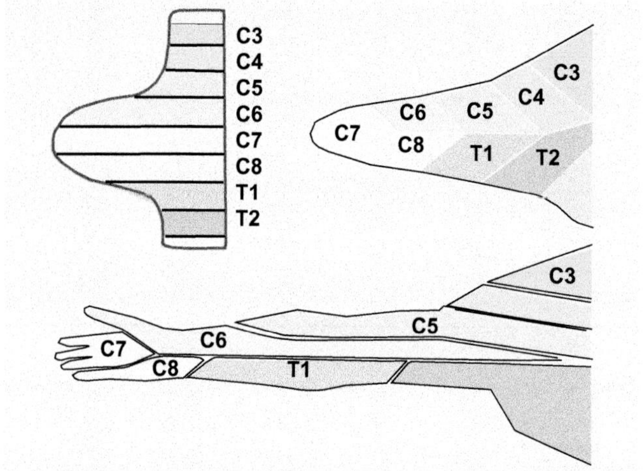

A Cutaneous nerve distribution The upper limb development clarifies the origin of the distribution of the segmental distribution of the upper limb. Redrawn from Moore (1982).

Age	Hand Function
1 Month	Hand clenches
2 Months	Opens hand
3 Months	Holds objects
5 Months	Primitive finger grasp
9 Months	Early finger pinch
12 Months	Picks up large objects
18 Months	Piles blocks
3 Years	Buttons clothing
4 Years	Can throw a ball
5 Years	Can catch a ball

B Hand function by age Hand function becomes progressively more skilled with advancing age.

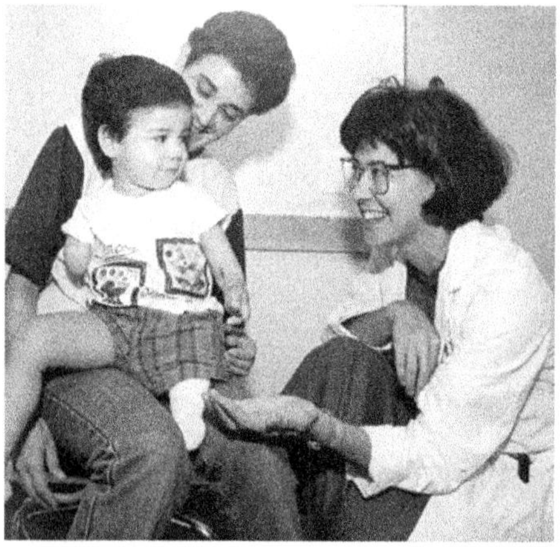

C Screening examination Examine whole child before focusing on the hand problem.

During the seventh gestational week, the upper limb flexes at the shoulder and elbow and rotates around a longitudinal axis and accounts for the cutaneous nerve distribution [A]. Cutaneous nerve distribution in the hand arises from C6, C7, and C8.

During infancy, hand function progresses in an orderly fashion [B]. Bimanual function becomes refined during the second year. Both fine and gross motor skills improve with age. The function of each upper limb is more independent than that of the lower limbs. Thus, a short arm causes less functional difficulty than a short leg.

Optimum hand function is achieved by the dominant hand possessing both strength and the ability to manipulate small objects. The nondominant hand should grasp and release effectively. Function ideally requires intact sensation, tactile surfaces free of scars, motor strength, and a good range of motion of the wrist and fingers.

Evaluation

The physical examination should follow the standard sequence of inspection, palpation, range of motion evaluation, and a careful neurological examination. Imaging should start with conventional radiographs.

Screening Examination

First perform a screening examination of the child, as hand problems are commonly part of a syndrome or association. Examine the whole child [C] to avoid missing other problems that may be important in establishing the diagnosis, as well as other problems that may require treatment. This examination is often best performed with the child on the parent's lap.

The Infant may be developmentally delayed but without any obvious deformities. Examine the head and trunk and look for associations that might involve the spine, heart, and kidneys. Also screen the lower limbs, as hand and foot problems may occur in the same syndrome or association.

Associations

Certain deformities of the upper extremity are often associated with specific syndromes [D, E, and F]. Examples include nail dysplasia in nail–patella syndrome and the various conditions associated with radial and ulnar deficiencies and syndactyly. Carefully examine the whole child. Look for dysmorphic features, and shortness of stature, and assess the child's general health. Inquire about medical problems in the family. Certain findings indicate the need for additional studies. For example, the finding of torticollis is an indication for a radiograph of the pelvis to rule out hip dysplasia. The finding of radial dysplasia is an indication for a hematologic, cardiac, renal, and spine evaluation. Check for a sacral dimple.

Syndrome	Comment
Goltz	Bone, skin, eye, anus, retardation
Mammary aplasia	Associated with ulnar hypoplasia

D Syndromes associated with ulnar defects These syndromes should be considered if an ulnar defect is present.

Syndromes with syndactyly
Apert
Carpenter
Noack
Pfeifer
Poland
Summit
Waardenburg
Oculodentodigital
Orofaciodigital

E Syndromes associated with syndactyly

Syndrome	Comment
Fanconi anemia	Radial dysplasia, skin, hematologic defects
Holt-Oram	Radial dysplasia and cardiovascular
Ladd	Radial dysplasia and craniofacial
Nagar	Radial dysplasia and craniofacial
Thrombocytopenia (TAR syndrome)	Associated with radial aplasia

F Syndromes associated with radial defects These syndromes should be considered if radial defects are present.

Upper Limb

Head and neck Observe the head and neck for abnormalities and asymmetry. The head is normally held in a vertical position by the vestibular and ocular righting mechanisms. Head tilt is common in "wryneck," or torticollis. Describe the deformity in terms of the three planes, flexion-extension, lateral head tilt, and rotation. Observe the shape of the head. Plagiocephaly is common in torticollis and includes a flattening of the malar prominence and a lowering of the position of the eye and ear on the involved side. The ipsilateral occiput is flattened.

Limbs Start with observation of the relationship of the neck and limbs. Note any asymmetry [A]. Observe differences in spontaneous movement. Loss of movement may be due to true paralysis from a nerve injury or more likely from pseudoparalysis due to trauma or infection. The infant with a clavicular fracture or septic arthritis of the shoulder or elbow will avoid active arm movement.

Observe the *carrying angle*, the alignment of the arm and forearm as viewed with the child in the anatomic position. The carrying angle is normally 0°–10° of valgus. A varus carrying angle causes the so-called *gun stock deformity*, which is usually due to a malunited supracondylar fracture [B]. An increase in carrying angle is seen in Turner syndrome.

Look for asymmetry or masses and note any finger or nail abnormalities [C]. Nail dysplasia is seen in the nail–patella syndrome. Other syndromes have characteristic finger deformities such as the "hitchhiker's" thumb in diastrophic dysplasia.

Palpation Palpation is most important if the child complains of pain. Exact localization of the point of maximum tenderness is very important in establishing the cause of pain. This is most feasible about the elbow, wrist [D], and hand, where the bone and joints are subcutaneous.

Range of Motion Describe the motion of the neck in three directions. The normal child is able to flex the chin to the chest. Lateral head tilt should allow the ear to touch the shoulder. Normal head rotation allows about 90° of motion to the right and left. Assess forearm rotation with the elbow flexed to a right angle. Supination and pronation are each about 90° in the normal child.

Joint Laxity The upper limb is readily examined to assess joint laxity. Assess the elbow, wrist, and fingers for the ability to hyperextend [E].

Pain

Pain is usually due to trauma , infection, or neoplasm. Pain is often manifest by pseudoparalysis in the infant and young child. Localization of the site of tenderness is very helpful in narrowing the diagnostic possibilities and in deciding what should be studied radiographically. Sometimes a bone scan is necessary to localize the problem.

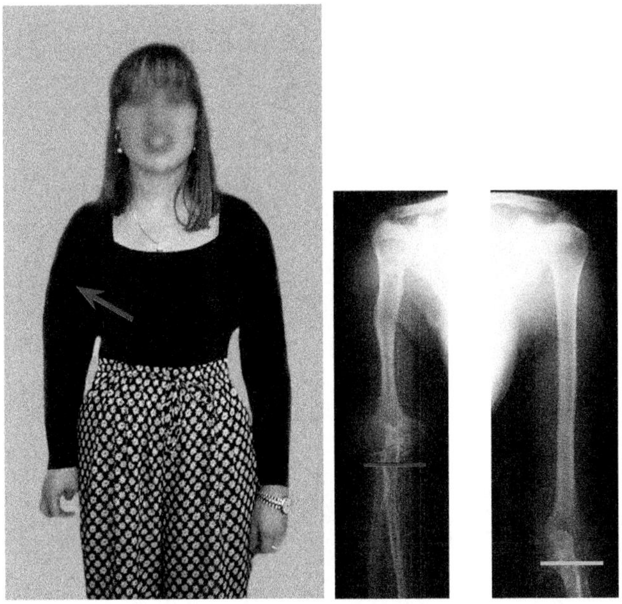

A Upper limb length inequality This girl's right arm is shortened due to a cyst of the proximal humerus. Her function is normal.

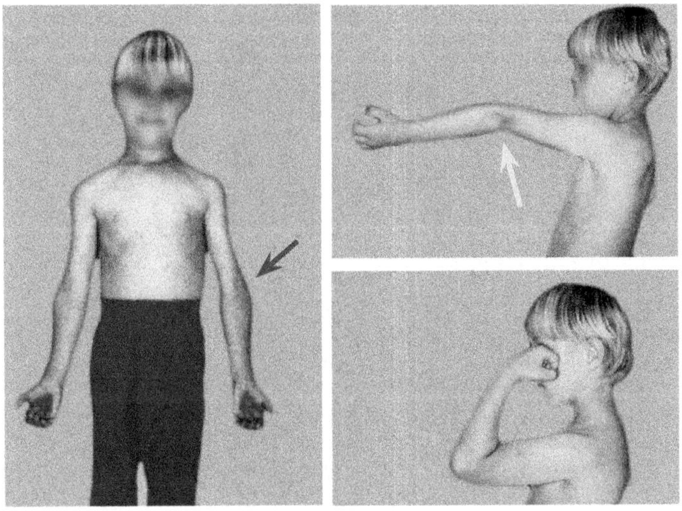

B Cubitus varus This child has a malunion following a supracondylar fracture. In the anatomic position, the child has a cubitus varus deformity (red arrow). Hyperextension deformity (yellow arrow) and limited elbow flexion (orange arrow) are also present.

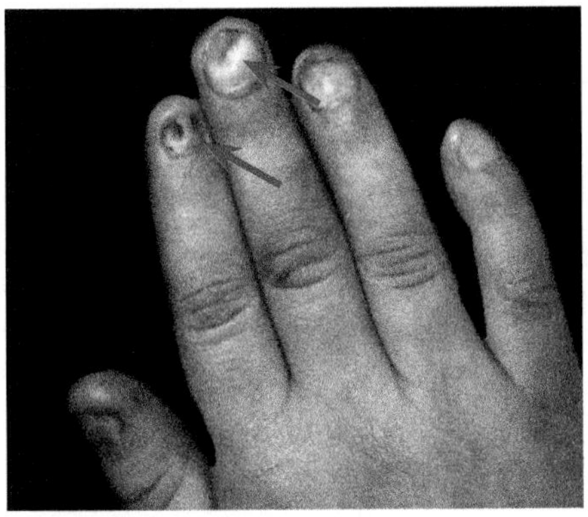

C Nail-patella syndrome Nail dysplasia is seen in the nail-patella syndrome.

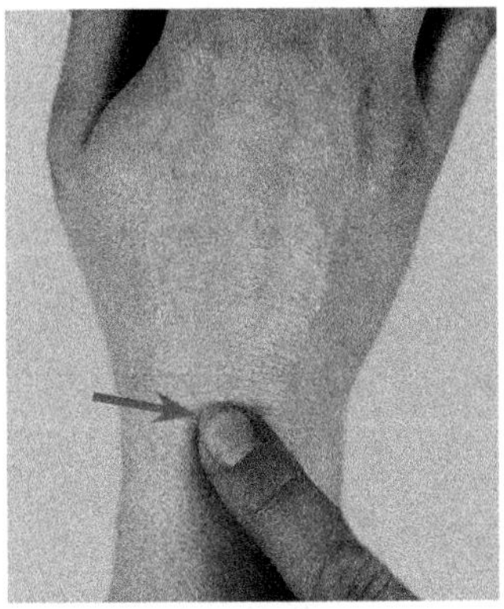

D Localize tenderness Correlate tenderness with anatomic structures.

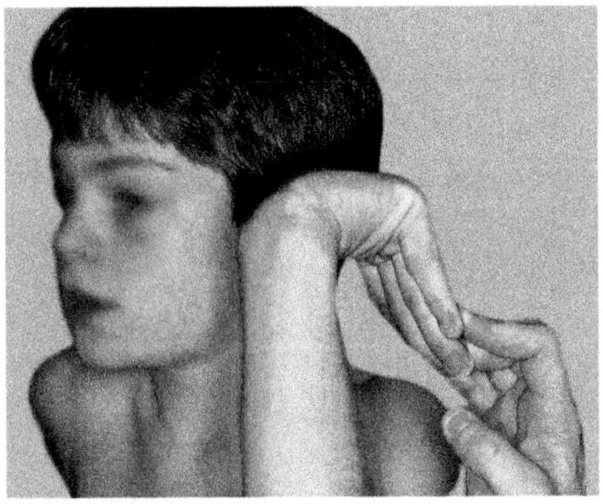

E Joint laxity Joint laxity is commonly assessed in the upper limb.

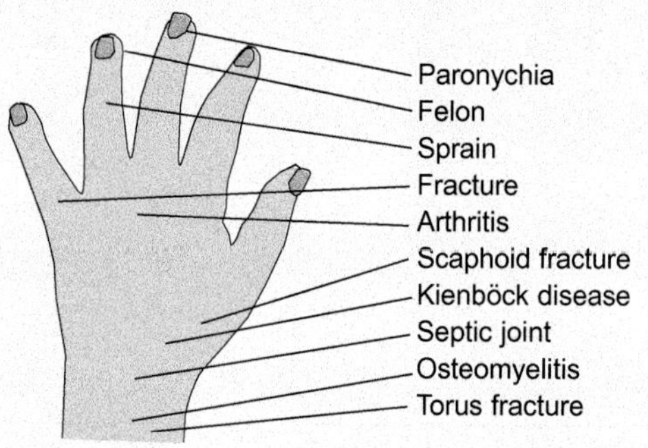

A Hand and wrist pain by location Often the diagnosis is suggested by the location of the tenderness or swelling.

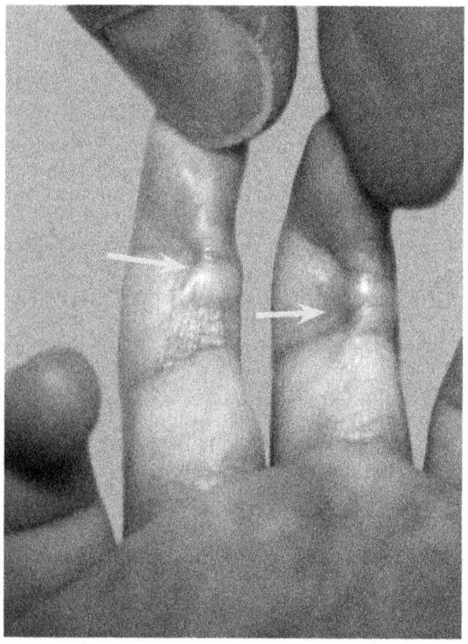

B Hypertrophic scar Friction burns in a toddler. Note the thickness of the scars. Reconstruction will require full-thickness skin grafts.

Age	Procedures
0 to 6 months	Floating polydactyly Strangulating amniotic bands
6 to 12 months	Border syndactyly Complex osseous syndactylies Aperts Macrodactyly needing amputations Broadbased polydactyly Thumb duplications
24+ months	Simple syndactyly Pollicization Angular deformities requiring osteotomy and fixation Thumb-index web reconstructions Hypoplastic thumbs, hands with ulnar dysplasia and complex polysyndactyly.

C Timing of procedures This table provides some generalizations for timing of operative procedures. Each indication should be individualized.

Hand Examination

Observation Observe the resting position of the hand as well as how the hand and fingers move. This is often best done from a distance to avoid frightening the child. Observe the position of the fingers. The resting position is altered by tendon lacerations or contractures.

Sensation Assess sensation by observing the texture for trophic changes, the presence of sweat, and the use of the hand. Ask for the parents' opinion about hand sensation. Parents usually know. In the older child, differentiating coins by feel alone may be useful.

Motor function Observe the child playing with a toy to assess the use of the hand. Observe how the dominant and nondominant hands are used. Be aware that bimanual hand function develops after an infant acquires sitting balance.

Pain A number of conditions that are unique to the hand and wrist may be the source of pain [A]. Among these are nonunion of the radial styloid, unrecognized fractures or idiopathic avascular necrosis of the scaphoid, and overuse syndromes. Most gymnasts experience wrist pain due to overuse. Gymnasts most at risk are older children who are new to the sport and participate many hours per week.

Management Principles

Because the hand is used in expression and is always visible, appearance is an especially important consideration in management.

Descriptions

Describe conditions by using the anatomic terms rather than words such as *clubhand* or *lobster claw* deformity.

Parents

Be aware of parents' feelings, especially if the child has a congenital or traumatic problem. Parents typically go through a series of stages in the grieving process that include first denial, then anger (which may be directed toward managing physicians), and then distress.

Healing

Because the skin of infants is prone to hypertrophic scar formation [B], be very careful about placement of surgical incisions, especially on the palmar aspect of the digits and in the web spaces.

Surgeon

Hand surgery in the infant or child is difficult due to the small size of the hand, the lack of cooperation of the patient, and the complexity of the problem. Seldom is there a need for the procedure to be done as an emergency, and because the best results are possible with the first attempt at repair, referral to a surgeon with special training and experience in managing hand problems in infants and children is best for the child.

Timing of Management

General guidelines have been established for optimum timing of various treatments.

Operative procedures are performed in general categories [C]. This timing is a rough guide. Individualize each procedure.

Management methods Apply treatment types to specific age groups. Some general guidelines are useful [A, next page].

Maturity

Consider the capacity of the child to cooperate with treatment and rehabilitation. Surgical dressings should protect the operated area from the child. Delay complex procedures requiring cooperation during rehabilitation until later.

Splinting

Splinting is a primary or adjective treatment method used for hand problems [B]. Many different types of splints have been developed for use on fingers, hands, wrists, and elbows as both static and dynamic splints. Most are made of plastic by therapists with a specific objective in mind.

Dressing

For most wounds, the following plan is appropriate [C]. If a tourniquet has been used, leave it inflated for the initial dressing application.

Wound closure Use 6-0 plain gut dyed blue with a marking pencil to make it visible and to make suture removal unnecessary. Use absorbable sutures.

Primary dressing Place a single layer of fine mesh gauze treated with petroleum jelly to prevent sticking directly on the wound. Over this, apply a saline-soaked dressing sponge to direct drainage from the wound.

Compression Apply gentle compressive dressing to secure the primary dressing, contoured and positioned not to restrict circulation. Apply the first layer of fluffed gauze between the digits, being careful to avoid excessive pressure. Then secure the gauze with roller gauze in 2- or 3-inch widths. This provides gentle compression, fits the hand well, and should hold the hand in a position with slight wrist extension and thumb abduction.

Padding Next, place cotton cast padding to protect the skin and bony prominences and to facilitate cast removal. A skin adhesive will help to maintain the padding in position.

Deflate the tourniquet and assess circulation to each digit. Elevate the hand for a few minutes during the post-tourniquet hyperemia phase before apply the cast.

Rigid outer dressing Apply a plaster or fiberglass cast that extends above the flexed elbow. This secures the dressing and prevents exploration and intrusion by the child and parents. Start the application with the elbow flexed slightly more than 90°.

In infants and young children, pad the digits and place a cast that becomes a mitten. This mitten prevents toys and food from entering the cast and further protects the wound and secures the dressing.

Sling Apply a sling made from 2-inch tubular stockinette placed around the neck and chest to hold the arm at the side.

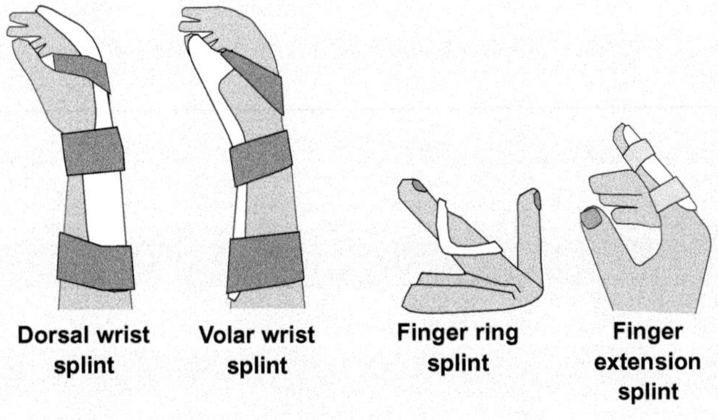

B Splints Many different types of splints are used for the hand. These are some examples.

Age	Treatments
0 to 6 months	Splinting well tolerated
6 to 12 months	Passive stretching
12+ months	Simple operative procedures
2 to 4 years	Complex procedures

A Timing of management Treatment is best tailored to the age of the infant or child.

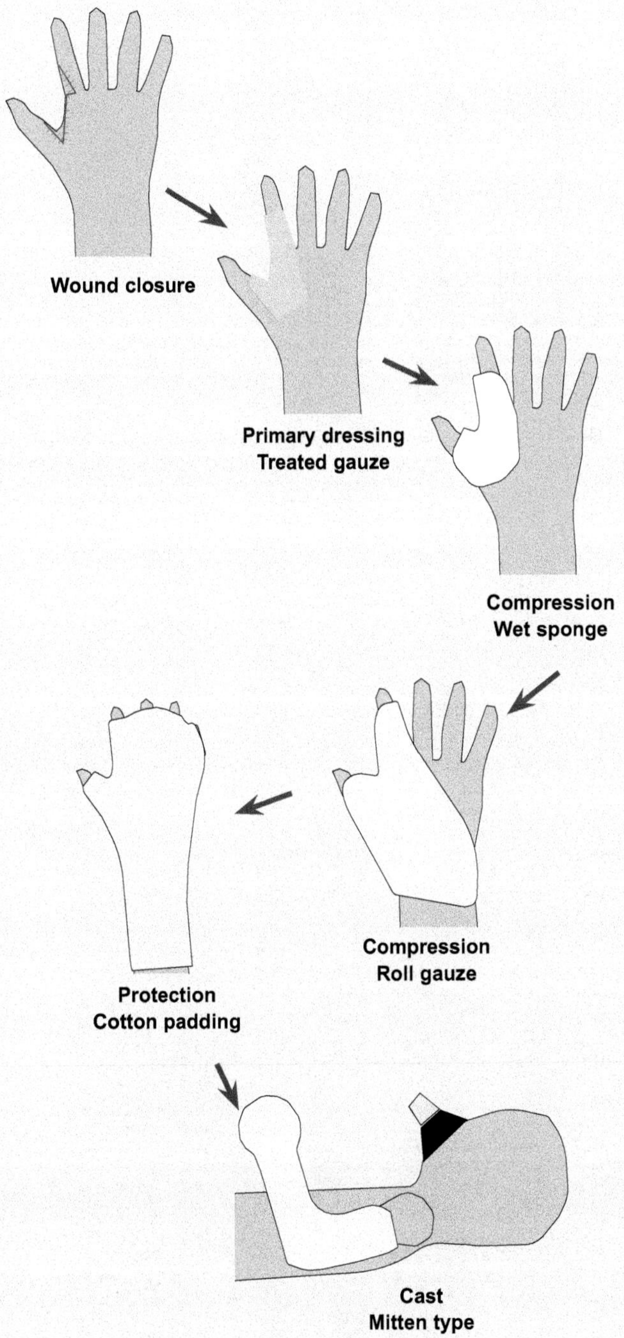

C Dressing sequence Dressings following surgery or injuries should be carefully applied.

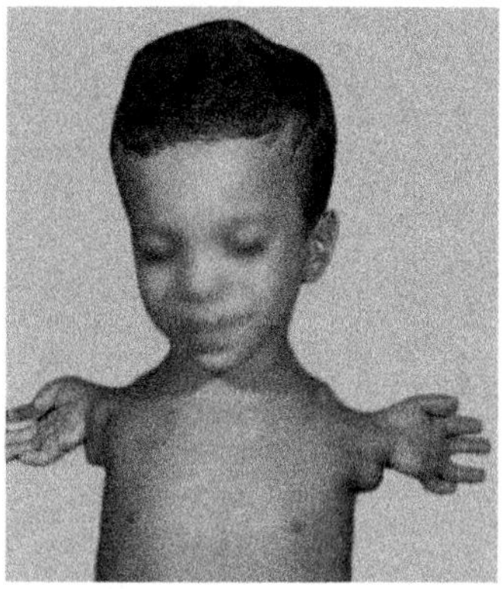

A Complete "phocomelia" This child has bilateral radial dysplasia due to the proximal form of TAR syndrome.

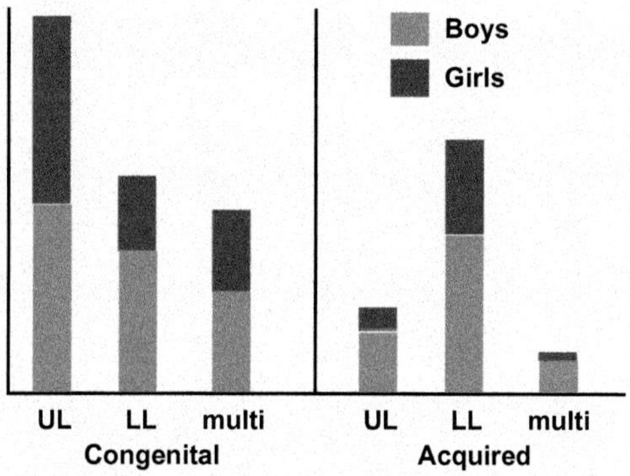

B Distribution of pediatric amputees Distribution for girls (red) and boys (blue) for UL (upper limb), LL (lower limb), or multi (multiple levels) are shown in 1,400 cases. From data of Krebs and Fishman.

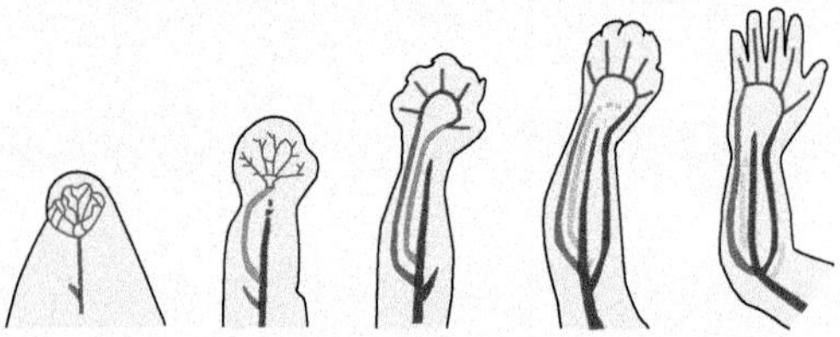

C Stages of vascular ingrowth and limb development Blood vessel ingrowth is essential to normal limb development, as shown in this sequence. Based on *Gray's Anatomy* (1973).

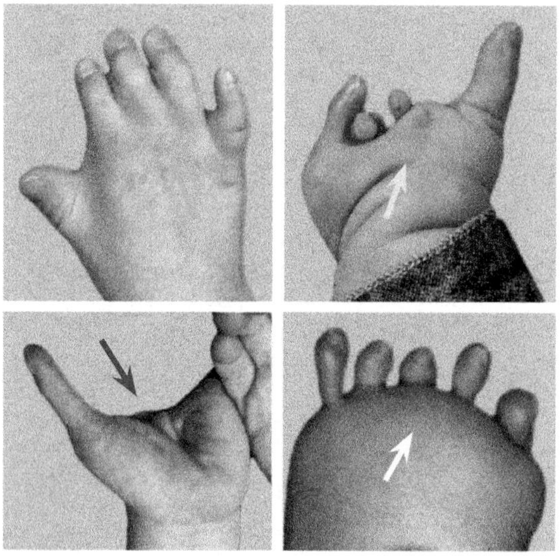

D Symbrachydactyly examples Short finger form (green arrow), cleft form (yellow arrow), monodactylous (red arrow), and peromelic form (white arrow).

Upper Limb Deficiencies

Upper limb deficiencies may be due to malformations [A] or disruptions, such as amniotic bands, from trauma, or as a result from resections of malignant tumors. Limb deficiencies are most common in the lower limb and in boys [B].

Etiology

Vascular ingrowth is needed to supply the progress zone [C]. Failure results in insufficient mesodermal substrate. In the *unifying theory of subclavian artery supply disruption sequence*, the type of deformity depends upon the timing of the disruption. These defects are referred to as symbrachydactyly.

Classification

The symbrachydactyly is a spectrum including the most common type of dysplasias [D].

Short finger form may be associated with Poland anomaly.

Cleft form previously called *atypical cleft hand.*

Monodactylous (thumb) form The thumb is the best preserved digit.

Peromelic–transverse arrest form This may occur at any level from shoulder to wrist. The feature that is always present is the nubbins at the end of the limb.

Evaluation

Although the diagnosis can usually be made by physical examination, obtain radiographs to document and classify the deficiency.

Screening examination is necessary to identify other abnormalities such as radial head dislocations or radioulnar synostosis.

Family situation should be evaluated carefully. Make certain that counseling is available for parents who are having difficulty dealing with the grief and guilt common in parents of limb-deficient children. Make a special effort to develop a warm and supportive relationship with the family because management is often difficult. Good rapport improves the child's compliance with treatment and the parents' acceptance of recommendations for management.

Management Principles

The following principles may be helpful in planning management.

Early prosthetics fitting is controversial Some physicians believe that covering the limb with a prosthesis prevents sensory feedback and slows development of bimanual function. Others recommend the fitting of a passive prosthesis between 3 and 6 months of age to promote the development of a more normal self-image by the infant. Most children reject prostheses.

First prosthesis is usually passive Convert to an active prosthesis based on the infant's developmental age.

Myoelectric power is inherently attractive to parents. Because these electrically powered limbs are expensive and difficult to maintain, long-term acceptance is poorer than for the simpler, body-powered prostheses.

Congenital and acquired amputations are different Congenital amputees have normal sensation at the end of the limb, and are not troubled by overgrowth, scars, or pain, in contrast to those with acquired forms. Congenital amputees also develop better techniques of compensation.

Modify prosthesis to facilitate activities of daily living. Make available an experienced occupational therapist to access the child's needs and make recommendations for modifications that enhance self care.

Family support groups are extremely valuable for both the parents and the child. Most childhood amputee clinics have ready access to these support groups and can help families make the necessary contacts.

Acceptance is usually less for upper than for lower limb prostheses. The lack of sensibility and fine movement control makes upper limb prostheses less useful than those for the lower limb. Children are most likely to accept an upper limb prosthesis when a specific functional need is recognized. This awareness usually occurs at about 8 years of age.

Bilateral deficiencies Rarely is prosthetic replacement useful or acceptable [A].

Most successful fittings are for children with proximal transverse forearm deficiencies [B].

Allow child natural adaptations Such adaptations are usually practical, effective, and energy efficient [C].

Replace prosthesis when destroyed, if it causes discomfort, or if it becomes suboptimal for function.

Discarding of prosthetics is most common when deficiencies are extensive, prosthetic devices are complex in design, and natural adaptations without a prosthesis are effective.

Operative Procedures

Procedures have limited indications.

Revisions for overgrowth may be necessary in both congenital and acquired transdiaphyseal amputations [D].

Krukenberg procedure This reconstruction separates the radius and ulna to allow grasp with sensibility [E]. The outcome is usually functionally good but cosmetically poor. The procedure is appropriate for blind patients with acquired amputations who cannot visually position items in their prosthetic hands or hooks.

Prosthetic Options

Terminal devices Options include several alternatives.

CAPP (child amputee prosthetic project) includes a closing spring and a frictional resilient covering that enhances control.

Hooks with elastic closures and plastic covering are durable and can be fitted with body-powered opening mechanisms.

Cosmetic hands may be passive, body-powered, or myoelectrically controlled.

Powering devices include several options:

Body power is commonly used for both opening of a terminal device and elbow flexion [B].

Myoelectric power may be provided by single or double electrodes placed over flexor or extensor muscles. Single controls are usually applied during the second year with sensors placed over extensor muscles to activate the opening device. The terminal device stays open as long as the muscle is contracted. A second sensor over the flexors may be applied about age 3 for active flexion. These fittings are experimental but children have a lower dropout rate as compared with adults.

Cosmetic passive hand is a commonly selected option due to its cosmetic advantage and simplicity.

Provide options Consider providing the child with a variety of prosthetic options to help with normal activities of daily living. About half of children use multiple prostheses based on the situation.

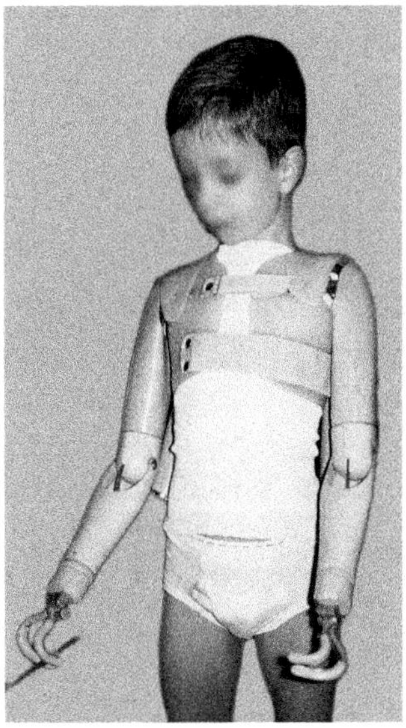

A Bilateral deficiencies Prosthetic replacement is seldom successful. Natural adaptations are more effective.

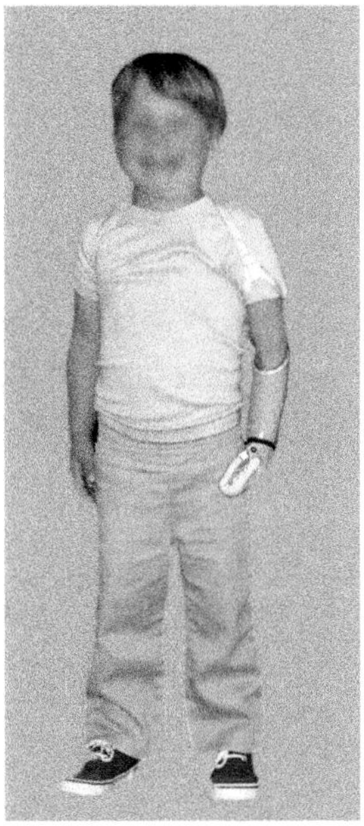

B Transverse forearm deficiencies Usually prosthetic fitting is successful.

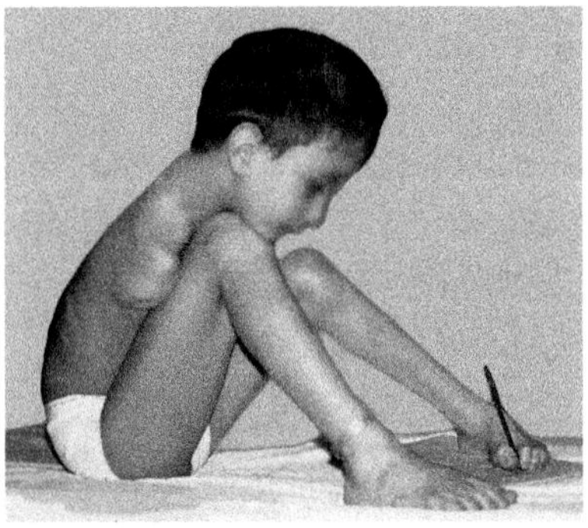

C Natural adaptation These children become surprisingly proficient in using the feet to duplicate hand function. The child preferred using the lower limbs rather than the prosthesis.

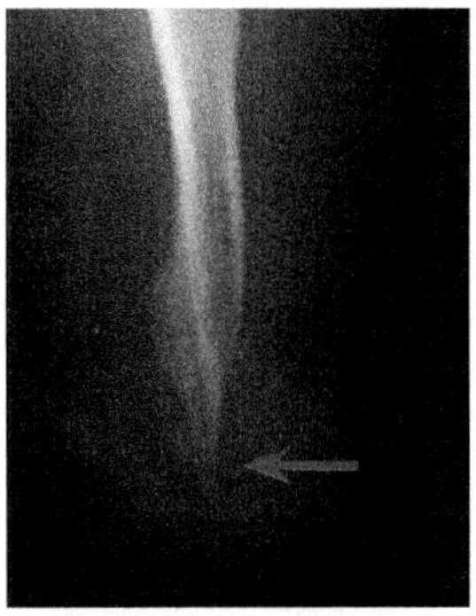

D Diaphyseal overgrowth This is a complication of through-bone amputations.

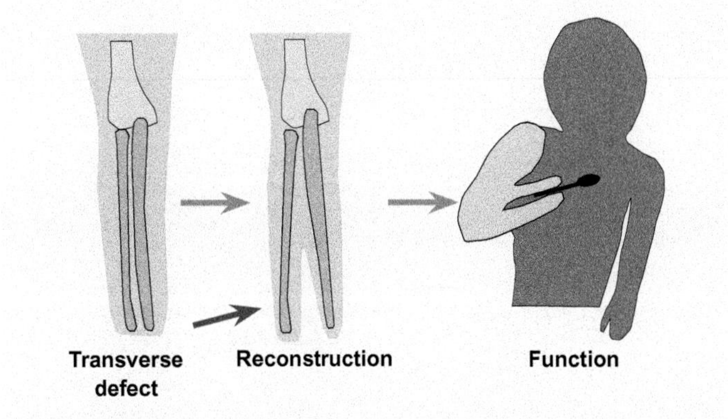

E Krukenberg reconstruction This separation of the distal radius and ulna (red arrow) and repositioning of forearm muscles provides the child with a functional grasp with sensibility.

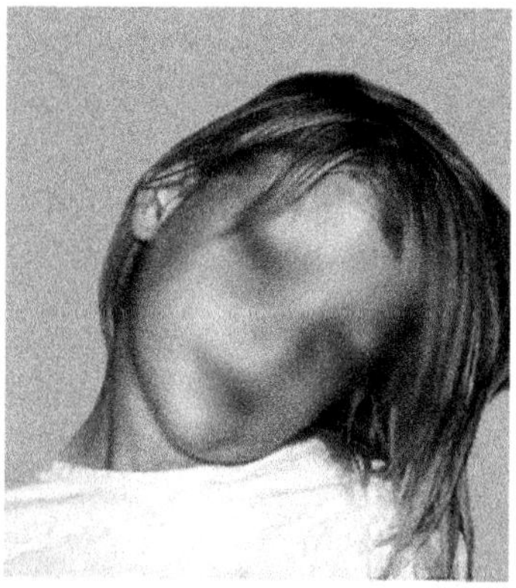

A Acute torticollis This form of torticollis develops suddenly in a previously normal child. Usually the deformity resolves spontaneously in a day or two.

Category	Comment
Muscular torticollis	Most common
Acute torticollis	Acute, resolves
Occipital cervical bony defects	Hemivertebrae
Miscellaneous	Neurogenic – tumors Inflammatory Traumatic Ocular: strabismus Hysterical Idiopathic: rotatory displacement

B Causes of torticollis The causes are many, but the vast majority of torticollis cases are due to disorders listed in the top three categories.

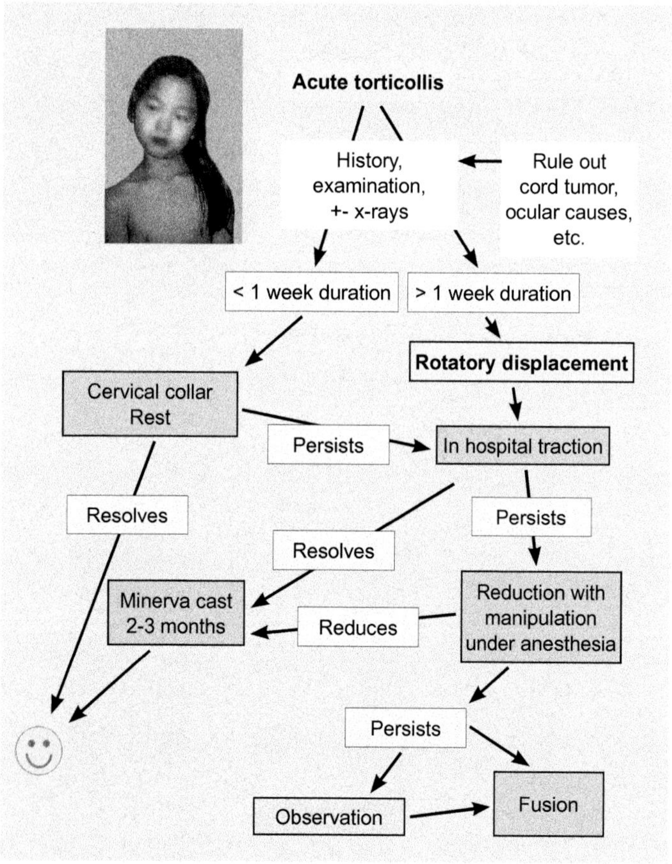

D Management of rotatory subluxation

Torticollis

Torticollis, or *wryneck*, includes a variety of conditions [B] that require different management.

Acute Torticollis

Acute torticollis is relatively common. It may occur spontaneously, follow minimal trauma, or occur after an upper respiratory infection [A]. Why the head tilts is uncertain. The tilt may be due to muscle spasm secondary to cervical lymphadenitis or possibly due to a minor subluxation of the cervical vertebrae.

Clinical features Acute torticollis causes the head to tilt, rotate to one side and become fixed. Radiographs of the cervical spine are difficult to assess because of the lateral flexion and rotation. Laboratory studies are normal.

Manage by immobilizing the neck with a folded towel and encourage rest. Early management is usually provided by the primary care physician. In most children, acute torticollis resolves within 24 hours. If the deformity persists longer than 24–48 hours, be more concerned and manage as rotatory displacement.

Rotatory Displacement

The more severe form of acute torticollis is called *rotatory displacement* or *rotatory subluxation*. This may be associated with severe pharangitis or otitis media, or follow head and neck surgery or trauma; in some cases, it occurs spontaneously. Treat rotatory displacement early to avoid permanent fixation and residual deformity [D].

Evaluate Determine the duration of the deformity and any associated history such as trauma or infections. Sometimes torticollis follows head or neck surgery. Patients with Marfan syndrome are susceptible. Examine the child for localized tenderness and neck range of motion. Perform a careful neurological examination. Be aware that spinal cord tumors may present with torticollis. Perform appropriate laboratory studies if infection is suspected. The value and reliability of conventional and dynamic CT scans are controversial and probably have little value in planning management.

Manage First apply traction. If early, head-halter traction is appropriate. In most children, the torticollis resolves with traction. If the deformity has persisted more than a week before resolution, consider extending the period of immobilization for 2 or 3 months using a Minerva cast [C]. For persisting deformity, halo traction or manipulation under anesthesia may be necessary. Should all these measures fail, operative repositioning and C1–C2 fusion may be necessary.

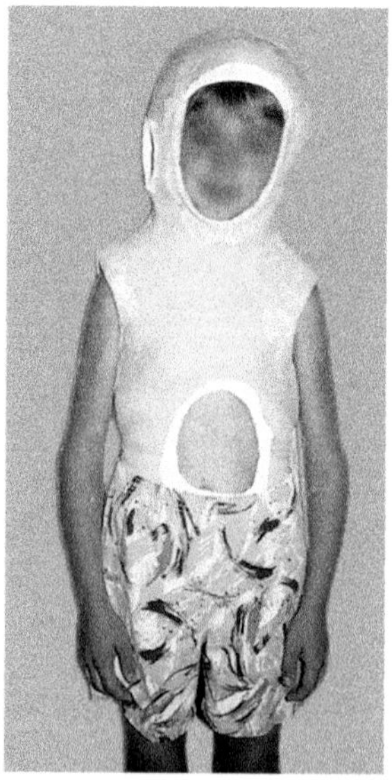

C Minerva cast This form of immobilization may be useful in children with delayed resolution of rotatory subluxation or requiring reduction. This type of cast is sometimes useful to provide immobilization following operative correction. The Minerva cast is better tolerated by the child than the parents. It is most easily applied with the child sitting or standing.

Chronic Nonmuscular Torticollis

In about 20% of children with chronic torticollis, it is due to nonmuscular causes. Radiographs may show conditions such as Klippel-Feil anomaly or hemivertebrae. If radiographs are negative and the sternocleidomastoid muscle is not contracted, consider an ocular etiology. Refer to an ophthalmologist for evaluation. Consider the other conditions that may cause torticollis, such as neonatal brachial plexus palsies and spinal cord tumors, before starting treatment.

Muscular Torticollis

Muscular torticollis is relatively common and presents in two age groups.

Infantile muscular torticollis The infant [A] is first seen because of a head tilt. Sometimes a history of a breech delivery is given and a firm tumor of the sternocleidomastoid muscle is palpated. Usually only a head tilt and limited neck motion due to a contracture of the muscle are found. Plagiocephaly (asymmetrical head) may be present [B and C].

Be certain to rule out developmental hip dysplasia. Even if the hip examination is negative, evaluate the hip by either ultrasound if the infant is seen in the neonatal period or by a single AP radiograph of the pelvis if the infant is older than about 10 weeks of age.

Infantile torticollis resolves spontaneously in about 90% of cases. The value of physical therapy by stretching is uncertain [A, right]. Of those that persist, operative correction may be necessary. Delay correction until about 3 years of age. Plagiocephaly rarely persists and is a cosmetic problem.

Juvenile muscular torticollis Sometimes muscular torticollis appears to develop during childhood [D]. In this juvenile type, usually both heads of the muscles are contracted, causing the head tilt and limiting neck motion. This type of torticollis usually is permanent and often requires operative correction.

Operative correction Bipolar release is the most effective procedure for correction of both infantile and juvenile forms of muscular torticollis.

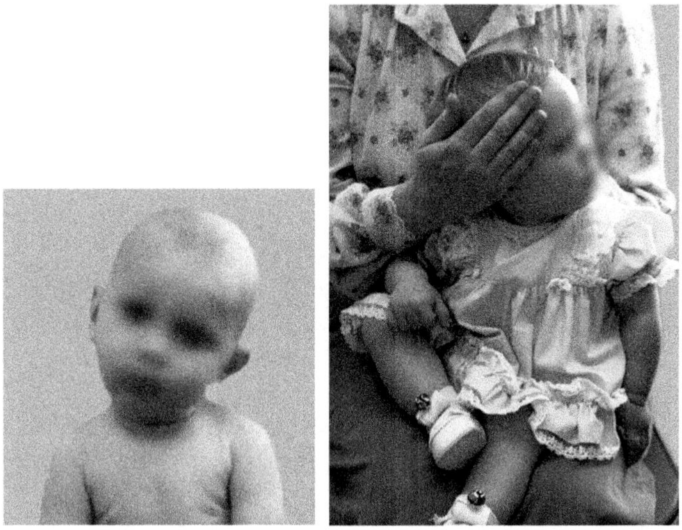

A Muscular Torticollis This is the most common neck problem in childhood. Torticollis is usually seen first in the infant (left). Some advocate treatment by stretching (right), but its value is uncertain.

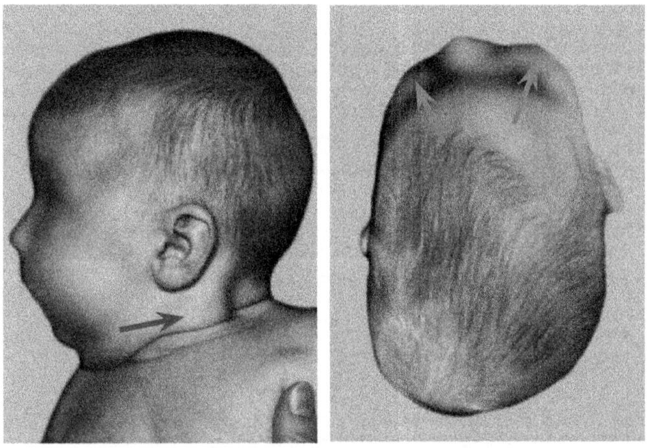

B Muscular torticollis and plagiocephaly The mass (red arrow) develops in early infancy and disappears spontaneously over a period of several months. The plagiocephaly (blue arrows) may persist longer.

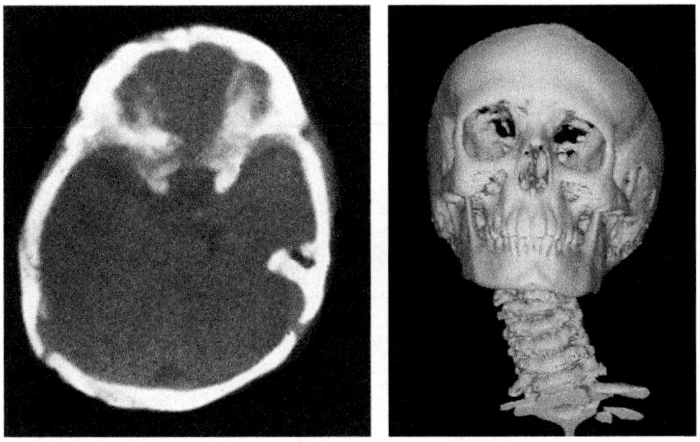

C Plagiocephaly torticollis Cranial deformity is readily shown by CT scans. 3-D reconstructions provide graphic documentation of the extent of the deformity.

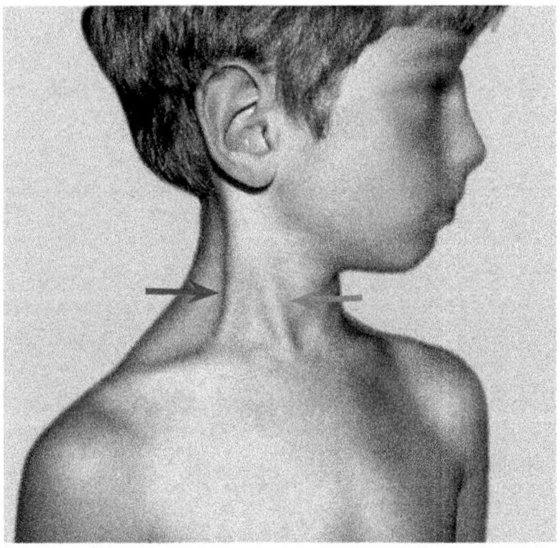

D Sternocleidomastoid contracture Both the clavicular origin (red arrow) and sternal origin (blue arrow) are contracted.

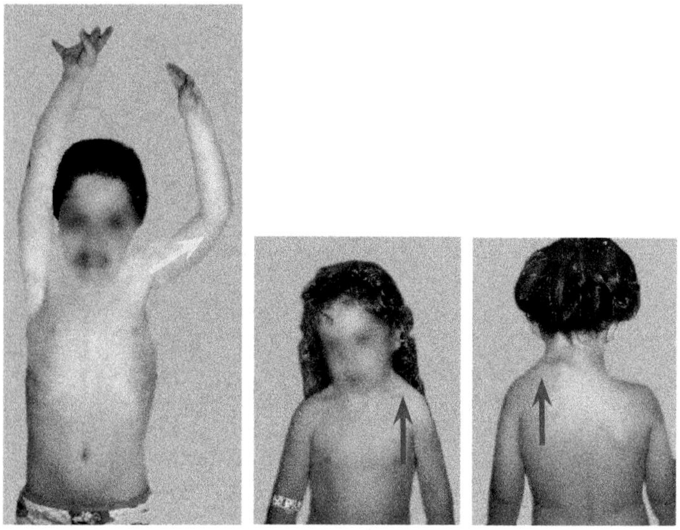

A **Sprengel deformity** Congenital elevation of the scapula causes a shoulder deformity (red arrows) that cannot be hidden by clothing. Some loss of abduction is a common mild disability (yellow arrow).

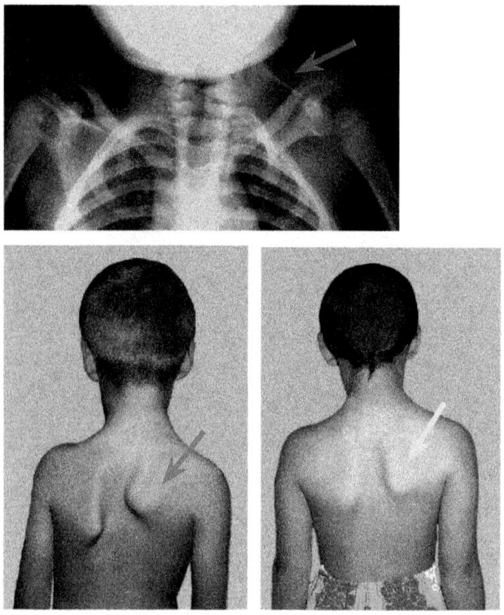

B **Spectrum of severity** Disability is proportional to the deformity. Shoulder elevation may be severe (red arrow), moderate (blue arrow), or mild (yellow arrow).

Sprengel Deformity

Sprengel deformity is a congenital elevation of the scapula [A]. The deformity results from a failure of migration of mesenchyme during the second fetal month.

Clinical Features

The deformity varies in severity [B], is usually unilateral, and is associated with other abnormalities in 70% of cases. These associated abnormalities include absent or hypoplastic parascapular musculature, abnormalities in the cervicothoracic vertebrae or thoracic rib cage, presence of an omovertebral bone, limited shoulder abduction, and multidirectional shoulder instability. Because of restricted scapulothoracic motion, most shoulder motion occurs through the glenohumeral joint.

Management

When the deformity is mild, correction is not appropriate because the operative scar is often more unsightly than the deformity. For moderate deformity, excise the superior pole of the scapula. For severe deformity repositioning of the scapula is necessary. This repositioning requires an extensive soft tissue release, caudad repositioning of the scapula, and sometimes excision of the superior portion of the scapula. Perform the correction in early childhood when the scapula is most mobile. This mobility allows maximum correction with the least risk of complications. For correction, several procedures have been described. The Woodward procedure is most widely used.

Green procedure Free all muscular attachments to the scapula, divide the omovertebral band, and rotate the scapula. Move the scapula caudad to a more normal position, and suture it into a pocket of the latissimus dorsi. In the original description of this procedure, traction was applied by a wire attached to the scapula and ilium to hold the scapula in the corrected position.

Klisic procedure This procedure includes performing an osteotomy of the clavicle, extensive muscle releases, excision of the superior scapular margin, and securing the repositioned scapula with sutures to a vertebral spinous process and rib with absorbable sutures [C].

Woodward procedure Exposure is made through a midline incision. Release the origins of the trapezius and rhomboid muscles, excise the omovertebral bone, and reposition the scapula [D]. Modifications include excising the superior and medial margins of the scapula.

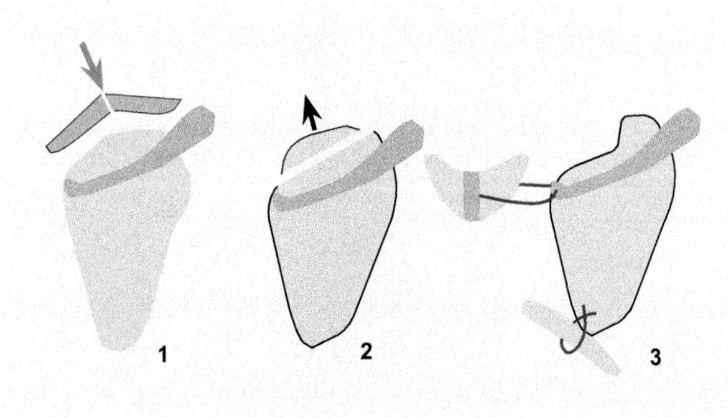

C **Klisic procedure** 1. The clavicle is divided (blue arrow). 2. The superior pole of the scapula is removed (black arrow) and the muscles are released. 3. The repositioned scapula is sutured to the rib and transverse processes (blue sutures). Based on Klisic (1981).

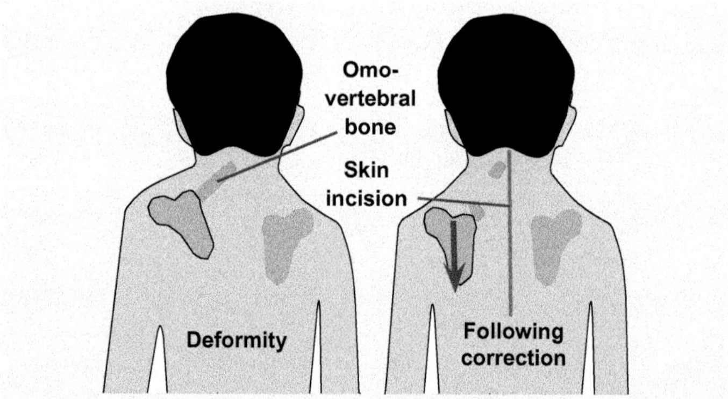

D **Woodward procedure** Through a midline incision, excise the omovertebral bone, release the soft tissue attachments, and reposition the scapula at a more distal location.

Neonatal Brachial Plexus Palsy

Neonatal palsy [A] is a traction injury to the brachial plexus that usually occurs during delivery. Risk factors include shoulder or fetal dystocia, obesity, and prolonged difficult labor. Despite improvements in obstetrical practices, the incidence of this palsy has not declined because of increases in birth weight and maternal obesity.

Natural History

Recovery depends upon severity. Overall, about half spontaneously completely resolve during the first year. Most improvement occurs in the first 3 months. Poor prognostic signs include the presence of a Horner syndrome, total plexus involvement, and a failure of return of function. Failure of recovery of elbow flexion by 3–6 months or, more accurately, failure of recovery of elbow flexion, wrist, and digital extension by 4 months correlates with a poorer prognosis. Common residual disabilities include loss of external rotation and abduction [C] and shoulder subluxation.

Evaluation

Note the resting position and spontaneous movement of each joint of the upper limb. Evaluate for Horner syndrome, and assess the range of passive and active joint motion.

Anatomic classification Severity is determined by the nature and extent of the lesion [B]. Mild lesions are stretch injuries of C5–C6. Severe injuries involve avulsion of nerve roots over multiple levels down to T1.

Residual deformity Use the modified Mallet classification. Five functions are assessed: hand-to-mouth, hand-to-neck, hand-to-spine, global abduction, and global external rotation. Each is graded from 1 to 4.

Management

Several forms of management may be useful.

Range of motion Maintain joint mobility with passive rotation of the shoulder (especially external rotation), elbow, and wrist. Instruct parents how to gently range these joints with each diaper change.

Brachial plexus exploration Evaluate those with severe injuries by CT and MRI studies. Plexus repairs are controversial, as results are unpredictable and should not compromise later reconstructive procedures. Consider early exploration in the first 3 months if Horner sign and a flail limb are present. Repairs of avulsion injuries are most uncertain and require transfers of intercostal or pectoral nerves. Direct nerve repairs are usually impossible, and sural nerve grafts to bridge a defect are needed. Reconstruction may again be considered between 4 and 6 months for less severe but persisting palsies.

Shoulder dysplasia Children with residual muscle imbalance often develop progressive glenoid hypoplasia and an increasing posterior subluxation of the humeral head. Monitor by sonography. In some, Botox (botulinum toxin) may be helpful in reducing muscle imbalance to protect the joint from increasing dysplasia. Manage by release of the insertions of the pectoralis major, latissimus dorsi, and teres major, followed by a closed reduction of the glenohumeral joint. Transfer the latissimus dorsi and the teres major to the rotator cuff.

Muscle procedures are indicated for children with disabling adduction and internal rotation contractures. The most common procedure is the Sever-L'Episcopo transfer. This procedure includes release of the pectoralis major, subscapularis, and joint capsule if contracted. The teres major and latissimus dorsi tendons are transferred from the anteromedial to the posterolateral aspect of the humerus. Axillary nerve palsy is a potential complication. This procedure is usually performed in early childhood.

Rotational humeral osteotomy is indicated for an internal rotation deformity that limits function. Delay the procedure until mid or late childhood. Rotate the humerus to provide about equal internal and external rotation. Results are predictable, correction is usually permanent, and complications are infrequent.

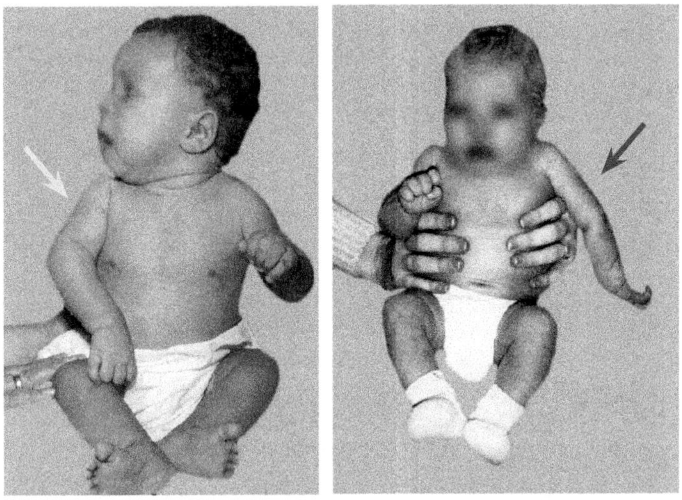

A Neonatal palsies These infants show moderate (yellow arrow) and severe (red arrow) palsies.

Type	Level	Function
I	C5 – C6	No elbow flexion
II	C5 – C7	No elbow flexion and extension
III	C5 – T1 no Horner sign	No elbow flexion or extension and poor hand function
IV	C5 – T1 Horner sign	Poor upper limb function + Horner sign

B Classification of brachial palsies Based on Narakas classification (1986).

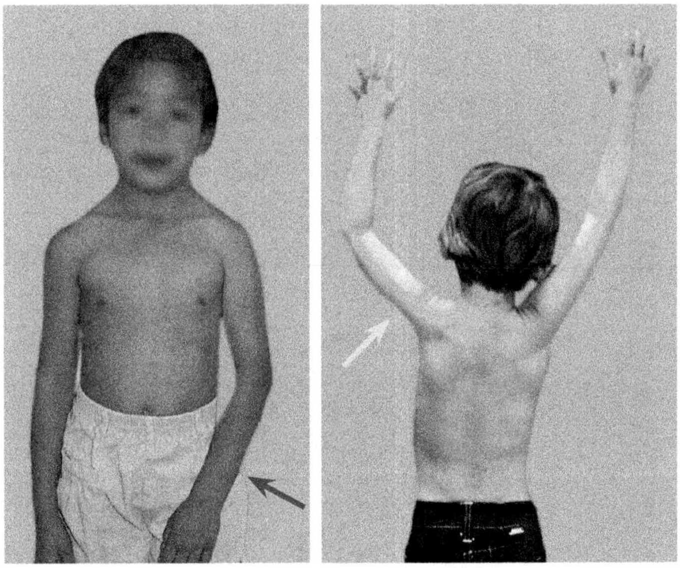

C Residual deformities in neonatal palsy Medial rotation (red arrow) and limited abduction (yellow arrow) are typical deformities that limit function.

Uncommon Upper Limb Conditions

Overuse Syndrome

Sometimes occurs in the shoulder involving the upper humeral epiphysis. The site is tender and radiographs may show widening of the physis [A].

Tumors

Lesions such as eosinophilic granuloma may cause shoulder pain [B].

Chronic Clavicular Osteomyelitis

The response of the clavicle to inflammation is unique [C], as the clavicle becomes enlarged, sclerotic, and tender, and may be confused with a malignant etiology. Evaluate with radiographs, a bone scan, biopsy, and culture. MRI and CT studies may be useful in assessing adjacent joints and soft tissue. Often the pathology is that of osteomyelitis but the culture is negative and the cause is chronic recurrent multifocal osteomyelitis (CRMO). The clavicular lesion may be solitary or one of several sites. Manage CRMO with nonsteroidal antiinflammatory drugs. Recurrence is common.

Less commonly, the cause is bacterial. Drain any abscess and treat with antibiotics. Extensive operative resection or debridement is not necessary. For both CRMO and bacterial osteomyelitis, the long-term prognosis is good.

Complex Regional Pain Syndrome

This syndrome is sometimes referred to as *reflex sympathetic dystrophy,* may occur in the upper extremities of children. Such causes as peripheral nerve injury, compression, entrapment, or tumors should be ruled out before making this diagnosis. The condition occurs most commonly in adolescent girls who complain of pain, stiffness, and limited function. Radiographs often show osteopenia, and bone scans may show normal, increased, or decreased uptake.

Poland Anomaly

This anomaly includes absence of the sternal head of the pectoralis major [D], other chest wall deformities, and usually finger or forearm abnormalities. This syndrome is part of the subclavian artery dysplasia syndrome. The disability is cosmetic, and chest-wall and breast reconstruction is often appropriate.

Cleidocranial Dysostosis

This rare congenital defect is transmitted as a dominant trait. The clavicles are so mobile that they may be approximated [E]. In others, the clavicles are simply dysplastic. Associated findings include a large head with a small face, drooping shoulders, coxa vara, narrow chest, and sometimes recurrent shoulder or elbow dislocations. Disability is minimal.

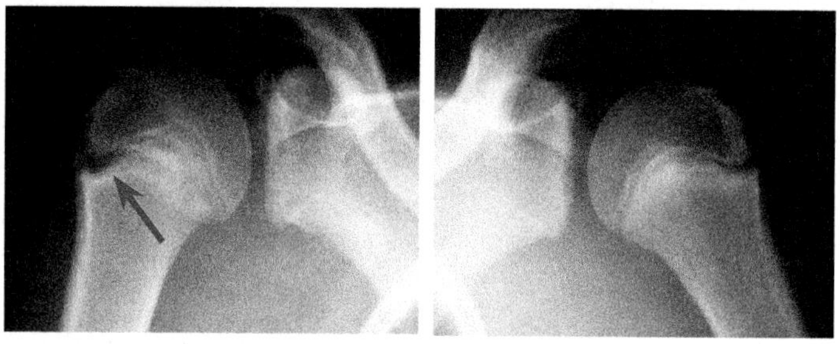

A Overuse syndrome shoulder Note the widening and sclerosis adjacent to the proximal humeral epiphysis in this baseball pitcher.

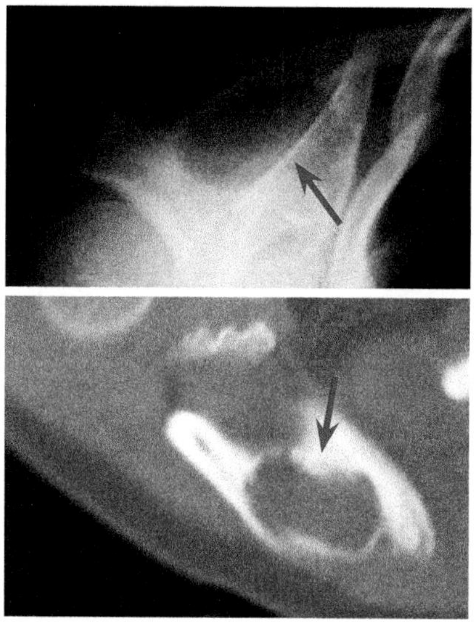

B Eosinophilic granuloma These lesions present in unusual locations such as the scapula (red arrows). They typically cause pain.

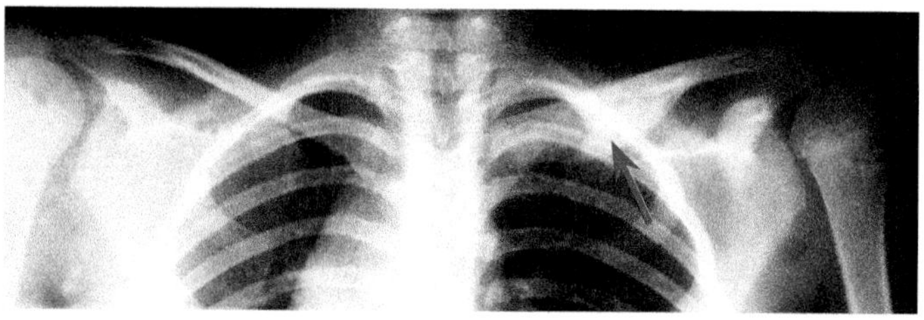

C Chronic osteomyelitis of the clavicle Note the swelling and sclerosis of the clavicle (arrow). A low-grade staphylococcal infection was found.

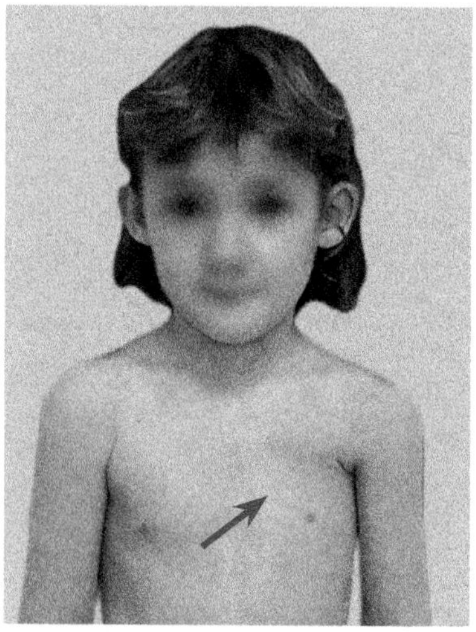

D Poland anomaly Note the deficiency in the pectoralis major muscle (arrow).

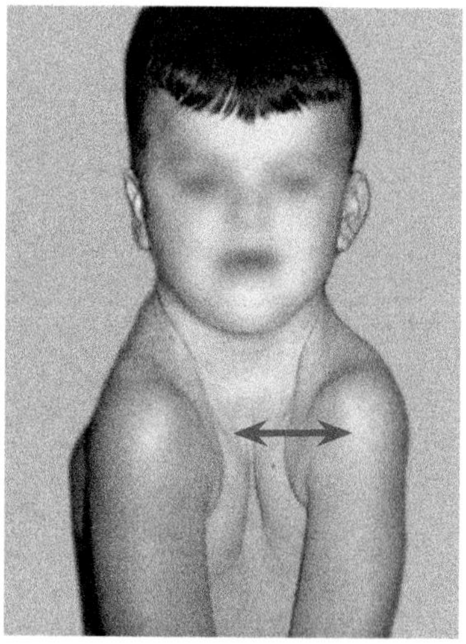

E Cleidocranial dysostosis Absent clavicles allow this boy's shoulders to narrow.

Shoulder

Congenital Pseudarthrosis of the Clavicle

Congenital pseudarthrosis of the clavicle is a rare defect of uncertain cause. The defect may be secondary to a failure of coalescence of the two ossification centers of the clavicle or to erosion of the clavicle from pulsation of the subclavian artery. The lesion practically always occurs on the right side.

Clinical features The pseudarthrosis produces a prominence over the clavicle [A], and narrowing and slight weakness of the shoulder. Radiographs show a midclavicular defect. Rarely, thoracic outlet syndrome is an associated problem. Long-term studies show little functional but some cosmetic disability.

Management Reasonable management options include either accepting or repairing the deformity [B]. Operative repair eliminates the prominence and improves shoulder symmetry but does leave a surgical scar. This scar may be minimized by positioning the incision below the clavicle, limiting its length, and utilizing a subcuticular closure technique.

Early operative correction may be performed in infancy or early childhood by resecting the sclerotic bone ends, careful dissection and preservation of the periosteal sleeve to maintain continuity, and approximating the bone ends using heavy absorbable sutures. No internal fixation or grafting is necessary. Remodeling corrects bony irregularity.

Late operative correction in mid or late childhood usually requires plate fixation and autogenous bone grafting to promote union.

Shoulder Dislocation or Subluxation

Congenital dislocations are very rare. Developmental dislocations may occur with neonatal brachial plexus palsies, or develop spontaneously during childhood. Most dislocations are traumatic.

Traumatic anterior dislocation in children usually recurs regardless of the initial treatment. Prepare the patient and parent for the probability that operative repair will be required.

Recurrent posterior dislocation may occur with minimal trauma, or it may develop spontaneously. If the deformity causes a significant disability, operative stabilization with a bone block or glenoplasty and capsulorrhaphy may be necessary.

Habitual dislocation occurs in loose-jointed older children or adolescents. One or both shoulders can voluntarily subluxate or dislocate [C]. Management is difficult. Shoulder exercise, avoidance of voluntary displacement, and counseling may be helpful. The child should be helped to find a more appropriate method of getting attention. Resolution usually occurs with time. Operative procedures may be necessary for persisting deformity, but recurrence poses a significant problem. The condition causes little long-term disability.

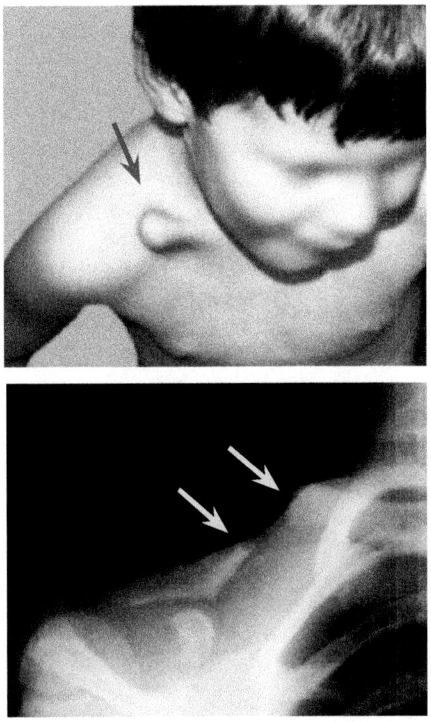

A Congenital pseudarthrosis of the clavicle This pseudarthrosis produced an unsightly lump on the shoulder (red arrow). Note the gap between the ends of the pseudarthrosis (yellow arrows). The defect was operatively corrected.

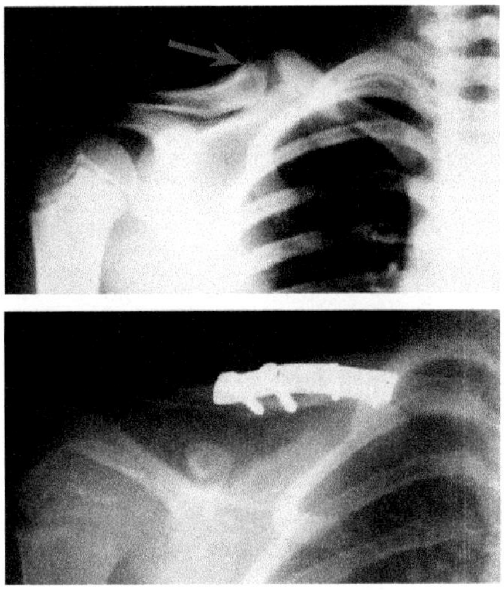

B Operative repair of congenital pseudarthrosis of the clavicle The repair involved excision, plating, and grafting.

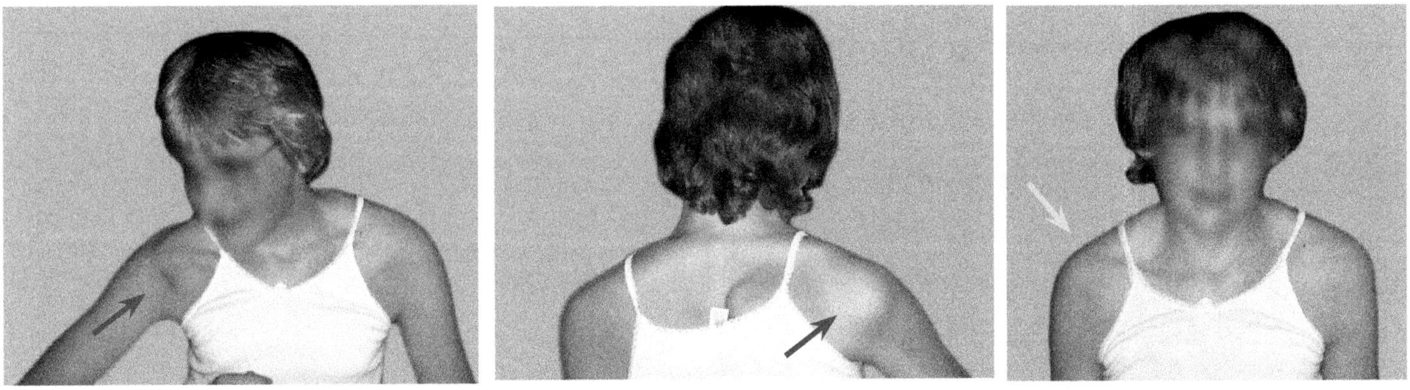

C Habitual posterior dislocation of the shoulder This girl is able to voluntarily dislocate her right shoulder (red arrows). Voluntary reduction occurs easily (yellow arrow).

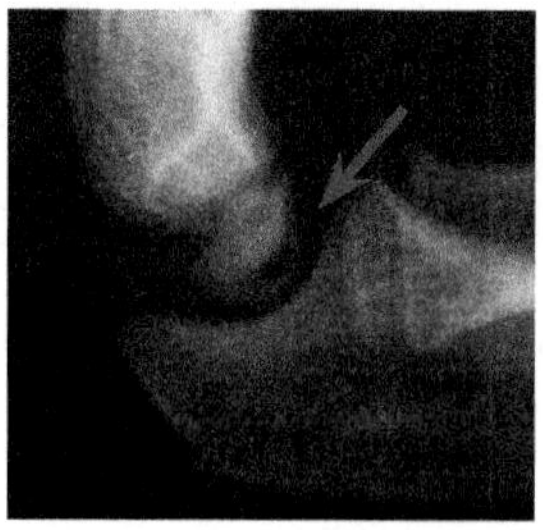

A Panner disease This 8-year-old has pain and tenderness over the capitellum.

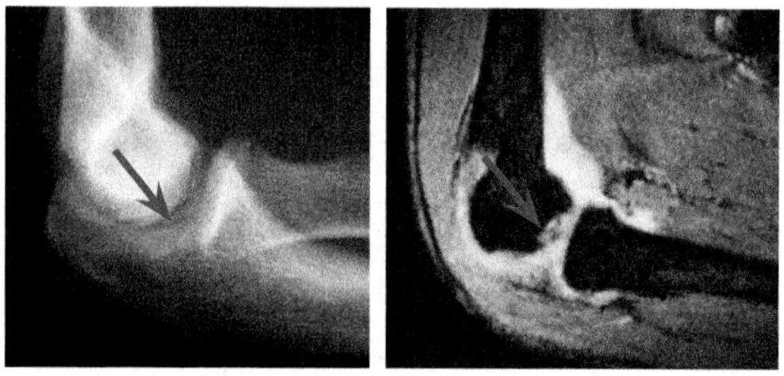

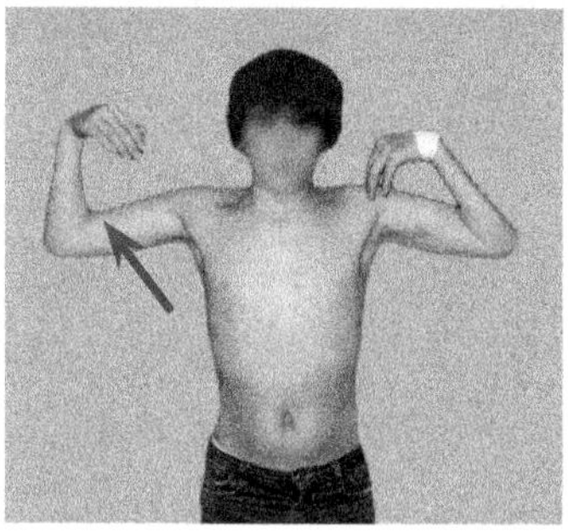

B Osteochondritis of the capitellum When this occurs in the adolescent, the problem is more serious and may cause limitation of motion. Removal of loose bodies is commonly necessary.

Elbow

Panner Disease

This is an osteochondritis of the capitellum that develops spontaneously during late childhood [A]. Clinical features include elbow pain, limitation of motion, and tenderness over the capitellum. Over a period of months, the capitellum fragments and then spontaneously reossifies. The process is usually benign, and complete recovery occurs with time. Treatment is seldom necessary.

Adolescent Capitellar Osteochondritis Dissecans

This avascular necrosis of the capitellum is often secondary to repetitive trauma and causes articular damage and often residual long-term disability [B].

Clinical findings include a history of stiffness, pain, and catching or locking. Examination usually demonstrates a decreased elbow motion and lateral tenderness. Radiography often shows loose articular fragments, flattening of the humeral capitellum, and subchondral cysts. MRI and arthroscopic examination may be helpful. Additional lesions of the radial head may be present.

Management depends upon the clinical findings. Remove loose fragments. The value of debridement and drilling is uncertain. Limit activities until healing is complete.

Prognosis Disability is common in adult life with about half showing joint stiffness and degenerative changes as well as enlargement of the radial head.

Recurrent Elbow Dislocation

Recurrent dislocations may be secondary to congenital hyperlaxity, as occurs in Ehlers-Danlos syndrome, a sequela from nonunion of a medial epicondylar fracture, or due to residual instability from a previous dislocation. Evaluate with radiography, MRI, and possibly arthroscopy. Tailor operative repair based on the pathology.

Elbow Flexion Contracture

Contractures may be congenital, as occurs with some forms of arthrogryposis, or acquired, as from burn contractures or elbow trauma with articular damage. Individualize management. Posttraumatic contractures may be improved by operative release. Release the anterior and posterior capsules, remove obstacles to motion, and provide a postoperative range of motion and splinting program.

Cubitus Varus Deformity

This deformity is usually due to a malunited supracondylar fracture. When severe, correct with a valgus osteotomy of the distal humerus [C]. The cosmetic result can be improved by translation of the distal fragment to avoid a residual lateral prominence.

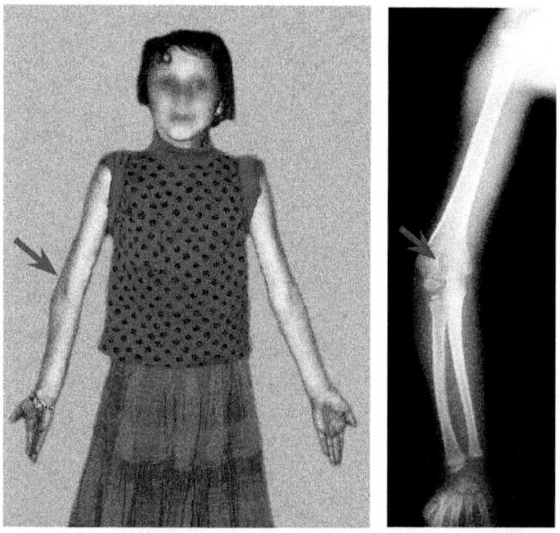

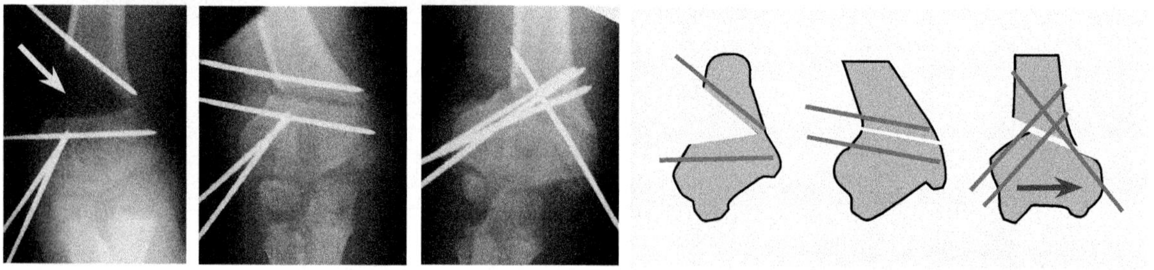

C Cubitus varus with operative correction This girl has cubitus varus (red arrows) secondary to malunion from a supracondylar fracture. This was corrected with a valgus osteotomy (yellow arrow). This correction resulted in a prominence on the lateral aspect of the elbow. This problem can be resolved by translating the distal fragment to a medial position (shown in drawing).

Forearm

Nontraumatic Radial Head Dislocation or Subluxation

Radial head dislocations may be congenital or develop gradually during infancy and childhood. Congenital dislocations are often associated with other defects.

Subluxation or dislocation limits forearm rotation and produces a palpable prominence over the displaced radial head [A]. Once dislocated, the radial head becomes progressively more prominent with growth. The radial head dislocation causes shortening of the radial side of the forearm, making the ulna more prominent at the wrist. Differentiate congenital and traumatic dislocations [B], as the management is different. Posterior dislocations are nearly always congenital. Congenital anterior dislocations are usually associated with other congenital defects.

Reduction of the nontraumatic radial head displacement has not been successful. If the radial head becomes unacceptably prominent or painful, excision may be necessary. When possible, delay excision until the end of growth. Excision may improve motion and reduce discomfort.

Radioulnar Synostosis

Radioulnar synostosis is usually congenital and occurs in the proximal forearm [C]. Synostosis may be unilateral or bilateral, complete or incomplete, and is usually an isolated defect. Synostosis rarely is familial. Sometimes synostoses develop after fractures of the proximal forearm.

Evaluation The defect may be found during infancy if a screening examination is performed. More often, the defect becomes apparent during early childhood when the loss of forearm rotation is recognized [D]. The position of forearm rotation is variable and determines the degree of disability.

Management is determined by the position of fixation. If rotation is fixed in a relatively neutral position, no treatment is required.

Rotational osteotomy is indicated for congenital synostosis if the forearm is fixed in more than about 45° of pronation or supination. Correct by a distal osteoclasis or subperiosteal osteotomy and immobilize in a cast with the forearm positioned in neutral or slight pronation.

Vascularized fat graft has been reported to be successful as an interposition tissue in preventing recurrence following resection of acquired synostosis [E]. Most other techniques of repair have been unsuccessful.

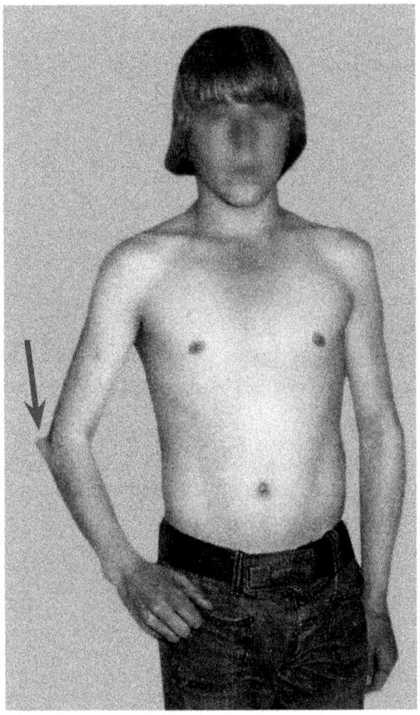

A Congenital dislocation of the radial head This 15-year-old boy has disability from this prominent radial head. The radial head was excised.

Feature	Traumatic	Congenital
Trauma history	Yes	No
Associated defects	No	Often
Direction	Anterior	Posterior
Radial head	Concave contour	Round contour
Capitellum	Normal	Convex
Ulna	Normal	Convex

B Differentiating congenital and traumatic radial head dislocation The differentiation can usually be made by the radiographic appearance of the elbow.

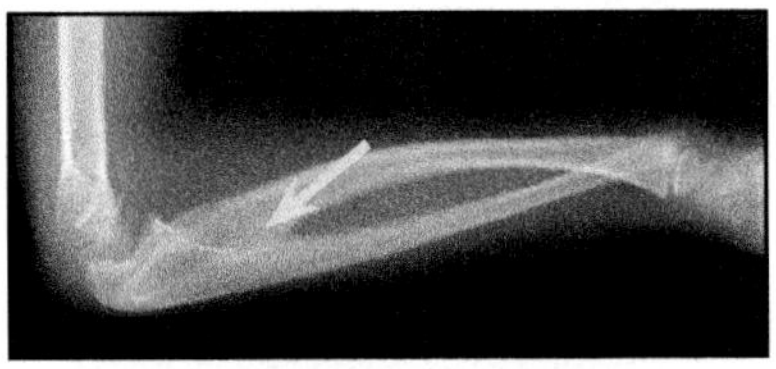

C Congenital radioulnar synostosis Note the proximal fusion and bowing of the radius.

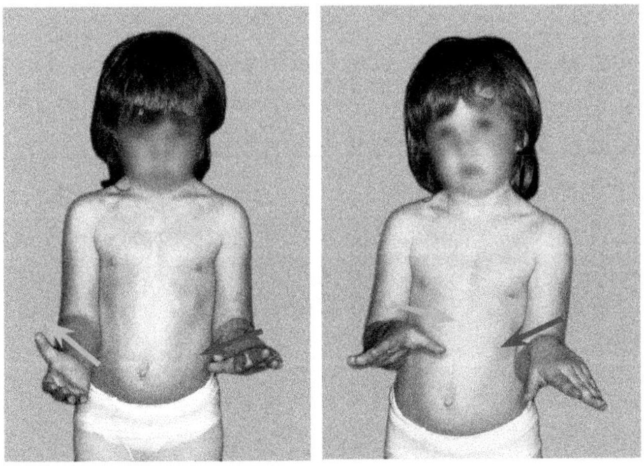

D Radioulnar synostosis limiting forearm rotation The left forearm is fixed in pronation (red arrows). The right forearm rotates freely (green arrows).

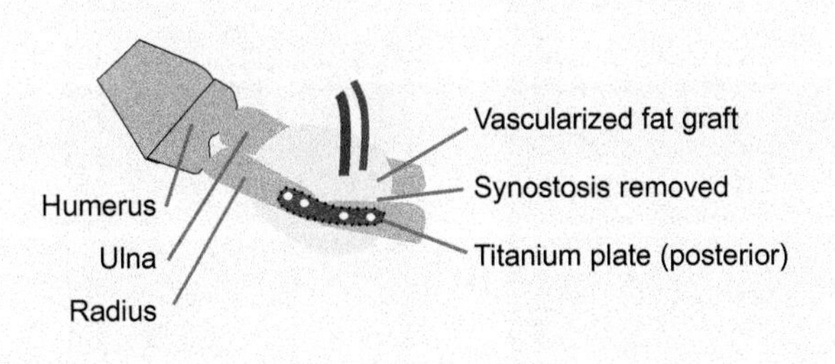

E Mobilization of radioulnar synostosis This technique utilizes a free vascularized fascio-fat graft. Based on Kanaya and Ibaraki (1998).

Primary bone tumors
Osteochondroma
Enchondroma
Osteoid osteoma
Aneurysmal bone cyst
Ewing sarcoma
Epidermoid cyst
Bone cyst
Osteoblastoma
Miscellaneous

A Primary bone hand tumors in children Based on Kozlowski et al. (1988).

Soft tissue tumors
Ganglia
Digital fibroma
Blood and lymph vessel
Giant-cell tumors tendon sheath
Tumeral calcinosis
Soft tissue chondroma
Synovial osteochondromatosis
Aggressive fibromatosis
Embryonal rhabdomyosarcoma

B Primary soft tissue hand tumors in children Based on data from Azouz et al. (1989).

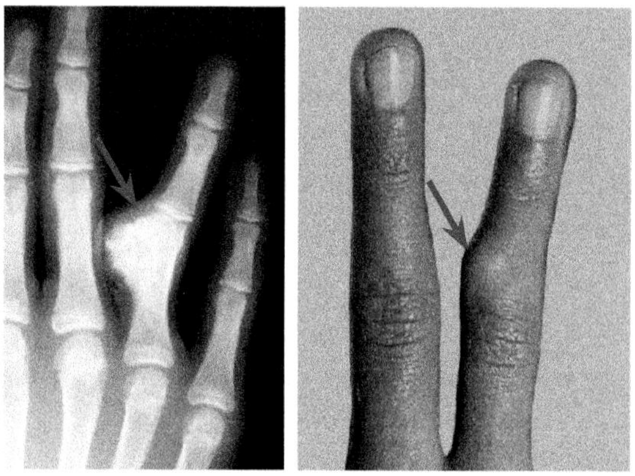

C Osteochondroma This large lesion interfered with function and was removed.

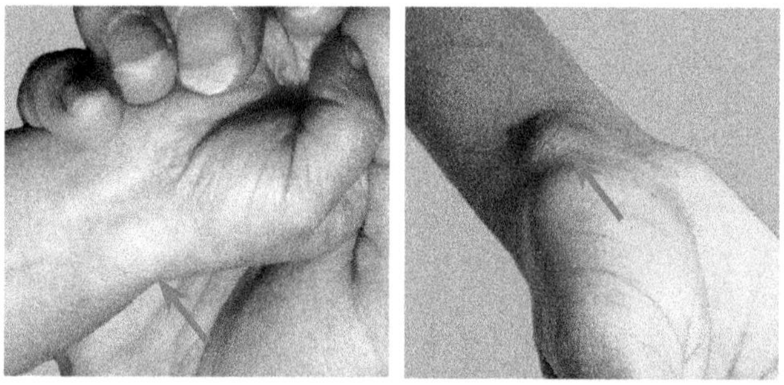

D Ganglia These are the less common volar ganglia (blue arrows).

Hand Tumors

Hand tumors in children include many different types that involve bone [A] and soft tissues [B]. Most tumors are benign and can often be followed unless they interfere with function [C] and require removal.

Wrist Ganglia

These cystic lesions arise from joints or tendon sheaths. They are most common on the dorsum of the wrist [D]. Ganglia may cause discomfort and an annoying prominence. Review wrist radiographs to rule out ligamentous injury.

Management First confirm the diagnosis by translumination or ultrasonography. One alternative is to aspirate the cyst. This confirms the diagnosis but only temporarily resolves the symptoms, as the cyst usually recurs. If the family and child are patient, allow the cyst to resolve with time. Most cysts will resolve spontaneously. Excise persistent or symptomatic cysts. Excision, especially of the volar ganglia, may be complex and involve much deeper structures than one might expect. Recurrence is common after all methods of treatment.

Osteochondromata

Multiple osteochondromata often involve the forearm, usually at the wrist [E]. Fingers and subungual areas may also be involved.

Clinical features Distal lesions of the ulna cause progressive shortening, bowing of the radius and/or ulna, increased ulnar tilt of the distal radial epiphysis, ulnar deviation of the hand, progressive ulnarward translocation of the carpus, and subluxation/dislocation of the proximal radial head.

Management is controversial. Surveys of adults suggest that the deformity causes little disability and is well accepted. Others recommend early excision of the lesions and ulnar lengthening. Be aware that operative gain in motion is usually minimal, recurrence is common, and repeated procedures are often necessary.

Enchondroma

Solitary enchondromas are common in the hand. When multiple, they may be part of the Ollier syndrome [F]. They may be treated by curettage and grafting if symptomatic.

Dysplasia Epiphysialis Hemimelica

Dysplasia epiphysialis hemimelica (DEH), or Trevor disease, is a rare developmental disorder causing asymmetrical epiphyseal cartilage overgrowth with accessory epiphyseal ossification centers [G]. This overgrowth causes angulatory deformity, shortening, and swelling. DEH of the hand is often confused with other tumors. Manage by excising the lesions and correcting secondary deformities by osteotomies. Expect recurrence as long as the child is still growing. These lesions are not premalignant.

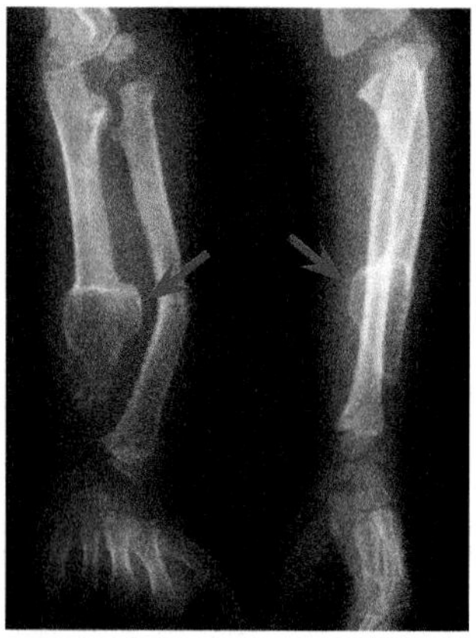

E Osteochondromata of the forearm These are the usual deformities of the typical distal ulnar lesions.

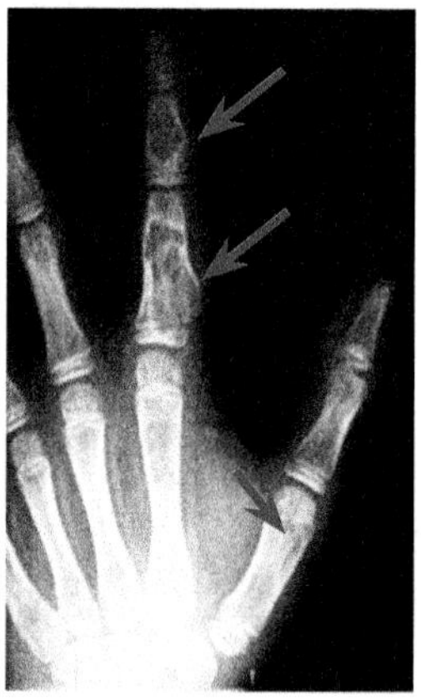

F Ollier syndrome involving the hand These lesions are often multiple, as shown (arrows).

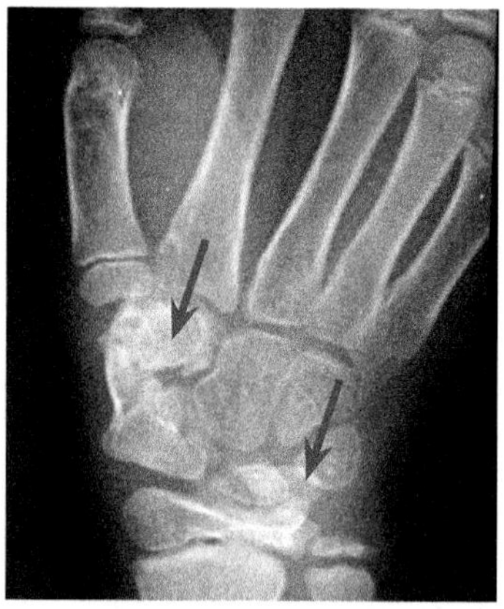

G Dysplasia epiphysialis hemimelica Intraarticular osteochondral tumors distort joint surfaces, causing deformity and swelling (red arrows). These lesions are often confused with other disorders.

Hand Infections

Hand infections [A] can be serious problems in children because they are varied, often difficult to assess, and sometimes cause long-term disability.

Penetrating Injuries

Penetrating injuries may cause infections of the soft tissues, bone, or joints of the hand. The organism is usually *Staphylococcus aureus*.

Animal Bites

Evaluate the injury by considering the animal, nature of the wound, circumstances of the attack, interval between injury and treatment, and location of the bite. Give rabies prophylaxis for bites from carnivorous wild animals, bats, and unvaccinated domestic animals. Update the child's tetanus immunizations. Administer a broad-spectrum antibiotic early. Leave deep contaminated wounds open and close secondarily.

Nail Infections

Paronychia is a localized infection of the nail base. Manage with soaks and antibiotics, or drain if suppuration has occurred [B].

Subungual infection is a more extensive infection that often requires elevation and excision of the involved portion of the nail.

Felons

Fingertip infections may be difficult to differentiate from injury. Make this differentiation by the history, examination, systemic manifestations, and laboratory studies. Operative drainage is necessary if suppuration has occurred [C].

Herpetic Hand Infections

Most herpetic hand infections occur in infants and young children who have oral lesions. Establish the diagnosis by clinical features, viral cultures, or Tzanck smears. Resolution occurs in 3–4 weeks. Antibiotic treatment is indicated only for superinfections. Cover the lesions to prevent spread.

Tenosynovitis

Inflammations or infections of tendon sheaths are not rare in children, and evaluation is more difficult due to the lack of cooperation during examination. The pattern of bursa and tendon sheaths of the hand are the same in children and adults [D]. Ultrasound imaging may be useful in establishing the level and extent of inflammation and purulence. Manage most cases first with elevation, splinting, and antibiotics for 24 hours, then reassess. If not substantially improved, consider operative drainage [E].

Dactylitis

The causes of dactylitis are numerous and include tuberculosis, sickle cell disease, congenital syphilis, psoriatic arthritis, and juvenile spondyloarthropathies. Most finger infections are due to osteomyelitis [F] or septic arthritis.

Hand Abscesses and Otopharyngeal Infections

Abscesses of the hand may be associated with inner ear or pharyngeal infections.

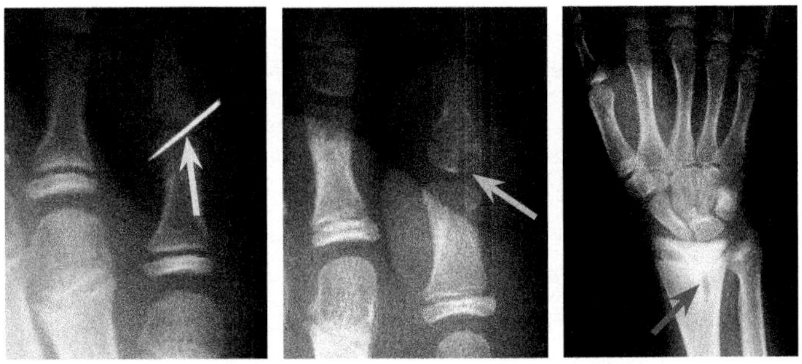

A Bacterial infections These include cellulitis from foreign body penetration (yellow arrow), osteomyelitis (orange arrow), and rarely, residual growth arrest secondary to meningococcemia (red arrow).

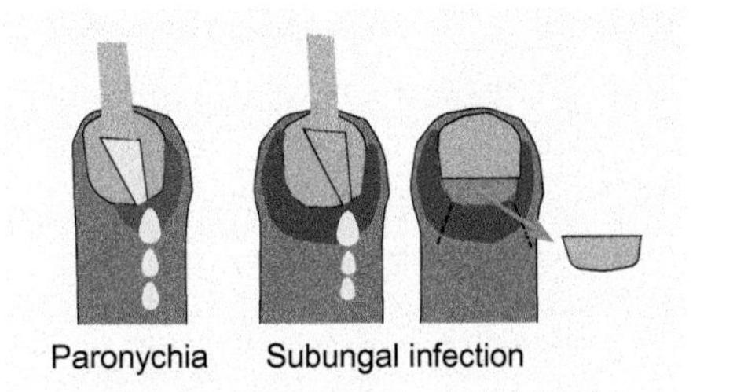

B Nail infections These may be treated with antibiotics, but if suppuration occurs, surgical drainage is required. Removal of the base of the nail may be necessary.

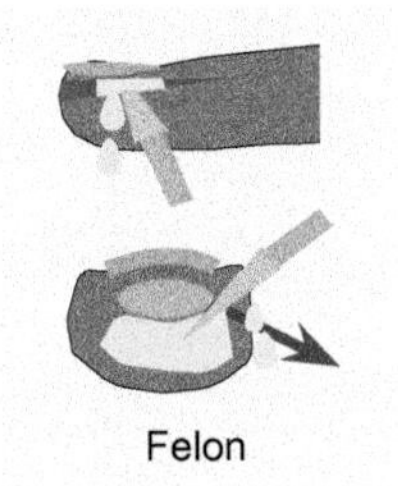

C Felon Drain pulp abscesses through a dorsolateral incision.

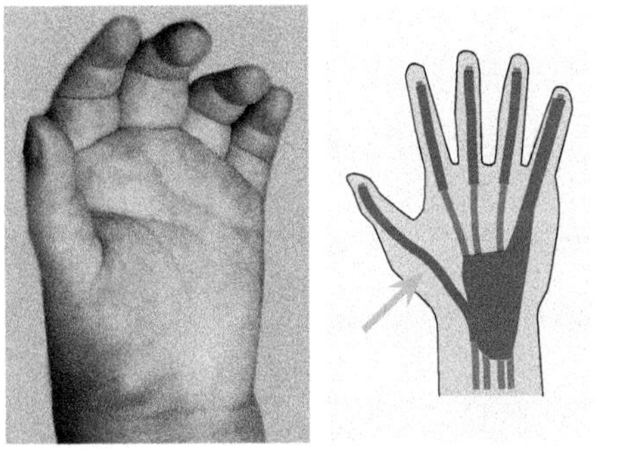

D Deep infections These may involve the tendon sheaths of the hand and cause diffuse swelling (arrow).

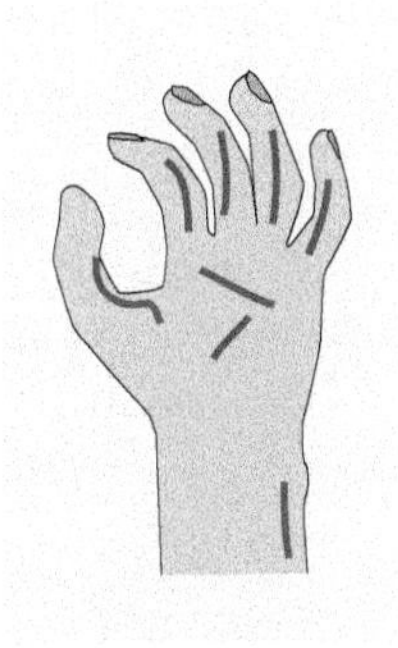

E Surgical drainage Follows the same principles as for adults.

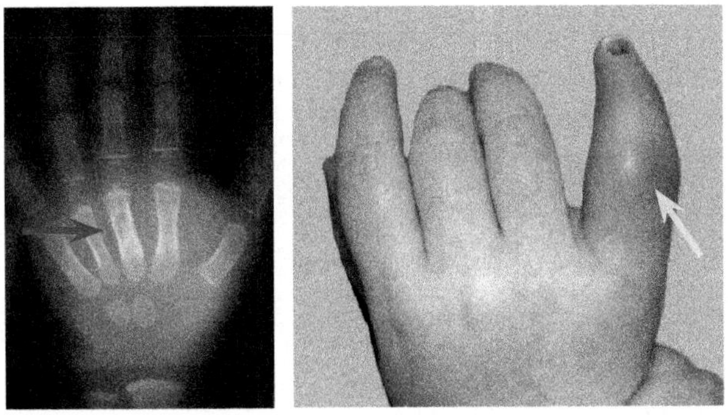

F Dactylitis Inflammation of the digits may occur from many causes. Metacarpal osteomyelitis (red arrow) or dactylitis associated with juvenile rheumatoid arthritis (yellow arrow) are common causes.

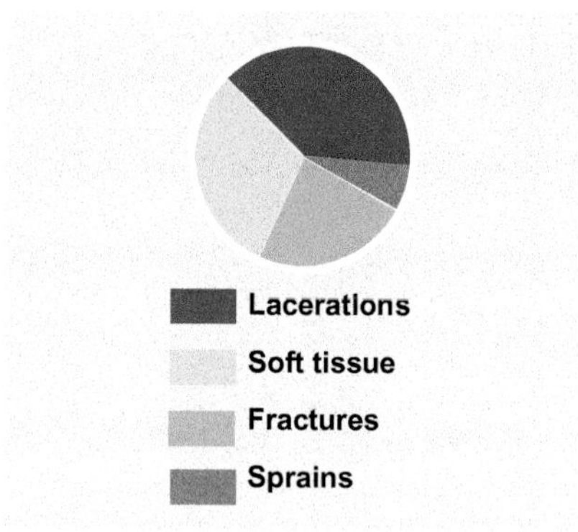

A Hand injuries in children The incidence of these injuries is shown in this pie chart. From data of Bhende et al. (1993).

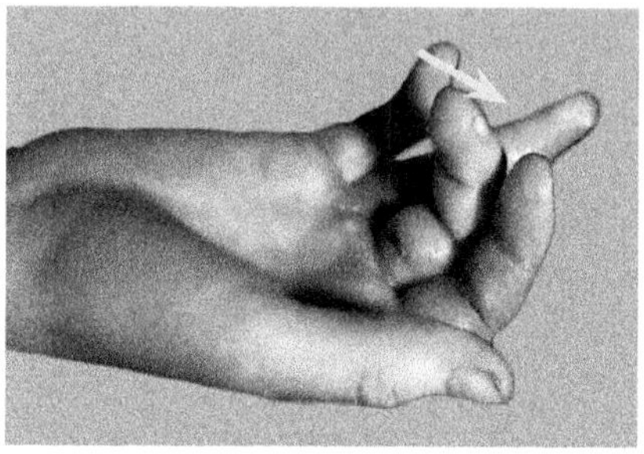

B Flexor tendon laceration Laceration of both tendons produces this characteristic finger position.

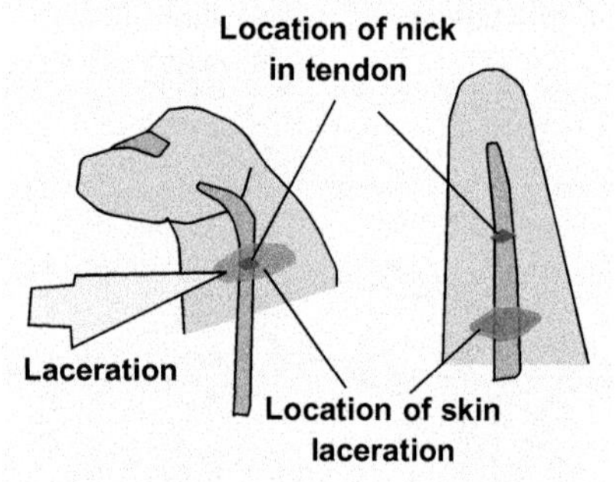

C Site of incomplete lacerations Partial tendon lacerations that occur with the finger flexed are likely to be well distal to the site of the skin laceration.

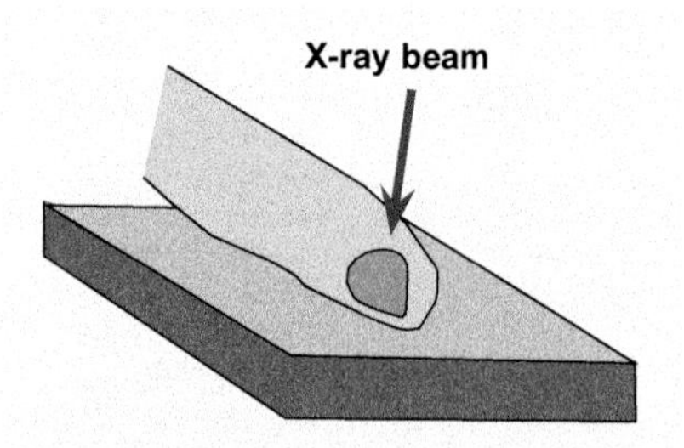

D Lateral radiographs For lateral radiographs of fingers, rotate the finger so the nail is in a vertical position.

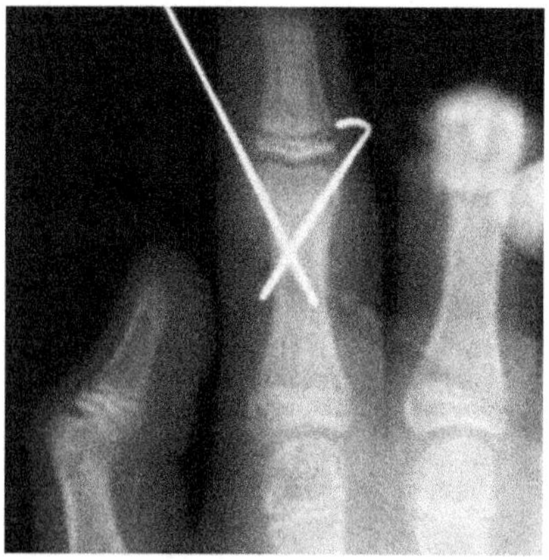

E K wire fixation Small, smooth K wires were used to fix this proximal phalangeal fracture.

Hand Injuries

Many hand injuries in children involve soft tissue [A]. Often these soft tissue injuries are most difficult to evaluate.

Principles of Acute Care

Consider these principles in management:

Emergency room evaluation is limited The distress of the child and family, ER noise, and confusion may preclude an accurate evaluation of the upset child with an injured hand. Some injuries may be apparent by simply observing the child's hand position [B]. Few conditions require emergency treatment. Dislocations and gross fracture deformity require reduction. Vascular problems need to be addressed. Consider the possibility of child abuse. Prioritize treatment of all injuries but do not neglect the hand.

Child abuse The presence of finger fractures in the infant should bring to mind the possibility of abuse. Order high-resolution radiographs of the hands and feet in suspected abuse cases as part of the skeletal survey.

Anesthesia Delay the anesthetic until the child has been fasting and the staffing situation is optimal for a repair. The skin wound may be closed and definitive treatment delayed a few days without jeopardizing the outcome.

Early reevaluation Schedule a reevaluation the next day in the clinic, where a calmer situation may make an accurate diagnosis possible.

Consider structures at risk Base this on the site of the laceration and the nature of the bleeding.

Tendon lacerations more distal If the finger is flexed during the laceration, the site of tendon laceration may be well distal to the skin lesion [C].

Arterial bleeding The presence of arterial bleeding means the possibility of a nerve injury, as the artery and nerve often lie adjacent to one another. Partial lacerations of vessels make bleeding most difficult to control.

Fracture evaluation usually requires only a careful physical examination and radiographs.

Make AP and true lateral radiographs of the individual digits to accurately determine the extent of malalignment. Use the nail as a guide in making the lateral radiograph [D].

Comparison views of the opposite hand may be helpful if the diagnosis is uncertain.

Evaluate rotational status by assessing the alignment with the finger flexed, if possible.

Fracture treatment Manage most fractures by immobilization for 3–4 weeks. Some fractures require reduction with or without fixation.

Displaced articular fractures require reduction and fixation.

Malrotated fractures require reduction because rotational deformity does not remodel.

End of growth Avoid overestimating remodeling potential at or near the end of growth.

Physeal fractures, especially crushing fractures of the distal phalanx, may show physeal arrest with deformity and shortening.

Indications for open reduction Perform open reduction on irreducible dislocations and articular fractures of the small joints. Any fracture where reduction cannot be obtained or maintained by closed means requires open reduction, and fixation if necessary.

Fixation Fix most fractures with small transcutaneous smooth K wires [E]. Consider absorbable fixation as an alternative.

Healing fractures Avoid operating on healing fractures. Allow most to heal, and correct any late residual deformity that causes a functional disability by osteotomy.

Soft Tissue Injuries

Fingertip crush injuries These injuries can occur at any age [A], but are especially common in the toddler. Protect the finger for comfort. Consider draining subungual hematoma for pain relief.

Fingertip amputation Manage these common injuries [B and C] by leaving the wound open to allow healing by secondary intention. Outcomes in children are excellent even if bone is exposed. When the tip is available, it can be sutured back in place as a composite graft and stabilized with a 25# needle.

Interphalangeal joint sprains These injuries are common, sometimes referred to as baseball fingers. Rule out fracture or tendon injury. No special treatment is necessary. Advise the child and family that these injuries resolve slowly over a period of a few months [D].

Tendon lacerations take several forms:

Complete flexor tendon lacerations alter the resting position of the hand [E], making the diagnosis simple. Repairs are based on the same principles as with adults. Immobilize for 3–4 weeks. Some improvement in motion will occur over a period of several years. Outcomes can be excellent in children.

Partial flexor tendon lacerations are more difficult to diagnose. If the tendon sheath is lacerated, a tendon injury is likely. If the tendon is lacerated while the finger is in flexion, the tendon injury will be well distal to the skin lesion once the finger is extended. Because partial tendon lacerations may become complete, unload the tendon by immobilizing the hand with the fingers and wrist in slight flexion for a period of three weeks. Repair the tendon if the laceration exceeds 30% of the cross section of the tendon.

Extensor tendon injuries Manage closed injuries by immobilizing the finger in extension for 4–6 weeks. Open lacerations require repair.

Nerve injuries Nerve transection should be repaired with magnification and microsurgical techniques. Outcomes are better in children than in adults.

Replantation Replantation should be considered unless the lost tissue is distal and severely crushed. The amputated digit should be cooled but not frozen. In children, about two-thirds of replanted digits survive. Replacement of digits with clean-cut injuries fare best. Results are better when the body weight is over about 25 pounds. Function and sensation return in most. Expect about one-third to have cold intolerance and another one-third to show fingertip atrophy. Growth is slightly retarded, but the shortening is seldom a significant problem.

Burns Most burns occur on the palm. Fortunately, most burns are minor, requiring only a nonadherent dressing. More serious burns [F] require extensive treatment, including debridement and skin grafts, and later reconstruction.

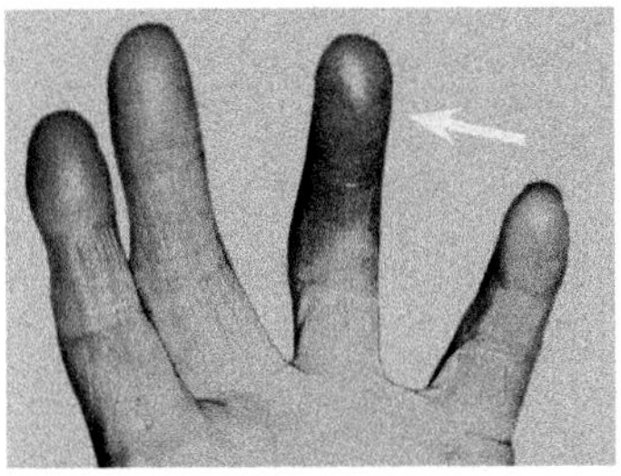

A Finger crush injury Note the extensive discoloration and swelling.

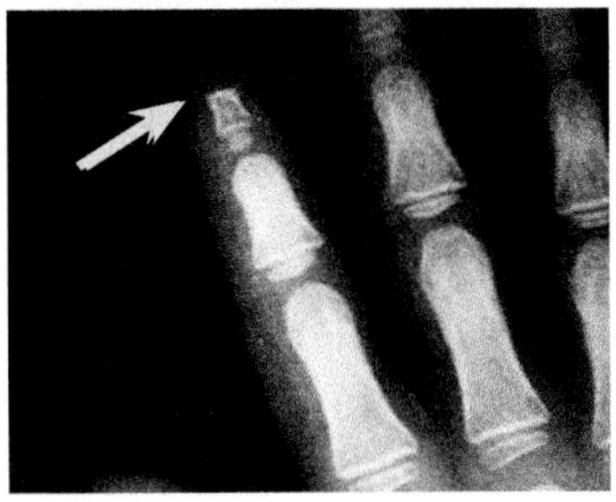

B Fingertip amputation The terminal portion of the index finger is missing.

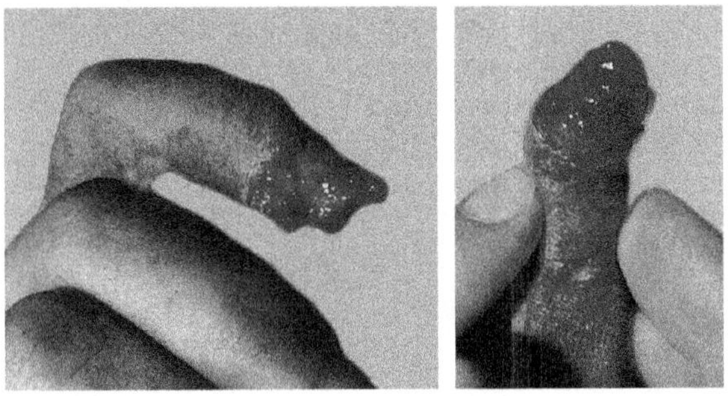

C Fingertip amputation Note the loss of the fingertip in this 12-year-old boy (orange arrows).

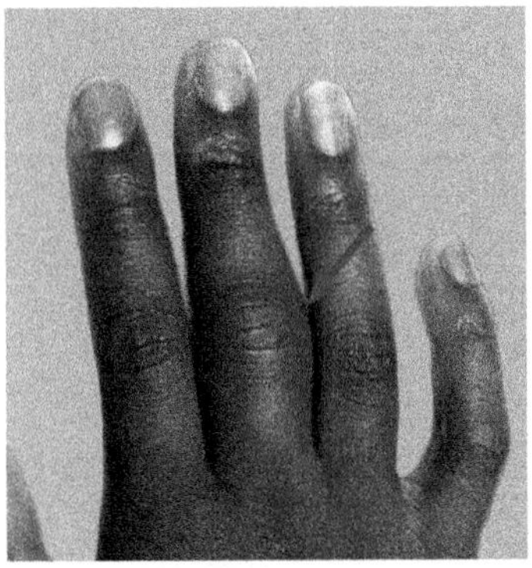

D Finger sprain This boy sustained this injury from a ball strike on the end of the finger.

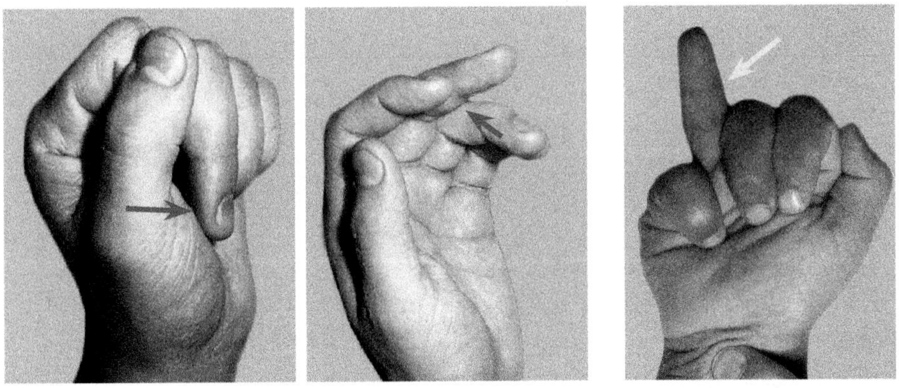

E Tendon lacerations Profundus tendon laceration of the long finger with the characteristic extension of the distal phalanx (red arrows). Laceration of both flexor tendons create a finger position that is more obvious (yellow arrow).

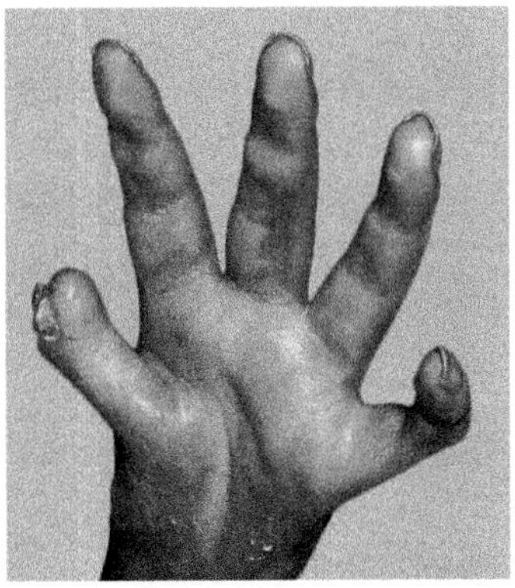

F Burned hand This severe injury resulted from an open flame.

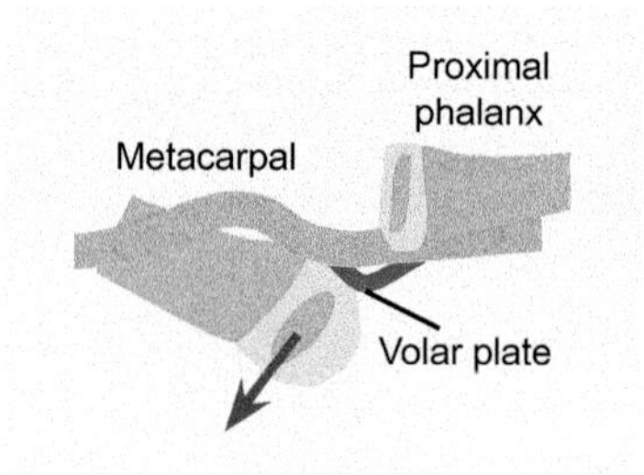

A Complex dislocation of index finger This drawing demonstrates the pathology of dorsal displacement of the volar plate and proximal phalanx. This injury requires open reduction. Based on Light and Ogden (1988).

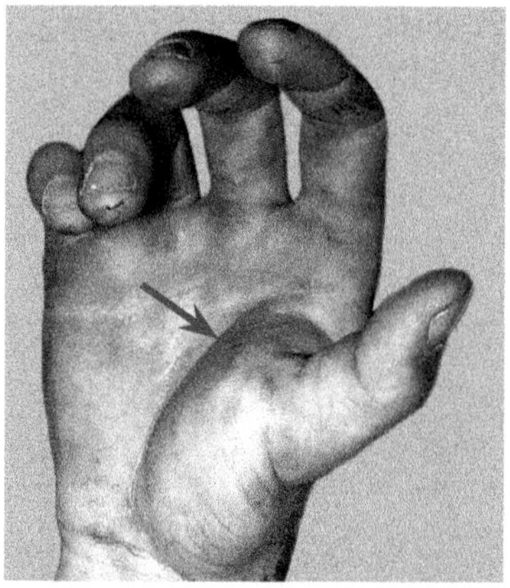

B Dislocation of thumb This dislocation was reduced by manipulation.

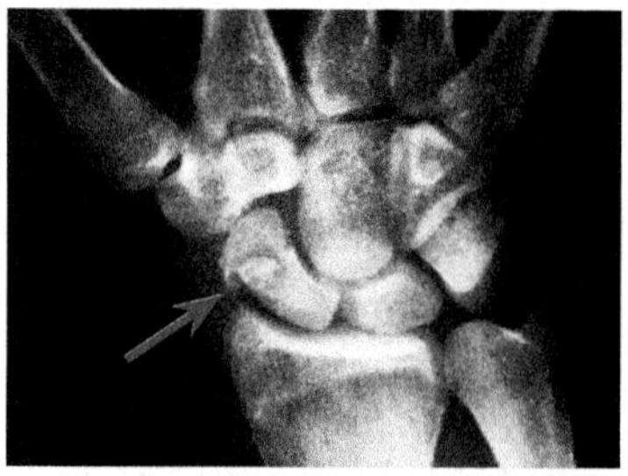

C Scaphoid fracture This 15-year-old boy sustained this injury in an auto accident.

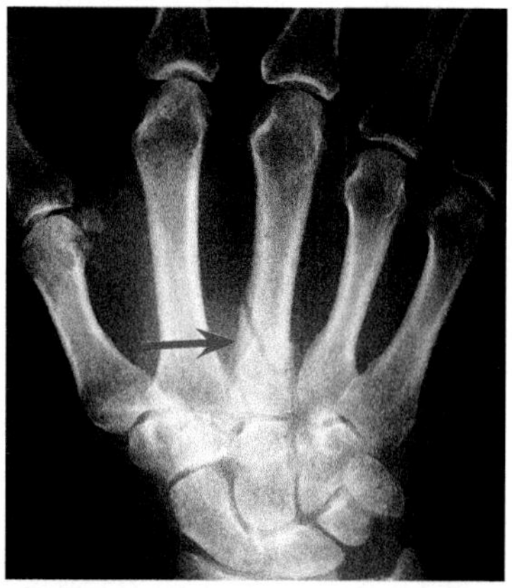

D Metacarpal diaphyseal fracture Order a true lateral radiograph of the metacarpal to be sure that this satisfactory alignment is present in the sagittal plane. This fracture (arrow) was managed in a short-arm cast with a long finger extension for 3 weeks.

Joint Injuries

Metacarpophalangeal joint dislocations These dislocations usually involve the index finger [A] or little finger. They usually require open reduction. This should be done early to avoid vascular compromise.

Thumb dislocations Manage by closed reduction [B]. Splint for 2–3 weeks, then allow active motion. Return to full activity in 6 weeks.

Interphalangeal joint dislocations Manage most with closed reduction. Open reduction may be necessary if articular fracture is present or if reduction is incomplete and the joint unstable.

Carpal Fractures

Scaphoid fractures These are relatively uncommon injuries in children. Tenderness is localized to the anatomic sniff box, and radiographs usually show the fracture. Order a scaphoid view in addition to AP and lateral studies. If the radiographs are negative, consider repeating the study in two weeks. Fractures occur in the waist in two-thirds of cases [C], and distal in one-fourth of cases. Proximal fractures are the least common. Manage acute non displaced fractures by immobilization in a thumb spica cast for about 7 weeks. Displaced fractures or nonunions are managed by operative reduction and grafting. For children with tenderness but without radiographic changes, immobilize for 2 weeks and repeat the radiographs.

Other carpal fractures The capitate, triquetrum, hamate, and trapezoid are very rare injuries in children. Most can be managed by cast immobilization.

Metacarpal Fractures

Diaphyseal fracture Obtain true lateral radiographs to assess the degree of angulation. Assess the rotational status with fingers in flexion. Correct rotational malalignment. If reduction is unstable, augment fixation with a smooth K wire. Immobilize with a finger-to-forearm cast with finger extensions in a functional position for 3 weeks [D].

Distal metacarpal fracture This fracture, also called boxer's fracture [E], is a pure flexion fracture that will remodel with spontaneous return of range of motion. If the angulation exceeds 60°, reduce with an ulnar nerve block with the finger flexed to 90°. Immobilize for about 3 weeks with the finger flexed to control rotation. Anatomically reduce and fix intraarticular fractures.

Base of thumb metacarpal fracture This fracture, also called a Bennett fracture, extends through the proximal thumb metacarpal. It requires reduction. Be certain that rotational alignment is correct. If unstable, fix with a transcutaneous K wire and supplement with a thumb spica cast.

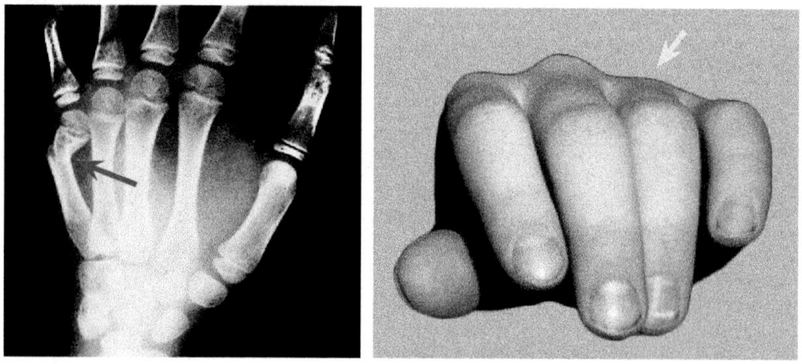

E Boxer's fracture Assess this fracture (red arrow) with a true lateral radiograph to determine the full extent of angulation. Make certain the finger is aligned in flexion. Some depression of the metatarsal contour was apparent on physical exam in another patient with a ring finger fracture (yellow arrow).

Phalangeal Fractures

Proximal phalanx epiphyseal fractures These are common injuries [A]. Assess rotation in flexion. Use internal fixation if unstable [B].

Mid and distal phalanx epiphyseal fractures These injuries are uncommon but may cause growth arrest and deformity or instability. Reduction and fixation are needed for displaced or unstable fractures [B].

Diaphyseal fractures Assess with true AP and lateral radiographs [C]. Assess for rotational alignment. Align and fix internally if unstable.

Mallet finger This may occur as a Salter-Harris Type I fracture in the young child or often a Salter-Harris Type II fracture in the adolescent [D]. Reduce in hyperextension. Stabilize in a finger splint for 6 weeks. The less common Salter-Harris Type III fractures require anatomic reduction.

Tuft fractures These fractures are commonly associated with crush injuries [E]. As these are open fractures, manage with antibiotics, soft tissue care, and follow-up. Complications include osteomyelitis and nail damage.

Growth disturbances These are rare injuries in the fingers [F]. Correct angulation by osteotomy.

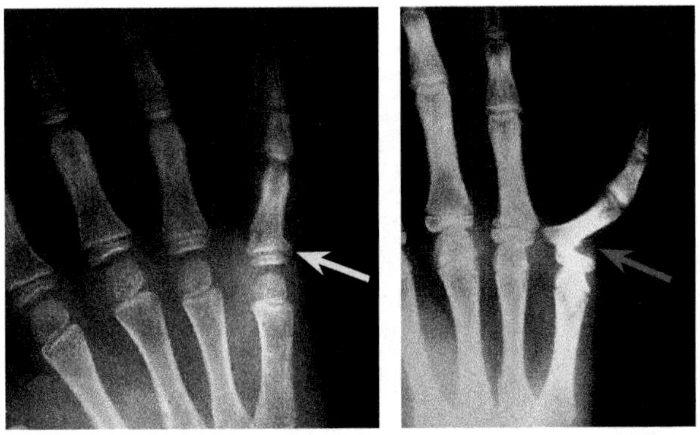

A Physeal fractures of the first phalanx These common injuries include those with minimal displacement (yellow arrow) and those with severe angulation (red arrow) that require reduction. Place an ulnar nerve block, manipulate, and pin if unstable.

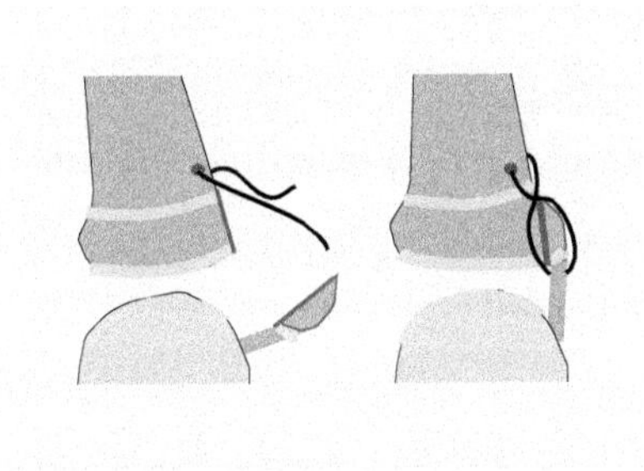

B Figure-eight tension band wiring One method of fixation of avulsed epiphyseal fractures. Based on Stahl and Jupiter (1999).

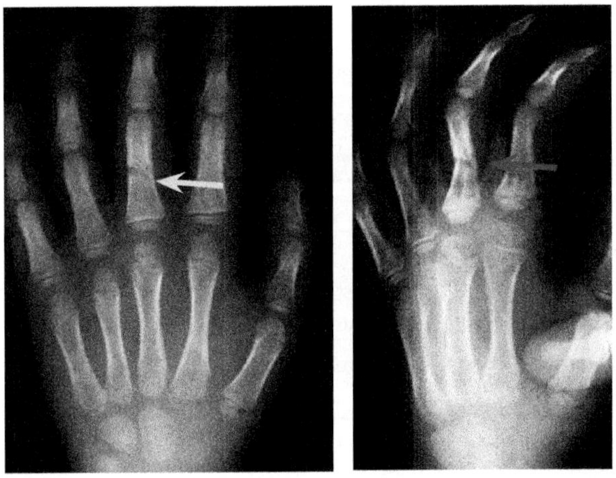

C Proximal phalangeal diaphyseal fracture. In this fracture, (yellow arrow), the degree of angulation is apparent only on the true lateral radiograph (red arrow).

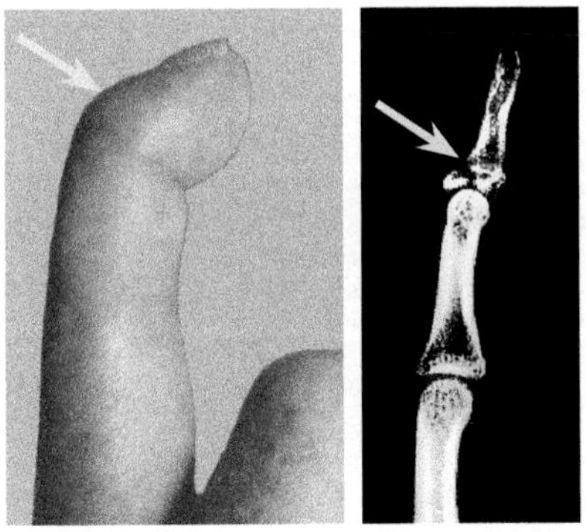

D Mallet finger This fracture requires anatomic reduction and fixation.

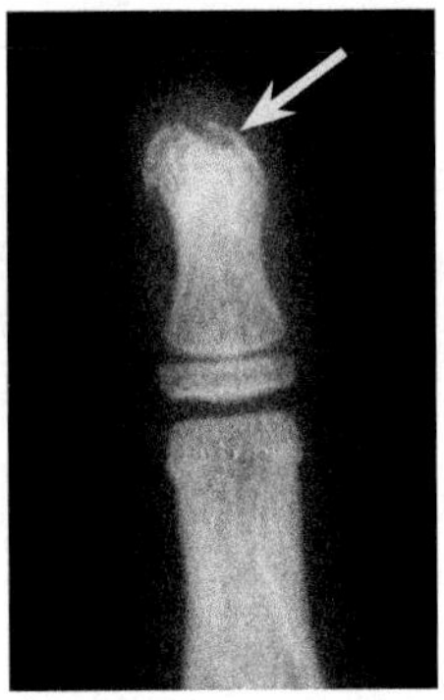

E Tuft fracture This open injury is more serious than often appreciated.

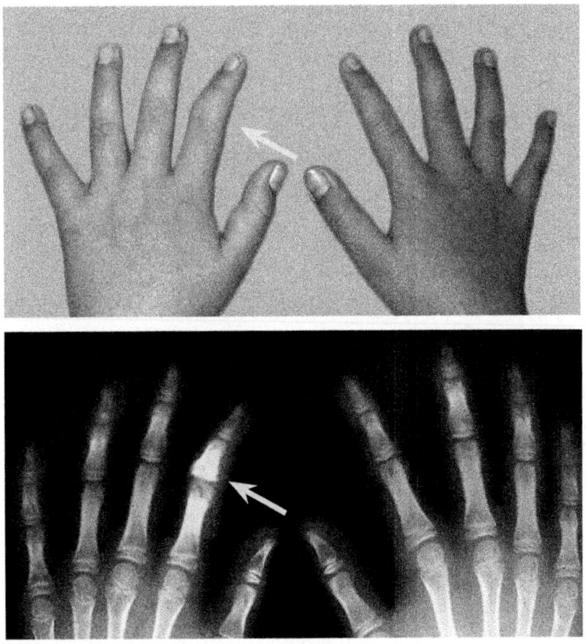

F Growth disturbance This child sustained an epiphyseal injury to the midphalanx. It was not anatomically reduced. Mild shortening and angulation were noted (arrows) 2 years later. This outcome is rare.

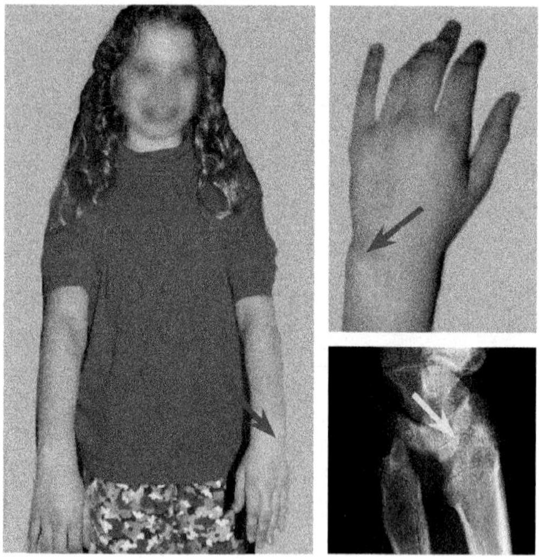

A Madelung deformity This deformity is more common in girls and produces limited wrist motion, prominence of the distal ulna (red arrows), and radial shortening (yellow arrow).

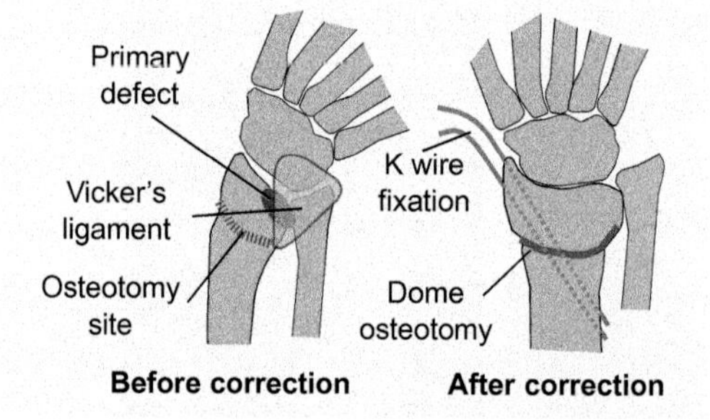

B Correction of Madelung deformity This correction is performed through a volar approach. Vicker's ligament is released and reflected distally. A dome osteotomy is performed, the deformity corrected, and the fragments fixed with 2 K wires. Based on recommendations by Ezaki (2002).

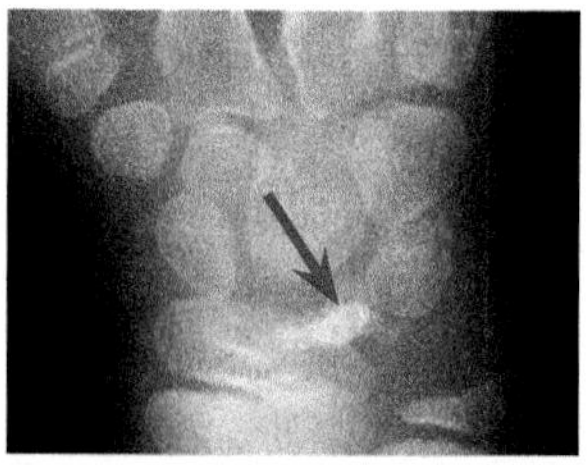

C Kienböck disease This 9-year-old gymnast developed wrist pain. The sclerosis of the lunate is obvious (arrow). This disease usually occurs in adolescence, producing pain and stiffness.

Category	Disorder
Primary	Proportionate growth pattern Accelerated growth
Secondary	Hemangiomata Lymphangioma Neurofibromatosis Fibrous dysplasia Lipomata Desmoid tumors Fibromatous hamartomas of nerve

D Classification of macrodactyly Secondary overgrowth may involve a variety of tissues.

Madelung Deformity

Madelung deformity is a defect in the volar and ulnar portion of the distal radial physis, producing a progressive deformity.

Clinical Features

The deformity, when associated with short stature, is often inherited as an autosomal dominant defect. It is associated with Leri Weil dyschondrosteosis and a Shox gene abnormality. Most cases are idiopathic. It is most common in girls, usually first noticed during mid to late childhood [A]. The physeal defect causes radial shortening and a tilt of the epiphysis. The deformity is characterized by a decreased radioulnar angle, lunate subluxation, and various degrees of dorsal subluxation of the distal ulnar. The deformity is often bilateral but asymmetrical in severity.

Management

If the deformity is mild, no treatment is necessary. For more severe deformities, operative correction is necessary to prevent progression or to correct established deformity [B].

During growth Consider either closure of the distal ulnar growth plate and resection and fat interposition of the radial physeal bridge or closure of both the radial and ulnar growth plates to prevent increasing deformity.

End of growth Consider a corrective osteotomy of the radius and shortening of the ulna. This often improves grip strength, increases range of motion, and reduces pain.

Kienböck Disease

Osteochondritis of the lunate is rare in children. It is thought to be due to repeated minor trauma together with negative ulnar variance (short ulna). The condition sometimes occurs in children with tension athetosis type of cerebral palsy, which combines increased tone and excessive motion. Clinical findings include localized pain and tenderness over the lunate, and typical radiographic features [C]. Manage with rest, NSAIDs, and time. Rarely, symptoms may persist, making operative treatment to reduce stress on the lunate necessary.

Macrodactyly

Overgrowth of the hand [E] may be secondary to a variety of disorders [D] or occur as a primary problem. In primary macrodactyly, tissues are normal but growth is accelerated. In secondary macrodactyly, tissues are abnormal. In some, the tissue type is obvious, as with hemangiomata. In others, MRI and biopsies may be required to establish the diagnosis. Management is often difficult. Operative procedures include soft tissue resections, epiphysiodesis, shortening osteotomies, or bone resections, and sometimes amputation of digits. Recurrence is distressingly frequent.

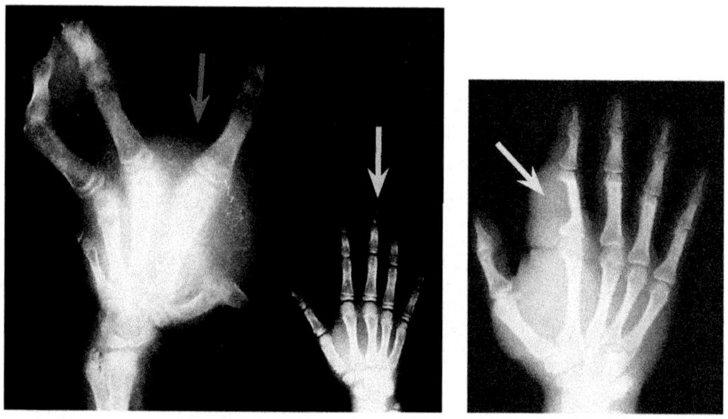

E Hand hypertrophy Note the massive hypertrophy of the left hand (red arrow) as compared with the normal hand (green arrow). In another child, hypertrophy is associated with neural hamartoma, producing soft tissue hyperplasia (yellow arrow).

Chronic Arthritis

Pauciarticular arthritis, seropositive rheumatoid arthritis, autoimmune disorders, leukemia, sickle cell disease, child abuse, and infections are causes of joint problems in the child's hand. Juvenile chronic arthritis is most common.

Management Principles

Several principles guide management.

Accurate diagnosis Make an accurate diagnosis and refer the patient to a rheumatologist. New disease-modifying agents are potent and require close, experienced medical supervision.

Family education Explaining management principles with the family improves compliance and reduces anxiety. Describe the basic features of joint anatomy, including the synovium. Describe the disease, the synovial inflammation [A], and the effect of inflamed synovium on the joint and muscle function and how it can cause joint damage.

Role of splinting Prescribe resting splints when the disease is active and joints are swollen and hot.

Therapy Exercises are important but should only be performed within the range of comfort. *Pain is not gain*—it is a warning sign.

Intraarticular steroids Inject steroids into the small joints of the wrist and hand when medical treatment fails to reduce the inflammation. Improvement is often dramatic and long lasting. Single injections are usually adequate. Apply gentle traction to open and find the joint. Inject triamcinolone, or another depot form of steroid, into the joint using a 26-gauge 3/8-inch needle [B].

Surgery

Operative procedures are much less commonly required because of the increased effectiveness of systemic care and steroid injections. If deformity develops, surgery may be required.

Synovectomy Medical care has largely replaced synovectomy for both the wrist and fingers. Rarely, when repeated injections fail to reduce the synovitis, synovectomy may be indicated.

Wrist Fusion or resection arthroplasty are effective. Avoid joint replacements in the child. Surgery provides pain relief, deformity correction, and preservation of muscle function.

Arthrodesis is indicated for severe malalignment about the wrist [C]. The procedure is reliable when performed in late childhood or adolescence. Small implants may be needed.

Carpal resection may be necessary to align the wrist before fusion.

Darrach resection arthroplasty of the distal radioulnar joint is effective and often combined with wrist fusion procedures.

Metacarpal phalangeal joints Deformity is now seldom severe enough to require treatment. If severe, fusion of the joint may be helpful if the IP joint motion is adequate. Implant arthroplasty may be appropriate in some cases.

Fingers Arthritis in children causes stiff joints. Deformities severe enough to require operative correction are uncommon. Problems include swan neck [D] and boutonnière deformities. Boutonnière deformities are most likely to cause disability.

Boutonnière deformities, or flexion contractures of the PIP joints, cause little functional problems when less than about 60°. If the deformity is more severe and limits function, fusion of the IP joint in about 30° of flexion may be helpful.

Thumb deformity usually consists of fixed flexion of the MCP and adduction contracture. If disabling, MCP arthrodesis combined with a adductor release is effective treatment. If only the IP joint is involved and symptomatic, consider arthrodesing this joint.

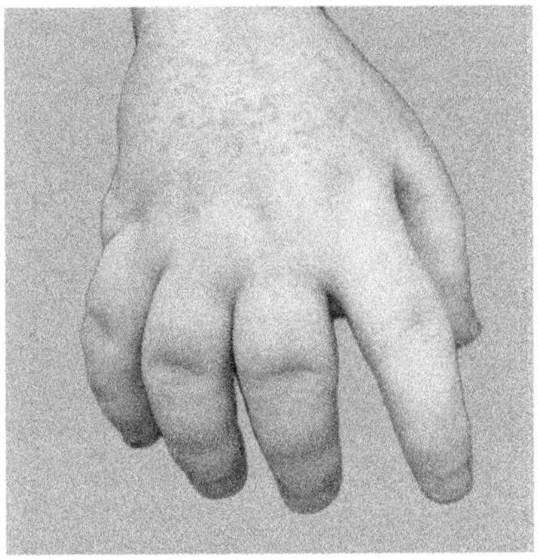

A Hand deformities in JIA Deformity may be due to synovitis or muscle imbalance. Most may be prevented by systemic and local treatment.

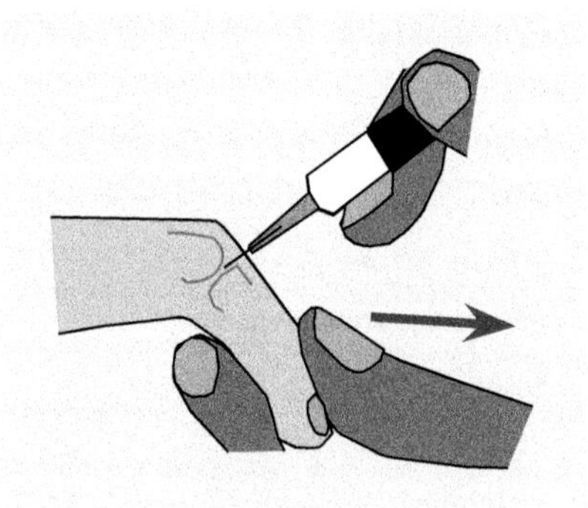

B Steroid injection Inject small joints of the fingers by first applying traction (red arrow) to open the joint and then injecting the steroid using a small needle.

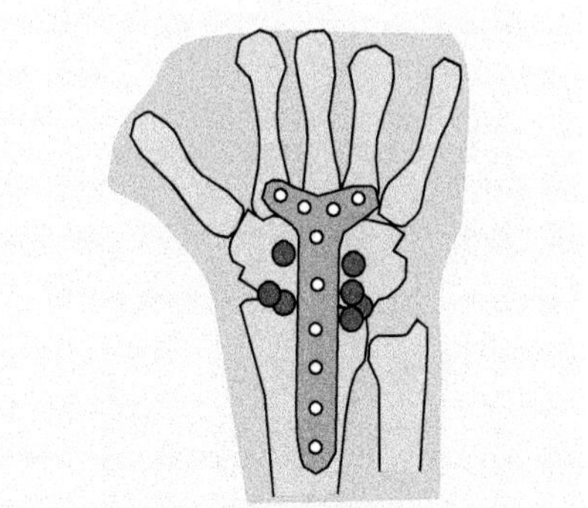

C Arthrodesis Deformity is corrected, bone graft applied (brown), and a plate is placed to hold position during healing.

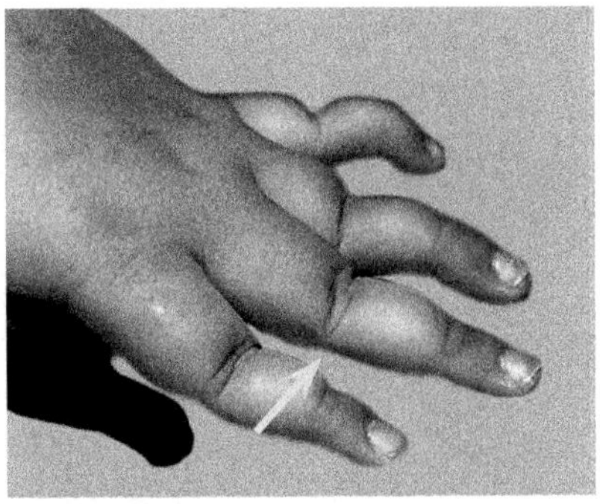

D Swan neck deformity This deformity is uncommon and seldom severe enough to require treatment.

	Ulnar Dysplasia	Radial Dysplasia
Prevalence	Rare	Uncommon
Visceral anomalies	Rare	Common
Musculoskeletal anomalies	Occasional	Occasional
Proximal limb anomalies	Occasional	Occasional
Total absence of bone	Uncommon	Common
Elbow	Unstable	Stable
Wrist	Stable	Unstable
Hand anomalies	Variable, severe	Thumb may be absent

A Comparison of ulnar and radial dysplasia Although both conditions involve forearm bones, they are very different.

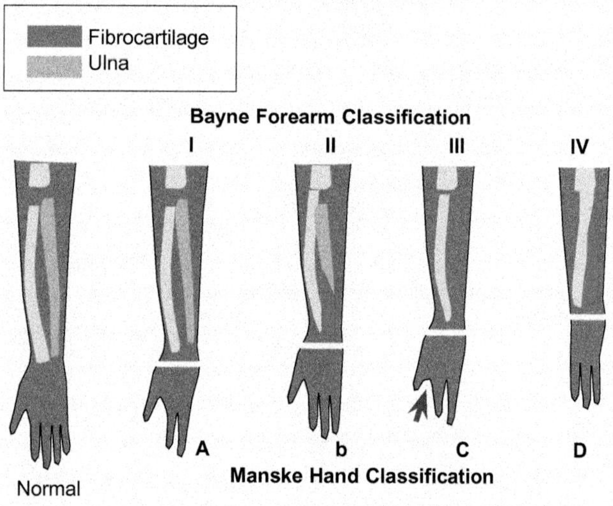

B Classifications of ulnar dysplasia Note that the Bayne classifies the forearm bony dysplasia, and the Manske classifies the hand dysplasias. The classifications are often used together to describe the dysplasia.

Hand Deformities

Radial and ulnar dysplasia show major differences [A].

Ulnar Dysplasia

Ulnar dysplasia includes an absence or hypoplasia of the ulna that is usually associated with anomalies of the hand. The deformity is often classified by the Bayne classification for the ulnar deficiency and the Manske classification for the hand anomalies [B]. Often the radius is shortened and bowed and the radius may be fused with the humerus. Finger deformities are common. Look for associated skeletal problems.

Management Most improvement can be made by focusing on the hand.

Wrist If ulnar deviation exceeds about 30°, consider resection of the ulnar analogue and corrective osteotomy in Bayne II and IV forearms.

Hand Deepening on the thumb-index web space and rotational osteotomies of the metacarpals may improve hand function.

Forearm and elbow Consider creating a one bone forearm in Bayne II or osteotomies to improve elbow position in Bayne IV.

Cleft Hand Deformity

Cleft hands include a spectrum of deformities that are inherited, usually bilateral, and usually involve the feet. Function is good but appearance may be distressing [C]. The clefts may be surgically reduced to improve appearance while preserving function.

Radial Dysplasia

Radial club hand includes an absence or hypoplasia of the radius and associated musculature, producing a radial deviation of the hand [D]. The deficiency may be isolated or part of a generalized skeletal dysplasia or syndrome. Look for other problems by performing a screening evaluation, giving special attention to the hematologic, urinary, and cardiac systems as well as the spine.

Management depends upon the severity of the deformity and the presence of associated defects.

Mild hypoplasia may not require any treatment.

Complete aplasia Stretch out the soft tissue contracture with casts and splints during the first year. This may be followed by operative correction.

Operative correction may include soft tissue release or lengthening and centralization of carpals on the ulna.

Follow-up throughout infancy and childhood shows that recurrence of the deformity is likely.

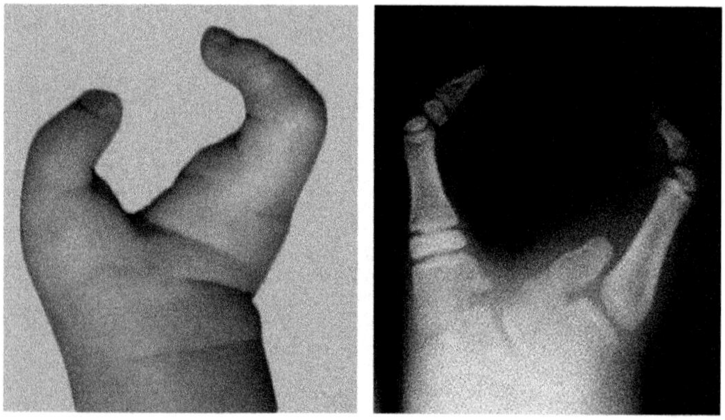

C Cleft hand deformity The child also had deformities of the feet. The condition was familial.

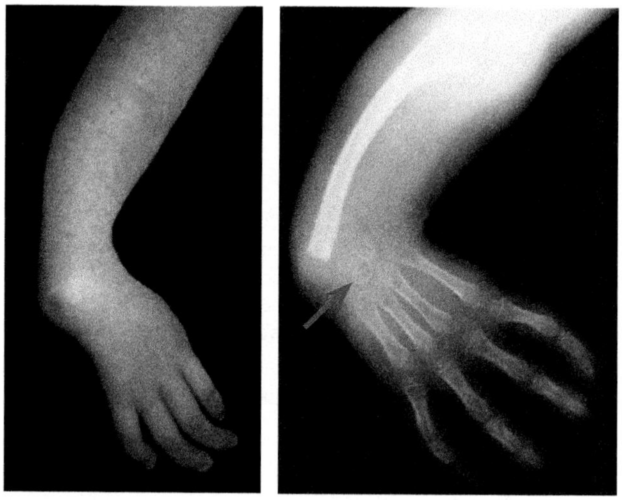

D Radial dysplasia This deformity causes a serious cosmetic as well as functional disability. The hand shifts to the radial side (arrow).

Thumb Deformities

Thumb Hypoplasia

Thumb hypoplasia is usually part of the radial dysplasia spectrum and accounts for about 5% of congenital hand anomalies. Management is determined by the type of dysplasia [A] and associated syndromes or anomalies.

Aplasia is treated by index pollicization.

Floating thumb, or *pouce flottant*, is usually managed by amputation and index pollicization late in the first year.

Short thumb may be associated with a variety of syndromes. If the shortening is excessive and interferes with function, consider performing a lengthening osteotomy, or deepening the web space. Tailor correction to facilitate function.

Adducted–abducted thumb deformities with shortening require tailored reconstruction that includes both soft tissue and bony reconstruction.

Congenital Clasped Thumb

This deformity is part of the spectrum that often includes a congenital absence of the extensor tendon combined with intrinsic tightness of the thumb. Correct between 3 and 6 months of age with serial casting. If this fails, operative reconstruction is necessary.

Thumb Duplication

Thumb duplications are radial or preaxial and are common. Thumb polydactyly can also be further classified by the pattern of deformity into seven types [B and C]. Type IV is most common. Types I–VI are usually unilateral, sporatic, and most common in boys. Type VII may be inherited, is often bilateral, and may be associated with other abnormalities. Treatment involves reconstruction of all bony and soft tissue elements, to preserve a stable, well-aligned, and functional thumb.

Trigger Thumb

Trigger thumbs are secondary to an acquired nodular enlargement of a segment of the flexor tendon [D]. Large nodules usually become wedged at the pulley, causing the digit to lock in flexion. Smaller nodules pass through the pulley, producing a snapping sensation. Initially manage by observation. Consider release if the problem is bilateral, extension is locked or improvement fails to occur with time. Operative release of the flexor A1 pulley restoring free movement of the thumb.

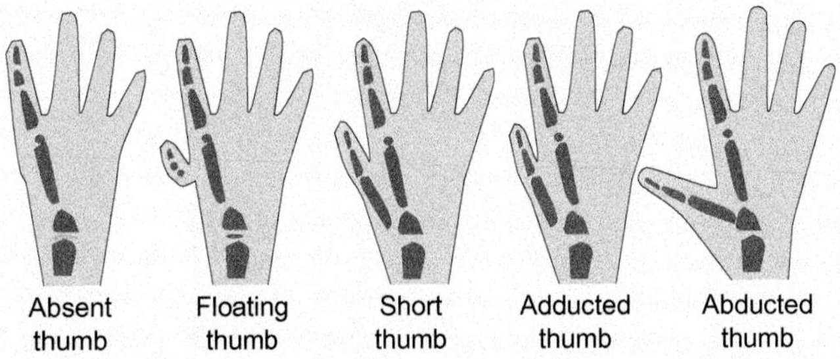

A Thumb deformities These deformities may be classified into very general patterns.

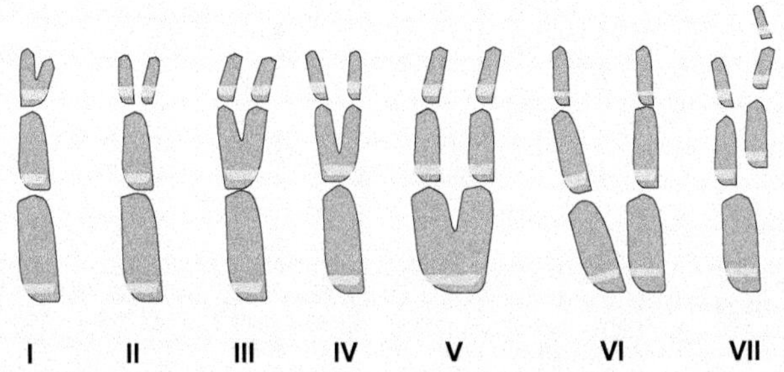

B Thumb polydactyly Wassel classification. From Gallant and Bora (1996).

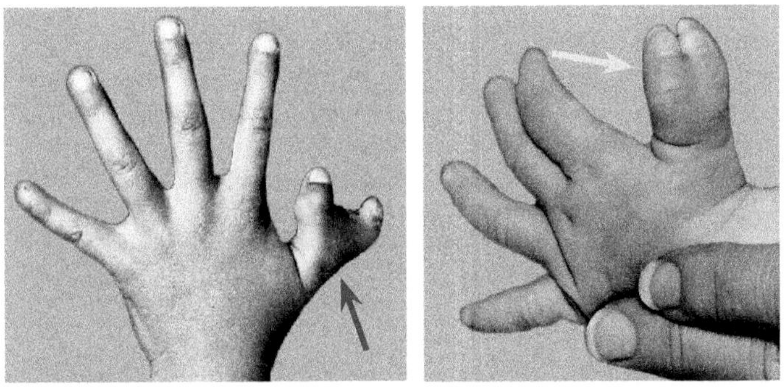

C Thumb duplication. Type IV (red arrow) and type III (yellow arrow) are shown.

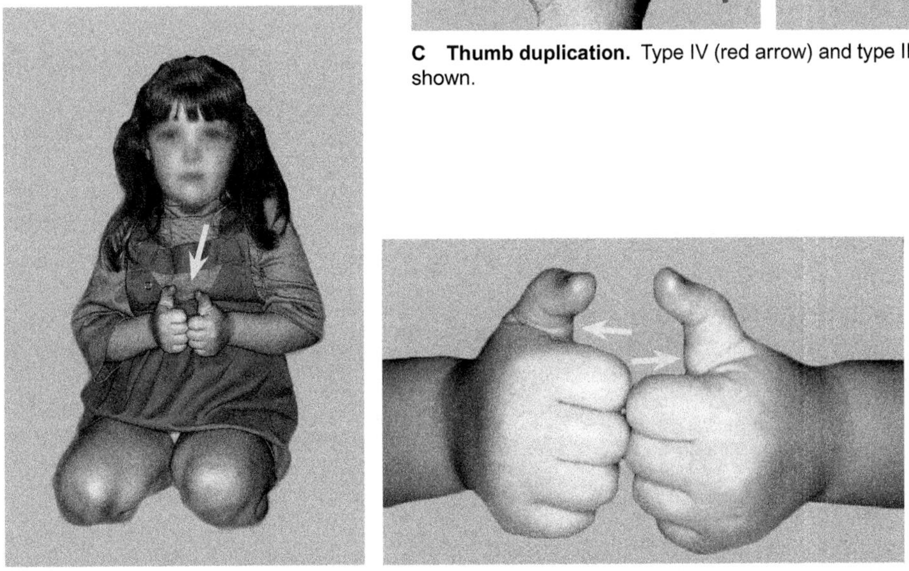

D Trigger thumbs Bilateral trigger thumbs locked in flexion. Operative release of the A1 pulleys allowed free movement of the tendon and extension of the thumbs.

Finger Deformities

Finger deformities can be grouped into general categories [A]. Finger deformities are often genetic, and the genes responsible for preaxial polydactyly, cleft hand and foot malformations, synpolydactyly, and types of brachydactyly have recently been identified.

Hypoplasia of the Digits

Types of hypoplasia of the digits are numerous and varied. This makes it necessary to individualize management with the objective of improving function, sensibility, and mobility. Digital reconstruction by toe-to-finger transplants or elongation of digits are examples of extraordinary reconstructive procedures.

Polydactyly

Polydactyly, or *duplication,* a failure in segmentation, accounts for 5–10% of all hand deformities. Polydactyly can be classified by the tissue involved [B and C] or by location. The locations include radial, central, and ulnar categories [D]. Central and ulnar polydactylies involve the fingers. Remove or ligate simple duplications in early infancy. Delay correction of complex duplications until late in the first year.

Syndactyly

Syndactyly [E] is a common deformity. The syndactyly may be complete or partial. It is described as *simple* if only the soft tissues are involved, or *complex* if bones are fused [F]. Syndactyly is most common between the middle and ring fingers. Syndactyly is seen in Apert, constriction band, and Poland syndromes. Correct by operative separation and full-thickness skin grafting [A, next page]. This correction is technically demanding, and revision rates are high if attention to detail is not meticulous.

Trigger Fingers

Trigger fingers are usually due to congenital abnormalities of the flexor mechanism. Surgical release may be necessary.

Deformity	Description
Hypoplasia	Small digits
Polydactyly	Too many digits
Syndactyly	Fusion of digits
Finger deformities	
Camptodactyly	Flexion contracture of the IP joint
Clinodactyly	Radial or ulnar angulation
Delta phalanx	Interposed delta-shaped ossicle
Kirner deformity	Progressive palmar, radial deviation of the distal phalanx of the little finger

A Classification of finger deformities These deformities occur in the transverse or sagittal planes.

Category	Classification
Simple	Soft tissue only
Complex	Bony duplications
Complete	Entire digit with metacarpals

B Classification of duplications A simple method of classification is described.

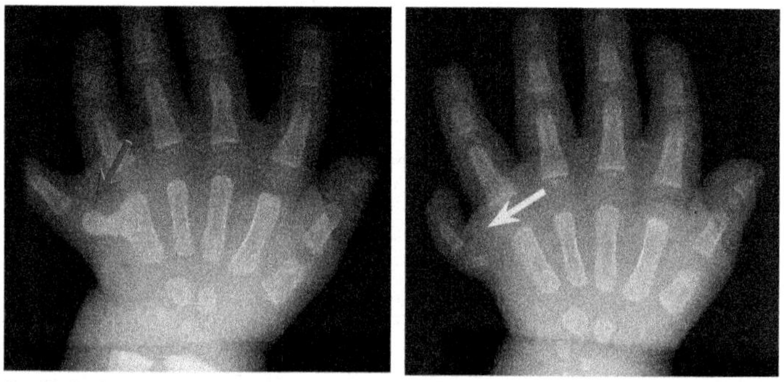

C Polydactyly In contrast with simple polydactyly (yellow arrow), complex polydactyly (red arrow) is much more difficult to repair.

	Radial	Central	Ulnar
Location	Preaxial	Central	Postaxial
Prevalence	Common	Rare	Common
Inheritance	None	Dominant	Dominant
Associated conditions	Often	Often with syndactyly, foot anomalies	Uncommon
Surgical repair	Complex	Very difficult	Less complex

D Polydactyly of the digits show differences in the categories of duplications.

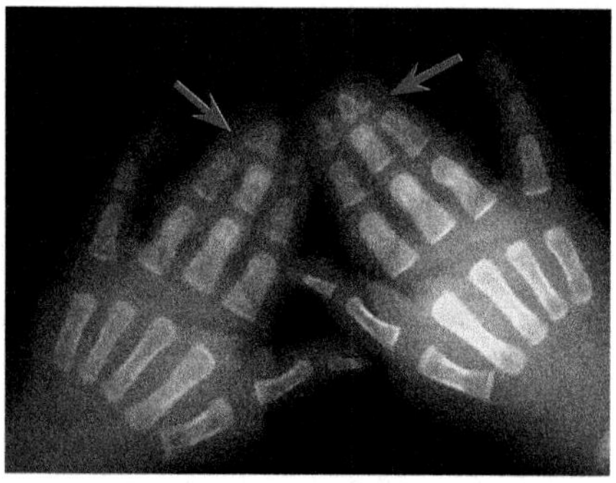

E Syndactyly Syndactyly is readily identified. Radiographs are useful in determining the degree of bony involvement.

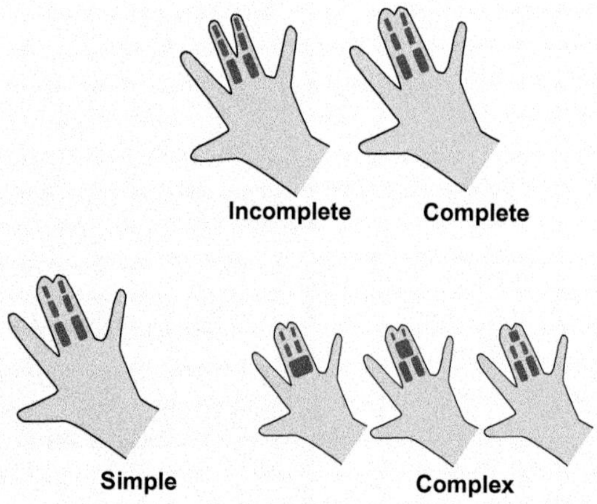

F Classification of syndactyly Syndactyly may be complete or incomplete, simple or complex.

Bent Fingers

Bent or curved fingers occur in the frontal or sagittal planes. Except for camptodactyly, all have an underlying bony deformity. Many are associated with a variety of generalized disorders.

Clinodactyly is a radial deviation of fingers, is often bilateral, and most commonly affects the little fingers [B]. The deformity is usually considered as a variation of normal, causes no disability, and seldom requires treatment. The deformity rarely is severe enough to require correction. Correct by performing a physiolysis of a delta phalanx or a wedge osteotomy of the trapezoidal phalanx when sufficiently large in mid childhood. Delay correction until late childhood or early adolescence to reduce the risk of recurrent deformity.

Camptodactyly is the common flexion deformity of the fingers [C] that is divided into infantile and adolescent forms. The deformity is often progressive. Disability is usually mild. Treatment includes splinting and, rarely, operative correction.

Delta phalanx is an abnormal interposed triangular ossicle [D] in the finger, producing an angulatory deformity. Correct by osteotomy, or resection of the bridging physis. Following physeal resection, fill the defect with autogenous fat to prevent recurrence.

Kirner deformity This is a rare, progressive curving of the terminal phalanx of the little finger. The etiology is unknown. The deformity is characteristic in appearance, usually causes little disability, and seldom requires treatment. If the lesion is painful, immobilize the finger with a splint. Rarely is the deformity severe enough to require correction by a phalangeal osteotomy [E].

Brachydactyly

Shortening of the metacarpal or fingers is often inherited as an autosomal trait or may be associated with a variety of conditions such as Poland, Holt-Oram, Cornelia de Lange, or Silver syndromes. Finger lengthening procedures are rarely appropriate.

Symphalangism

Fusions may involve the proximal or distal interphalangeal joints. The deformities are often inherited and are varied in pattern. Sometimes an osteotomy is necessary to reposition the finger in a more functional position.

Reconstructive Procedures

Finger osteotomies are often appropriate to correct deformity and to position the finger in a more functional position. Fix most finger osteotomies with K wires. Osteotomies are commonly performed.

Toe-to-finger transfers Toe transfers are the most effective means of improving grip function of the hand in children with absent digits. Second toe transfer is usually made. Operative indications are rare.

Finger lengthening of up to 10 mm in single-stage and 30 mm by gradual distraction may be achieved. Metacarpal lengthening improves pinch function in children with either transverse deficiency or constriction band syndromes. Finger lengthening may improve appearance in children with brachydactyly. These lengthening procedures are only rarely indicated. The decision involves a careful assessment, considering the risks and the aesthetic and functional benefits.

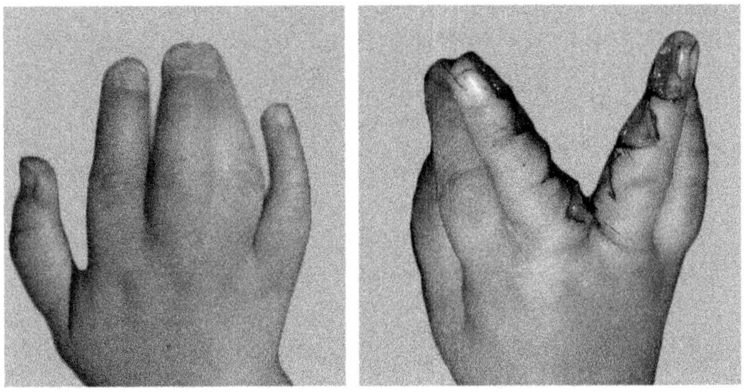

A Operative repair of syndactyly Repair is usually effective with good functional outcomes.

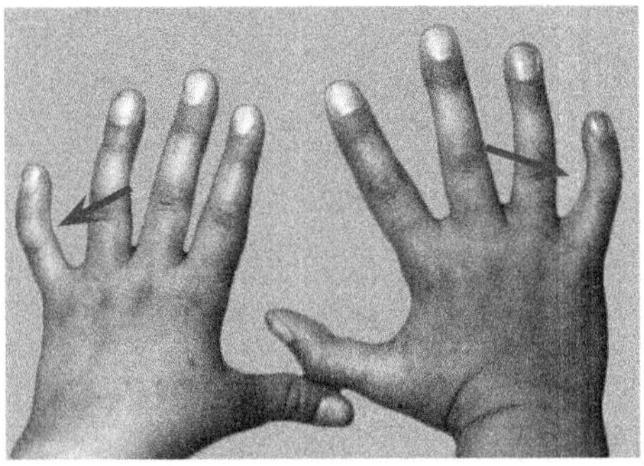

B Clinodactyly This classic deformity involves both little fingers.

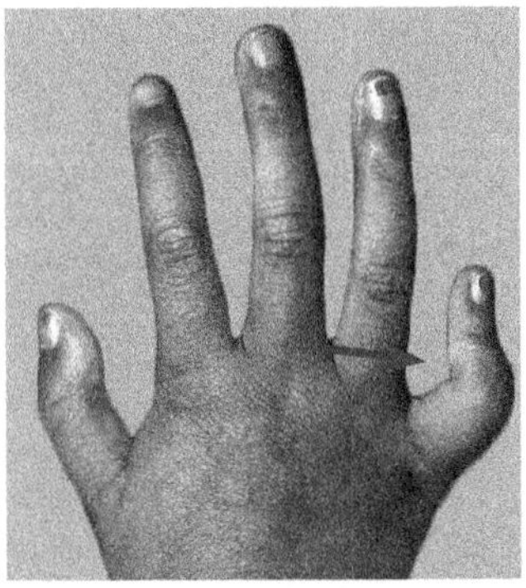

C Camptodactyly Note the flexion deformity of the proximal interphalangeal joint (arrow).

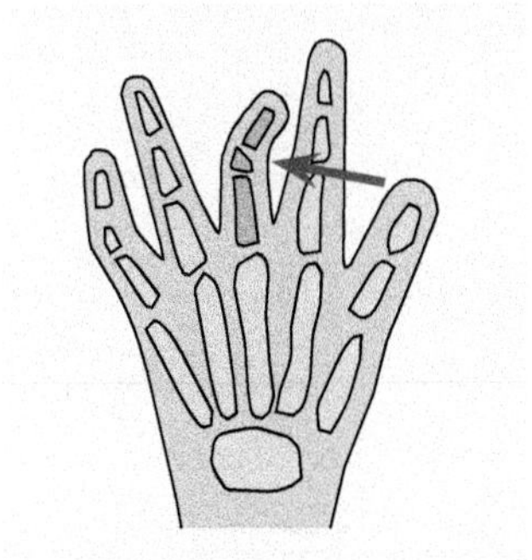

D Delta phalanx The delta phalanx sometimes requires operative correction.

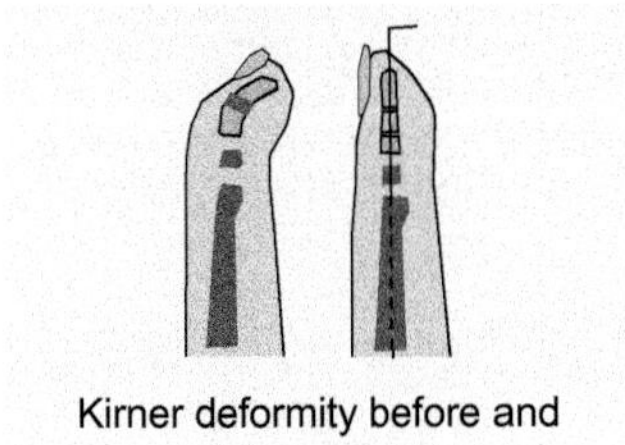

E Kirner deformity Kirner deformity corrected by osteotomy.

GENERAL

Ekblom AG, Laurell T, Arner M. Epidemiology of congenital upper limb anomalies in 562 children born in 1997 to 2007: a total population study from Stockholm, Sweden. J. Hand Surg. 35(11)-A:1742-1754, 2010.

Manske PR, Oberg KC. Classification and developmental biology of congenital anomalies of the hand and upper extremity. J. Bone Joint Surg. 91(Suppl. 4)-A:3–18, 2009.

Swanson AB, Swanson GD, Tada K. A classification for congenital limb malformation. J. Hand Surg. 8(5-2)-A:693-702, 1983.

DEFICIENCY

Bayne LG, Klug MS. Long term review of the surgical treatment of radial deficiencies. J. Hand Surg. 12(2)-A:169-179, 1987.

Bayne LG. Congenital hand deformities: ulnar club hand (ulnar deficiency). In Operative Hand Surgery, Green DG, ed, Churchill Livingston, New York, 1982.

Eaton CJ, Lister GD. Toe transfer for congenital hand defects. Microsurgery. 12(3):186-195, 1991.

Goldfarb CA, Manske PR, Busa R, Mills J, Carter P, Ezaki M. Upper-extremity phocomelia reexamined: a longitudinal dysplasia. J. Bone Joint Surg. 87(12)-A:2639-2648, 2005.

James MA, McCarroll HR Jr, Manske PR. The spectrum of radial longitudinal deficiency: a modified classification. J. Hand Surg. 24(6)-A.1145-1155, 1999.

Miura T, Nakamura R, Horii E. The position of symbrachydactyly in the classification of congenital hand anomalies. J. Hand Surg. 19(3)-B:350–354, 1994.

O'Rahilly R. Morphological patterns in limb deficiencies and duplications. Am. J. Anat. 89(2):135-193, 1951.

FAILURE of DIFFERENTIATION

Baek GH, Kim JH, Chung MS, Kang SB, Lee YH, Gong HS. The natural history of pediatric trigger thumb. J. Bone Joint Surg. 90(5):980-985, 2008.

Hefner RA. Inheritance of crooked little fingers. J. Hered. 20(8):395-398, 1929.

Kemp T, Ravn J. Über erbliche Hand-und Fussdeformitaeten in einem 140-koepfigen Geschlecht, nebst einigen Bemerkungen ueber Poly-und Syndaktylie beim Menschen. Acta Psychiat. Neurol. Scand. 7:275-296, 1932.

Kjaer KW, Hansen L, Eiberg H, Utkus A, Skovgaard LT, Leicht P, Opitz JM, Tommerup NA. 72-year-old Danish puzzle resolved--comparative analysis of phenotypes in families with different-sized HOXD13 polyalanine expansions. Am. J. Med. Genet. 138A:328-339, 2005.

Kirner J. Doppelseitige verkrummungen des kleinfingerendgliedes als selbstandiges krankheitsbild. Fortschritte auf dem Gehiete der Rönigenstrahien, 36:804-806, 1927.

Larner AJ. Camptodactyly: a 10-year series. Eur. J. Dermatol. 21(5):771-775, 2011.

DUPLICATION

Frazier TM. A note on race-specific congenital malformation rates. Am. J. Obstet. Gynec. 80:184-185, 1960.

Furniss D, Lettice LA, Taylor IB, Critchley PS, Giele H, Hill RE, Wilkie AOM. A variant in the sonic hedgehog regulatory sequence (ZRS) is associated with triphalangeal thumb and deregulates expression in the developing limb. Hum. Molec. Genet. 17:2417-2423, 2008.

Tupper JW. Pollex abductus due to congenital malposition of the flexor pollicis longus. J. Bone Joint Surg. 51(7):1285-1290, 1969.

Wassel HD. The results of surgery for polydactyly of the thumb. A review. Clin. Orthop. 64:175-193, 1969.

OVERGROWTH

Cerrato F, Eberlin KR, Waters P, Upton J, Taghinia A, Labow BI. Presentation and treatment of macrodactyly in children. J. Hand Surg. 38(11)-A:2112–2123, 2013.

Tsuge K, Ikuta Y. Macrodactyly and fibro-fatty proliferation of the median nerve. Hiroshima J. Med. Sci. 22(1):83-101, 1973.

UNDERGROWTH

Blauth W. The hypoplastic thumb. Arch. Orthop. Unfallchir. 62(3):225–246, 1967

Buck-Gramcko D. Congenital Malformations of the Hand and Forearm. Churchill Livingstone, London,1998.

Poland, A. Deficiency of the pectoral muscle. Guys Hosp. Rep. 6:191, 1841.

CONSTRICTION

Patterson TJ. Congenital ring-constrictions. Br J. Plast. Surg. 14:1-31, 1961.

SKELETAL ABNORMALITIES

Gschwind C, Tonkin M. Surgery for cerebral palsy: Part 1. Classification and operative procedures for pronation deformity. J. Hand Surg. 17-B:391-395, 1992.

House JH, Gwathmey FW, Fidler MO. A dynamic approach to the thumb-in palm deformity in cerebral palsy. J. Bone Joint Surg. 63-A:216-225, 1981.

Tonkin M, Freitas A, Koman A, Leclercq C, Van Heest A. The surgical management of thumb deformity in cerebral palsy. J. Hand Surg. 33(1)-B:77-80, 2008.

Tonkin M, Gschwind C. Surgery for cerebral palsy: Part 2. Flexion deformity of the wrist and fingers. J. Hand Surg. 17(4)-B:396-400, 1992.

Zancolli EA, Zancolli ER Jr. Surgical management of the hemiplegic spastic hand in cerebral palsy. Surg. Clin. North Am. 61:395-406, 1981.

WRIST

Carter PR, Ezaki M. Madelung's deformity. Surgical correction through the anterior approach. Hand Clin. 16(4):713-721, 2000.

Dannenberg M, Anton JI, Spiegel MB. Madelung's deformity. Am. J. Roentgen. Radium. Ther. Nucl. Med. 42(5):671-676, 1939.

Laffosse JM, Abid A, Accadbled F, Knör G, Sales de Gauzy J, Cahuzac JP. Surgical correction of Madelung's deformity by combined corrective radioulnar osteotomy: 14 cases with four-year minimum follow-up. Int. Orthop. 33(6):1655-1661, 2009.

Vickers D, Nielsen G. Madelung deformity: surgical prophylaxis (physiolysis) during the late growth period by resection of the dyschondrosteosis lesion. J. Hand Surg. 17(4)-B:401-407, 1992.

ELBOW

Almquist EE, Gordon CH, Blue AI. Congenital dislocation of the head of the radius. J. Bone Joint Surg. 51(6):1118-1127, 1969.

Blodgett WE. Congenital luxation of the head of the radius. Report of two cases. Analysis of fifty-one cases. Am. J. Orthop. Surg. 3:253-270, 1905.

Green WT, Mital MA. Congenital radio-ulnar synostosis: surgical treatment. J. Bone Joint Surg. 61(5)-A:738-743, 1979.

Kanaya F, Ibaraki K. Mobilization of a congenital proximal radioulnar synostosis with use of a free vascularized fascio-fat graft. J. Bone Joint Surg. 80(8):1186-1192, 1998.

SHOULDER

Cavendish ME. Congenital elevation of the scapula. J. Bone Joint Surg. 54(3)-B:395–408, 1972.

Eulenberg M. Casuistische mittelheilungen aus dem gembeite der orthopadie. Arch. Klin. Chir. 4:301-311, 1863.

Fawcett J. The development and ossification of the human clavicle. J. Anat. Physiol. 47:225–234, 1913.

Gilbert A, Tassin JL. Surgical repair of the brachial plexus in obstetric paralysis. Chirurgie 110:70-75, 1984.

Green WT. The surgical correction of congenital elevation of the scapula (Sprengel's deformity). J. Bone Joint Surg. 39-A:1439-1448, 1957.

Haerle M, Gilbert A. Management of complete obstetric brachial plexus lesions. J. Pediatr. Orthop. 24(2):194-200, 2004.

Hale HB, Bae DS, Waters PM. Current concepts in the management of brachial plexus birth palsy. J. Hand Surg. 35(2)-A:322-331.

König F. Eine neue operation des angeborenen schulterblatthochstandes. Beitr. Klin. Chir. 94:530-537, 1914.

L'Episcopo JB. Tendon transplantation in obstetrical paralysis. Am. J. Surg. 25:122-125, 1934.

Lloyd-Roberts GC, Apley AG, Owen R. Reflections upon the aetiology of congenital pseudarthrosis of the clavicle. With a note on cranio-cleido dystosis. J. Bone Joint Surg. 57:24–29, 1975.

Mallet J. Obstetrical paralysis of the brachial plexus. Rev. Chir. Orthop. Reparatrice Appar. Motil. 58(Suppl 1):166–168, 1972.

Matsuoka T, Ahlberg PE, Kessaris N, Iannarelli P, Dennehy U, Richardson WD, McMahon AP, Koentges G. Neural crest origins of the neck and shoulder. Nature 436(7049):347-355, 2005.

McBurney CH, Sands A. Congenital deformity due to malposition of the scapula. NY Med. J. 47:582-583, 1888.

McMurtry I, Bennet GC, Bradish C. Osteotomy for congenital elevation of the scapula (Sprengel's deformity). J. Bone Joint Surg. 87-B: 986-989, 2005.

Narakas AO. Brachial plexus surgery. Orthop. Clin. North Am. 12(2):303-323, 1981.

Sever JW. Obstetric paralysis: report of eleven hundred cases. JAMA 85:1862-1865, 1925.

Sprengel RD. Die angeborene verschiebung des schulterblattes nach oben. Arch. Klin. Chir. 42:545-549, 1891.

Woodward JW. Congenital elevation of the scapula: correction by release and transplantation of muscle origins. J. Bone Joint Surg. 43-A:219-228, 1961.

INFECTION

Doyle JR. Anatomy of the finger flexor tendon sheath and pulley system. J. Hand Surg. 13(4)-A:473-484, 1988.

Kanavel AB. Infections of the Hand. A Guide to the Surgical Treatment of Acute and Chronic Suppurative Processes in the Fingers, Hand, and Forearm. Lea & Febiger, Philadelphia and New York, 1912.

REFERENCE

CHAPTER 14

Questions Parents Frequently Ask

1. What are developmental variations?

These are common problems many infants and children develop during normal growth. These include flexible flatfeet, in-toeing and out-toeing, bowlegs, and knock-knees.

2. Why do infants and children develop these variations?

These variations are simply part of normal development that occurs in some children. It may be a pattern that is inherited or can occur for the first time in a family. Unfortunately, they may mimic deformities that are secondary to some underlying disease. Your physician will make certain the condition is not abnormal.

3. If I am concerned about the future, what should I do?

It is best to follow the advice of your physician. Your pediatrician or family physician will guide you. As they see many children with this problem, they are ideally qualified to advise you.

4. What are the features of these developmental variations?

They are very common. They occur in healthy infants and children. They resolve naturally over time.

5. How should these variations be managed?

It is best to allow the variation to resolve on its own.

6. Should we try to hasten the resolution by requiring my child to walk or sit in a corrected position?

No. This will not hasten the resolution and will simply frustrate your child.

7. Are corrective shoes or inserts useful?

No. Shoes and inserts do not hasten the resolution.

8. Is there any harm in such treatments?

Yes. Our studies have shown that adults who used these orthopedic devices as children remembered the experience as negative. Furthermore, the users had significantly lower self-esteem than adults who did not wear devices. This study suggests that the use of unnecessary treatment is not neutral but actually harmful.

9. Some doctors recommend shoe inserts, back manipulations, and other treatments. What should I do?

For a treatment to be imposed on your child, it should be both necessary and effective. We have not found any scientific evidence to support the use of these interventions.

10. My parents (grandparents) are insisting that we do something. What should we do?

If something must be done, do something that will clearly help your child. Follow these recommendations:

a. Do not focus attention on the variation because this may give your child a sense of being defective.

b. Encourage your child to be physically active.

c. Provide a healthy diet and avoid overeating to prevent childhood obesity.

d. Provide your child with flexible shoes that allow full mobility of the foot.

Handouts

The following pages may be photocopied and given to families to help them to understand their child's condition.

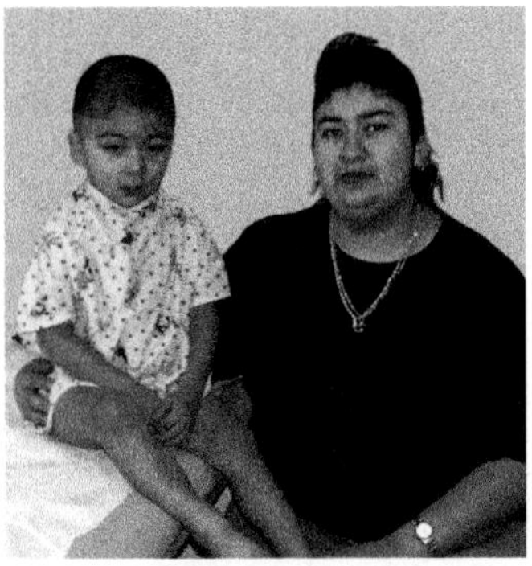

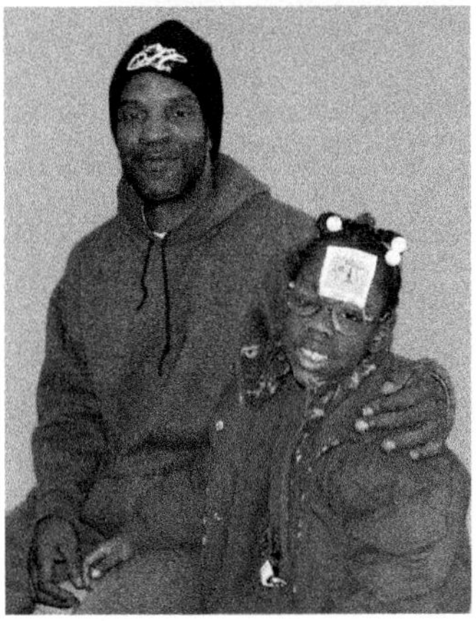

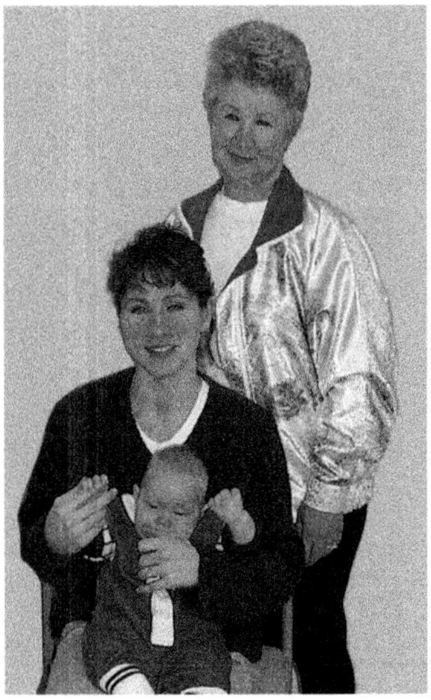

A Families These are typical families that, because of their concern, often ask questions about their child's problem.

What Parents Should Know

About flatfeet, in-toeing, bent legs, and shoes for children

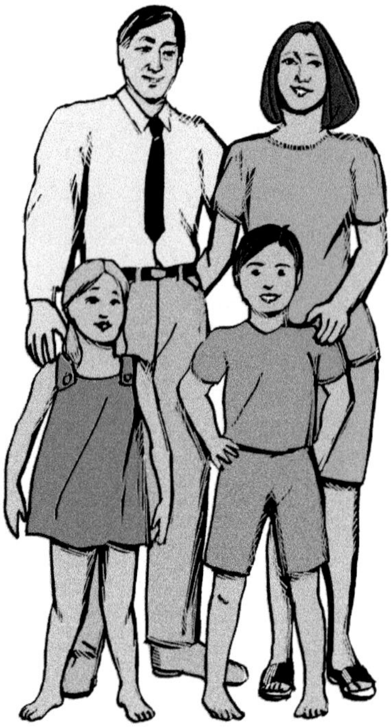

Most variations of normal childhood are outgrown.

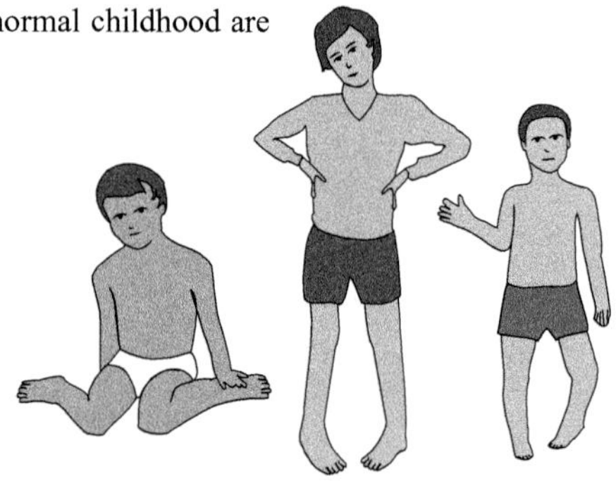

Your doctor will make sure things go well for your child.

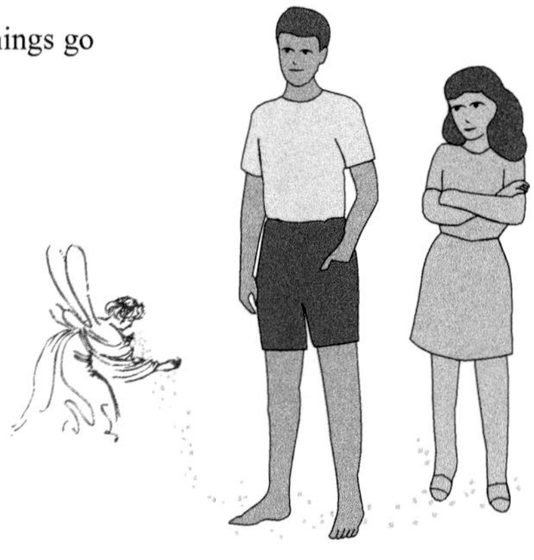

Mother Nature's treatment is safe, inexpensive, and effective. Let the magic of time and growth correct the problem.

Bowlegs and Knock-knees

During their normal development, infants often have bowlegs. With growth, the child may then become knock-kneed by about 18 months of age. Special shoes, wedges, inserts, or exercises only make the child feel bad and do not correct the shape.

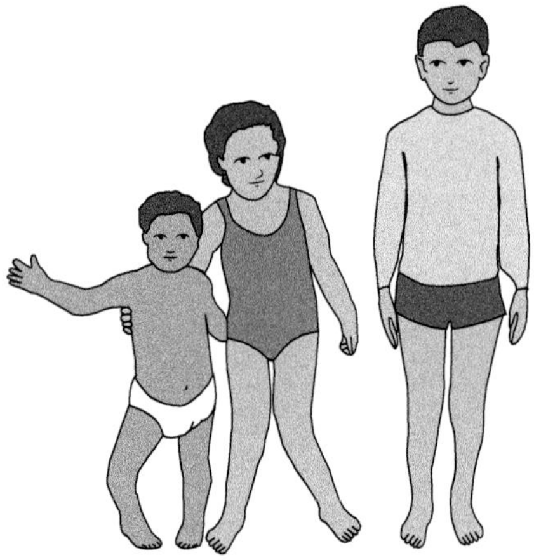

Your doctor will decide if your child's legs are normal. If normal, the condition will correct with time.

Your doctor may be concerned if the condition is:

severe,

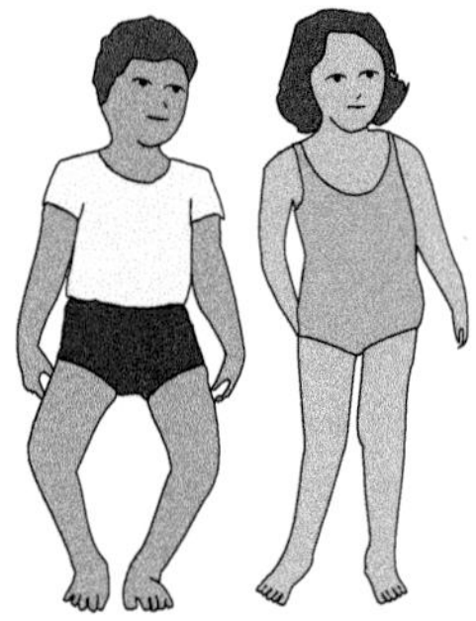

occurs only on one side,

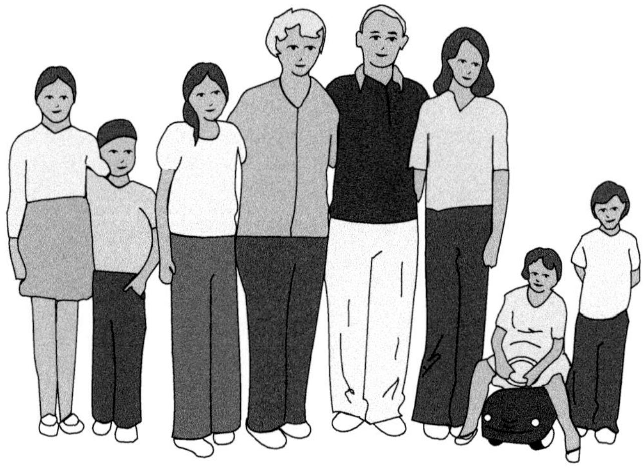

or runs in the family—especially if the family tends to be unusually short in stature.

Torsion

In-toeing is common in childhood and is usually outgrown.

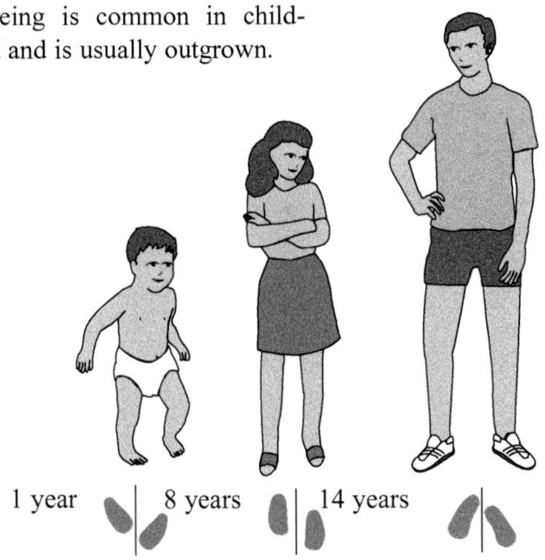

There are three causes of in-toeing that your doctor can determine:

1. Hooked foot
2. Tibial torsion
3. Femoral torsion

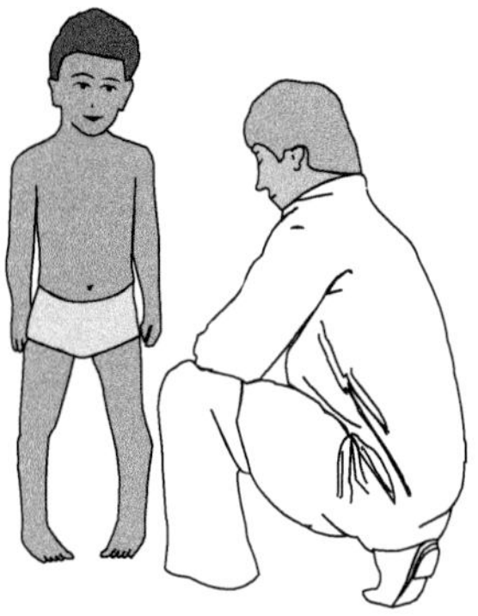

Hooked Foot

Hooked foot is caused by the position of the baby before birth.

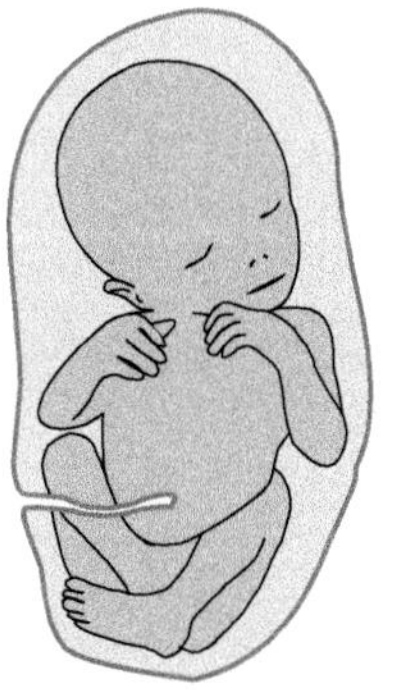

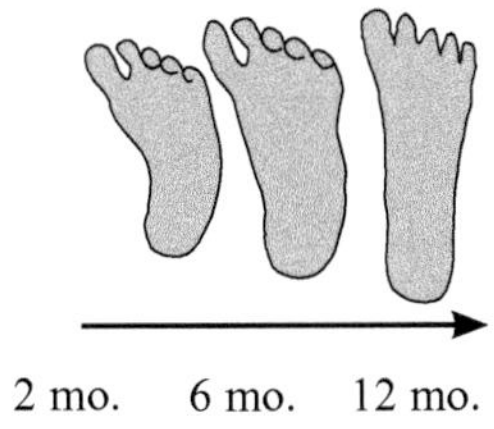

Most hooked feet get better without treatment during the baby's first months, although improvement may be seen throughout the first three years.

Rarely, the hooked foot is stiff, persists, and may require treatment with a cast or splint. Special shoes do not correct this condition.

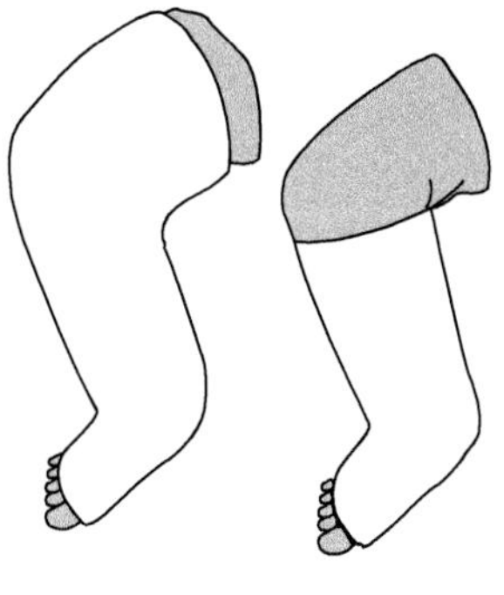

Tibial Torsion

Tibial torsion is an inward twist of the lower leg. It is a variation of normal that is very common during infancy and childhood.

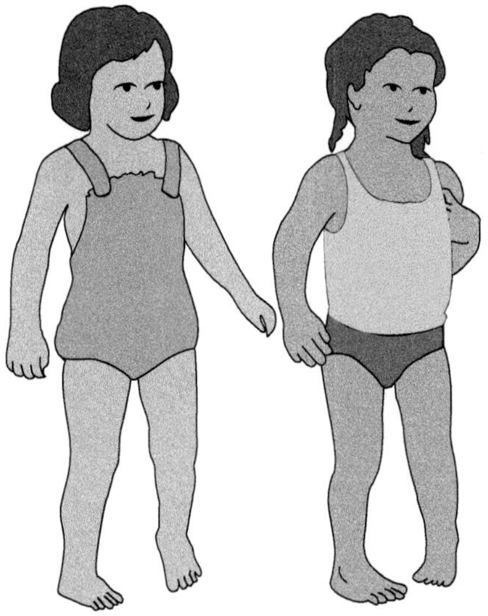

Splints, exercises, braces, or shoe modifications do not correct the twist and may, in fact, be harmful. Most legs with tibial torsion straighten without treatment during infancy and childhood.

Femoral Torsion

Femoral torsion is a twisting of the thigh bone, causing an inward rotation of the leg. The cause of femoral torsion is unknown. Femoral torsion is most severe when the child is about 5 or 6 years old. Most children outgrow this condition by the age of 10 years.

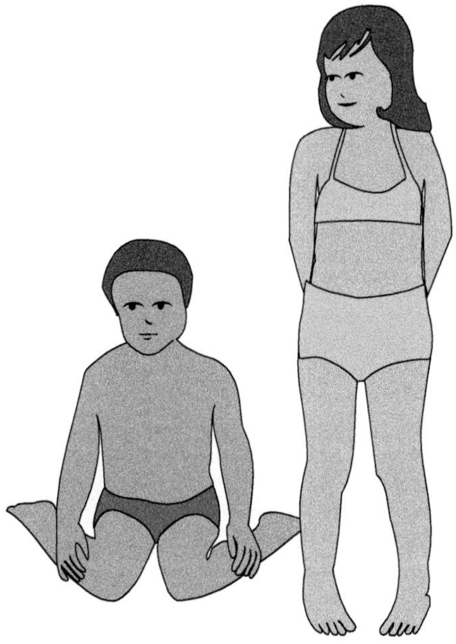

Shoe inserts, modifications, or braces do not correct this condition. They may make the child uncomfortable and self-conscious, and may hamper play.

Flatfeet

Parents worry about flatfeet, but...

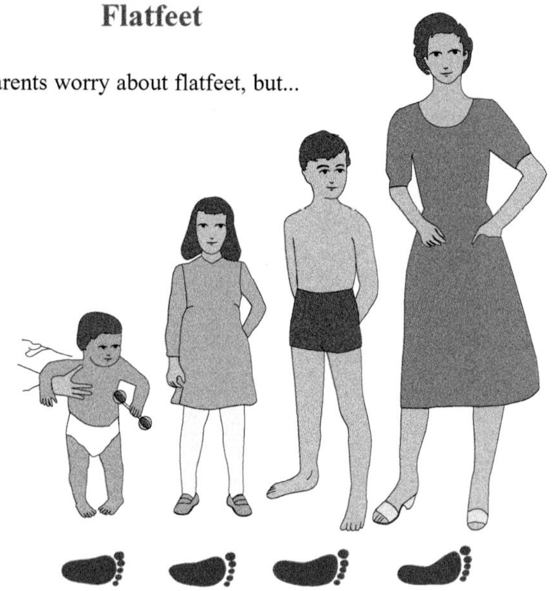

...flatfeet are normal in infants, children, and adults. Special shoes, inserts, wedges, or exercises do not create an arch in a child with a flexible flatfoot.

Did You Know?

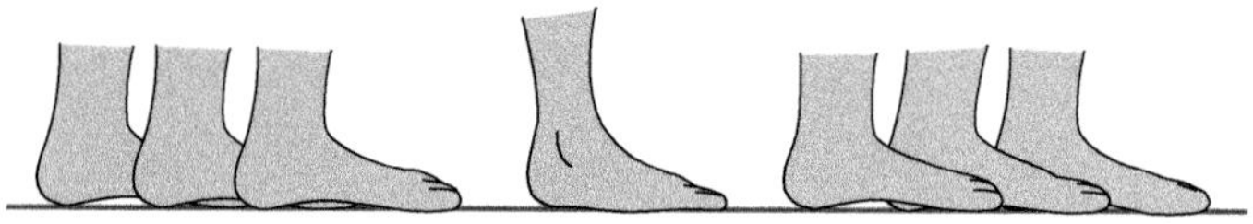

One in five children never develops an arch. Most adults with flexible flatfeet have strong, pain-free feet.

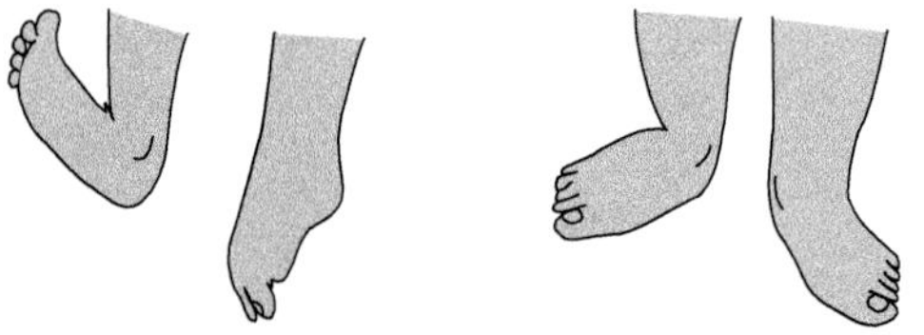

Most children have low arches because they are loose-jointed. The arch flattens when they are standing, and their feet seem to be rolled in and pointed outward.

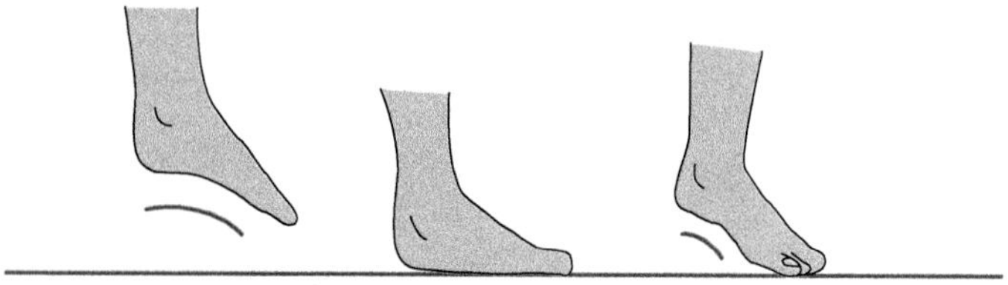

The arch can be seen when these feet are hanging free or when the child stands on his or her toes.

Just as normal children are of different heights ...

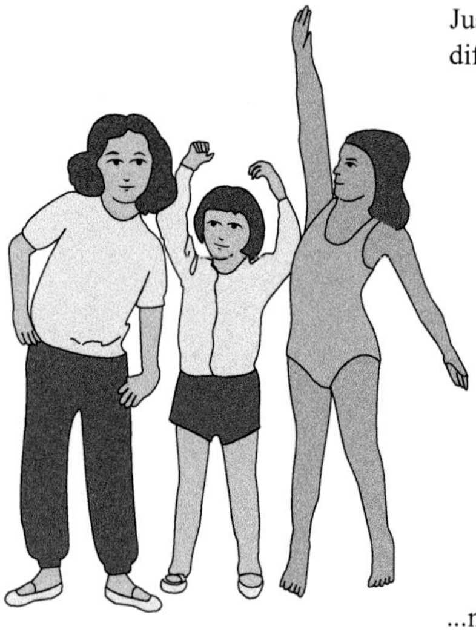

...normal arches have different heights, too!

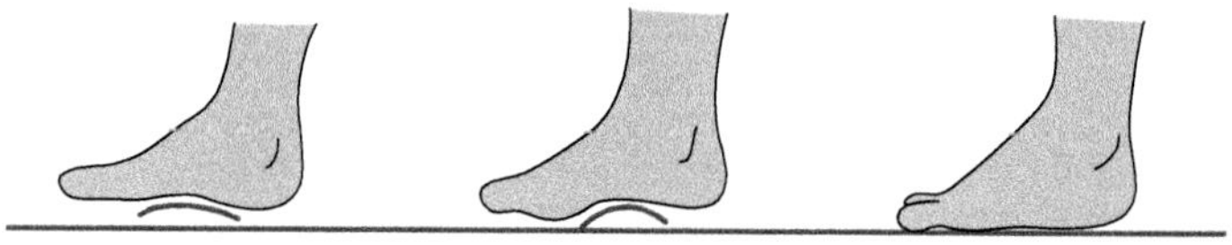

Wearing a pad or insert under the arch of a simple flexible flatfoot can make the child less comfortable...and it's a waste of money!

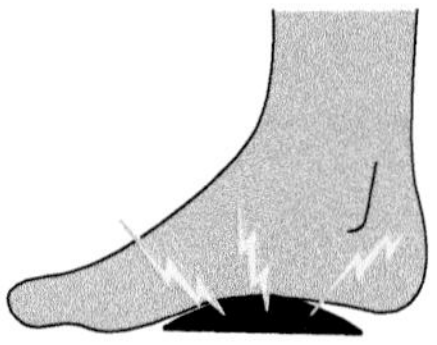

The physician is concerned if the flatfoot is:

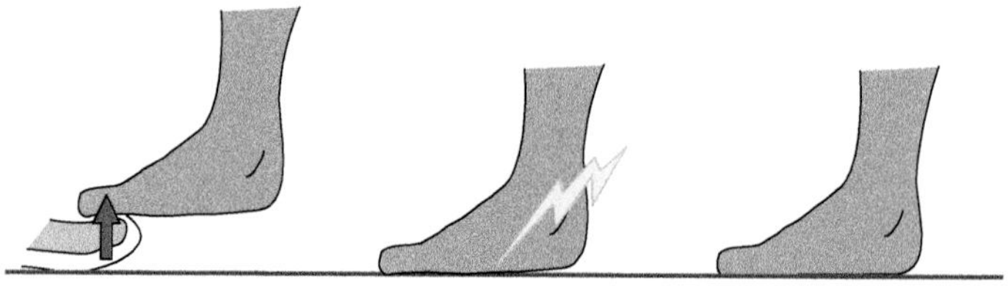

But the physician is most concerned about a high arch because it is most likely to cause pain later.

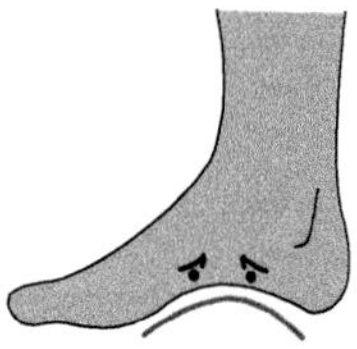

Shoes for Children

Barefoot people have the best feet! Your child needs a flexible, soft shoe that allows maximum freedom for the foot to develop normally.

Size

Shoes are much better a little large than too small.

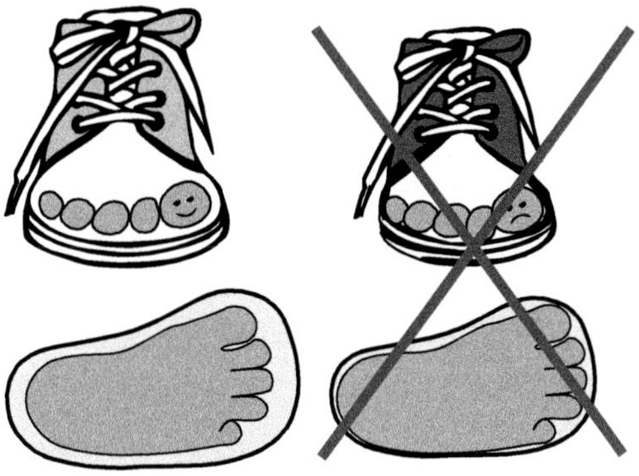

Flexibility

Stiff, "supportive" shoes are not good for feet, because they limit movement, which is needed for developing strength and retaining foot mobility. A child's foot needs protection from cold and sharp objects and freedom for movement.

Children's falls cause many injuries. A flat sole that is neither slippery nor sticky is best.

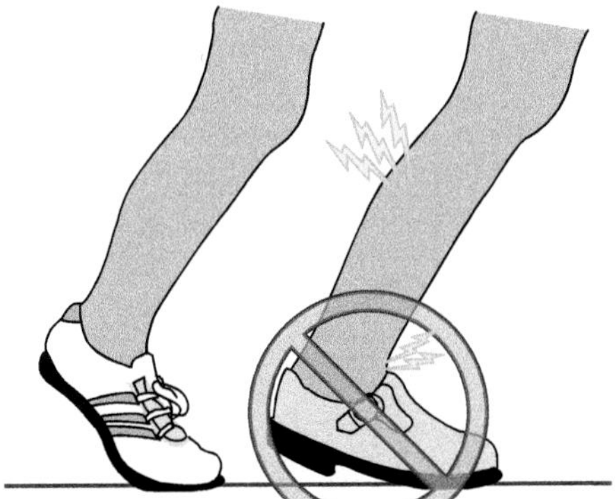

Material

A material that breathes may be best, especially for warm climates.

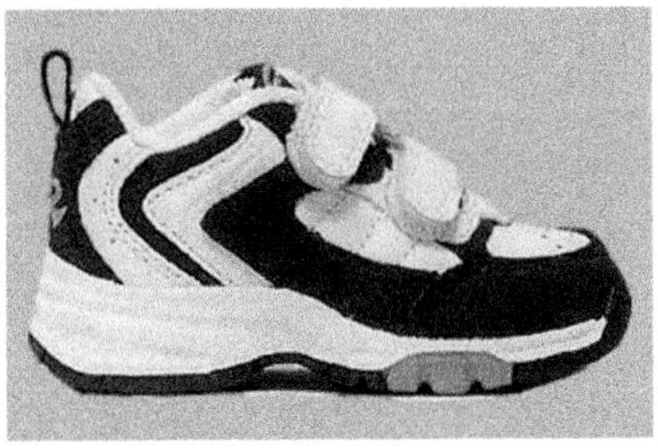

Avoid odd shapes

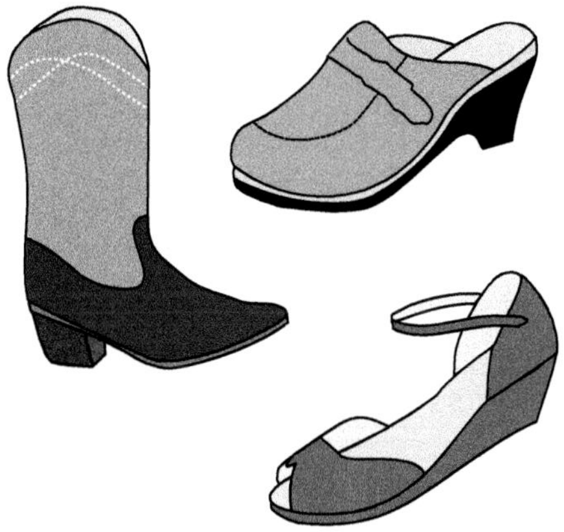

Pointed toes, elevated heels, and stiff soles are bad for the foot.

Remember...

The best things you can do for your child are to encourage physical activity and be sure your child doesn't overeat.

So-called corrective shoes, inserts, wedges, or braces are ineffective and only make your child unhappy.

This cannot be overemphasized: Let the magic of time and growth correct the problem. Mother Nature's treatment is safe, inexpensive, and effective.

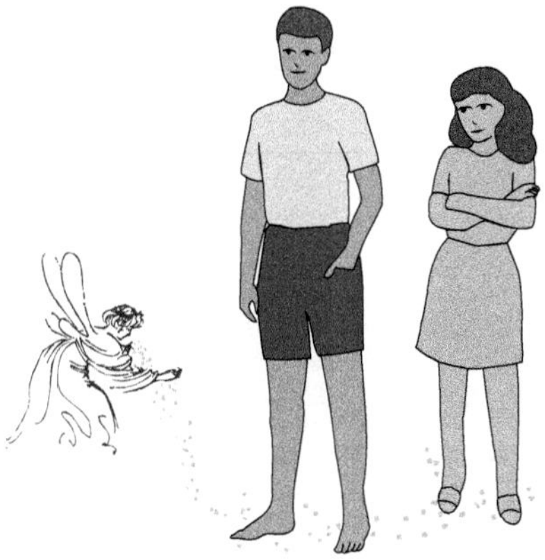

"Play is the occupation of the child"

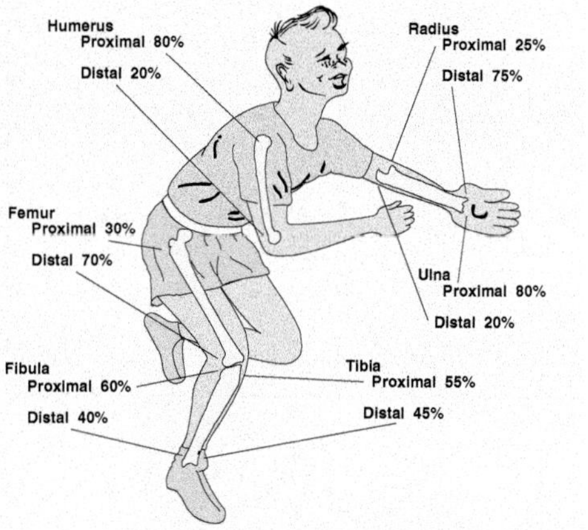

A Growth plate contribution of long bone growth From Blount WB. Fig. 147, *Fractures in Children.* Williams & Wilkins, Baltimore, 1955.

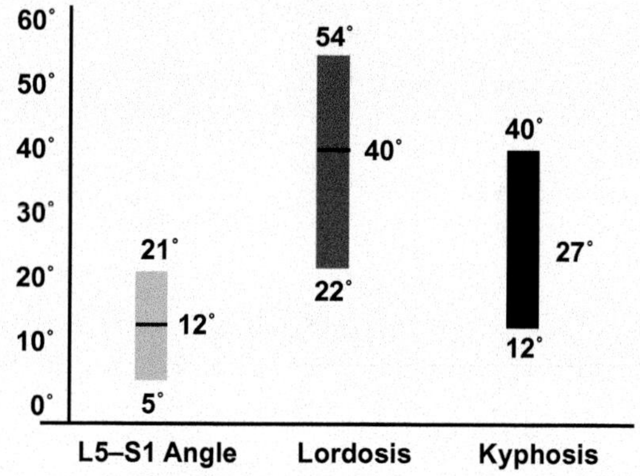

B Normal values of sagittal measures of the spine in children The range includes values from the 10th to the 90th percentiles. The L5–S1 angle includes measures between the inferior surface of L5 and the superior surface of S1 (green). Lordosis is measured using the Cobb method between L1 and L5 (red). Kyphosis is measured using the Cobb method between T5 and T12 (blue). From Propst-Proctor & Bleck. JPO 3:344, 1983.

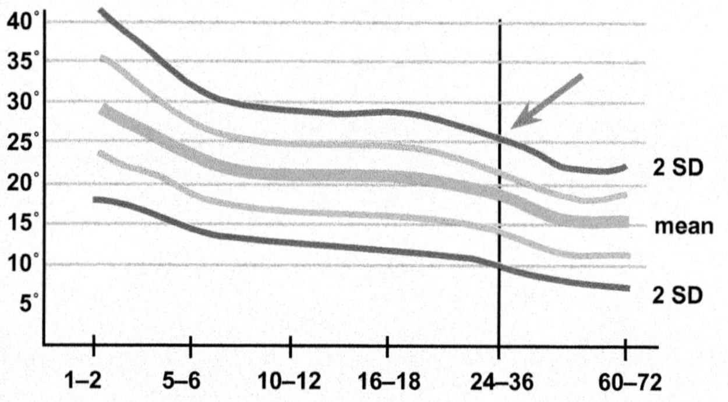

C Acetabular index Illustration shows normal values by age group in months. Mean values (green line), 1 SD (orange) and 2 SD (red) are drawn. Note that at about 25 months, the acetabular index should be below 25° (blue arrow). Redrawn from Tönnis D. Clin Orthop 119:39, 1976.

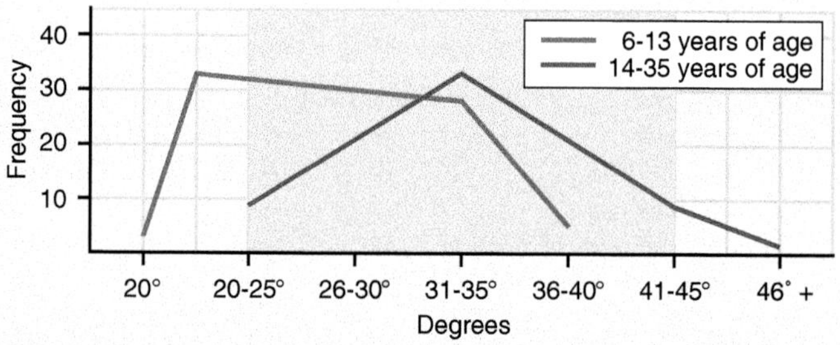

D Center-edge angle Illustration shows mean values by age group. Green shaded area shows the normal range for adults. From Severin E. Acta Chir Scan 84:93, 1941.

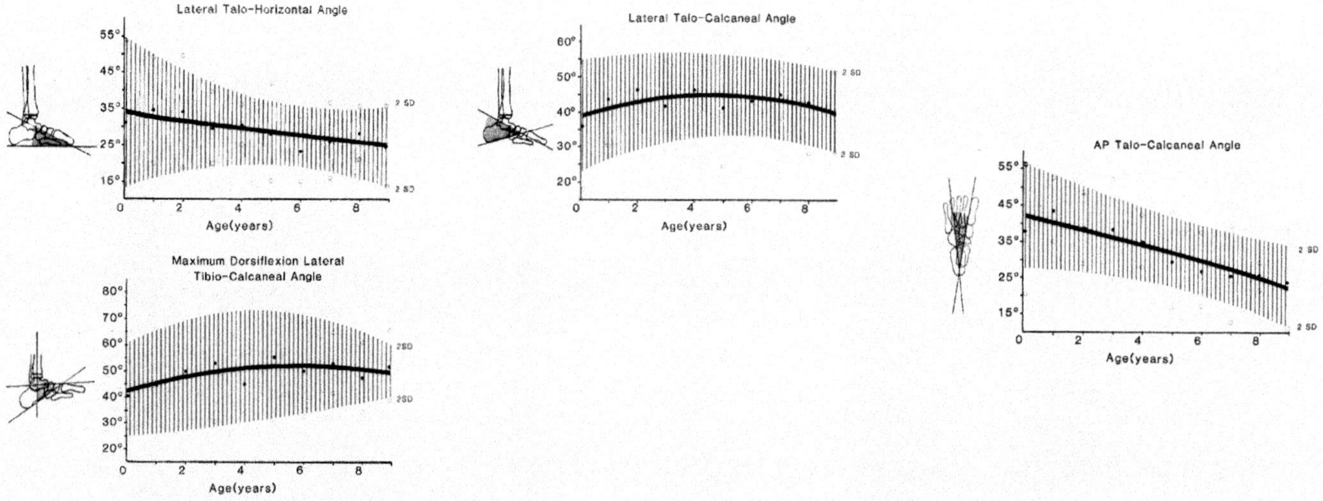

E Normal values for standing foot radiographs in infants and young children These illustrations show mean values and normal range (plus or minus two standard deviations) in shaded areas. From Vanderwilde R, Staheli LT, Chew DE and Malagon V. JBJS 70A:407, 1988.

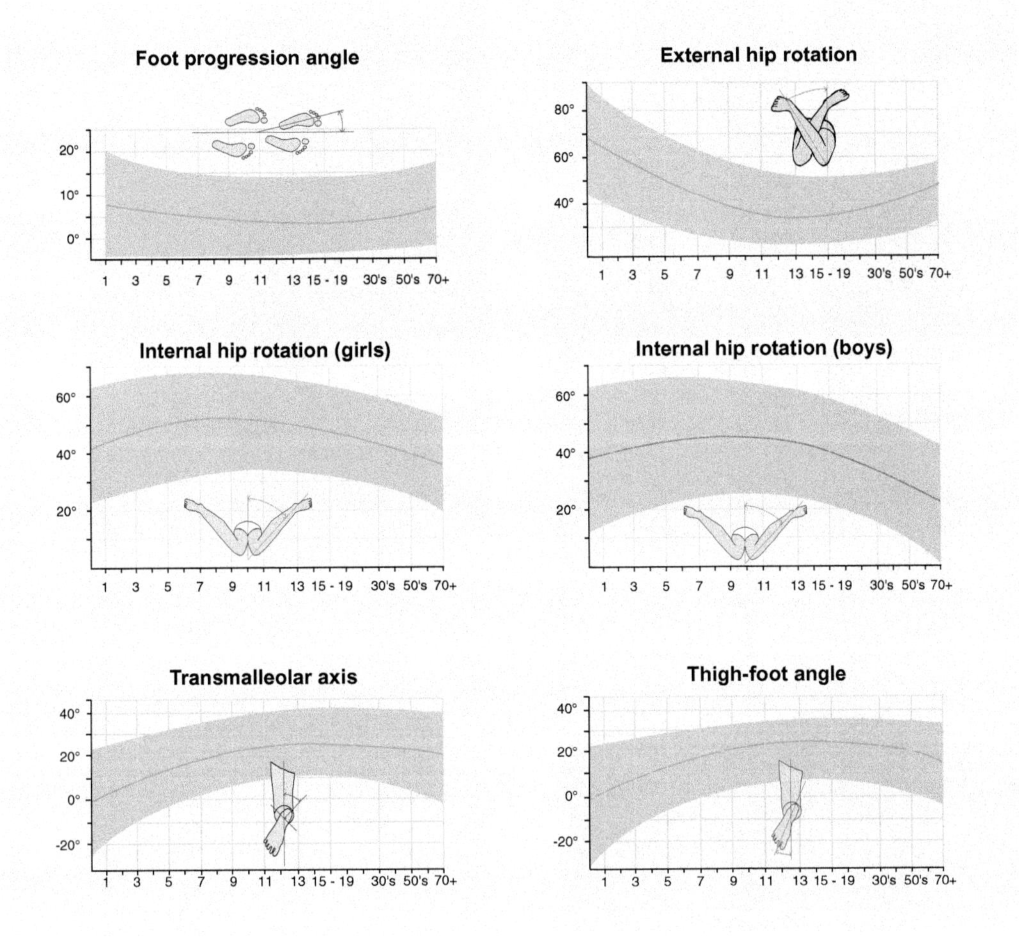

A Rotational profile normal values These charts show mean and normal ranges (plus or minus 2 standard deviations) in green. Because internal rotation is different for girls and boys, separate charts are shown. Redrawn from Staheli et al. JBJS 67:39, 1985.

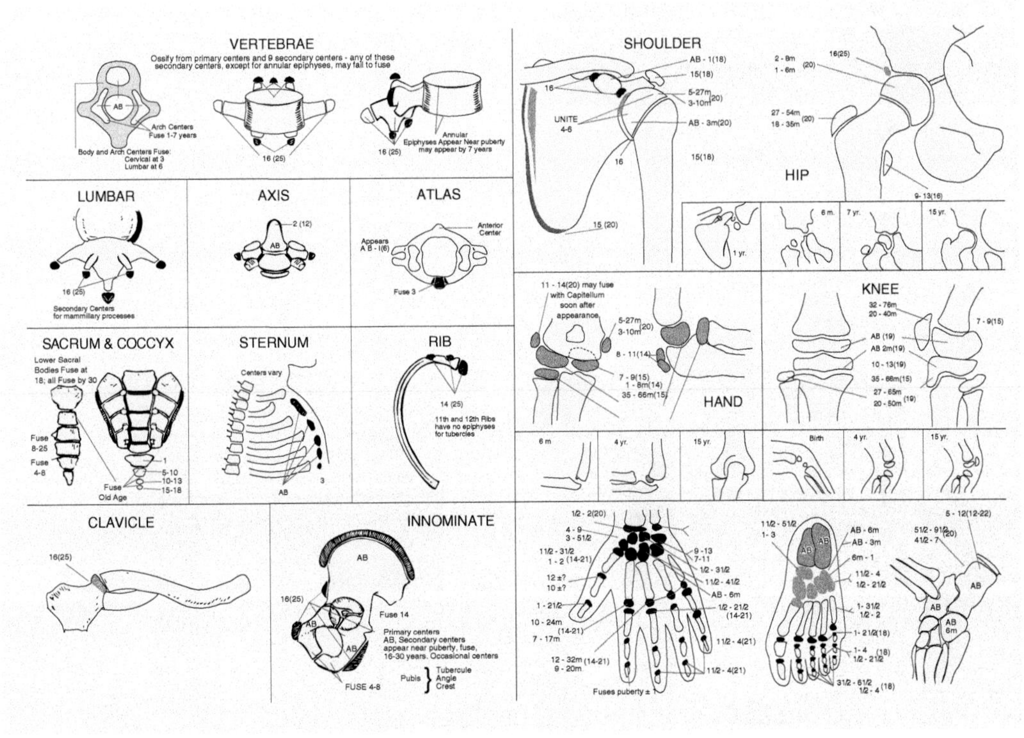

B Ossification centers Redrawn from Girdany BR and Golden R. AJR 68:922, 1952.

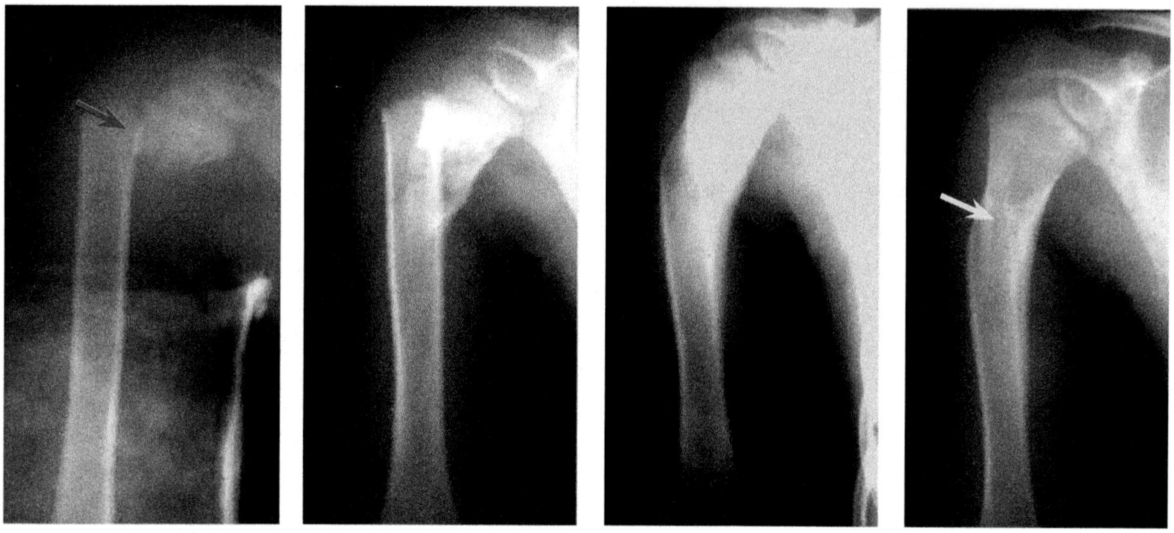

A Remodeling of the humerus This 8-year-old boy shows a complete loss of apposition (red arrow). Note the remodeling over the next two years (yellow arrow).

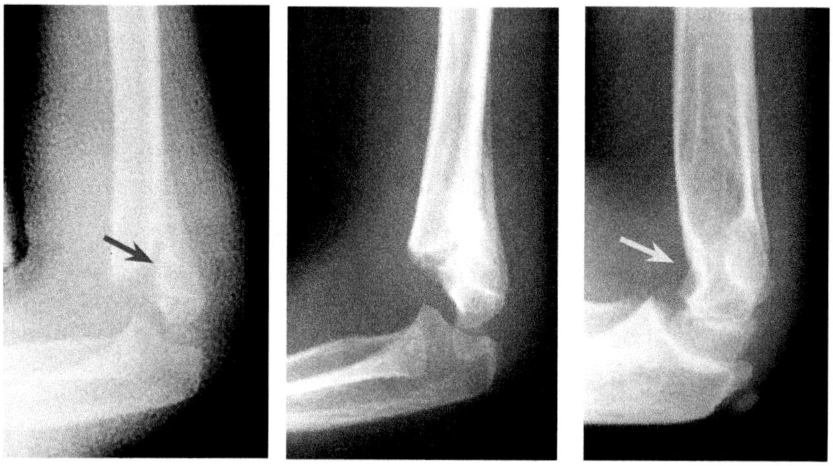

B Remodeling of sagittal plane in a supracondylar fracture This fracture (red arrow) remodeled over a period of four years (yellow arrow). Remodeling about the elbow is much slower than in the proximal humerus.

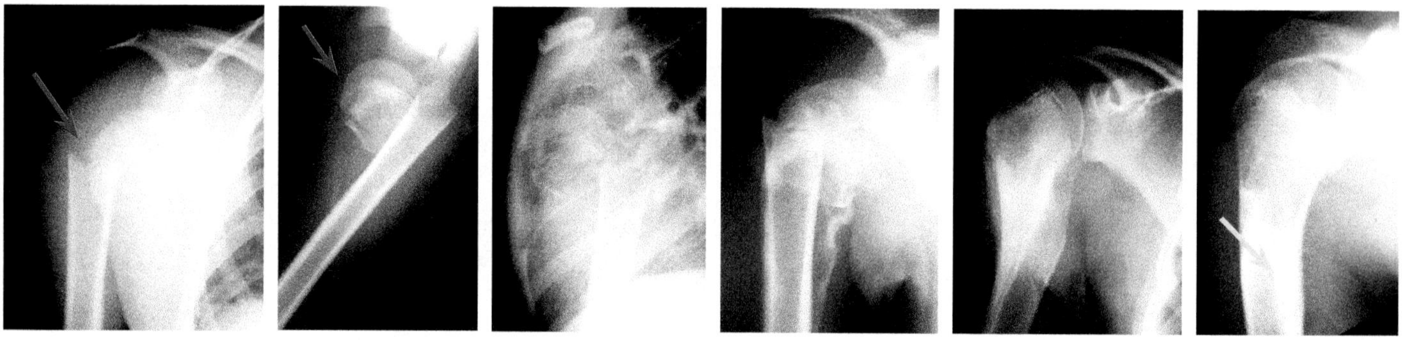

C Remodeling of the humerus This sequence shows a fracture (red arrow) in a 12-year-old boy over a period of two years. The fracture was left unreduced with side-to-side apposition and shortening. Note the remodeling within the intact periosteal sheath (yellow arrow).

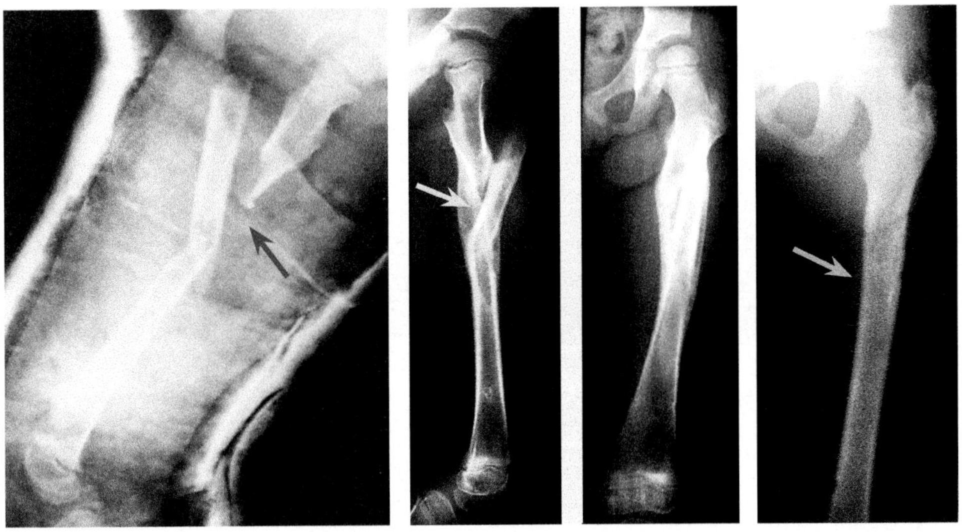

A Remodeling of femoral shaft fracture This segmental fracture in an 8-year-old girl was managed in traction and in a cast (red arrow). Note the filling in of the periosteal sheath after six months (yellow arrow) and restoration of normal femoral shape at age 13 years (orange arrow).

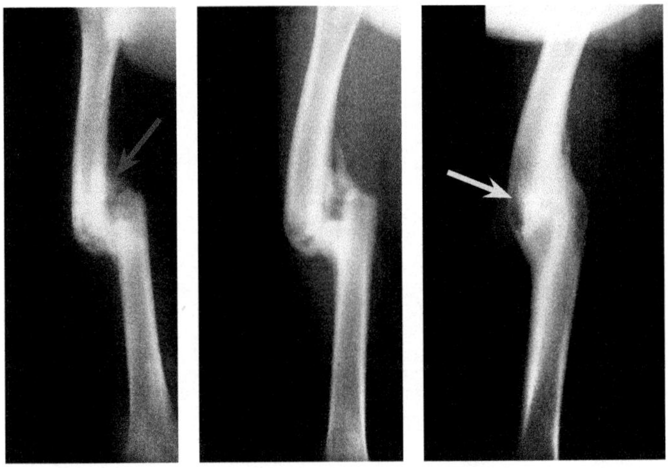

B Limited remodeling in adolescent This transverse fracture of the midshaft of the femur (red arrow) in a 15-year-old boy healed but showed limited remodeling (yellow arrow) due to the limited remaining growth.

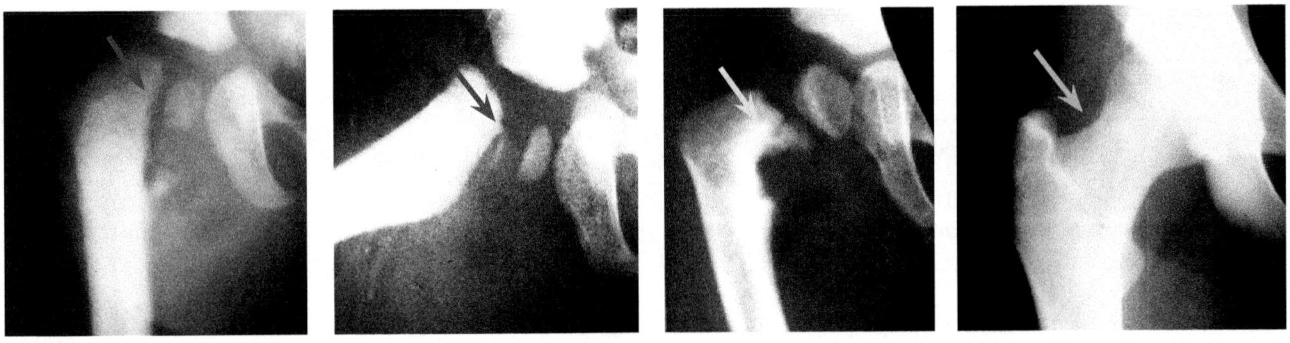

C Remodeling of proximal femoral physeal fracture in an infant Note the remodeling of the completely displaced femoral head (red arrows) throughout childhood (yellow arrow). Normal appearance is shown at age 15 years (orange arrow). Courtesy E. Forlin.

INDEX

15